KNOWLEDGE AND TECHNOLOGY INTEGRATION IN PRODUCTION AND SERVICES

Balancing Knowledge and Technology in Product and Service Life Cycle

IFIP - The International Federation for Information Processing

IFIP was founded in 1960 under the auspices of UNESCO, following the First World Computer Congress held in Paris the previous year. An umbrella organization for societies working in information processing, IFIP's aim is two-fold: to support information processing within its member countries and to encourage technology transfer to developing nations. As its mission statement clearly states,

IFIP's mission is to be the leading, truly international, apolitical organization which encourages and assists in the development, exploitation and application of information technology for the benefit of all people.

IFIP is a non-profitmaking organization, run almost solely by 2500 volunteers. It operates through a number of technical committees, which organize events and publications. IFIP's events range from an international congress to local seminars, but the most important are:

- The IFIP World Computer Congress, held every second year;
- open conferences;
- working conferences.

The flagship event is the IFIP World Computer Congress, at which both invited and contributed papers are presented. Contributed papers are rigorously refereed and the rejection rate is high.

As with the Congress, participation in the open conferences is open to all and papers may be invited or submitted. Again, submitted papers are stringently refereed.

The working conferences are structured differently. They are usually run by a working group and attendance is small and by invitation only. Their purpose is to create an atmosphere conducive to innovation and development. Refereeing is less rigorous and papers are subjected to extensive group discussion.

Publications arising from IFIP events vary. The papers presented at the IFIP World Computer Congress and at open conferences are published as conference proceedings, while the results of the working conferences are often published as collections of selected and edited papers.

Any national society whose primary activity is in information may apply to become a full member of IFIP, although full membership is restricted to one society per country. Full members are entitled to vote at the annual General Assembly, National societies preferring a less committed involvement may apply for associate or corresponding membership. Associate members enjoy the same benefits as full members, but without voting rights. Corresponding members are not represented in IFIP bodies. Affiliated membership is open to non-national societies, and individual and honorary membership schemes are also offered.

KNOWLEDGE AND TECHNOLOGY INTEGRATION IN PRODUCTION AND SERVICES

Balancing Knowledge and Technology in Product and Service Life Cycle

IFIP TC5/WG5.3 Fifth IEEE/IFIP International Conference on Information Technology for Balanced Automation Systems in Manufacturing and Services (BASYS'02)
September 25-27, 2002, Cancun, Mexico

Edited by

Vladimír Mařík
Czech Technical University in Prague
Czech Republic

Luis M. Camarinha-Matos
New University of Lisbon
Portugal

Hamideh Afsarmanesh
University of Amsterdam
The Netherlands

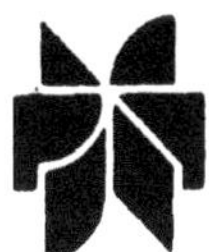

SPRINGER SCIENCE+BUSINESS MEDIA, LLC

DOI 10.1007/978-0-387-35613-6

Library of Congress Cataloging-in-Publication Data

A C.I.P. Catalogue record for this book is available from the Library of Congress.

Knowledge and Technology Integration in Production and Services:
Balancing Knowledge and Technology in Product and Service Life Cycle
Edited by Vladimír Mařík, Luis M. Camarinha-Matos and Hamideh Afsarmanesh
1-4020-7211-2

Printed on acid-free paper.
www.springer.com/mycopy

TABLE OF CONTENTS

BASYS 2002 – 5th IEEE/IFIP International Conference on Information Technology for Balanced Automation Systems in Manufacturing and Services

Cancun, Mexico, September 25-27, 2002

INTERNATIONAL PROGRAMME COMMITTEE

General Chair: V. Mařík (CZ)
Co-Chair (workshop): C. Bremer (BR)
Co-Chair (panel): E. Garcia (MX)
Co-Chair (track 1): H. Afsarmanesh (NL)
Co-Chair (track 2): L. M. Camarinha-Matos (P)
Co-Chair (track 3): E. H. Van Leeuwen (AUS)
Co-Chair (track 4): J. J. Pinto-Ferreira (P)

H. Adelsberger (D)
A. Adlemo (S)
R. Baggen (D)
R. Bernhardt (D)
P. Bernus (AUS)
D. Brandt (D)
J. Browne (IRL)
W. Cellary (PL)
J. Cernetic (SLO)
J. Christensen (USA)
Y. Demazeau (F)
A. Dogac (TR)
H. Erbe (D)
A.F. Filip (RO)
H.T. Goranson (USA)
P. Grefen (NL)
R. Groppetti (I)
P. Groumpos (GR)
W.A. Gruver (CAN)
M. Hannus (FIN)
B. Katzy (D)
B. Koelmel (D)
P. Kopacek (A)
K. Kosanke (D)
D. Kotak (CAN)
G. Kovacs (H)
J. Lažanský (CZ)
I. Mazon (CR)
D. McFarlane (UK)
E. Merchant (USA)
A. Molina (MX)
L. Nemes (AUS)
D. Norrie (CAN)
E. Oliveira (P)
G. Olling (USA)
L. Osorio (P)
V. Ouzounis (D)
J. Prieto (D)
G. Putnik (P)
R. Rabelo (BR)
I. Rudas (H)
J. Rykowski (PL)
G. Schreck (D)
W. Shen (CAN)
Q. Sun (PRC)
S. Tamura (J)
A. Tjoa (A)
S. Tzafestas (GR)
E. Ulich (CH)
H. Van Brussel (B)
F. Van Houten (NL)
P. Verissimo (P)
F. Vernadat (F)
T. Vlček (CZ)
G. Vossen (D)
R. Wagner (A)

STEERING COMMITTEE

Chair: L. Camarinha-Matos (P)
H. Afsarmanesh (NL)
H.-H. Erbe (D)
V. Mařík (CZ)

ORGANIZING COMMITTEE

Chair: A. Molina (MX)
M. Martinez (MX)
M. Velaudia (MX)
M. Zeithamlová (CZ)
Z. Hochmeisterová (CZ)
H. Krautwurmová (CZ)

PREFACE

The BASYS'02 conference, co-organized by IFIP WG 5.3 and WG 5.5, under the technical co-sponsorship of IEEE Robotics and Automation Society, is the fifth BASYS conference in line. The first conference, BASYS'96, was held in Vitoria, Brazil, BASYS'97 in Lisbon, Portugal, BASYS'98 in Prague, Czech Republic, and BASYS'00 in Berlin, Germany.

This series of conferences, having the title "Balanced Automation Systems", was originally intended to discuss the balance between the technical aspects of automation and the human and social points of view. But each new event has – as a rule - highlighted several new topics that required a certain degree of balancing in automation, manufacturing and services. The BASYS'02 conference is aimed mainly at *balancing knowledge and technology in manufacturing, services and the product life-cycle.* Namely, a balance between *local knowledge-intensive solutions* and global performance in highly distributed systems, *based on diverse technologies* (such as virtual organizations, holonic manufacturing systems or multi-agent systems for design and diagnostics) is considered. The proceedings content is focused much more than before on the interoperability and standardization issues, open architectures as well as the knowledge-based integration paradigms with special attention being paid to product-service integration, customer-production integration, and product life-cycle stages integration. The organizers tried to challenge the professional community to present *novel application scenarios for balanced distributed and integrated systems.*

One of the main goals of the BASYS'02 conference is to promote discussions and interactions among researchers and specialists from industrial practice within four tracks:

Track 1 is aimed at systems interoperability and enterprise modeling. Considering the wide spectrum that this track covers, and the many emerging approaches in these two areas, papers included in this track cover a number of different challenging aspects, as described here. Some research effort address advanced product and process modeling approaches and constraint based information integration. Flexible interoperability for manufacturing and self-governing working groups is addressed by some papers. Two papers describe Distributed web-based scheduling and distributed production modeling and systems. The use of simulation services for training and education is suggested. An e-contracting approach and the use of a "recommender" for the e-commerce personalization are introduced. Finally two papers provide example applications of enterprise modeling and service information integration in Tourism and Health Care sector.

Track 2 focuses at all aspects of networked enterprises, including different virtual organization models, infrastructures for virtual organizations as well as at distributed business processes connected with the virtual enterprising, collaboration support services, organizational structure and behavior, and performance metrics.

Track 3 was organized in a tight cooperation with the HMS (*Holonic Manufacturing Systems*) consortium working within the frame of the international IMS (Intelligent Manufacturing Systems) program. This track gives a floor to presentations of the results of the HMS results and thus creates a natural "overture" to the HMS-20 consortium meeting, taking place in Cancun in the days after the BASYS'02 conference. Several papers summarize the current results in the holonic real-time control and in the corresponding standardization efforts. Many papers document the shift of attention in the holonic area from low-level real-time control towards agent-based, higher-level distributed decision-making. Papers aimed at production agent-based planning and scheduling document not only the viability, but also a huge potential of applications of the multi-agent systems in manufacturing.

Track 4 is strongly oriented to system integration aspects. As a rule, the multi-agent paradigm is widely used for integration purposes and represents the philosophical or theoretical background for many aspects of many types of integration-oriented solutions. The papers included in this track tackle different approaches to the product-services integration, design-manufacturing integration, market-search and manufacturing integration, etc. A wide spectrum of up-to-date optimization and optimal resource allocation techniques can be found, some of them connected with quite diverse application areas like medical care or robotics.

The BASYS conferences provide a great opportunity for discussion of concepts, models, methodologies, technological developments, case studies, new research ideas, and other results among specialists - researchers, industrial managers, practitioners, developers, users or technology transfer experts - working in quite different fields like in automatic control, systems planning and integration, enterprise architecture, planning and scheduling, flexible manufacturing, knowledge engineering, business processes management or in the field of social impact studies. The openness, broadness and multi-disciplinarity of the conference topics together with its clear intent to concentrate the attention on the novel, inspiring approaches based on knowledge and up-to-date technology gives the event a really unique flavor.

Such an open and multi-disciplinary forum is highly needed also for summarizing and consolidating existing trends and for creating roadmaps and designing future scenarios as an objective background for encompassing the future research and its foundation. The BASYS conference is at present considered as one of the information sources for the THINKcreative and VOmap European projects, aimed at designing the virtual enterprises research roadmap towards the 6th Framework Program.

Prague, Lisbon, Amsterdam
June 12, 2002

Vladimír Mařík
Czech Technical University in Prague
Czech Republic

Luis M. Camarinha-Matos
New University of Lisbon
Portugal

Hamideh Afsarmanesh
University of Amsterdam
The Netherlands

PART 1

SYSTEMS INTEROPERABILITY AND ENTERPRISE MODELING

1

METHODS AND TOOLS FOR CONSTRAINT BASED INFORMATION INTEGRATION

Sven Kleiner and Reiner Anderl
Technical University Darmstadt
Department of Computer Integrated Design
kleiner@dik.tu-darmstadt.de

An analysis of today's data exchange processes and product data integration technologies expose a lack of continuous computer aided methods during product development. This document outlines a new approach for the integration of product models based on constraints. A parametric product data model is presented which offers the possibility to link interdisciplinary product model structures and properties in order to allow interoperability among applications in design departments. A first software prototype illustrates the realized integration infrastructure and demonstrates the functionality of the constraint based information integration concept.

1. INTRODUCTION

The ever increasing pressure towards lower costs, shorter development cycles and more product quality requires the use of computer aided methods and software tools in engineering departments. Today, innovative products are complex and include mechanical, hydraulic, pneumatic, electric, controller, and even software components. From this it follows, that different CAx systems support engineering work.

In virtual product development processes, product models of the involved engineering domains are characterized by incomplete information and have to be modified many times within iterative processes. Provided that different CAx systems can have access to all relevant data and data can be kept consistent during engineering processes, design activities can be processed quicker and more adaptive according to customer's requirements and change requests. Therefore, the involved engineering domains, CAx systems, and partial product models need to be integrated in an environment, which supports necessary product model integration and data exchange. A new approach for the integration of product data models using constraints of product model parameters and structures is presented in order to enhance system integration and Concurrent Engineering.

2. TECHNOLOGIES OF INTEGRATION IN VIRTUAL PRODUCT DEVELOPMENT PROCESSES

A holistic approach, which is based on integrating product development processes comprises a three-level-architecture (Gausemeier et al., 1999). The integration of processes, systems and models. The integration of processes means supporting engineering methods and work within departments, companies and co-operations as well as workflow management. The main objective of system integration is a spanning communication in CAx environments providing communication and network services. Model integration signifies that different tools using proprietary product data models are sharing data using a common data base or an integrated digital product master model. The result of model integration is a discipline overlapping product model. To limit the scope of a general product model, a number of special purpose models modularize the common product data model and are tailored to certain design aspects.

2.1 Integration of Systems

Regarding communications between engineering tools and sharing of engineering data the following system architectures are popular.

Firstly, tools are connected directly. This architecture implies one-to-one interfaces between tools using data access methods of provided application programming interfaces (API). APIs depend on software programs and software releases. Hence, operation and service of one-to-one interfaces is very expendable. Secondly, the interconnection of tools is indirect. The communication between engineering tools is supported by Product Data Management systems (PDM) using physical files or a data base. Last but not least, the continuing evolution of standards like CORBA (Common Object Request Broker Architecture) and the specified CAD services from the OMG (Object Management Group), the DCOM (Distributed Common Object Model) or .NET technologies from Microsoft will drive architectures to flexible integrated platforms in future, where software applications even in engineering domains will exchange product data in an active way.

2.2 Integration of Product Models

With the assistance of a common product data model, data mapping mechanism between product data models in CAx tools can be provided. For the integration of different model views a defined data model structure is crucial and entails efficient methods for data mapping between all interesting views. The idea of ISO 10303 - STEP (Standard for the Exchange of Product Model Data) is based on a single, standardized product model, that captures and retrieves all relevant product data. But common neutral and standardized data models support geometric based engineering processes only. For example, ISO 10303-214 (STEP Application Protocol 214, AP 214) is used for data exchange between CAD systems or between CAD and FEA systems only. Furthermore, the missing of parametric, constraint-based, and feature-based model characteristics is a handicap of STEP AP's. The required relations between design and simulation models are not realized in any STEP AP until now.

3. INTEGRATION OF PRODUCT MODELS USING CONSTRAINTS AND REFERENCES

3.1 Interdisciplinary Constraints in Product Development

Product models for design, analysis and simulation are usually built up parametrical and hierarchal in multiple ways by specific software packages for design (CAD), finite element analysis (FEA), multi body system simulation (MBS), controller design (CACD), etc. In order to define and analyse product attributes different product models such as design models, kinematic models, hydraulic models, electrical models, and system models are needed. The total number of the mentioned partial models in product development represent the holistic structure and characteristics of the intended product. The process of modeling is specific in each engineering discipline and the resulting product models are not connected tight enough to form an integrated digital master model. Nevertheless, properties of the mentioned product models need to be shared and differing product model structures must be comparable to each other (Anderl et. al, 2001).

Except for geometry based data transfers (e.g. CAD-FEA, CAD-MBS) there is neither exchange nor integration of product model data for interdisciplinary product development (e.g. design of mechatronic systems) available. Hence, a new approach has been researched, which links product models using constraints between parameters and model structures. The integration concept is based on parametric product models, which share their properties using constraints and are connected using logical links between model nodes.

Figure 1 shows the concept of interdisciplinary constraints representing relationships between product models.

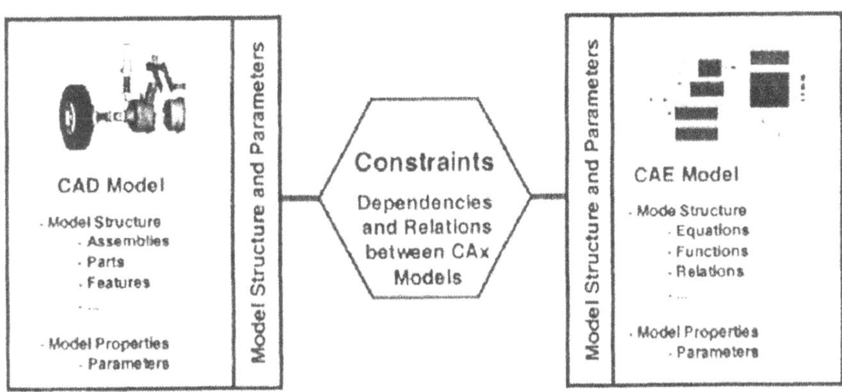

Figure 1: Interdisciplinary Constraints between Product Models

3.2 A Framework for a Constraint Based Information Model

The information model which integrates CAx models is the blueprint of a virtual product model and a repository for interdisciplinary knowledge. Concerning information modeling the paradigm of parametric is still in research. The short-term approach has already led to the definition of constraints in ISO 10303-50 (STEP Part 50) and parametrics ISO 10303-108 (STEP Part 108). Furthermore, the suggested approach can act as a framework for parametric in virtual product development. The defined information model is specified using the Unified Modeling Language (UML) and is based on the mentioned concepts of ISO10303 and parametrics.

The fundamentals for the development of neutral, parametric information structures for the integration of product models are provided by existing product data models or data models from ongoing research and development [Donges et al. 1999], [Gräb, 2001] as well as concepts from constraint logic programming [Frühwirt and Abdennadher, 1997]. The design of an extended, parametric information model could consider only few basic entities of STEP data models, for example units of functionality (UoF). The following information model containing parameters and constraints has been developed because standardization activities in the area of parametrics are still in work and are restricted on relations between geometrical information only.

Figure 2 illustrates the main classes and the structure of the developed parametric information model. The information model allows the integration of CAx models using interdisciplinary constraints restricting attributes of product model properties represented by scalar parameters, vectors, and matrices as well as model nodes represented by items, which are linked by interdisciplinary references.

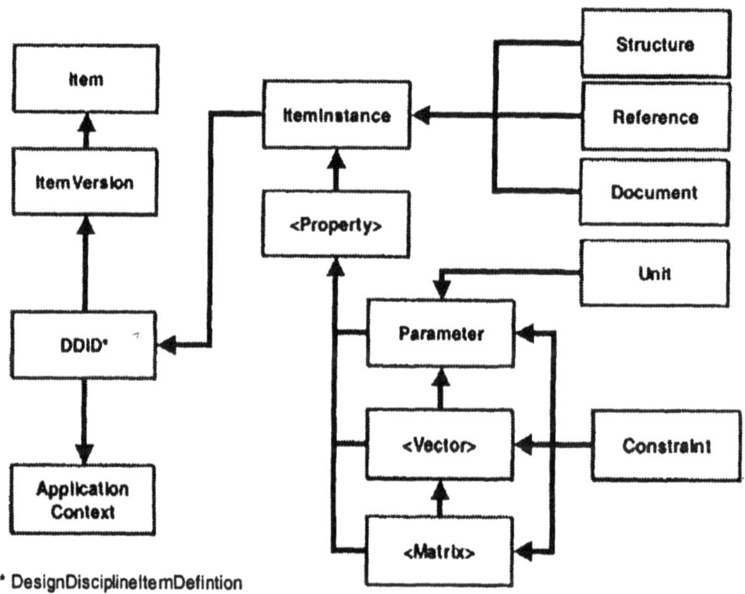

Figure 2: Schematic structure of the extended, parametric information model

The information model is containing the class Item, which represents real or virtual objects such as parts, assemblies, and models. Every object Item has a version (class ItemVersion) and specific views (class DesignDisciplineItem Defintion). A view is relevant for the requirements of one or more life cycle stages and application domains and collects product data of the Item and ItemVersion object. The extension of STEP product data models considers the inclusion of general product characteristics (class Property), attributes (class Parameter) and restricted relationships (class Constraint and Reference). The developed information model is based on the integration of independent CAx models using its structures and properties. The links between CAx models are implemented using the classes Constraint and Reference, which can set properties or structures of different product models in relationship to each other.

3.3 A Realization of the Constraint Based Integration Concept

Using the Java programming language, the information model and necessary methods are implemented in a software prototype which is called X-Portal. The X-Portal enables the management and the exchange of structures and parameters of CAx models.

The software system links different CAx systems (e.g. CAD system CAE system) and imports and exports product data of CAx models, which are stored in a PDM system. The architecture of the X-Portal is illustrated in figure 3. The main components of X-Portal are

- a neutral product data model based on ISO 10303 (STEP) and extended by parametrics (data representation schema),
- interface components to CAx Systems (CAx Connectors) and a PDM System,
- a graphical user interface for the analysis and synthesis of CAx models and interaction.

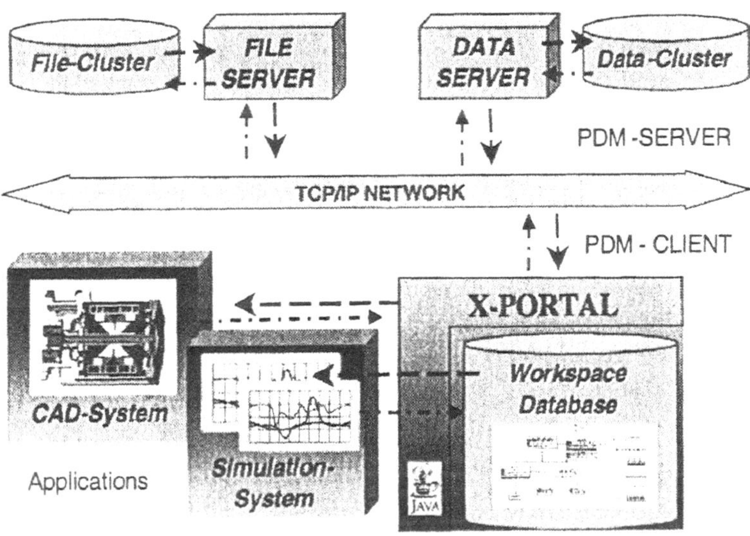

Figure 3: System Architecture of X-Portal

The X-Portal is based on conventional methods for data exchange and on new concepts for the integration of parametric product data. The management of CAx models and data exchange between different application systems are supported by linking directly CAx systems as well as using import and export functions based on XML. In order to link product models and support data exchange between different CAx models, parallel representations of different model structure trees were implemented. Different views on product models, for example function structure view, product structure view, simulation model structure view, enable an interdisciplinary modeling process under consideration of specific conditions and requests of users. Relations and constraints between model structure trees and properties can be defined using simple "drag and drop" mechanisms.

Figure 4 shows how the X-Portal shall be used during product development. The mode of operation in principle can be described as follows: The X-Portal starts up a connection between different CAx systems (e.g. CAD system Pro/Engineer, CAE system Matlab/Simulink). Subsequently, those CAx models are loaded into the X-Portal, which are needed for modeling reasons and serve as data sources. The user identifies the relevant data in accordance with his specification regarding data provision. Data provision and data preparation are supported by a defined discipline-spreading function structure, which facilitates the access to unknown model information. Last but not least, the identified model data are transferred to a target system (e.g. CAE system Matlab/Simulink) or exported into a digital file for further data processing.

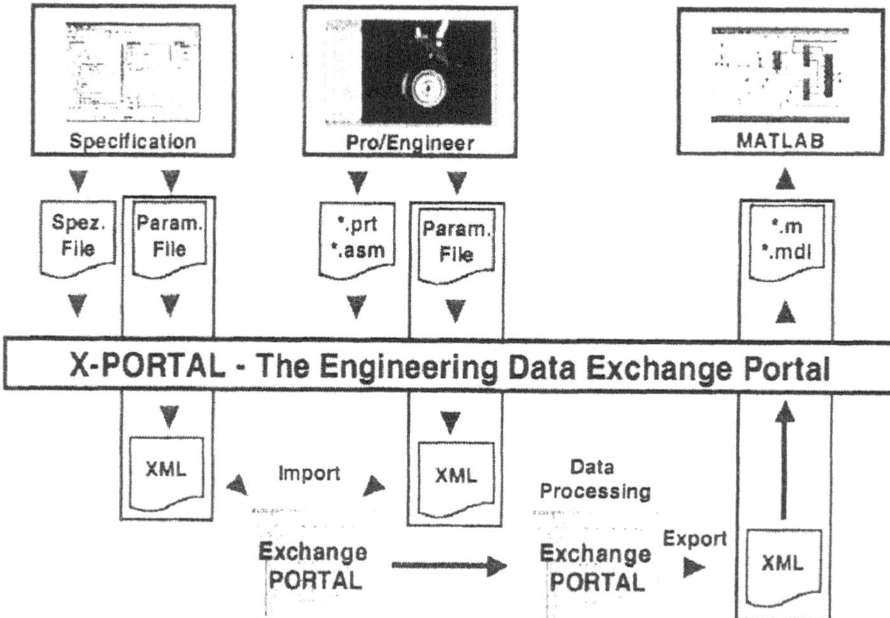

Figure 4: Data Processing during Product Development supported by X-Portal

For the determination of correlations between CAx models, the definition of a neutral system structure (e.g. function structure of the intended product) is important, which sets the models and model items (nodes) in relationship to each other. The application of system structure operations permit the representation, analysis, and synthesis of relations between different model structures, such as CAD (structure of building and assembly) or CAE (structure of physical and mathematical behavior). The system structure indicates references between CAx model nodes and serves as an integrative structure for interdisciplinary modeling in design, computation, and simulation. It was shown that this methodology particularly meet the need of developers, since the spreading use of a system structure supports the working method of engineers from any domain.

Figure 5 shows the graphical user interface of the X-Portal. The panels represent different product models and model nodes (Structure Browser Panel) as well as model properties (General Property Panel) using views defined by application contexts. Relations between model structures and model transformations can be executed using context menus and mouse operations.

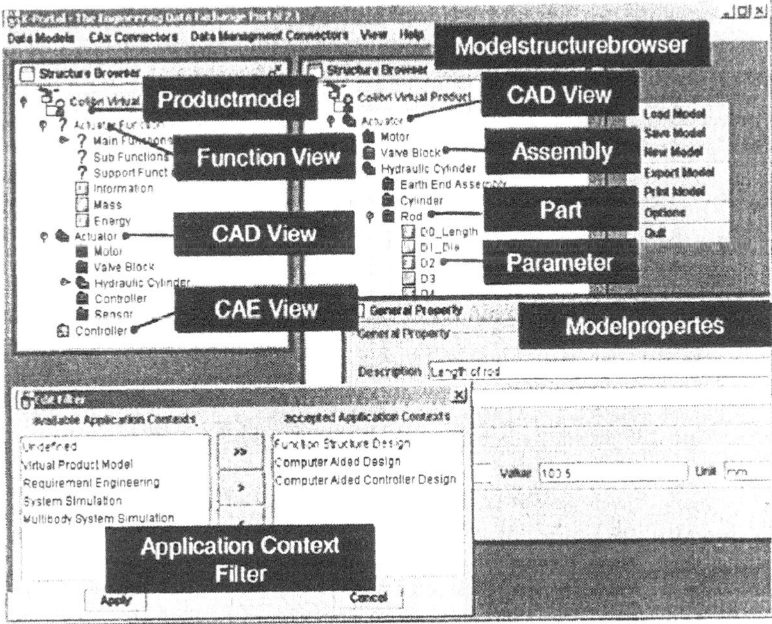

Figure 5: Screenshot of X-Portal

4. ENGINEERING OF MECHATRONICS PRODUCTS SUPPORTED BY X-PORTAL

In the following, the development of an integrated wheel suspension of an innovative service vehicle will be described as a use case scenario in order to show how mechatronic product development could be supported by X-Portal.

The development of an integrated wheel suspension was originally motivated by a research project (Anderl et al., 2000). In this project, a vehicle for the distribution of goods in cities has been designed in order to check interactions between different engineering disciplines during the product development process. The final physical DMU of the service vehicle is illustrated in figure 6.

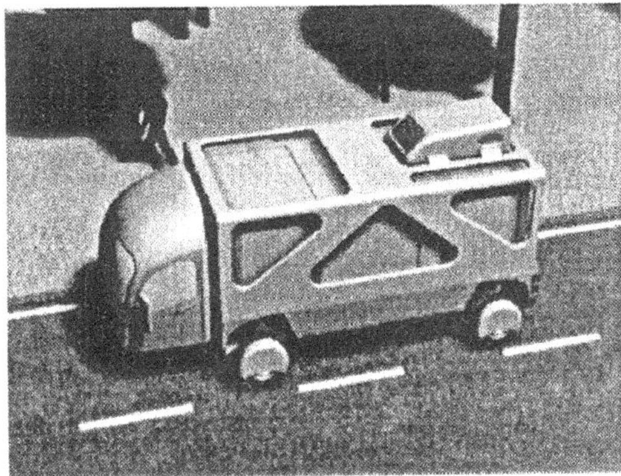

Figure 6: DMU of the innovative service vehicle

New engineering design methods for mechatronic products as well as CAx systems were used during development and optimisation without having any hardware prototype of the wheel suspension in early design stages. Students of mechanical engineering, industrial engineering, and electrical engineering were involved to support researchers during design of selected vehicle components and optimisation of system behaviour, for example vertical dynamics of the vehicle. One specific task was to design the structure and shape of passive components of the active wheel suspension using a CAD system and to model and to analyze dynamical system behavior of passive components using CAE systems.

Parametric CAD models of the wheel module have been designed with the CAD system Pro/ENGINEER and the dynamics of the passive wheel module have been investigated using MATLAB/Simulink. The X-Portal supported the virtual product development according to design methodology and the mentioned constraint based integration concept (Kleiner and Anderl, 2002). Further, it was used to extract geometrical, functional, and dynamical parameters from CAx models and to link them to parameters of other CAx models in order to keep data consistent across the domain specific product models. X-Portal imported and exported data in order to set up and parameterize models for dynamic system simulation in MATLAB/Simulink.

5. FINDINGS

The conception of an extended parametric product data model and the implementation of the software prototype X-Portal have validated a new approach of constraint based product data integration. It is possible to integrate different CAx models by linking model properties and structures using constraints and references in order to specify their relationships for product development reasons. In addition, it is important to incorporate PDM functions such as version, configuration, and change management for the management and data exchange of product models in the next releases of X-Portal for its application in the entire product life cycle.

6. REFERENCES

1. Anderl, R. et al. "Computer Aided Design of Mechatronic Systems exemplified by the Integrated Wheel Suspension of an Innovative Service Vehicle". Proceedings of the 1st IFAC-Conference on Mechatronic Systems, VDI-Verlag, Düsseldorf, Germany, 2000.
2. Anderl, Reiner, Gräb, Robert, Kleiner, Sven. „Integration parametrischer Produktdaten als Grundlage der virtuellen Produktentwicklung". In Industrie Management 3/2001, GITO, 2001, pp 76-80.
3. Anderl, Reiner, Kleiner, Sven. „Interdisciplinary Methods and Tools for the Design of Mechatronic Products". In Proceedings of the Design 2002. 7th International Design Conference, May 14-17, 2002. Dubrovnik, Croatia. pp. 515-520.
4. Donges, Christian, Krastel, Marcus, Anderl, Reiner. „MechaSTEP – STEP Datenmodelle zur Abbildung mechatronischer Systeme". In Produktdatenjournal Nr. 1/1999, ProSTEP, 1999, pp. 30-34.
5. Frühwirt, T., Abdennadher, S. Constraint-Programmierung. Berlin, Springer, 1997.
6. Gausemeier, J., Grasmann, M., Kespohl, H.-D.. „Verfahren zur Integration von Gestaltungs- und Berechnungssystemen". In VDI Berichte Nr. 1487, VDI, 1999, pp. 71-87.
7. Gräb, Robert. Parametrische Integration von Produktmodellen für die Entwicklung mechatronischer Produkte. Aachen, Shaker, 2001.

2

FEATURE DRIVEN ASSOCIATIVE PART AND MACHINING PROCESS MODELS

László Horváth
Budapest Polytechnic
John von Neumann Faculty of Informatics
lhorvath@zeus.banki.hu

Imre J. Rudas
Budapest Polytechnic
John von Neumann Faculty of Informatics
rudas@zeus.banki.hu

János F. Bitó
Budapest Polytechnic
John von Neumann Faculty of Informatics
jbito@zeus.banki.hu

Aniko Szakal
Budapest Polytechnic
szakal@bmf.hu

This paper describes a research for associative integration of part and part manufacturing modeling. In order to gain associative models, the authors analyzed effects of changes of part models on manufacturing process models. Also they analyzed how part manufacturing and production constrain part design. The applied modeling is based on generic Petri net representation of manufacturing models that facilitates handling of process variants by using of the same process model. The modeling assumes unified solid model with topology controlled identification of surfaces and reorderable form feature based part model. The paper is organized as follows. Firstly basic concepts and objectives of the integrated modeling research are introduced. Following this, relationships between part and part manufacturing processes are detailed. Next handling of effects of part model changes and implementation of the proposed modeling are discussed. Finally, contribution to enhancement of capabilities of present day CAD/CAM is concluded.

1. INTRODUCTION

Continuous development of products can be realized only by the application of advanced modeling techniques as form features as building elements of part models, variational geometry and constraints. Traditional lack of manufacturing process modeling for this purpose is the main obstacle to integrated application of flexible design, manufacturing planning and manufacturing technologies.

Changes in a part model are often deteriorate part manufacturability [6]. Correct analysis of manufacturability is a difficult and complex task because manufacturing and production aspects are to be handled together with economical and financing considerations. Effects of a change of a model on manufacturing are hard to be foreseen. Quick assessment of this effect and quick repeated evaluation of the manufacturing process are main objectives of this research. As preliminaries of this research, a generic manufacturing process model [1], an integration of the manufacturing process model in a Virtual Manufacturing (VM) environment [3] and an application of knowledge based methods in manufacturing process modeling [2] have been proposed by the authors. The main contribution of this paper is integrating a manufacturing process modeling methodology with form feature based part modeling by the using of relationship and constraint definitions. Constraints posed by the manufacturing process model restrict the range of allowed modifications of the part model. Generic manufacturing process modeling has been conceptualized taking into consideration recent achievements in generic product modeling [7].

The paper is organized as follows. Firstly basic concepts and objectives of the integrated modeling research are introduced. Following this, relationships between part and part manufacturing processes are detailed. Next handling of effects of part model changes and implementation of the proposed modeling are discussed. Finally, contribution to enhancement of capabilities of present day CAD/CAM is concluded.

2. OBJECTIVES AND CONCEPTS

Customer demanded continuous improvement and variant creation of products are challenges in early 21st century. Quick response of product design for customer demands is a basic requirement that also assumes quick response of manufacturing process planning, production planning, production control and production. While flexible product design and flexible production resources are available, present day manufacturing process planning technology can not cope with these requirements. Prevailing process for physical shape creation is still machining.

Figure 1 summarizes the causes and effect of main changes in part models. Changes in actual orders including changes in customer demanded product features demand changes in design of parts. Other part design changes are decided during continuous product development. The above-mentioned changes of part models affect the related manufacturing processes. Scheduled and unforeseen changes the job shop level as breakdowns, damages and shortages of production equipment, devices and tooling, including electronic control units and devices affect manufacturing processes. Minor changes of part models are often solutions for serious shop floor problems. Using associativity driven relationships between models, modification of a parameter of a model entity initiates a chain of modifications of other parameters of other model entities. Results of earlier decisions are protected by constraint definitions. Relationships of the constrained parameter with other model entity parameters propagate the constraint.

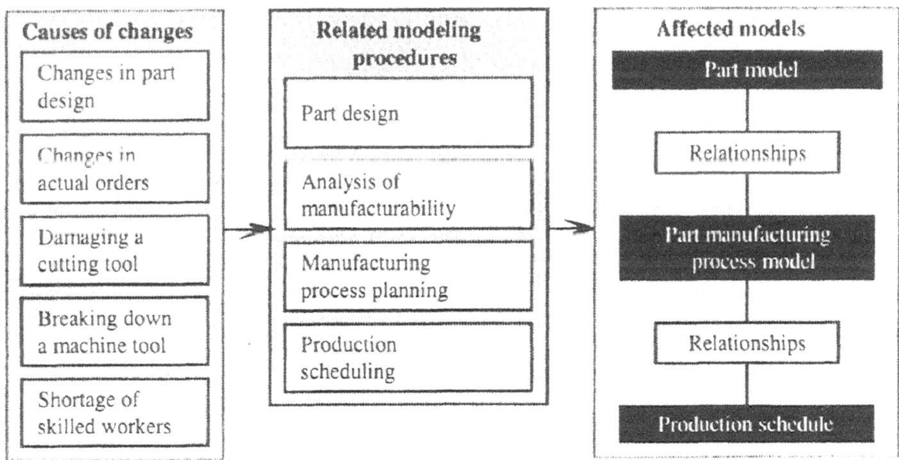

Figure 1 - Engineering activities in changing environment

Let's consider part manufacturing. Manufacturing engineers still use traditional process structure and process elements. This is why the authors considered the same structure and process elements for their modeling as applied by conventional manual planning of part manufacturing processes (Figure 2).

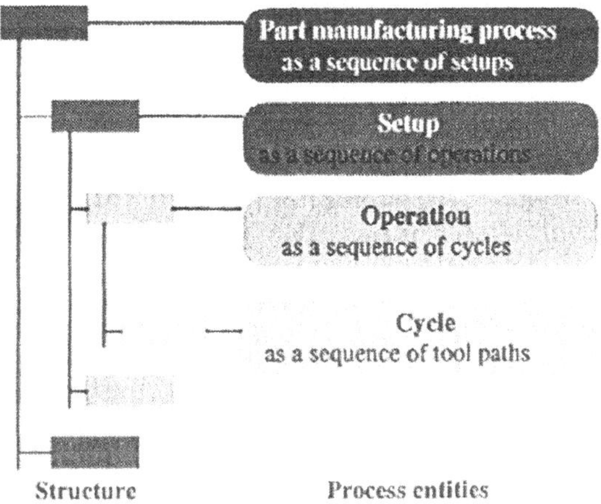

Figure 2 – Entities in the structure of part manufacturing process

The Authors earlier investigated application of Petri net as representation in the demanded generic, multiple leveled manufacturing process model. As a continuation of that research, the authors are working on an integrated modeling approach and methodology where relationships govern and constraints control mutual modification of models as required in flexible engineering and production systems. Figure 3 shows the structure of the proposed generic manufacturing process model in accordance with the structure of part manufacturing process (Figure 2). More details about the model can be read in [2]. Petri nets are well proved for solving large number of problems in the manufacturing engineering [4]. Various concepts are applied for handling the variant nature of manufacturing process [5].

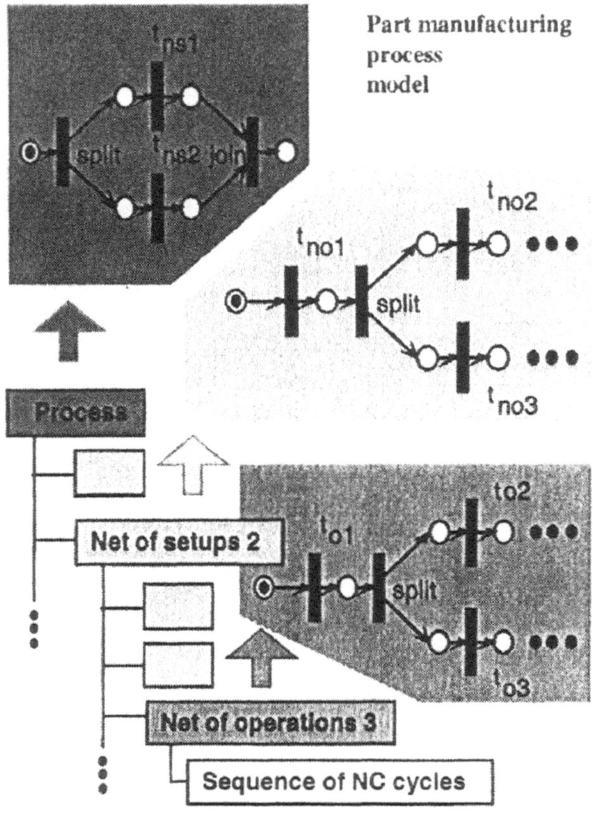

Figure 3 - The part manufacturing process model

3. ASSOCIATIVITY DEFINITIONS BY RELATIONSHIPS

Feature based part model is created by a series of modifications of a basic shape with form features. Sequence of these modifications is recorded in the part model. If a shape modification effect of the form features is the same as of the related machining operations then manufacturing process model entities can be mapped to part model entities directly.

The sequence of shape modifications can be reordered for machining process planning reasons. As a result, two sequences of shape modifications are created, representing construction and manufacturing shape aspects. Reordering of shape modifications is available in feature driven modeling systems. Using relationships between part and part manufacturing process models, manufacturing process model entities can be related to part model entities (Figure 4a). The sequence of shape modifications is reorderable according to the requirements of operation sequences within setups. The result is a tree of shape modifications in which a branch describes a manufacturing task for a setup. A form feature is mapped to an operation or a cycle. Geometric entities are accessed through topological entities in boundary representations.

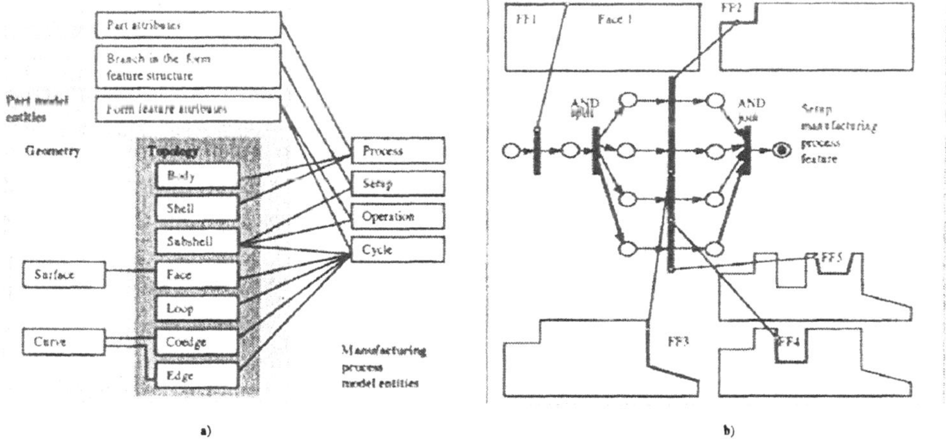

Figure 4 - Possible relationships between part and manufacturing process model entities

Figure 4b illustrates modeling of a setup when shape modifications during creation of the part model are the same as shape modifications of the part during manufacturing. A setup consists of a sequence of operations. A transition represents a machining operation for a shape modification. Machining of *Face 1* is represented by a transition then all shape modifications are mapped to appropriate transitions in the manufacturing process model. Repeated execution of a Petri net takes into consideration machining of the newly created form features in the manufacturing process. If an operation is proved to be suitable and available in the shop floor level, it gains an *in process* status. This method support handling of variants because omitted or suppressed form features will not be taken into account in the process model. Suppression, omitting or deleting a form feature results *out of process* status of the affected operation.

4. EFFECTS OF PART MODEL MODIFICATIONS

Changes in a part model are handled as follows. When an entity or one of its parameters is involved in the part model, this information is communicated with the appropriate manufacturing process model creating procedures immediately. Then these procedures react to the change and do as they can by processing the new model information. Using relationships (associativities) does this by between model entities or their attributes. Breaking of constraints is not allowed but revision of constraints can be initiated.

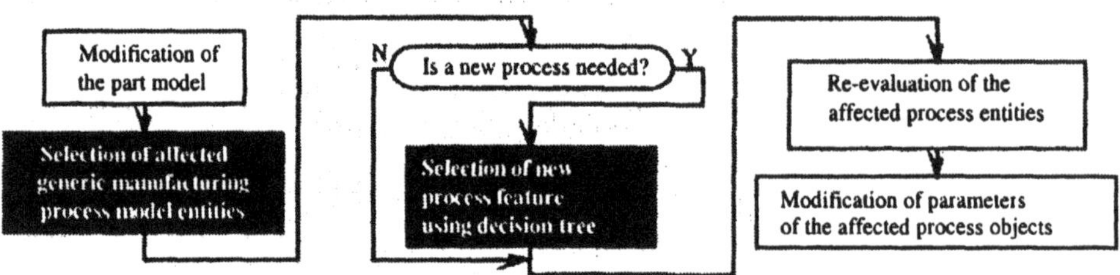

Figure 5 - Modification of the process

Any modification of a part model initiates analysis of its effect. Then modification the process model can take place (Figure 5) if necessary. The affected generic manufacturing process model entities are selected by using of relationships between part and process models. Needs for modifications are analyzed level by level within the manufacturing process model. If a new process is needed, its selection should be repeated. The new process is selected on the basis of modified part model attribute values by using of decision tree then evaluated in the way that is detailed in [3]. If an old process is to be modified then the affected process features are repeatedly evaluated and a new process variant is created. Evaluation of a process model entity includes checking the involved process objects for suitability and availability then execution of the Petri net. Sometimes a modification of the part model needs only repeated calculation some manufacturing process object attribute values as diameter or length of a cutting tool.

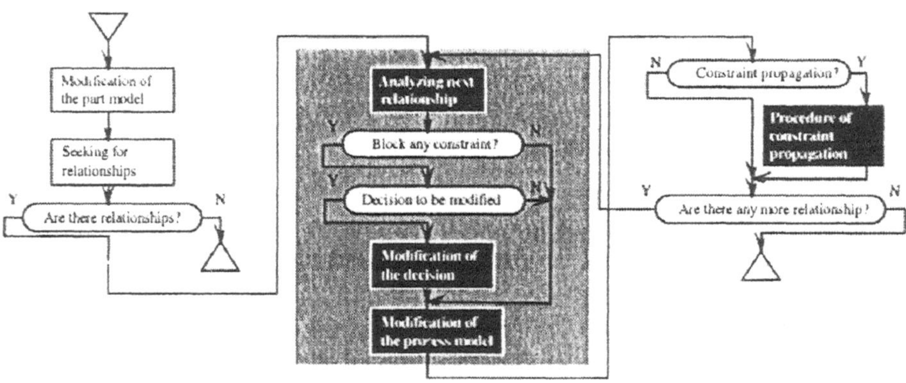

Figure 6 - The mechanism of manufacturing process modification

Effect of part modification is governed by relationships between part and manufacturing process models (Figure 6). If a relationship points to a constraint, it can be modified only by modification of the related decision by an authorized engineer. Reverse application of a relationship can be used for making proposal for part model modification. Modified constraints are propagated in the manufacturing process model.

Form feature dimensions in a part model often govern manufacturing process variants. A detail of a net of operations feature for a setup is represented in Figure 7. An OR split and join pair handles three variants of operations. The decision on variant is done at the place P_d using IF-THEN-ELSE rules. These rules are attached to the place P_d. Rules define relationships between part and process models. Modification of dimension h_2 can reverse an additive type feature to a subtractive type feature in the part model (Figure 7). The resulted shape contains a slot that requires an additional slot milling operation *(branch=V2)*. Substantial increase in length l_1 results exceeding the upper limit of the end milling (ULEM), an additional face milling operation *(branch=V3)* is to be included. After firing of the transition that represents the OR split tokens at the places in the two unnecessary branches are made inactive before firing of the first transition on the selected branch.

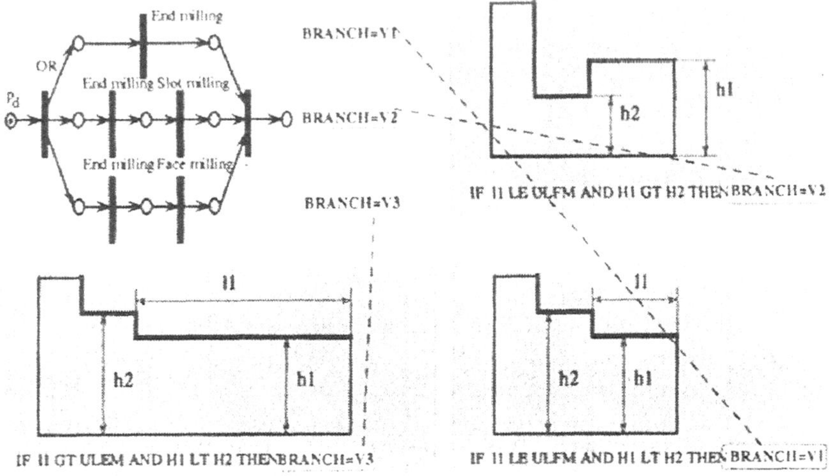

Figure 7 - Feature dimension driven creation of manufacturing process variants

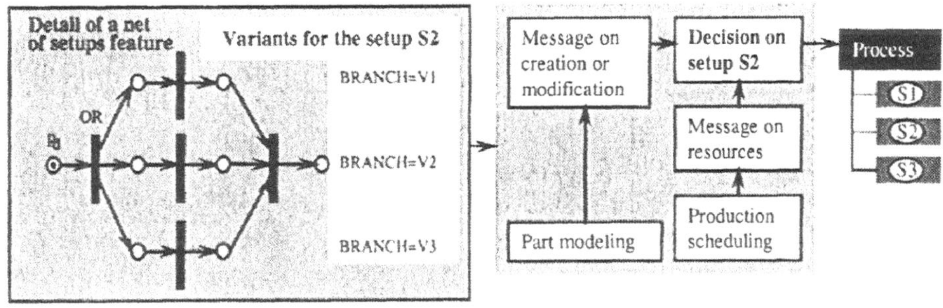

Figure 8 - Decision on setup variants

A detail of a generic net of setups manufacturing process feature on the Figure 8 shows that three setup variants are offered to choose from. A variant is selected as a solution on the basis of groups of form features that can be manufactured in a single clamping position on a single machine tool.

5. CONCLUSIONS

A feature relationship driven integration of manufacturing process model and part model has been proposed in this paper by the authors. They intend to fill the conventionally existing gap between these models. Generic process model entities are proposed that are full associative with form feature based part models. An actual process variant is created by evaluation of generic manufacturing process model entities. This evaluation is automatically repeated as an effect of part model feature changes. The authors proposed application of their earlier developed Petri net based manufacturing process model as generic description of part manufacturing processes. Integration of the proposed manufacturing process model by using of relationships can be used for communication part model modification information with a generic process modeling system and initiating repeated evaluation of the process model in order to creating a modified manufacturing process. The proposed method is intended as a contribution to research on integrated product information modeling. A higher level of integration of product and manufacturing engineering has been introduced in this paper.

6. ACKNOWLEDGMENTS

The authors gratefully acknowledge the grant provided by the OTKA Fund for Research of the Hungarian Government. Project numbers are T026090 and T037304.

7. REFERENCES

1. Horváth, L., Rudas, I. J.: Emerging Intelligent Technologies in Computer Aided Engineering, *Journal of Advanced Computational Intelligence*, Vol 4, No. 4 2000, pp. 268-278

2 Horváth, L., Rudas, I. J.: Modeling of Manufacturing Processes Using Petri Net Representation. *Engineering Applications of Artificial Intelligence.* ,Vol. 10, No. 3. pp. 243-255, 1997

3 Horvath, L., Rudas, I. J.: Evaluation of Petri Net Process Model Representation as a Tool of Virtual Manufacturing, *Proceedings of the 1998 IEEE SMC International Conference,* San Diego,California, USA, 1998, Volume 1, pp. 178-183

4 Desrochers, A. A., Al-Jaar, R. Y.: *Applications of Petri Nets in Manufacturing Systems*, IEEE PRESS, New York, 1995

5 Kruth, J. P., Detand, J: A CAPP System for Non-linear Process Plans, *Annals of the CIRP*, 1992/1. pp. 489-492

6 Shah, J. J., Mantyla, M., Shah, J. J.: Parametric and Feature-Based Cad/Cam: Concepts, Techniques, and Applications, John Wiley & Sons;1995

7 Männistö, T., Peltonen, H., Martio, A., Sulonen, R.: Modelling generic product structures in STEP, Computer-aided Design (30)14 (1998) pp. 1111-1118

3

MODELLING OF AN ALSTOM ELECTRICAL ENGINE MANUFACTURING LINE ACCORDING TO PROCESS APPROACH ADVOCATED BY STANDARD ISO9000:2000

Benoît Iung*, Jacques Richard*, Marjolaine Dellea*, Gianni Ragni**
*Centre de Recherche en Automatique de Nancy (CRAN) Faculté des sciences BP 239
F-54500 Vandoeuvre-lès-Nancy cedex
Benoit.iung@cran.uhp-nancy.fr
**Alstom Moteurs SA, Chemin Rompure
F- 54250 Champigneulles Nancy
Gianni.ragni@powerconv.com

The customer's satisfaction in term of time, cost and quality of the product is today the major concern of the company. To optimise this satisfaction, the company has to master in best way, its processes and to decentralise its decision-making levels closed to the field components to react quickly and to anticipate the quality drift. A contribution to this challenge is proposed in this paper by developing a methodology based on the process approach. This approach is formalised with UML for a manufacturing process as advocated by the ISO9000:2000 to lead first to a meta-model in which some quality modelling constructs are integrated. Then, the meta-model is specialised based on the quality requirements for an ALSTOM manufacturing line of electrical engines in order to validate all the methodology and to obtain a reference model to be particularised and usable in operation.

1. INTRODUCTION

The customer satisfaction in terms of time, cost and quality of the product is today the major concern of the companies. To optimise this satisfaction, the company has to master in best way, its processes and to decentralise its decision-making levels closed to the field components to react quickly and to anticipate the quality drift. In that way, the quality standard advocated by the ISO9000:2000 (ISO/CD1 9000, 2000) proposes an approach different from the version 1994. Indeed in the precedent version 1994, the quality document composed of the twenty chapters imposes, on the company, a repository with rigid functioning but without specific method in the continual improvement of the quality.

In the opposite way, the new version 2000 defines general frame enabling continual improvement by the approach called "Process" approach. This approach requests the company to identify the whole of its activities under shape of processes, to establish the processes cartography by the relations which connect them and to master them by the continuous improvement of their performances (processes, interactions between processes). Process characterising a transformation between an "input" product and an "output" product, everything is then process in the company because the transformed products can be of service, software, mechanical, or informational as a variable of the manufacturing system to be controlled.

In this context of process approach, the paper presents CRAN works done in relationships with the group ALSTOM[1], of which the major concern of its subsidiary implanted in Nancy (East of France) is better to master quality at the level of the manufacturing lines of its electrical engines. Indeed short-term objective on these manufacturing lines within the new factory site, is to operate autonomous teams (responsible for a process) which will have the capacity and the means to observe process, to define and to implement adequate corrective actions (minimisation of unavailability and no quality) and especially preventive actions to master the manufacturing process. This has to succeed a decisions decentralisation (aiding in monitoring, diagnosis, prognosis and decision-making phases) in closer processes of manufacturing (Pétin *et al.,* 1998) to be locally reactive and to anticipate so as soon as possible the quality drift (logic of continuous improvement and of tracability by having the good information, at the right time and in the good place). Our contribution to these works within Enterprise modelling approach context (section 2) is mainly methodological by exploring on the foundation of Information and Knowledge technologies, an approach integrating collectively the product and the production process all along its manufacturing life. It is mainly based on two first steps:

- A modelling of the process approach for a manufacturing process under the shape of a loop **Plan-Do-Check-Action** (Deming, 1986) (figure 1) as advocated by standards ISO 9000:2000 to lead to a meta-model (section 3) of the approach process for the manufacturing processes.
- The integration of "modelling constructs" (section 4) in the meta-model by mainly considering the concepts issued from the General System Theory, from the maintenance standards and from failure cause analysis (method 5M).

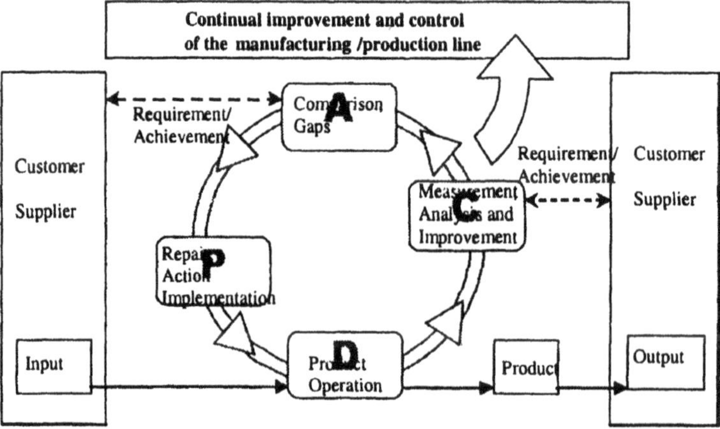

Figure 1 - Entities conceptual view of process approach for a manufacturing/production process (ISO/CD1 9000, 2000)

On the base of these two steps, the continuation of the methodology consists in specialising the meta-model in the context of an ALSTOM manufacturing line of electrical engines (section 5) and more precisely to the assembly process of rotor ALSTOM to build a partial model of the product class "assembled rotors" manufactured in Nancy. The global result of this methodology gives rise, on one hand, to tools which support its engineering and operation, and on the other hand, to conclusions and prospects for this work (section 6).

2. QUALITY CONTROL IN ENTERPRISE MODELLING

Quality Control strategies and operations should be considered as complete Enterprise process which the goal is to provide confidence that customer needs and requirements for product will be met while interworking with other shop-floor and business processes to carry out the global Enterprise goal. Engineering such a Quality Control system within an Enterprise system states a holistic approach for integrating views and evaluations, not only of the systems themselves, but also for their mutual interactions and their interactions with the environment (Morel *et al.*, 2001). It is so necessary in the sense where today, several companies are certified or in phase of certification, that Enterprise modelling framework (Vernadat, 1996) such as CIMOSA (Amice, 1993), GERAM (IFAC/IFIP, 1998) supports concretely methods, models and tools to integrate also the product quality and quality control points of view.

In that way, works were already led on the process modelling (Spur *et al.*, 1996) (Mertins *et al.*, 1999) in a context of Enterprise modelling. For example, a process model based on the approach CIMOSA, was developed allowing the implementation, the use and the maintenance of a quality control system at the company level and which fulfil the requirements of standards ISO 9000:1994 (Kosanke and Zelm, 1997). The application of this model guarantee an easy management of the quality documentation system but without taking into account the modelling of the life cycle of quality continuous improvement at the manufacturing/production process level in terms of PDCA loop. The integration of this PDCA loop within a flexible manufacturing cell was tested, in CRAN, on the basis of functional and informational modelling but without taking into account the requirements of the standard ISO9000:2000 (Richard *et al.*, 1994).

From these works, it results that the quality control as developed in the precedent version of the ISO9000 standard can be already integrated within the Enterprise modelling framework by means of models, while numerous works have to be done to integrate this point of view at the process level as advocated by the new version.

A first contribution to the integration at the process level is proposed in this paper by means of a new methodology for quality control which is based on the process approach defined in the standard ISO9000:2000. This methodology fits within the CIMOSA framework because :

- the meta-model of the process approach for the manufacturing process (generic object model) is supported by the information view of the view generation axis, at the generic level of the instantiation axis and at the requirements level of the model derivation axis.

- the partial model is supported by the same information view and at the same derivation level but at the partial level of the instantiation axis.

This partial model can be particularised (particular level) with various types of rotors made in Nancy. All the models are formalised by means of the language UML (UML, 1999) supported in our case by the MEGA Suite[2]. It allows defining, thanks to the uses cases concept, the quality product at the manufacturing process level among complementary points of view proposed by the standard (e.g. quality control at the Enterprise level).

3. META-MODEL OF THE PROCESS APPROACH

The first phase of the methodology consists in modelling the process approach for the manufacturing process as defined in the standard ISO 9000:2000 and in the way to be consistent with the "Enterprise - Control System Integration" principles proposed by (Isa/ds95, 1999). The modelling aims at :

- formalising in an explicit way all the normative text concerning the process approach for the manufacturing processes (quality control at the shop-floor level). The modelling leads to create a meta-model of the process approach for the manufacturing processes. It represents the object (data) of this process approach, their interactions and the constraints between these objects. This meta-modelling principle is already used in "application protocols" standardisation of STEP ISO/10303[3].
- integrating the standards at the first step of the design of company process model,
- allowing the company to obtain the certification ISO9000:2000 more easily because the manufacturing processes work and are organised so as to fulfil the requirements of this standard.

The meta-model is developed from the conceptual view of the entities represented in the figure 1. That means on one hand, to take into account the input and output in terms of product quality requirements and the satisfaction of these requirements by the supplied product, and on the other hand, to implement the manufacturing process under the shape of a PDCA loop. It is so necessary to extract from the standard all the terms with their definitions, all the parts of the concepts diagrams (these diagrams show the links existing between the terms of the standard), all the requirements of the standard related to conceptual view of the entities and to interpret them so as to delete all the ambiguities of the standard. On these bases, the meta-model formalisation has been realised (with UML) by specifying first the use case diagram for the standard ISO9000:2000 with the external actors who interact with it. Then, for this use case, a class diagram is elaborated by modelling :

- the terms of the standard in relation to this use case. Each term is materialised with a meta-class.
- the links existing between these terms. It is done on the basis of the relationships already defined in the concept diagrams, of the term descriptions but also of a "justified" interpretation of the normative text. Each link between

two meta-classes is materialised with an association relationship having a name, a role and multiplicities.

- the constraints between relationships defined by justified interpretation of the normative text. Each constraint is materialised with a link between meta-classes or between association relationships.

The figure 2 shows a part of the meta-model of the process approach for the manufacturing process as advocated by the standard ISO9000:2000.

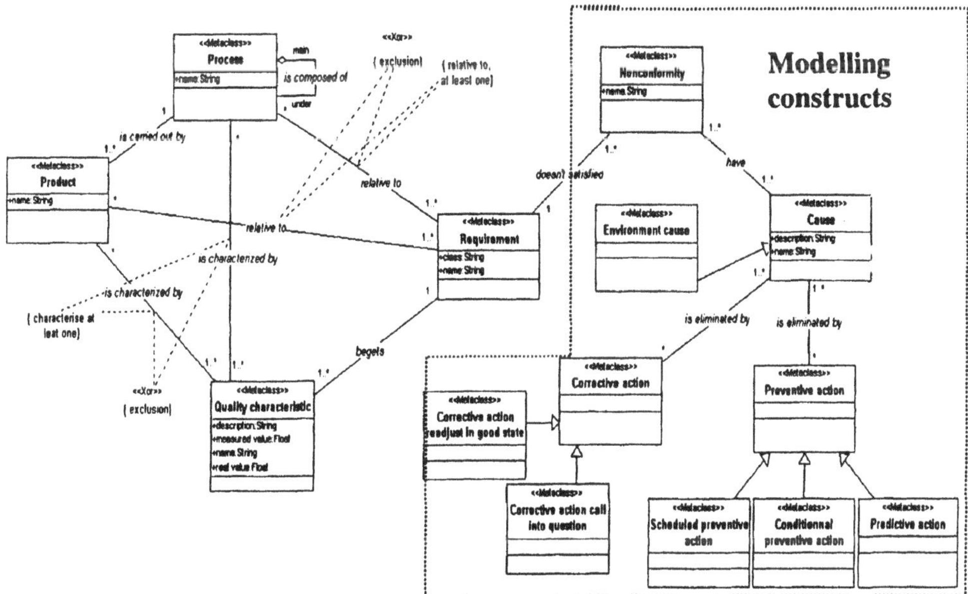

Figure 2 – Part of the meta-model of the process approach – and some quality modelling constructs

4. INTEGRATION OF QUALITY MODELLING CONSTRUCT

From the formalisation of the normative text, the second phase of the methodology consisted in integrating quality modelling constructs into the meta-model by considering other concepts such as :

(a) The general system theory already used in Manufacturing Engineering by (Mayer *et al.*, 1995),

(b) The maintenance standards as defined by IEC-50(191)[4],

(c) The principle 5M (Ishikawa, 1963).

(a) One aspect of the general system theory is to define a mechanical object by three attributes (shape, space, time) knowing that one process transforms **at least** two of these attributes whose one is mandatory **time** (time - shape or time - space). So, we made the assumption that a process, which transforms **only** two of the object attributes, is an **elementary process**. This implies for the meta-model that a process can be defined as a elementary process if it transforms only two attributes or can be decomposed in relation to the attributes transforming into several sub-processes until elementary processes (activities). Due to this principle and as an object has these three attributes, a product must have its requirements defined related to these three attributes. It leads to add to the meta-model, subtypes related to the meta-class Requirements (Product requirements, Process requirements) and with a disjunction constraint between these two subtypes. Moreover it allows adding stereotypical subtypes (Time, Space, Shape) related to the meta-class Product Requirement with totality and junction constraints between these three subtypes. Indeed a "Product Requirement" is necessarily described as Time, or Shape or Space type (by integrating also the rule that Time is required to characterise any Transforming) and a same product can have one or several requirements with regard to these three types.

(b) The principles and definitions issued from the maintenance standards are meta-modelled by specialising subtypes (Figure 2) related to the meta-class Preventive Action : scheduled preventive action, conditional preventive action, and predictive action. The subtypes are constrained in the way to ensure that a preventive action is necessary linked with one and only one of these types.

(c) The principle resulting from the 5M is meta-modelled by specialising the meta-class Cause with five subtypes M : Machine, Method, Material, Man power, environMent. The subtypes are constrained so as to ensure that a cause is necessarily a cause related to one and only one of these 5 types. All these subtypes (exhaustive way) have to be checked in relation to a nonconformity of the product.

5. SPECIALISATION PROCEDURE OF THE META-MODEL

On the base of these two first steps, the continuation of the methodology consists in specialising the meta-model in the context of an ALSTOM manufacturing line of electrical engines. In our case to demonstrate feasibility and interest of such methodology vis-à-vis of ALSTOM, we developed a specialisation procedure related to the assembly process of the rotors ALSTOM to build a partial model of the product class "assembled rotors " manufactured in Nancy.

Specialisation consists in developing, in a chronological way, seven stages allowing to specialise all the meta-classes of the meta-model due to "engineering" questions that translate, in a pragmatic way, the association relation-ships, the constraints and the multiplicities of the meta-model. Every specialisation is represented with the modelling language by a sub-class of the meta-class of the meta-model. These seven stages are : 1 - definition of the context of the study (Sub-classes Product, Process, Customer and Provider); 2- qualification and characterisation of the product (Sub-classes Requirements and Quality Characteristics); 3- identification of the means to determine the quality characteristics (Sub-classes Test, Observation, Measure); 4- identification of the means to determine the conformity or the nonconformity (Sub classes Validation, Verification, Objective Evidence, Inspection); 5- identification of the conformities and nonconformities (Sub-classes Conformity and Nonconformity); 6- processing of the nonconformities (Sub-classes Scrap, Regrade, Rework, Repair); 7-processing of the nonconformity causes (Sub-classes Cause, Preventive action, Corrective action).

For example, in relation to the ALSTOM manufacturing line, the first instantiation phase allows to define the study environment in terms of creating (a) the sub-class "rotor assembled" of the meta-class Product, (b) the sub-class "to assemble rotor" of the meta-class Process and all sub-classes related to the sub-processes (elementary processes such as to pile sheet metal, ...), (c) the sub-class "autonomous team in charge of rotor assembling" of the meta-class Provider, and (d) the sub-class "autonomous team in charge of rotor assembling calibration" of the meta-class Customer. Every elementary process has been, in another step of the process approach methodology, the starting point for the new application of the seven stages of the specialisation procedure in order to have, at last, the partial model of rotor products assembled in Nancy. It leads to master the quality of the ALSTOM manufacturing line by a process approach imbricating a set of sub-processes formalised with the PDCA loop. This partial model (figure 3) can be considered as a reference model that can be particularised with various types of rotors made in Nancy and usable directly in operation on the manufacturing line.

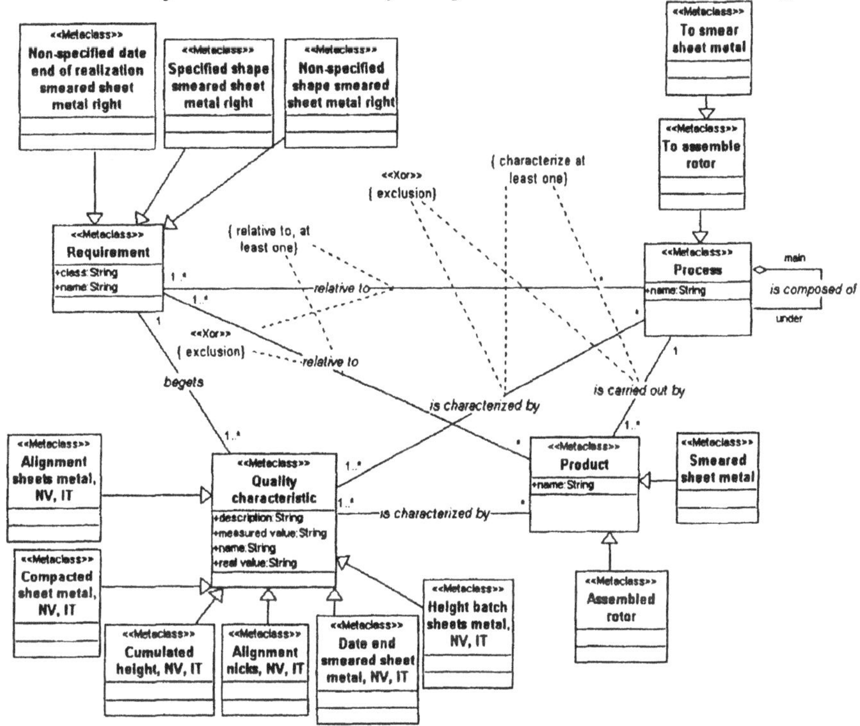

Figure 3 – Part of the partial model of the product class "assembled rotors "

6. CONCLUSION

The contribution developed in this paper led to the development of a generic methodology for manufacturing processes modelling. It is generic, first at the partial level, because a new global process related to a product application class (e.g. assembled rotors) is developed from a specialisation procedure of the normative model (meta-model) whatever the process is, and second at the particular level, because a particular process related to a specific product of the application class (e.g. rotors made in Nancy) is developed from a particularisation procedure of the partial model.

The feasibility and efficiency of this methodology is tested today until end of this year, from an engineering and operation levels, on the rotor assembling line in Nancy. Indeed, a software prototype supporting all the methodology has been developed (from UML models towards data base SQL-Server, from questions towards Access interrogation forms of the data base), on the hand, to help the engineers to inventory all the required knowledge on these line processes (to fulfil the partial model in accordance with the meta-model), to underline where are the quality mastering problems (what is missing to fulfil the models) and then, by exploiting the knowledge encapsulating in the prototype data base, to propose on site to each unit responsible of one line process, some help (document or screen views) to make correct diagnosis (knowledge on causes) and actions (preventive or corrective actions) in relation to the anticipation of a non-conformity product.

In addition to the operational tool, one work in progress is to integrate methods such as SPC, FMEA, HAZOP, with this methodology in order to define more precisely each of the causes and preventive actions. Finally a step towards the use in UML 2.0. of formal language SDL (Specification Design Language) has to be envisaged to allow the verification of the model UML.

7. REFERENCES

1. AMICE. CIMOSA : Open System Architecture for CIM. Research report of ESPRIT project 688/5288 AMICE. Springer Verlag, Berlin, 1993.
2. Deming W.-E. Out of the crisis, Ed. The Massachusetts Institute of Technology, ISBN 0-911379-01-0, 1986.
3. IFAC/IFIP Task Force, GERAM : Generalised Enterprise Reference Architecture and Methodology. ISO WD 15704, Requirements for Enterprise-Reference Architectures and Methodologies, 1998.
4. Isa/ds95.01. Enterprise - Control System Integration Part 1: Models and Terminology. Isa/ds95 standard. Draft 14, November 1999.
5. Ishikawa K. Cause and effect diagram. In: Proceedings International Conference on Quality Control, pp 607-610, Tokyo, 1963.
6. ISO/CD1 9000. Quality Management System, Work of the ISO/TC 176, Sub-Committee SC1 Concepts and Terminology. 2000.
7. Kosanke K., Zelm M. CIMOSA and its application in an ISO 9000 process model. In: Proceedings of the IFAC Workshop on Manufacturing Systems: Modelling, Management and Control (MIM'97), Vienne, 1997.
8. Mayer F., Morel G., Lhoste P. Towards manufacturing Engineering based on semi-formal Systemic Engineering. In: Proceedings of the 14th International Congress on Cybernetics, Namur, Belgium, August 21-25, 1995.
9. Mertins K., Jochem R. Quality-Oriented Design of Business Processes, Kluwer Academic Publishers Group, ISBN 0-7923-8484-9.1999.
10. Morel G., Zaremba M. Information system paradigm for agile manufacturing automation. In : 10th IFAC INCOM'01 Symposium on Information Control problems in Manufacturing. (Vienna, Austria). ifacpubs@elsevier.co.uk: Elsevier Sciences. IFAC Publications. 2001
11. Pétin J.F., B. Iung, G. Morel. Distributed Intelligent Actuation and Measurement System within an integrated shop-floor organisation. Computers in Industry. 37 (3), pp. 197-211. 1998.
12. Richard J., Rondeau E., Bajic E. Quality management of the manufacturing process in a CIM architecture. Computer Integrated Systems, pp 179-190, 1994.
13. Spur G., Mertins K., Jochem R.. Enterprise Integration Modelling, Beuth Verlag, Berlin, 1996.
14. UML. Unified Modelling Language Specification. v1.3, OMG. 1999.
15. Vernadat F.-B. Enterprise Modelling and Integration, (principles and applications), Eds Chapman & All, ISBN 0-412-60550-3, 1996.

---

[1] http://www.alstom.com
[2] MEGA SUITE is a software provided by the MEGA International company – http://www.mega.com
[3] http://www.pdtsolutions.co.uk/standard/papers/pdtag/paper.htm#infounit
[4] IEC-50(191) International Electrotechnical Vocabulary - Chapter 191 "Dependability and quality of service".

4

IMPLICIT HIERARCHICAL META-MODELING IN SEARCH OF FLEXIBLE INTER-OPERABILITY FOR MANUFACTURING AND BUSINESS SYSTEMS

Ricardo Jardim-Gonçalves and Adolfo Steiger-Garção
Dep. de Eng. Electrotécnica e Computadores da Fac. de Ciências e Tecnologia da Univ. Nova de Lisboa, UNINOVA., rg@uninova.pt and asg@uninova.pt

There are numerous proposals worldwide to represent data models and services for the main business and manufacturing activities. This paper suggests an architecture and methodology for the design and development of new integrated models, extending the use of existent standard-based protocols as a basis for the development of implicit models, avoiding "yet another model". These models are built on top of existent components, supported by a hierarchical architecture developed at a model's meta-level and offering several degrees of flexibility. The work results from the Research and Development done by the authors during the last years under the umbrella of a cluster of R&D international projects.

1. INTRODUCTION

When searching for integrated product and services life cycle, enterprises are facing a major problem regarding the explosion of the number of heterogeneous interfaces and data models the software applications need to handle (Ducroux, 1999) (Cofurn, 2001) (ATLAS, 1995) (e-Construct, 2000) (PDES Inc., 2002) (SUMMIT, 1998) (Jardim-Goncalves, 2001a). To have all software applications integrated and achieve compatibility in interfaces and data, it is required that each application develop one dedicated translator for each other application not compatible it would like to operate. This is a very complex situation considering the effort required to develop each translator and the unpredictable number of incompatible platforms that could exist (Camarinha-Matos, 1999) (Davalcu, 1999) (Poyet, 1999) (VEGA, 1999) (Umar, 1999) (Jardim-Goncalves, 2001b).

The scenario to seek out is the one where all applications could be easily integrated independently of the platform in use by each application as if all platforms were equal, interoperating in flexible and configurable enterprise environments. This could conduct to an open platform able to support full integration of systems, promoting the adequate use of the multiple existent and emerging standards like Application Protocols (APs) and Business Objects (BOs), providing an adequate environment for integrated modeling (Arsanjari, 1999) (Radeke, 1999) (Lazcano, 2000) (Nayak, 2001) (Chen, 2000) (Jardim-Goncalves, 2002a).

The manufacturing enterprises have identified this problem even bigger, regarding the large and varied number of product and business life cycle activities they have to support and integrate. In this scenario, a possibility could be to search for a unique standard model that covers the complete spectrum of an enterprise needs. However, this solution is not realistic, and a balanced approach needs to be found (West, 2001) (Alonso, 1999) (CECOM, 2001) (Clements, 1997).

Today, several APs and dedicated models have been developed to cover the main industrial application activities, from design to production and business. Most of these models were designed and developed using standard methodologies and techniques, and some of them are registered as International Standards, e.g., ISO10303 STEP APs (ISO10303, 2002) (SOAP, 2001). Others, although not developed directly under the umbrella of International Organizations for Standardization, were developed by international consortia and associations, like W3C, and due to its impact in the real world and large acceptance by the users, they are broadly in use and considered *de facto* standards ("standards and *de facto* standards" will be referenced hereinafter by "standards").

An example is ebXML (ebXML, 2001). ebXML is a modular suite of specifications that enables enterprises to conduct business over the Internet. Using ebXML, companies can have a standard method to exchange business messages, conduct trading relationships, communicate data in common terms and define and register business processes. One of the technical foundations of ebXML is the Extensible Markup Language (XML) (XML, 2001) that allows parties to exchange structured data.

In spite of the large number of existent and emerging standards for enterprise data exchange, most of them have been developed using divergent methodologies and without concern to have their models interoperable with other standards, in the same or complementary scopes of usage (Jardim-Goncalves, 2000). Since most of these standards were developed in an isolated way, there is not any global plan to be interoperable with others. And to achieve it, it is needed to develop additional methodologies to support the integration of these models. Some international research projects are in course to help in this aim, as is the case of the European IST-2001-37368 project IDEAS: Interoperability Developments for Enterprise Application and Software - Roadmaps.

However, companies have to conduct habitually operations embracing horizontally several specialized domains, making necessary their applications to interoperate with others vertically specialized in each field. A challenge could be to reuse the existing standard models, finding and selecting reference models for each range of activities. Then, for the set of applications to be integrated and interoperable according to the scope of activities, to develop and implement an integrated model through harmonization and mapping based on the adoption and extension of the selected standard models in each application's platform (AP236, 2002).

This approach promotes the reuse of the existent application protocols and business objects, through a methodology that saves all the effort experts already spent when developing the standard models in reuse, admitting flexibility in the construction of new integrated models and avoid "yet another model".

This is a very important aim in face of the rapidly changing business and manufacturing requirements, and the scientific community researches looking for further proposals that could enable the immediate reuse of the available standardized models. The objective is to propose a framework for the implementation of an open business-oriented integrated platform, where Product Life Cycle activities and services can take place between trading parties using different platforms, in the same way as using the same platform (CECOM, 2001)(West, 2001)(Jardim-Goncalves, 1999).

This paper presents part of the Research and Development done by the authors during the last years under the umbrella of a cluster of international projects (i.e., ECOS, FSIG, Cofurn, funStep AP-DIS, prodAEC) resulted in a set of prototypes and in a framework to develop meta-models on top of standardized existing components (FSIG, 2002) (prodAEC, 2002). This proposal uses an inter-related meta-modeling mechanism as the basis for the design and development of new integrated components, appearing as an implicit model built on top of existent ones, and is part of the core of the first author's PhD thesis.

2. FRAMEWORK FOR META-STANDARD APs

Nowadays, a key question when searching for a model to be used as the support for an integration task is about the languages that describe and implement the model.

For instance, ISO10303 developed and has in development 38 APs, covering a large scope of the industrial needs. These APs are described following the STEP methodology (STEP-1, 1994), and its Application Schemas described using the EXPRESS language (STEP-11, 1998). Other standards have developed normative models for data exchange, e.g., VdDK, ebXML registries, OMG, WfMC, OAG, EDIFACT)

For data exchange based on these models it is expected to be used one of the standard's recommended Implementation Methods, as is the case of STEP's Neutral Format in Part 21 or XML in Part 28. However, the available tools to assist the implementation of such models are generally of very low functional and semantic level, and not so much spread in the market. STEP describes its Standard Data Access Interface (SDAI) in its part #22, specifying its functionalities in a general and neutral way independently of a programming language.

Also, the Document Object Model (DOM) is an API to access data represented in XML format (XML, 1998). This API understands the XML data described as a tree-based representation, and defines the mechanisms required to navigate across such tree in width and depth. They enable access and handle of its elements and attribute values as tree data nodes, allowing insert and delete of such nodes, and the conversion of the tree structure back into XML data format. These mechanisms provide a very flexible way of access and produce XML data format output, usually easier than simply writing or reading directly to a file in that format.

Nevertheless, there are in the market several tools for system's design and model development with a large acceptance by the users and software developers. Most of these tools have also facilities to automatically generate the data structures and interfaces for most of the popular programming and database languages, which are very convenient for implementation purposes. Examples are those from Rational Rose (www.rational.com) and Mega Suite (www.mega.com).

Facts:

- On one hand there is a huge investment developing models using standard-based methodologies.
- On the other hand, there is a technology very well accepted by the market, using methodologies like the Unified Modeling Language (UML) that, besides the modeling features provided, it also offers others like process design or system's deployment (OMG, 2001) (OMG, 2001a) (Starick, 1999) (DSTC Pty, 1999).

Question:

How to avail the large number of existent models described in languages like EXPRESS or XML, and reuse them and put them in the market in popular format like UML or any other?

One immediate answer could be to develop model translators to UML. But the core of the problem still persists, once UML models are represented in proprietary internal formats depending on the tools managing them, not existing an established neutral way to represent them.

2.1 XML Meta-Data Interchange (XMI)

The Object Management Group (OMG) released very recently a proposal named XML Metadata Interchange (XMI), intended to provide a general methodology for interchange of models, at first instance covering the OMG standards (e.g., MOF, UML, Corba) (OMG/XMI, 2001).

Today, XMI has been accepted universally as a standard for meta-model representation. Major groups for electronic data exchange, and most of the popular toolkits available in the market, have been adopting XMI as the standard for import/export of modeling information, supporting direct translation for major modeling technologies like UML, UMM and STEP (Starzyk, 1999).

To have mappers and translators between XMI and all major standard modeling languages, as is the case of EXPRESS for the STEP APs (STEP-25, 2001) or the several registered DTDs, would be an important achievement to assure reusability and acceptance of these models by the market.

The key issue in this case is to assure an accurate translation in terms of semantics and rules, what is not always simple to achieve. The mapping between modeling languages and semantics are not at all times realized through the identity operation, and transformation functions sometimes are complex to define (Parent, 2000)(Arsanji, 1999).

2.2 The STEP25 Tool

A major objective of the COFURN project (COFURN, 2001) is to demonstrate to industry the integration of several applications adopting the emerging standard ISO10303 AP236: Application protocol for furniture product and project decoration.

Its Application Reference Model is described in EXPRESS, and several software houses are in charge to develop interfaces to make their applications (e.g., CAD systems for decoration, electronic catalogue management systems, CAD for furniture design) interoperable among them using it. A public demonstration of this integration task using AP236 happens during the first week of July 2002 in Brussels.

Further than to prove the interoperability and automatic data exchange among these applications, the demonstration shows that the traditional effort required for the development of the translators can be significantly reduced when using standards for meta model representation associated to automatic code generators.

The new XMI language was adopted for the meta-model representation, and to achieve the aim as the proof of the concept, UNINOVA developed the STEP25 tool that translates EXPRESS-based model to XMI following the emerging ISO10303 Part25 directives (STEP-25, 2001)

This tool is a first that we know that implements and proofs this concept for EXPRESS to XMI binding, validating the Application Reference Model of AP236.

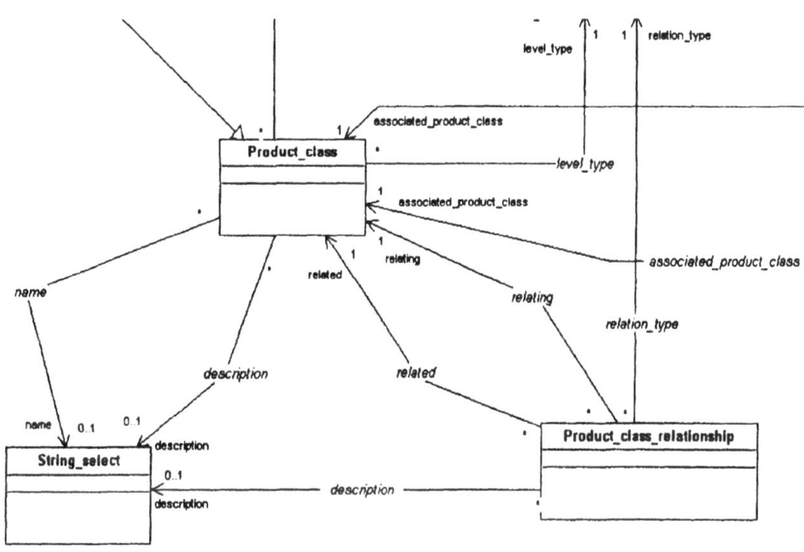

XMI:

```
 (* ENTITY product_class; *)
<Foundation.Core.Class xmi.id="product_class.CLASS">
 <Foundation.Core.ModelElement.name>product_class</Foundation.Core.ModelElement.name>
 <Foundation.Core.ModelElement.visibility xmi.value="public"/>
 <Foundation.Core.ModelElement.isSpecification xmi.value="false"/>
 <Foundation.Core.GeneralizableElement.isRoot xmi.value="false"/>
 <Foundation.Core.GeneralizableElement.isLeaf xmi.value="false"/>
 <Foundation.Core.GeneralizableElement.isAbstract xmi.value="false"/>
 <Foundation.Core.Class.isActive xmi.value="false"/>
</Foundation.Core.Class>
(* END_ENTITY product_class; *)
```

EXPRESS:

```
ENTITY product_class;
 name : OPTIONAL string_select;
 id : undefined_object;
 description : OPTIONAL string_select;
 level_type : OPTIONAL undefined_object;
```

DTD:

```
<!ELEMENT Product_class EMPTY>
<!ATTLIST Product_class
        id ID #REQUIRED
        name IDREF #IMPLIED
        description IDREF #IMPLIED
```

version_id : OPTIONAL undefined_object;	level_type IDREF #REQUIRED
END_ENTITY;	version_id IDREF #IMPLIED>
ENTITY product_class_relationship;	Product_class_relationship EMPTY>
relating : product_class;	<!ATTLIST Product_class_relationship
related : product_class;	id ID #REQUIRED
description : OPTIONAL string_select;	description IDREF #IMPLIED
relation_type : undefined_object;	relation_type IDREF #REQUIRED
END_ENTITY;	relating IDREF #REQUIRED
	related IDREF #REQUIRED>

Figure 1 - Extract of EXPRESS to XMI mapping, and subsequent translation to UML and DTD.

With the ARM model described in XMI, it is used commercial Mega Suite platform to import such model to UML, and afterwards using the facilities of this platform to automatically generate code ready to assist in the implementation of the translators and repositories compatible with the reference model. Also the tool was tested with subsets of ISO10303 AP214, AP225 and ISO13584 part 20.

Figure 1 depicts a subset of the ARM AP236 and the respective meta-model representation in XMI resulting from the output of the execution of the developed STEP25 tool. Also it depicts the UML representation when imported the XMI representation in the MEGA Suite platform.

STEP25 is available for any one interested to use it. Authors will be very pleased to receive EXPRESS input files to help validate the tool.

3. ARCHITECTURE FOR INTER-MODELING

The integration of standard models can be executed by a platform for inter-modeling, based on standardized meta-level descriptions of the integrating model components and mapping rules. The authors propose the platform depicted in Figure2.

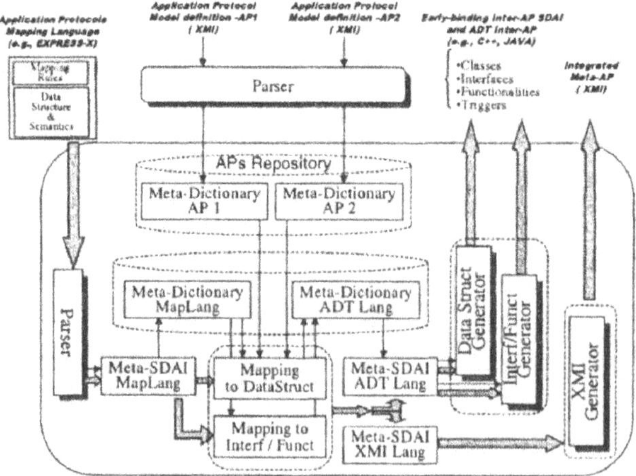

Figure 2 - Internal architecture of a platform for inter-modeling

The inputs for the platform are:

1) The models to be combined and integrated. These models should be described at a meta-level adopting in this case the XMI format. Those models not yet available at meta-level should be translated from its native modeling language (e.g. EXPRESS, XML) using for instance the framework proposed by (Jardim-Goncalves, 2001b). The translation process also includes a classification procedure of all model's components, to enable immediate search and reuse of the models' sub-schemas in the repository.
2) The mapping description to rule the integration, for example described in EXPRESS-X or XLST. This input describes the transformations needed to apply to a model component to be syntactically and semantically connected with the others. The general rule could be defined as:
   entityA.attribL = f(entitityV.attribK, entitityW.attribL,...)
   In the practical cases implemented, the use of the Identity operator was enough for most of the situations. Only a few required more complex transformations, as for instance the decomposition of an attribute in a set of them in the mapped model.

The outputs are:

1) The integrated model, described at meta-level using XMI, and resulting from the immediate reuse and extension of the selected model's components after the proper mapping.
2) A set of facilitators for implementation. These facilitators are libraries of Abstract Data Types (ADTs) generated automatically by the platform to assist in the implementation of the integrated model. These libraries can result available in many programming languages (e.g., C++, Java) and they are ready to be linked with the software applications. They will be a major part of the interfaces that enable the applications to adopt the new model (Jardim-Goncalves, 2001a), saving development effort to the implementers.

An analysis of the questionnaire filled by the Software Houses that participated in the development of the pilot demonstrators and used these facilitators, concluded that they saved about 60% of the implementation resources, if they did not use them.

3.1 Dynamics of the Platform

The first entry point of the platform are the input models (e.g., AP1 and AP2) in XMI format. Using a parser, the models are compiled to populate the Meta-dictionary according a meta-level structure in the APs repository, acting as a warehouse with all models' components classified and ready to be reused, extended and integrated.

This parser was developed based on the *ExParser* developed at the National Institute for Standardization and Technology (NIST) (www.nist.gov), with the inclusion of assertions in JAVA to produce the XMI translation.

In this architecture, the repositories for the meta-dictionary storage can be physically separated or be the same, using or not the same structure for dictionary data representation. However, for uniformity the interface to the repositories is normalized, through a unique Meta-SDAI's interface. In the implemented prototypes only one unique repository was adopted.

A meta-SDAI is a library of services that provides a set of pre-established functionalities needed for the translation at meta-level and repository access. Its existence in the architecture of the platform is of major importance to keep the platform flexible and independent of the modeling languages adopted. When substituting a meta-SDAI module by another, a new modeling or mapping language can be adopted by the platform using the same interface, without any further change.

The second platform's entry point is the mapping description. This input is also parsed and stored at a meta-level in the MapLang repository, to enable a neutral operation of the mapping information.

The platform outputs are generated by the execution of the mapping module, resulting from the interpretation of the mapping rules between the models, through the direct access to the models' meta-data repositories. To fit the requirements of the integrated meta-model, each selected component from the standard repositories could be reused, extended or reduced. The result is the new integrated model, together with the set of generated implementation facilitators.

For implementation of the new generated model, an early or late binding approach can be adopted. In the early binding case, the resultant integrated model is described standalone in XMI. In the late binding case, the integrated model is implicit. This means the mapper engine provides the interface for the integrated model, dynamically mapping the components' structure represented in XMI at different levels of abstraction, i.e., Semantics, Dynamics and Syntax. In this case, the mapper should be implemented using one of the technologies supported by the applications willing to adopt the new integrated model, offering the interface that virtualizes the integrated model to the implementer. The developments done were based on the early-binding approach.

The presented architecture is modular and open, making easy its adaptation to adopt any other modeling language, than EXPRESS, XML or XMI. Intending to translate to or from any other language, it means to consider new Meta-SDAIs, and plug them in the presented architecture.

3.2 Standard-Based Catalogue for Platform Setup and Model Description

To facilitate the search and decision support in the selection and usage of the models' components, these should be classified and described by standard catalogues (Figure 3). Moreover, the modular approach in the design of the proposed platform, results that a general system for inter-model integration can be dynamically adjusted using a plug-and-play mechanism, selecting the suitable modules (i.e., Meta-SDAIs and Mapping) from a catalogue, and link them to the platform according to the kind of integration required.

ISO13584 PLib (PLib, 1998) is a standard for representation of libraries of parts and catalogues, and was selected to support the platform for representation of catalogues of components and modules (i.e., Units of Functionality, Application Objects and Assertions, Integrated Resources, Data Access Interfaces, Object Business Data Types, etc.).

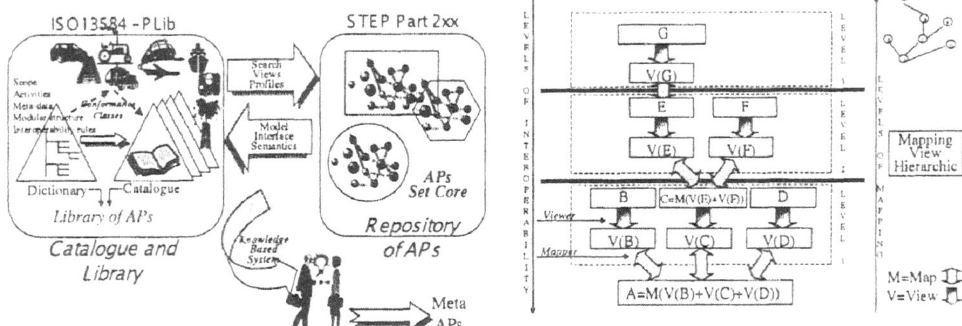

Figure 3– Framework for assisted management of inter-modeling platforms and meta-data

Figure 4 – Hierarchical meta-modeling in multi layer architecture

These libraries are defined jointly with a common ontological system, for classification and harmonization on the semantics of the classified elements (Sardet, 1997)(Fowler, 2000). It should support multi-language description in order to avoid semantically misunderstandings when using native language for search and use of the components to be included in the meta-protocol. With this possibility, anyone willing to develop an integrated model can search the available resources in a standard format catalogue, and select the best fit.

In COFURN project, it was developed an on-line dictionary using php technology on top of an Oracle RDMBS, where terms can be searched, inserted and translated on-line including related terms, synonyms, pictures and movies.

Additionally, a Knowledge Based System can offer intelligent support to the modeler for the selection of the better component according to search criteria and aims for reuse. In the developed case, mechanisms for synonyms and related terms are implemented, offering an integrated dynamic through references system.

4. HIERARCHICAL META-MODELING - APPROACH

For more complex cases, multi-layer architectures could be considered to implement the integrated model. This requirement conducts to the development of a hierarchical mapper, and multi-level implicit modeling. In this case it will be also needed to support an upper-level ontology structure, implementing the inter-relationships between the several ontologies used in the internal architecture of each meta-model component, as described in the previous section. Should this multi-standard integration comprises a multi-level hierarchical methodology, the complete integrated model will be materialized in the root of a resultant n-ary tree (figure 4).

Each node of the tree represents an already integrated model with a wider scope of coverage and interoperability than any of its children nodes, which could be another node or a standard-based model. One node can be used directly by the application, or reused as source for the construction of a new level of the integrated model. This methodology makes possible to construct in many levels the full integrated model ready to support the interoperability between all the application's activities, where the top level represents the complete integrated model, and each intermediate level is constructed using standard models (the atomic elements of the tree) or an already defined node. Each node is represented by a meta-model definition that describes the integrated model at its level. The integrated description results from the mapping procedure between all children nodes, also defined in a meta-model level. This example demonstrates the necessity to develop standards for meta-model representation, where the interchange and integration of models could be done in a neutral format. The expectative is to have available soon descriptions of APs and BOs in a standard meta-level format, and XMI has been identified as a very plausible candidate. While this is not globally achieved, it is necessary to use translators for the standard modeling languages.

Achieving a meta-modeling standardized description, universal catalogues, browsers and intelligent editing systems for development of integrated models can be developed. If these meta-model representations and catalogues become available through Internet using the presented framework, one can search using the web for existent models, or update and extend them. Furthermore, using this approach and in case of updates in the model's components, catalogues will be automatically updated reflecting promptly to the integrator.

The creation of a new layer in this hierarchical methodology should not be forced through a rigid methodological rule. Otherwise, it is up to the user to decide based on the available modules, those to select to link. For instance, during the development of AP236 it was identified the case of the link of a catalogue of furniture module with a room representation one, creating a new layer for project decoration. Afterwards, the shipbuilding industry would like to see project decorations included in the space of a ship. Therefore, a new layer could be created joining the previous joined one with the shipbuilding's.

Nevertheless, the documentation of the new integrated hierarchical model can be developed assisted by an intelligent system based on the existent information collected from the several components reused when constructing the new model. The developed methodology MetaDOC can be used for this purpose (Jardim-Goncalves, 2002b)

5. SUMMARY AND ACKNOWLEDGEMENT

Companies have been searching for flexible integrated environments to better manage their services and product life cycle, which their software applications could be easily integrated independently of the platform in use. Ideally, they would like to see open platforms based on a full-interoperable model covering the complete spectrum of their necessities. Because there are available today a large number of standard models developed to cover specialized domains of a company's needs, a global integrated model could be constructed based on the reuse, extension and assembly of these.

To contribute for this aim, this paper proposes a platform for inter-modeling based on standardized meta-level descriptions of the integrating model and mapping rules, and suggests the use of XMI for the meta-model representation. The major risks for the adoption of XMI identified in this context are twofold: 1) difficulties that can be find in the mapping rules for the translation from the input model to XMI, and 2) the degree of acceptance worldwide of XMI, that could be reduced on the emergence of a new standard for meta-model representation released by a more powerful group or organization.

To keep the platform flexible and independent of the modeling languages, the interface with the core of the platform's architecture is done through Meta-SDAIs, assisted by standard-based catalogues for platform's setup and model description. For implementation of the new generated model, an early or late binding approach can be adopted. In the early binding case, the resultant integrated model is described standalone in XMI. In the late binding case, the integrated model is implicit, handled by the mapper engine. For more complex cases, multi-layer architectures could be considered to implement the integrated model. The developed methodology MetaDOC can be used to document the new integrated model.

The authors would like to thank all the national and international organizations that supported the international projects that resulted in the development of the prototypes and framework presented in this paper, the European Commission, CEN/ISSS, Ministry of Industry of Portugal, Portugal/USA Foundation for Development, IPQ - Portuguese Standardisation Body, ISO TC184/SC4. Also, the authors express recognition for the project partners and our colleagues that work and contribute in the mentioned projects and in the development of ISO10303 (STEP) AP236.

6. REFERENCES

1. A. Lazcano et al. The wise approach to electronic commerce. International Journal of Computer Systems Science & Engineering, special issue on Flexible Workflow Technology Driving the Networked Economy, Vol. 15, No. 5, September 2000.
2. Alonso et al, "WISE: Business to Business E-Commerce", 9th International Workshop on Research Issues in Data Engineering - IT for Virtual Enterprises, RIDE-VE'99, IEEE Computer Society, pp 132-139, 1999
3. AP236, 2002, ISO10303 Part 236, Application Protocol: Furniture product and furniture project decoration data.
4. Arsanjari, Ali, 1999, Service provider: A domain patern and its business framework implementation, Proceeding of Pattern Languages of Programs (PLoP'99).
5. ATLAS, 1995, http://www.marchland.com/piebase/project/atlas.htm
6. Camarinha-Matos, L. and Afsarmanesh, H., 1999, Tendencies and general requirements for virtual enterprises, IFIP Working Conference on Infrastructures for virtual enterprises, Porto 1999, Chapter 2, Kluwer Academic Publishers, ISBN 0-7923-8639-6.
7. CECOM, 2001, http://www.cenorm.be/isss/Projects/c-ecom/default.htm
8. Chen, Q, Inter-enterprise collaborative business process management. Technical report, HP Labs Palo Alto, http://www.hpl.hp.com/techreports/2000/HPL-2000-107.pdf, 2000.
9. Clements, P., Standard support for the virtual enterprise, International Conference on Enterprise Integration Modeling Technology - ICEIMT'97, 1997, Torino, Italy. http://www.mel.nist.gov/workshop/iceimt97/pap-cle2/stdspt2.htm
10. COFURN, 2001, http://www.funstep.org/right/projects/cofFs.htm
11. Davulcu, H., Modeling and analysis of interactions in virtual enterprises. 9th International Workshop on Research Issues in Data Engineering – IT for Virtual Enterprises, pages 12–18. IEEE Computer Society, 1999.
12. DSTC Pty Ltd. Uml profile for enterprise distributed object computing (edoc), initial submission by dstc. Technical report, DSTC Pty Ltd, ftp://ftp.omg.org/pub/docs/ad/99-10-07.pdf, 1999.
13. Ducroux, F., The IT integration supporting the extended enterprise, 1999, pp. 137-145, ICE'99 - 5th International Conference on Concurrent Enterprising, The Hague, Netherlands, CCE-DMEOM, UK, ISBN 0-9519759-8-6.
14. ebXML. ebxml technical architecture specification v1.0.4. Technical report, www.ebXML.org, 2001.
15. e-Construct, 2000, http://www.econstruct.org
16. Fowler, Julian, 2000, "Co-operative use of STEP and PLib". http://www.nist.gov/sc4.
17. FSIG, 2002, funStep Interest Group, www.funstep.org
18. ISO10303, 2002, , www.tc184-sc4.org
19. Jardim-Gonçalves, R., et.al., 1999, Integrating manufacturing systems using ISO 10303 (STEP): An overview of UNINOVA projects, IJCAT, pp. 39-45, Vol.12, No 1,[2] ISSN 0-952-8091
20. Jardim-Gonçalves,R;Steiger-Garção,A.,2000,A framework for adoption of Standards for Data Exchange, 7th ISPE Int. Conf. on CE: Research and Applic.- CE'2000, pp.333-342, Technomic, ISBN 1-58716-033-1.
21. Jardim-Gonçalves, R., Steiger-Garção, A., 2001a, published in book: Agile Manufacturing: 21st Century Manufacturing Strategy, Chapter 48: "Putting the pieces together" using standards. Elsevier Science Publishers, pp. 735-757, ISBN: 0-08-043567-X.

22. Jardim-Gonçalves, R., Steiger-Garção, A., 2001b, Supporting Interoperability in Standard-based Environments, 8th ISPE Int. Conf. on CE: Research and Applic. CE'2001, ISBN: 0-9710461-0-7.
23. Jardim-Gonçalves, R. and Steiger-Garção, A., 2002a, Implicit multi-level modelling for integration and interoperability in flexible business environments, submitted to Communications of ACM, special issue on Enterprise Components
24. Jardim-Gonçalves, R., Steiger-Garção, A., 2002b, METAdoc: a framework for development of meta-protocol documents, Ricardo Jardim-Gonçalves and Adolfo Steiger-Garção, 6th WSEAS International Conference on SYSTEMS, Rethymna Beach, Rethymnon, accepted to be published.
25. Nagi, L., Design and Implementation of a Virtual Information System for Agile Manufacturing, IIE Transactions on Design and Manufacturing, special issue on Agile Manufacturing, 1997, Vol. 29(10), pp. 839-857
26. Nayak, N., et al, Virtual Enterprises - Building Blocks for Dynamic e-Business, In Proceedings of the workshop on information technology for virtual enterprises ITVE 2001, IEEE Computer Society, pp 80-87, 2001
27. OMG, 2001, Object Management Group, http://www.omg.org
28. OMG. "A UML profile for enterprise distributed object computing" Joint final submission. Document number ad/2001-06-09, June 2001
29. OMG/XMI, 2001a, Object Management Group/XML Meta Data Interchange, http://www.omg.org/technology/xml/index.htm
30. Parent, C. and Spacapietra, S., 2000, Issues and Approaches of Database Integration, Communications of ACM.
31. PDES, Inc., 2002, http://pdesinc.scra.org/
32. Plib, 1998, ISO TC184/SC4 DIS - ISO13584, Part1 - Parts Library: Overview and Fundamental Principles.
33. Poyet, P., A framework for distributed information management in the virtual enterprise: the VEGA project, The PRODNET communication infrastructure, IFIP Working Conference on Infrastructures for virtual enterprises, Porto 1999, Chapter 19, Kluwer Academic Publishers, ISBN 0-7923-8639-6
34. prodAEC, 2002, http://www.prodaec.net.
35. Radeke, E. et al. Distributed information management in virtual engineering enterprises by GEN. 9th International Workshop on Research Issues in Data Engineering - IT for Virtual Enterprises, RIDE-VE'99, pages 36–43. IEEE Computer Society, 1999.
36. Sardet, Eric; et.al, 1997, Formal Specification, Modelling and Exchange of Classes of Components according PLib. Global Network Engineering 97, pp 179- 201.
37. SOAP, 2000, http://www.mel.nist.gov/sc5/soap/
38. Starzyk, D., 1999, STEP and OMG Product Data Management specifications – A guide for decision makers, OMG Document mfg/99-10-04 and PDES Inc. Document MG001.04.00.
39. STEP-1, 1994, ISO10303 STEP Part1 - Overview and Fundamentals Principles
40. STEP-11, 1998, ISO TC184/SC4, IS - ISO 10303, Part11 – EXPRESS Language reference manual
41. STEP-25, 2001, ISO10303 STEP Part25: EXPRESS to XMI binding, www.nist.gov/sc4
42. SUMMIT, 1998, Project summary, http://exnorm.com/r&d/summit/pages/summary.html
43. Umar. A framework for analyzing virtual enterprise infrastructure. In Proceedings of the 9th International Workshop on Research Issues in Data Engineering - IT for Virtual Enterprises, RIDE-VE'99, pages 4–11. IEEE Computer Society, 1999.
44. VEGA, 1999, http://cic.cstb.fr/ILC/ecprojec/vega/home.htm
45. West, M., 2001, ISO/WD 18876-1 Integration of industrial data for exchange, access and sharing – Part1: Architecture overview and description, ISOTC184/SC4/WG10 N333.

5

AN ACTIVITY-BASED MODEL OF CONCURRENT ENGINEERING SYSTEM

Goran D. Putnik[*], Antonio José Caulliraux Pithon[**]
[*] *Universidade do Minho, Department of Production and Systems Engineering, Portugal*
putnikgd@dps.uminho.pt
[**] *Centro Federal de Educação Tecnológica – RJ, Brazil*
pithon@cefet-rj.br, pithon@dps.uminho.pt

The Concurrent Engineering (CE) concept is an advanced organizational concept based on idea of parallel/simultaneous and concurrent processing of the requirements of different business/enterprise's functions such as marketing, CAD, CAM, PPC, manufacturing, etc. which application leads to radical shortening of the total production process time as well as quality improvement. The CE based organization is oriented to product and, further, it is characterized by the much higher organizational dynamics than the traditional organizational models due to frequent products change. To support this dynamics effectively, and efficiently, it is necessary to develop corresponded models of the CE process that would serve as the base for the CE based organization design. The paper presents an activity-based model of CE System, using IDEF0 diagrams as the representation class, covering the concrete CE system's life cycle, that is composed of two basic global processes: the CE system design and the CE system operation. The model refers, as well, the CE tools and control (management) processes for the CE processes presented.

1. INTRODUCTION

Presently, with the appearance of new technologies, enterprises are seeking a better positioning in the market by means of a slimmer production process that allows them to become more competitive in the launching of new products in less and less time spaces. One of the solutions found by companies at the beginning of the 80' was the migration of traditional organization (organization characterized by sequential processing), whose capacity of fast reconfiguration, high productivity and low cost no longer reached the parameters of the present demanding market, for the increase of parallelism among development activities, i.e. activities that were performed solely after final approval of previous activities are anticipated in such manner that they no longer depend on prolonged approval cycles.

This concept is called Concurrent Engineering (CE). Thus, the Concurrent Engineering (CE) concept is an advanced organizational concept based on idea of parallel/simultaneous processing of the of different business/enterprise functions' requirements such as marketing, CAD, CAM, PPC, manufacturing, etc. which application leads to radical shortening of the total production process time as well as quality improvement. The basic mechanisms for the implementation of parallel/simultaneous processes are the multifunctional teams (called also the "taskforce"), that work together simultaneously, and the corresponded information technologies and tools for the CE process support. As the team works simultaneously it is not possible to process more than one single product at the time. From the other hand, changing to the new products implies reconsideration of the team structure as well as it may imply other CE support tools. Therefore, the traditional "functional" organization of the enterprise is affected and it is imposed a new product (project) oriented organization, based on product (project) oriented engineering teams to perform necessary tasks. This kind of organization sometimes is called the "orthogonal organization" (as opposite to the functional organization), "matrix organization", "horizontal organization", and similarly, and it is characterized with the much higher organizational dynamics than the traditional one.

To support this dynamics effectively, and efficiently, it is necessary to develop corresponded models of the CE process, or processes, that would serve as the base for the CE based organization design and, further, it's effective and efficient implementation and operation. In the paper it is presented an activity-based model[1] of *CE System*, using IDEFO diagrams as the representation class, covering the concrete CE system's life cycle, that is composed of two basic global processes: the CE system design and the CE system operation. The CE system design process is further decomposed in five sub-processes, covering the design of CE groups, selection of CE tools, etc., and the CE system operation processes are decomposed in eight sub-processes, covering the product life cycle. The processes are supported by/use corresponded CE tools as well as the processes are subjected to control (management).

Before we introduce our model of CE System, it is worth mentioning that the authors who work in area of Concurrent Engineering, e.g. (Causing 1989), (Pawar 2000), (Prasad, 1997), approach the theme only so far as it deals with definitions, principles, never referring to a model aimed at a CE Systems Project. Actually, we find only in (Ranky 1994) a CE specified explicitly from the system point of view.

IDEFO, used for the CE model representation proposed herein, is a graphic modelling language, which is a semi formal representation of sequences and hierarchy of processes, consisting of activities and functions in as many levels deemed necessary. The IDEFO basic construct is an activity, or process, represented (graphically) by a box, Input and Output of the activity/process and Mechanisms that an activity/process uses. Additionally, each activity/process is subjected to Control. Input, Output, Mechanisms and Control are represented (graphically) by arrows.

The IDEFO is also a representation class for the system's/enterprise's "workflow" representation.

---

[1] A model of a system/organisation/enterprise is created in order to represent a system/organisation/enterprise that serves as reference common to all its members, whether people, systems or resources. Based on the model of the system/organisation/enterprise, any person can acquire a general view of the operations of the system/organisation/enterprise, thereby enabling a deeper analysis and identification of points for improvement.

A strict definition of the model is (Ebbinghaus et al., 1996): "For a given formula, a model of this formula is any interpretation taken as true".

The advantages of this diagram can be summarized by: 1) easy use, because a quick reading can provide a view of the entire process; 2) it permits the use of texts and glossaries, which results in a complete understanding of the processes and eliminates misinterpretations. The disadvantage of IDEF0 is that it is not able to represent the simultaneity and concurrency of processes.

The model described covers the activities of a traditional enterprise, but may also be applied to virtual enterprises with some alterations.

2. CONCURRENT ENGINEERING

The concept of CE defines that various activities are developed in parallel, interactively and concurrently, involving professionals from different specialties, covering the entire product development cycle, as opposed to the traditional sequential stage method. Thus, one activity is re-fed by another. Additionally, the activities/functions concur among themselves in order to achieve the best possible solution. This new manner of working is very beneficial in that it avoids possible losses of time and resources, as well as it minimise the design and manufacturing processes changes, caused by a lack of complete involvement of the different sectors in all stages of development that form part of the project, besides the improvement of development quality. To the contrary, the time and resources spent in the performance of tasks that would later have to be re-done would never be recovered (Pithon, Putnik; 2001).

The Concurrent Engineering Reference Model proposed (Putnik, 2000a) is multidimensional. On the figure 1 is presented a three-dimensional CE subspace where the first dimension presented is a CE application domain dimension, i.e. the product domain. In principle, the CE can be applied to any kind of product: "traditional" tangible products, services (e.g. client relationship), processes (e.g. manufacturing processes), information, (enterprise) system, etc. The second dimension is the EC process dimension that defines three types of CE processes, the CE process planning (or design), the EC processes themselves and the EC processes control (or management). The third dimension is the technology dimension i.e. the third dimension refers the methods (algorithms, procedures) and Hardware/Software (concrete) tools for the process support.

Other dimensions are considered too, e.g. the dimension of the CE system components and their relationship that represents the CE system organisation dimension.

Regarding this dimension, the CE concept is characterised by use of the multifunctional teams (also known as taskforces) that are the basic mechanism for the installation of parallel/ simultaneous and concurrent processes. The team/group leader, besides its leadership function (that includes group management and other aspects of the group leadership), serves also as the linking element between the directors and the group (members), figure 2 (Pithon, Putnik; 2002).

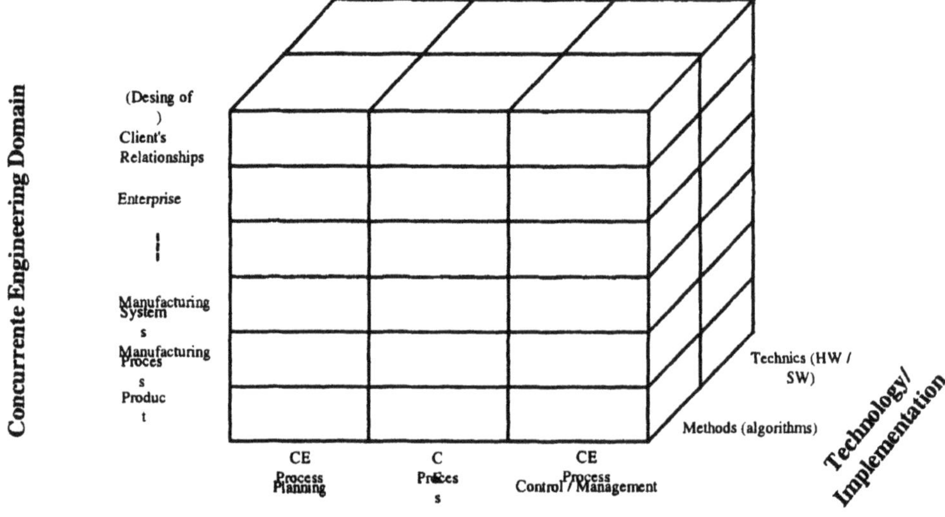

Figure 1 - Concurrente Engineering Reference Model

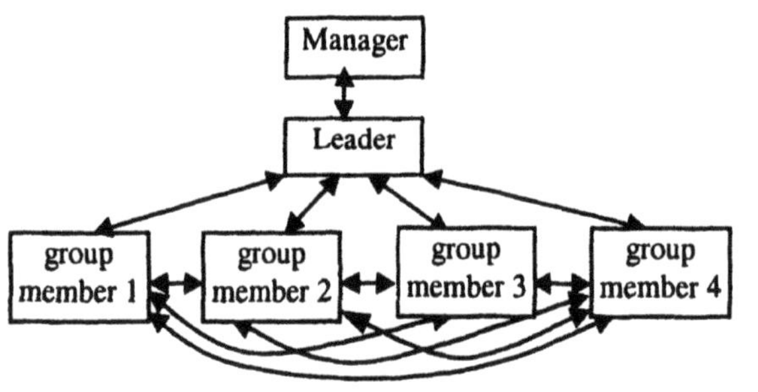

Figure 2 – Management Model of Concurrent Engineering Group

The model described in section 3 is oriented to the first layer of the reference model but can be applied to any other layer considering particularities of the concrete layer.

3. CE SYSTEM MODEL

There are various definitions of a system. One says that a (general) system is a relation over (set of) objects while another adds operations to the system specification, etc. For our purposes, our definition should satisfy the CE Reference Model (figure 1) as well. In accordance with the CE reference model, at the figure 1, to define a CE system it is necessary to define (1) CE domain, (2) CE processes and (3) technology (methods and techniques).

Considering the CE reference model referred and the following use of IDEF0 technique it is easy to find a correspondence between these two representations. In IDEF0 the CE domain is represented by the Input/Output arrows, (2) CE processes are represented by the activity/process box and the Control arrow (as the Control itself is a process), and (3) technology (methods and techniques), i.e. tools, is represented by the Mechanism arrow.

The section 3.1 presents the CE System model aimed primarily at "traditional" enterprise. The model is also applicable to the Virtual Enterprises (VE) with some additional specific information flow that is represented on the same figures by the thick grey dashed line. In section 3.2 are presented some specific sub processes regarding CE in VE.

3.1 CE System Model Aimed at "Traditional" Enterprises

In order to describe the model at its highest level, an A0 context diagram has been created (figure 3) where by the box A0 is presented the global CE process (Pithon, Putnik; 2001).

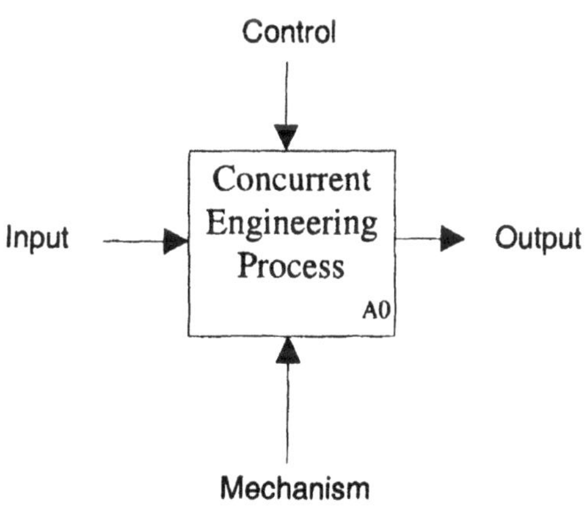

Figure 3 – CE System global model – (Diagram of A0 context)

Decomposition of the process A0 is shown in diagram on the figure 4. We have two global sub processes which are: the *CE System design* (A1), which corresponds to the CE process planning from the CE reference model at the figure 1, and of the *CE System operation* (A2), which corresponds to the (objective) CE process and the CE process control, or management, from the CE reference model at the figure 1.

It is important to notice that the diagram on the figure 4 serves as a model for the "traditional" enterprise as well as for the VE with the difference in the information flow represented by the thick grey dashed line (that will be explained in the section 3.2).

The A1 process, i.e. the CE System design process, is consisted of five sub-processes, see figure 5, that cover CE team design (A11), selection of software/tools for CE teams (A12), CE team management methodologies (A13), development of (software) tools for CE teams (if necessary) (A14), and the training of the CE team in the use of new tools (if necessary) (A15).

The A2 process, i.e. the CE System operation process, is consisted of eight sub-processes, see figure 6, that cover all aspects of the entire life cycle of product, from Market Research (for new products to be produced by the enterprise with the objective of meeting the client's needs) to After Sales service. These are: market research for a new product (A21), product specification (A22), product project and development (A23), refinement and construction of prototype (A24), pre-production (A25), production (A26), distribution (A27), and after sales service (A28).

It is worth to notice that eight sub-processes referred correspond by the names to the general product life cycle, which is, in fact, the objective of the CE concept, but they are not the processes along the product life cycle. They are true CE processes that refer particular aspects of the product life cycle. CE approaches the product development by multifunctional team composed by experts for different aspects of the product life cycle. Each one of these experts perform one of the CE processes in accordance with its expertise, which is implicitly represented by CE processes which names associate to the particular general product life cycle. Consequently, more correctly, we could say that the processes A21-A28 are: CE process that considers market research for a new product (A21), CE process that considers product specification (A22), CE process that considers product project (A23), etc.

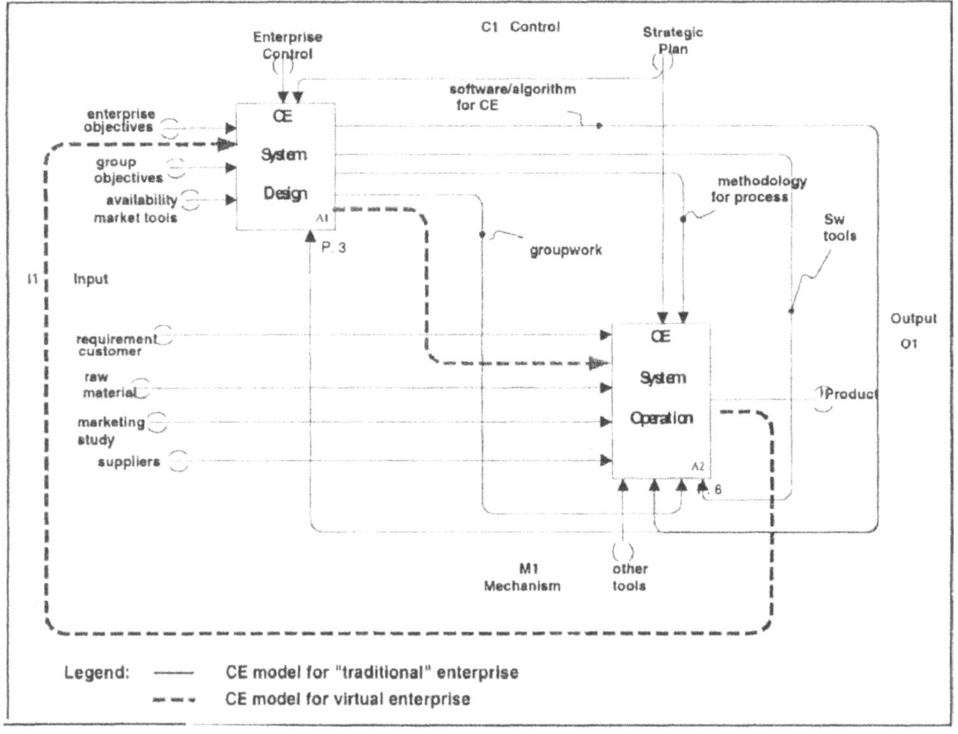

Figure 4 – CE System design and operation (decomposition of A0 diagram)

Naturally, there are other possible decompositions of the A2 process. Also, different association with the CE team members (CE operations definition[2], which is not the issue in this paper) are possible, e.g. one A2x process could be performed by one, two, or more EC team members as well as one team member could perform one, two, or more CE A2x processes.

The processes A21 to A28 should be performed simultaneously and concurrently, as it is the CE principle. However, the processes A21 to A28 are presented sequentially in the figure 6 due to the IDEF0 incapacity to represent correctly the simultaneity and concurrence of the processes. The simultaneity and concurrence of the processes could be represented in IDEF0 diagrams by the

[2] By the operation we consider the set of processes allocated to one resource. In the context of "Operation" one processes is called the "Operation element". For example, if we have to drill two holes and if we allocate drilling of each one hole to two different machines that we will have two operations, each operation with one operation element. If we allocate drilling of both holes to only one machine than we will have only one operation and this operation will have two operation elements. The similar concept is applied to services, in our case to the CE processes, where the "machine" is a human expert that performs one or more processes. Note: The CE processes in this paper do not consider the CE operations in the above sense as it is the issue of the concrete CE processes/CE team design solution.

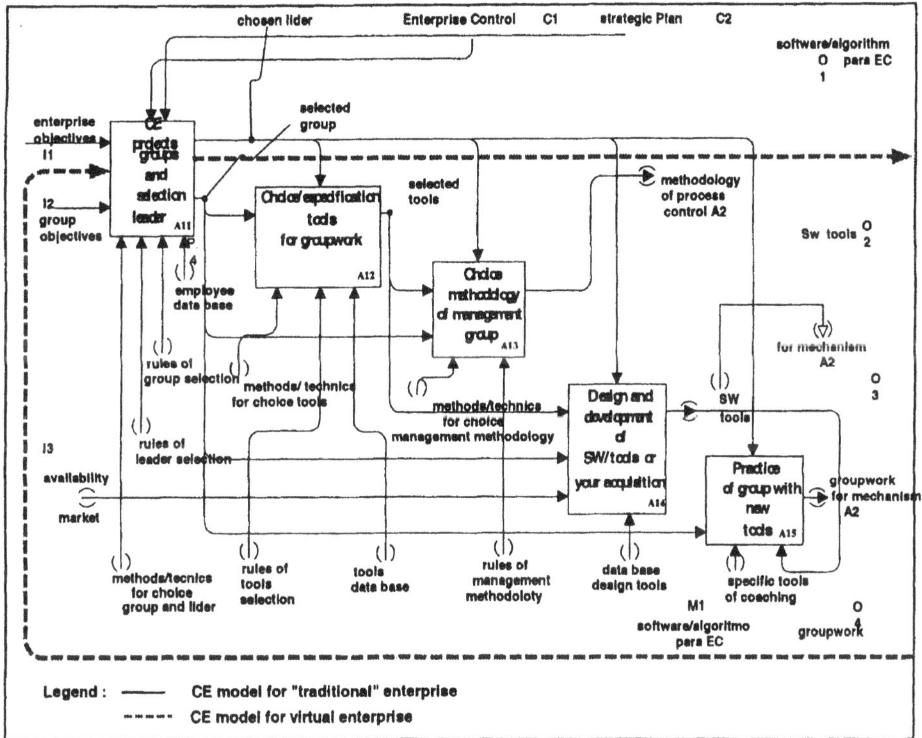

Figure 5 – CE System design processes (decomposition of A1 process)

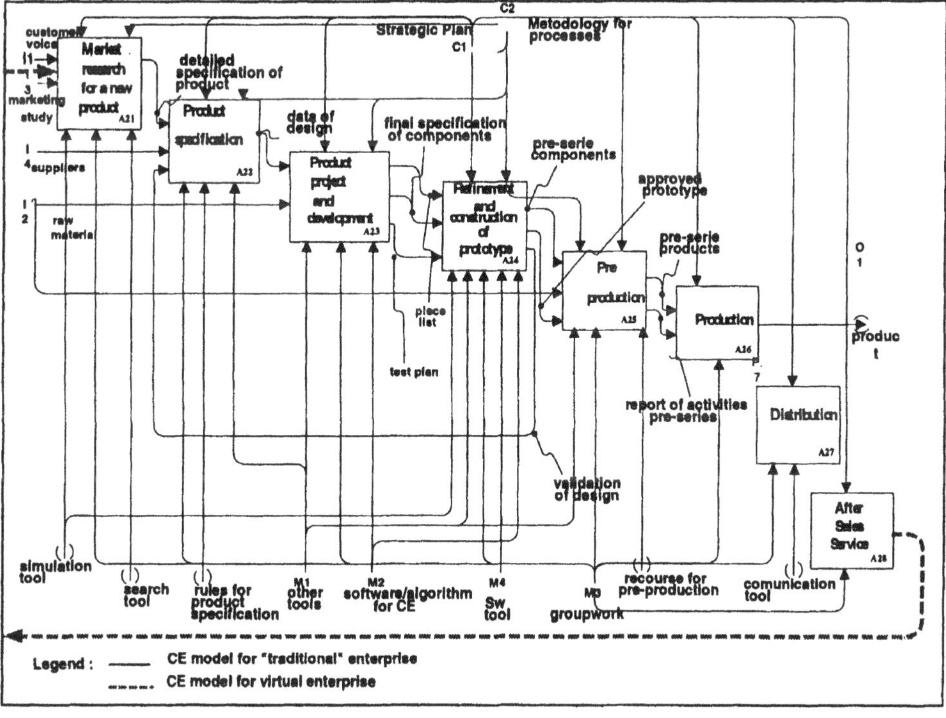

Figure 6 – CE System operation processes (decomposition of A2 process)

feedback information flow between each two processes together by the CE process control/ management that enters all sub process. Thus, the interpretation of the processes presented on the figure 6 and their relationship should consider their simultaneity and concurrence.

Due to the space limitation, of the further decomposition of processes it is presented only the decomposition of the A11 process, which, for the traditional enterprise, consists of the CE team leader selection (A111) and CE team constitution (A112), figure 7.

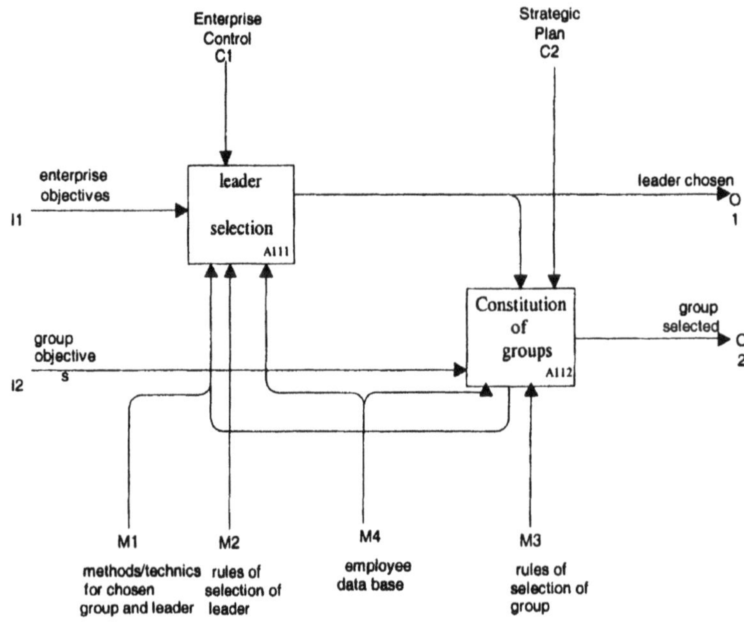

Figure 7 – CE team design processes in "traditional" enterprise (decomposition of A11 process)

3.2 The CE Model Aimed at Virtual Enterprises

The *elements* of the CE System model for Virtual Enterprises are already presented in figures 4, 5 and 6. The main particularity is that CE system design and operation are performed also simultaneously and concurrently (while in "traditional" enterprise these processes are sequential), represented by a closed circle in figures 4, 5 and 6 meaning that the CE system design has re-feeding from the CE system operation. In other words, the CE system is re-designed, or reconfigure, along the (objective and concrete) CE process. The principle agent of the CE system reconfigurability in VE is the broker (Putnik, 2000b), (Pithon, Putnik, 2002), as it is for the VE in general. The objective of this approach is improving the system's flexibility, through the CE team reconfigurability, i.e. the CE team members changes, figure 8 (Pithon, Putnik, 2002).

The further decomposition of the processes shows other particularities of the CE system model for VE. For example, the decomposition of the process A11 shows the broker selection process, figure 9, that doesn't exists in the CE system model for "traditional" enterprise.

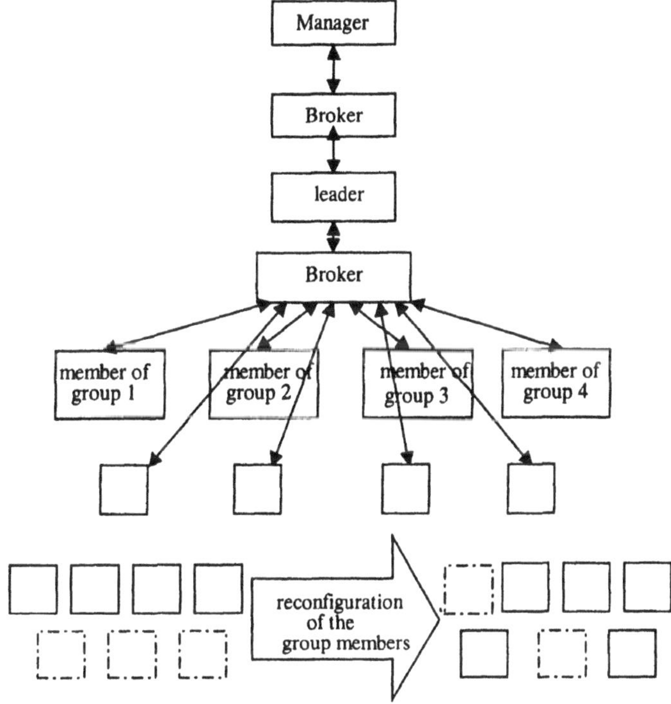

Figure 8 - Management model of CE teams in Virtual Enterprises

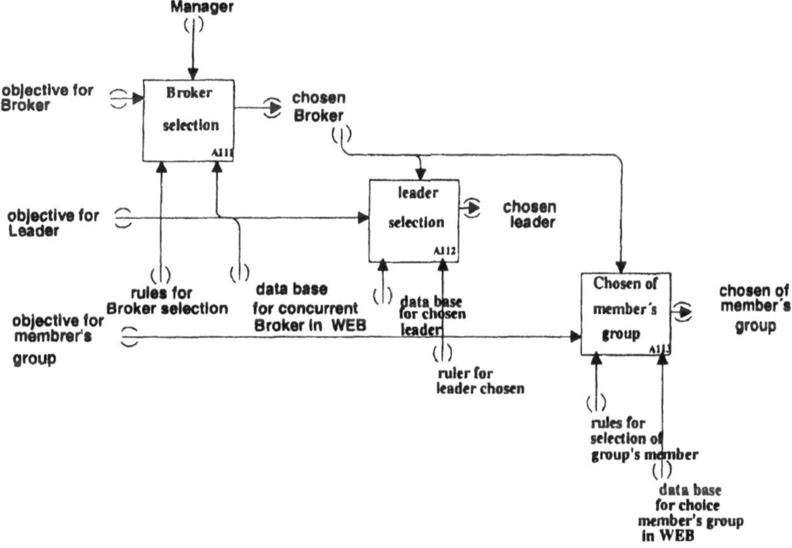

Figure 9 – CE team design processes in Virtual Enterprise (decomposition of A11 process for CE teams in Virtual Enterprise)

4. CONCLUSION

It is presented a model of CE system at the first place with the objective to serve as a reference for development and implementation of CE systems in "traditional" enterprises as well as in virtual enterprises. The model also represents a workflow for CE at a global/higher levels. On the second place, it is expected that it will contribute for further better understanding of the CE processes and systems.

The future work will aims at more detailed specification of the CE processes and systems, especially considering different application domains as well as the system's variability. It is planned application of some more formal specification languages, e.g. some of the Formal Description Techniques (FDT) as SDL, ESTELLE, LOTOS, or UML, in order to provide more efficient development and application of CE systems and CE system's tools and environments together with the issue of system's integrability. The author's special interest is development of CE systems in VE.

5. ACKNOWLEDGMENTS

We would like to thank FCT (Fundação para a Ciência e a Tecnologia – The Foundation for Science and Technology) of Portugal, for the financial support provided for this research.

6. REFERENCES

Causing, D. (1989). "Concurrent Engineering." American Society of Mechanical Engineers.

Ebbinghaus, H. (1996). Mathematical Logic, Springs

Pawar, K. S., Sudi (2000). "Virtual collocation of design teams: coordination for speed." International Journal of Agile Management Systems **Vol. 2, nº 2**: 104-113.

Pithon, A; Putnik, G. (2001). Concurrent Engineering and Groupwork . Introduction; Technical Report, CESP-GIS-01-01, University of Minho

Pithon,A; Putnik G. (2002). Team Work for Concurrent Engineering in Agile/Virtual Enterprise by BM_Virtual Enterprise Architecture Reference Model; PRO-VE 2002, Kluwer (to be published)

Prasad, B. (1997). Concurrent Engineering Fundamentals, V.2, Prentice Hall

Putnik G. (2000a). Notes on Concurrent Engineering, MSc course on Industrial Engineering, University of Minho, Guimarães, Portugal

Putnik, G. (2000b). BM_Virtual Enterprise Architecture Reference Model. In A. Gunasekaran (Ed.), *Agile Manufacturing: 21st Century Manufacturing Strategy* (pp. 73-93). UK: Elsevier Science Publ.

Ranky, P. G. (1994). "Concurrent Engineering and Enterprise Modelling." Assembly Automation **V.14, Nº 3 MCB University Press.**

6

SELF-GOVERNING PRODUCTION GROUPS: TOWARDS REQUIREMENTS FOR IT SUPPORT

Peter H. Carstensen and Kjeld Schmidt
The IT University of Copenhagen, Denmark, {carstensen, schmidt}@it-c.dk

Many manufacturing enterprises are introducing various forms of flexible work organizations on the shop floor. However, existing computer-based production planning and control systems pose serious obstacles for self-governing groups and other kinds of shop floor control to become reality. In order to understand and overcome these obstacles we have undertaken a series of six field studies in manufacturing companies. Based on our findings from these studies — and inspired by the research field of Computer Supported Cooperative Work — we present a first set of requirements and principles for IT-based systems for self-governing production groups. The intention is to support responsible workers in their situated planning, control and coordination of shop floor activities.

1. INTRODUCTION

For most of the 20th century, manufacturing has epitomized a work organization characterized by radically centralized and very detailed and rigid regulation of work in which the individual's sphere of activity is reduced to a small repertoire of monotonous movements (Blauner, 1964; Braverman, 1974). The result was a high rate of labor turnover. To deal with this problem, sociologists and ergonomists suggested radical changes to the work organization in the form of job enlargement and introduction of production groups on the shop floor that would have control over day-to-day task allocation and production planning and control. Over the following years, a number of 'socio-technical' experiments with work organizations based on higher degrees of local control were carried out, often successfully (Hirschhorn, 1984) but these principles were never implemented on a large scale. However, a series of fundamental changes over the last two decades have placed the issue of the work organization in manufacturing on the agenda again. Faced with turbulent markets, industrial enterprises are opting for strategies that involve shorter product life cycles and increasing product diversification, which in turn requires a reduction of inventories and buffer stocks, extremely short lead times, shrinking batch sizes, concurrent processing of multiple different products and orders, etc. (Gunn, 1987). To meet these requirements, industrial work organizations must be able to adapt rapidly and diligently to changing demands in a concerted and integrated way.

To cope with these demands, a large number of manufacturing enterprises are now trying to introduce various forms of flexible work organizations on the shop floor (Womack et al., 1990; Durand et al., 1999). While the precise organizational forms vary, they are basically characterized by local control over job allocation and day-to-day production planning and control, often called 'autonomous' or 'self-governing' production groups. When serious attempts at shop floor control are being made, it very soon becomes quite evident, however, that existing computer-based production planning and control systems pose severe obstacles for self-governing production groups and other kinds of shop floor control to become reality (Odgaard, 1994). They were designed for an entirely different world.

In view of these experiences we have initiated investigations with the objective of developing novel forms of production planning and control systems that would specifically address the requirements of self-governing production groups and other kinds of shop floor control. Our work has been heavily inspired by the field of Computer Supported Cooperative Work (CSCW). Here cooperative work is seen as inexorably distributed in the sense that actors are acting, and have to act, on partial knowledge of the state of affairs (Schmidt, 1991). There is thus, in principle, no all-knowing agent. Orderly coordination is accomplished through the local actions and interactions of actors who have only local control. The presumptions of MRP systems, that the planning department of the enterprise is able to predict and control, in essence, the manifold interdependent activities of a manufacturing enterprise, is illusory, and in flexible manufacturing the enormous systemic costs of maintaining this illusion have become evident. However, cooperating groups do cope with the enormous complexity arising from the fact that their activities interdependent and yet distributed — through organizational constructs such as plans, schedules, procedures, etc. Such constructs do not in every detail or determine local action; they are rather 'resources for situated action' (Suchman, 1987); they are normative constructs that, to competent members, specify the appropriate next step to be taken, unless the actors have reasons not to do so (Schmidt, 1999).

Even when faced with turbulent environments, the models of interdependencies underlying coordinative constructs are far from useless, but they are used in a quite different manner than simple plan execution. They may indicate the desirable end result of the effort, they may be provide reasonably useful insight into the likely effects of an action, or they may be modified temporarily and then used for coordinative purposes even if the system otherwise would be beyond its bounds (Carstensen and Sørensen, 1996; Grinter, 1997).

To investigate and inform this approach and these ideas further field studies were conducted at six different manufacturing companies in Denmark. The primary purpose was to provide a proper basis for a detailed discussion of requirements for IT support for self-governing production groups. This paper presents the central findings and conclusions from the field studies and briefly discuss overall requirements and principles for applicable IT support.

2. APPROACH

In order to obtain a coherent understanding of complex work settings and the work conducted there, field studies are essential (Yin, 1989; Orlikowski, 1993). This paper is based on data collected in six such studies of more or less self-governing groups of shop floor workers. The studies focused on planning and coordination activities of the members of the groups and the resources and techniques used by them in these activities.

Each of the six studies was performed over a period of a few months and was mainly based on qualitative interviews (Patton, 1980), observation studies, and analyses of various coordinative artifacts and other documents (e.g., weekly work plans, schedule boards, production plans, and log books). Each of the studies involved 5-10 in-depth interviews as well as observational and other studies.

The first study was conducted in 1998-99 and resulted in a set of preliminary requirements for IT support which were in turn expressed in the design of a 'horizontal prototype' (cf. Carstensen et al., 1999). As a follow-up to this study, five additional studies were undertaken during 2001. In May 2001 the initial findings and conclusions from the entire range of studies were summarized in a report that was discussed at a two-day seminar with group members, managers, and shop stewards from participating companies.

The studies were not ethnographies but were focused on a set of defined issues and were structured accordingly. In particular, the five second-stage studies focused on a number of topics that were identified from the first study. The research approach taken can be characterized as qualitative research heavily inspired by theories and conceptualizations from the field of CSCW and from other studies of complex work settings.

3. THE SETTINGS

In the process of selecting the six companies and groups, we aimed at covering a range of quite different types of production, different kinds of organization of work, different regimes of self-governance, etc.. These differences notwithstanding, there were some striking similarities in the problems the groups were facing in their daily struggle with planning their activities, monitoring progress, rescheduling, etc.

The six studies were conducted at:

- ABB Energy and Industry, a factory producing facilities for the distribution of electrical power from power plants to consumers. We studied a group of 15-20 workers processing metal plates. The core activities were punching, cutting, canting, welding, and surface treatment. This group had an internal planner (the role rotated among members). The planner was responsible for daily planning and interaction with the central planning department.
- Odense Steel Shipyard, one of the largest shipyards in Europe. We studied a group of 18 workers producing large steel profiles. The group was headed by an appointed foreman who conducted most of the planning, ordering of materials, etc.
- NKT Cables, a leading European cable manufacturer. We studied three groups with 12-24 members. The groups had been self-governing for a decade and handled most of the staffing and production planning.
- Blika. a medium-size manufacturing company producing steel wardrobes and steel wire products. We studied two groups (each having 11 members). The groups have been self-governing for more than eight years.

- Man B&W Alpha Diesel, a leading manufacturer of propulsion plants for smaller and medium-sized ship types. We studied two groups, a group in parts production and a group in assembly. The groups at Man B&W have appointed coordinators within the groups. The coordinators handle most of the production planning, materials procurement, etc. In peak situations the groups might appoint extra coordinators if necessary.
- Brüel & Kjær. a leading manufacturer of sound and vibration measurement equipment. We studied a group assembling small amplifiers for sound measuring equipment. This group had 17-20 members and they handled most of the production and staffing themselves. Group members were furthermore responsible for ordering materials and for quality assurance.

The workers in the cases represented different categories of skill and training, from engineers with specialized formal training to operators with no formal training. At ABB the distribution was fifty-fifty, at Lindø and Man B&W members generally were trained engineers, whereas workers Blika, NKT and Brüel & Kjær mostly did not have formal training. There was no correlation between the educational level in the groups and the degree of autonomy enjoyed by the groups. In fact, the members of the most autonomous group of the groups we studied (at Brüel & Kjær) had not formal training (with one exception).

4. OBSERVATIONS

As mentioned there were both similarities and differences among the groups. All of the groups were handling part of the planning activities themselves, although the degree of autonomy differed significantly. In the group at the shipyard a foreman had overall responsibilities, whereas the assembly group at Brüel & Kjær handled all activities relating to staffing, production planning and control, materials procurement, and quality assurance without even having formal roles.

Some of the groups used existing (centralized) IT systems for their production planning and coordinative activities. A key observation here was that the use of production planning systems caused significant problems, as these systems did not fulfil the users needs for local control, adequate levels of granularity of information, etc.

Although the degrees of autonomy differed among the groups, all groups had control of, and responsibility for, how the work was to be carried out, and thereby control of the division of activities among group members. In some situations this required accounting for who would be available when, who had the required skills for a specific task, etc.

In analyzing our observations we distinguished three general categories of tasks relating to self-governance: Staffing and work allocation, Production planning and control, and Information and experience exchange. In the following each of these will be presented in a little further details.

4.1 Staffing and Work Allocation

The activities under this category primarily served to establish a staffing plan indicating who would be working which shifts and, within that framework, who would be doing what when. The plans would account for general constraints such as vacations and other planned absences, and would take into account the competencies of the individual workers with respect to the work to be done (e.g., 'is he certified for driving the truck?' or 'is she trained for running the canting center?'). The plans would be updated continually to deal with contingencies such as workers calling in sick or absent for training purposes etc. In one of our studies coordinators would also engage in negotiations related to lending out personnel in situations with excess capacity (in order to ensure 'a proper salary for rest of the members') or, conversely, borrowing actors from other groups in production peak situations.

In most of the groups, staffing plans were established once a week, but they would be updated and re-organized on a daily basis due to changes. To cope with this an overview of the skills and competencies of group members was essential. In most of the groups, however, coordinators were not supported in this regard. The group at Brüel & Kjær, on the other hand, every year constructed a matrix representation that matched required tasks (and, implicitly, required skills) with members of the group and thus made it visible who had formal training in which tasks or processes.

Work was allocated in terms of a variety of categories, in terms of work stations or locations, in terms of tasks, in terms of time periods, or a combination of these. At ABB and NKT, for example, allocation was expressed in terms of time period and work station. At Brüel & Kjær, by constrast, work was generally allocated in terms of locations, but in this case the specific activities to be undertaken at which location was negotiated from situation to situation.

The work allocation and staffing activities also included establishment of plans for general work allocation and job rotation in the following period. Typically such plans were established once every six months or once a year. These plans in turn required plans for meeting the training requirements of members. In about half of our studies it was the groups who themselves established and negotiated these rotation and training plans.

4.2 Production Planning and Control

Production planning and control constitute a core set of tasks and a major challenge for many self-governing production groups. The groups must handle and interrelate many very different and yet mutually interdependent constraints and parameters when establishing the plans, such as, for example, deadlines (relative importance of conflicting deadlines), required and possible flows of materials and sub-products, required raw materials or components, required and possible sequences (routing), flexibility in choice of sub-processes and materials, effects of decisions downstream in the production, etc.

In most of the groups, production planning work was undertaken by the group themselves. Some groups had dedicated roles for planning, typically a role that was rotated among group members every second or third month. At Brüel & Kjær, planning was a separate task which was addressed every Thursday morning by practically all group members.

The initial production planning is typically done on the basis of production orders (requests) generated by some central planning department. Production orders to the groups can be at a very general level ('we need 500 BMR1798 pre-amplifiers produced by the end of week 27'), or as very detailed task lists in which each and every production process is specified in terms of sequence, workstation, fixtures, materials, components, amount (number, length), CNC-program, etc. The latter is typically lists produced by the central MRP systems. In most cases, however, the groups had to take local and temporary contingencies into account in adopting centrally generated plans, e.g., which of the optional workstations can deliver the required tolerance? how do we handle this member's absence? is there an alternative to this process?

A new version of the production plan was typically established on a daily basis or on a weekly basis. When the groups finished the planning, the plans were typically negotiated with actors from the central planning department. In some of our cases this negotiation took place before the detailed planning was done (i.e., to inform the planning process), whereas it in other cases was discussed after the detailed planning had illuminated potential problems.

As result of the planning activities, some of the groups had to identify needs for materials and components and order these from the storage or from internal or external sub-suppliers.

Production control, i.e., monitoring progress with respect to plans and rescheduling work in accordance with (previously) unforeseen events and changes, is of course equally important to self-governing groups.

Schematically, core activities of production control work of the groups would include:

Ensuring consistency between the plan and the actual work. This included monitoring progress. There are often major differences between what is foreseen in the plans (e.g. with respect to initial set-up time for a process) and reality. Hence, actors would monitor to what extent the plans were, or could be, fulfilled. Another aspect that the central planning systems did not and could not support was to take space requirements into account. We observed several situations were re-scheduling had to be done due to space requirements. For example, the assembly group next process downstream was two days behind schedule and had therefore no space available for the eight new plates to be produced; these therefore could not be delivered and would block for other processes in the planned flow.

Handling unforeseen events. Events like these occurred both due to defective equipment, lack of (or defective) materials and components, human errors, absence of members with key competencies, changes in demands and priorities from the rest of the factory, etc. In such situations the groups, or the coordinators in the groups, would re-schedule work or reroute work flow. Rescheduling and rerouting often involved negotiations with the central planning departments or production groups down- or upstream in the flow.

Monitoring the flow of materials. This included contacting other groups upstream in the production or suppliers of component or materials so as to ensure availability of components and materials when required. This kind of monitoring activities was of course also often essential internally in the groups, as members were often suppliers to other members. The monitoring activities were more or less undertaken by all actors, i.e., everybody was attentive to the issue of whether they could expect to have the materials required for their individual tasks.

Managing the local storage of materials and sub-components. This had to do with ensuring that the required components and materials were available when needed, and keep track of the consumption so that requests and purchase could be handled in time. Two of the groups had an internal storage in which their most common sub-components and materials were stored. The groups were responsible for ordering new materials for the storage when required.

Assuring product quality. Most of the self-governing production groups we observed were responsible for quality assurance of their own products. Some of the groups had a dedicated role responsible for organizing quality assurance work and implementing procedures fulfilling overall company requirements. It was usually a responsibility which the groups were proud of, but at the same time a set of tasks that were sometimes quite unstructured and that were not supported by any standard procedures or systems. We generally found only little systemacity in the collection and distribution of experience among group members.

Requesting assistance. In many situations a group might need support in their work from people outside the group (e.g., order a crane for moving very large components). In these situations the groups themselves would interact with the actors providing the service.

4.3 Information and Experience Exchange

In many groups a lot of energy was used on informing each other on changes in plans, material flows, etc. A general observation was that group members are heavily interdependent in their activities and that they, as a consequence of this, spend much time on coordinating and negotiating activities. This was also the case in relation to other groups (e.g., other groups down-stream, central planners, purchasing department, process support technicians, etc.). In many of the situations we have investigated, the members did not have effective and efficient means (or media) for coordinating with each other or with people outside their own group.

Many of the groups were also confronted with requirements regarding accounting for, or documentation of, the processes. Again few support tools were available.

Exchange of experiences and knowledge was a major challenge for all the self-governing groups. There was a strong need for collecting and expressing experiences (e.g., 'how long time does it take to produce 200 of the BMR1798?' or 'what is the alternative production process when the canting work station breaks down?'). Although the exchange of such experiences within the groups is important, no facilities currently support this. We have observed a number of 'private' log-books or photo albums, but such solutions cannot be scaled-up and are fragile over time, as they are not systematic and based on robust and agreed-to classification schemes. The most common means for exchanging experiences was 'war stories' exchanged during breaks, over lunch, etc.

In about half of the studies, production work was widely distributed (in space and time), so that group members could not easily interact with one another on an ad hoc basis. This exacerbated the problems with experience and knowledge exchange. In these cases log-books and note pads were used instead. This information was, however primarily status information, e.g., 'the bending II workstation is unstable - avoid complex processes'.

5. DISCUSSION: TOWARDS PROPER IT SUPPORT

As argued above, workers in self-governing groups face serious challenges and problems in handling the administrative, managerial, and coordinative tasks required for planning and managing their work.

5.1 The Nature of Manufacturing Work

Along the same line as authors like Harrington (1979; 1984) our studies have illustrated some central complexity aspects of manufacturing. In the following we will briefly characterize these and reflect upon the implications for the planning and control of the work.

Manufacturing is essentially and massively material. It's about changing the physical form of things – by changing the geometry of objects and by putting parts together in more or less complex configurations. Manufacturing work is thus not only materially embedded or situated, like all human behavior, and it is not merely materially constrained, like all work. Manufacturing work is fundamentally, inexorably, and continually faced with and dealing with an infinite array of physical, chemical, mechanical, thermodynamic, electrical, biological, etc. objects, processes, constraints, contingencies, inferences, breakdowns, etc.

The work to be planned and managed is therefore extremely variegated, even within the same department, or self-governing group (from one workstation to another, from one situation to another). Due to the different character of the materials, processes, parts, and tools and other equipment, the actors have to manage activities, problems, and challenges that are particular and unique to the setting or situation. Even highly sophisticated attempts at developing models of manufacturing processes (Todd et al., 1994b; Todd et al., 1994a) thus invariably turn out to be strikingly incomplete, in that they cover but a restricted set of processes or planning parameters. Trivial issues of space utilization may for example take precedent over other issues, such as delivery date, economy of scale, lead time, etc. Finished products may for instance take up so much space that the issue of keeping order in the shipping room may require the production plan to be rescheduled. Similarly, in a cable factory the same drum may house multiple pieces of cable and it may be more efficient to reschedule production than to unwind and rewind the drums. Current production planning and control systems (based on MRP technology) cannot express such issues. The actors have no dedicated means for taken these issues into consideration.

The inexhaustible material variety of manufacturing work also means that production planning and control activities cannot be conceived of in abstraction from the very transformation processes that are their target. Production planning and control and process control are both conceptually and practically in an 'internal relationship'. Production control activities are not external to but rather inexorably conceived of and expressed in term of the material transformation processes. Thus, if production planning and control systems and process control systems are designed in isolation of one another, radical and potentially disruptive impediments to production work are introduced.

Production planning and control systems must thus, at the very least, interface to a vast and open-ended array of other kinds of software systems: process control systems for different kinds of processes, CAD/CAM systems, accounting systems, payroll systems, etc.

Finally, most manufacturing processes involve a large variety of qualitatively different processes such as pressing, extruding, cutting, polishing, painting, screwing, assembling, etc., that are typically distributed over a large collection of more or less specialized workstations which, in turn, often will be specialized themselves. Due to the infinite variety of processes, the total process is radically distributed over specialized workstations. Moreover, because manufacturing work is radically distributed, manufacturing work is characterized by very complex interdependencies. Any local contingency may have repercussions up- or downstream, which, to the local decision makers, may be intractable. A system supporting the local planning and control work in the different groups might thus be running in different instances in different, but still interdependent, production groups. The repercussions up- or downstream will affect interaction across these instances of the local planning and control system.

5.2 Towards IT Support

Most planning, coordination and control of manufacturing operations are based upon centralized systems build upon models of bills of materials, routings, process specifications, etc. The master production schedule is thus 'the vital control center for the company's manufacturing planning and control system' (Gunn, 1981, p. 9). The enormously complex production control problem is thereby, in theory, reduced to executing this plan.

As argued above, the idea of having a complete model of manufacturing is chimerical, however. One could claim that most existing planning and control work at the shop floor is functioning okay, not because of the central planning systems, but because the human actors are highly flexible and adaptive to the situations occurring. Moreover, as soon as manufacturing companies launch on the course of flexible adaptation, entirely different production control strategies are required, and the kind of support required on the shop floor differs radically from what traditional MRP and similar systems are capable of providing.

Aiming at a centralized system based upon a 'complete model' of the activities is thus not a viable approach to building adequate IT-support systems for shop floor planning and control. Instead, we suggest, we should consider how IT could support the planning, managing, collaboration and coordination activities, and thereby assist intelligent and responsible workers in their situated coordination activities on the shop floor.

However, the radical and inexhaustible variety of manufacturing work takes manufacturing apart from typical application domains for IT. Accounting is essentially manipulation of representations of economic activities. The contingencies of the material world is of minor concern (except when invoices are lost, archives burnt or flooded etc.). More than that, accounting practices are regulated by law and accounting thus offers a large homogeneous market for software houses. The same applies, more or less, to so-called 'office work', that is, the construction and manipulation of documents, which also has been amenable to computerization by means of a limited suite of generic applications (e.g., word processing, spreadsheets and organizers).

By contrast to such domains, in which IT perhaps can be said to have experienced easy triumphs, manufacturing is not an appropriate domain for (more or less complex) monolithic applications or application systems (such as accounting) or for integrated suites of generic applications (such as 'office work' or desktop publishing). Manufacturing seems to require another, radically different software development strategy than that of the traditional areas of IT deployment. A monolithic application system will invariably create all sorts of problem on the shop floor, as workers strive to make the system fit. The dismal record of the existing monolithic MRP-based production planning and control systems in contemporary manufacturing seems to confirm that. Instead, an open-ended approach seems required.

An open-ended approach must provide a framework (architecture, platform) in which specialized software modules designed to deal with specific tasks of control, coordination, communication, process control etc. can be incorporated and interact in an orderly fashion. To assist intelligent and responsible workers in their situated coordination activities on the shop floor, the underlying models of MRP systems, etc. are not obsolete but must be used — and made useful — in a very different way: constraints that are not essential must be removed or relaxed, so that workers can circumvent or overrule the recommendations of the system when that is deemed appropriate. Furthermore, since it is unlikely that a conceptual model of manufacturing can be defined once and for all, new issues or processes will invariably emerge that need to be included as parameters or resources in the model. It therefore seems as if the framework must provide an abstract notation for defining functionalities, planning and control parameters, interfaces, protocols, etc.

It is beyond the scope of this paper to extend the discussion on architecture further here. We have, however from our studies, identified a set of overall principles for the design of this kind of systems. These can also be seen as an abstract summary of some of our findings:

- Plans are resources for action, not structures that are executed mindlessly. The systems supporting the planning and execution must allow deviations from plans.
- No system should aim at having a 'complete picture'. Our studies have clearly illustrated that situations at the shop floor are contingent. No matter how detailed we aim at registering the events in the production, there will always be 'white spots' in the databases, e.g., Jensen handling the canting machine is ill, Bending Workstation II is causing problems, etc. A large degree of flexibility in the planning in accordance with this kind of knowledge must be provided to the actors.
- The system should provide an open-ended overview of status to the actors. If the actors are to handle and coordinate the activities in a situated manner, they need to have a good overview of the state of affairs. Since it is not possible to foresee the borders (perspective) of the required information, the information must be provided in an open-ended manner, so that the actors themselves are in control of how much overview information they need.
- Actors should have ultimate control. Based on the core assumption that the relevant space of deviations is impossible to foresee — that has been documented many times in our studies — the systems should avoid automation of processes that cannot be overruled by the actors.

- The system should allow experimentation with plans. It is more or less difficult for actors on the shop floor (or anywhere else) to predict the consequences of changes to plans and schedules. It is therefore important, that planning support systems allow different kinds of experimentation with the plans.
- The perspective and level of detail should be variable and selectable. Our studies indicate that actors sometimes may need to investigate very detailed information, e.g., about a specific production process, whereas they in other situations need an overall picture with a different granularity.
- Education and training in the basic concepts and model are essential. In several of our studies we observed that members had serious problems in understanding and coping with the information provided from the central planning systems. One obvious reason was that key concepts (e.g:, bill-of-materials) were not fully understood by the actors, and using the information in the systems thus became quite difficult.
- A high degree of usability is self-evident. The fact that the user interface is easy to learn and use is still essential.

Most of these overall principles might appear 'obvious' and we perhaps do not require in-depth field studies to identify them. However, we have not come across shop floor support systems that adhere to these principles, and in most of the settings and situations we have studied it was quite clear that the requirements are far from fulfilled and that the principles are not adhere to at all. And we have no reason at all to expect it to be different in other settings. In fact some of the settings we studied have been carefully and systematically striving to improve the support for the self-governing groups for years.

Finally, after having suggested a key role for IT in planning and control of shop floor activities, it is important to emphasize that IT by no means is a panacea. There are a number of areas in which IT cannot support workers, but we believe that IT, combined with other initiatives, can provide a useful tool for self-governing groups

To test out some of the ideas and principles for IT support of self-governing groups, we designed a horizontal prototype of a manning and production planning system. The prototype was based on findings from the first of our six field studies. The prototype is illustrated and discussed in length in Carstensen et al. (1999). The reactions (both from managers and workers) were very positive. To investigate further we conducted the five extra field studies presented in this paper. We believe, that we now have a basis for starting discussions on requirements for IT systems for self-governing groups. We are however aware that much further work is required. For example, work on identifying how different characteristics of the production should be reflected, how the interaction with existing information systems and other technologies should be handled, how a proper IT architecture for this kind of systems should be designed, etc. etc. There is still a long way to go!

6. ACKNOWLEDGMENTS

The IDAK project is supported by Industriens Uddannelsesfond. The project was conceived and initiated by Irene Odgaard of the Central Organization of Danish Industrial Workers (CO-Industri) whose support is gratefully acknowledged. Hans

Jørgen Lynggaard, Alex Skandorff Vestergaard and Uffe Kock Wiil were involved in the six field studies. We are indebted to the workers and managers at the six companies for having given the project their support, their interest, and their time. Thanks to the anonymous reviewers for very relevant comments and suggestions.

7. REFERENCES

Blauner, R.: *Alienation and Freedom: The Factory Worker and His Industry*, University of Chicago Press, Chicago, 1964.

Braverman, Harry: *Labor and Monopoly Capital. The Degradation of Work in the Twentieth Century*, Monthly Review Press, New York and London, 1974.

Carstensen, Peter H., Schmidt, K., and Wiil, U. K.: "Supporting shop floor intelligence: A CSCW approach to production planning and control in flexible manufacturing," in S. C. Hayne (ed.): *GROUP'99 - International ACM SIGGROUP Conference on Supporting Group Work, Phoenix, Arizona*, ACM, 1999, pp. 111-120.

Carstensen, Peter H., and Sørensen, C.: "From the social to the systematic. Mechanisms supporting coordination in design," *Computer Supported Cooperative Work. The Journal of Collaborative Computing*, vol. 5, no. 4, 1996, pp. 387-413.

Durand, J.-P., Stewart, P., and Castillo, J. J. (eds.): *Teamwork in the Automobile Industry: Radical Change or Passing Fashion?*, Macmillan etc., 1999.

Grinter, Rebecca E.: "Doing software development: Occasions for automation and formalisation," in J. A. Hughes at al. (eds.): *ECSCW '97. Proceedings of the Fifth European Conference on Computer-Supported Cooperative Work, 7-11 September 1997, Lancaster, U.K.*, Kluwer Academic Publishers, Dordrecht, 1997, pp. 173-188.

Gunn, Thomas G.: *Computer Applications in Manufacturing*, Industrial Press, New York, 1981.

Gunn, Thomas G.: *Manufacturing for Competitive Advantage. Becoming a World Class Manufacturer*, Ballinger, Cambridge, Mass., 1987.

Harrington, Joseph: *Computer Integrated Manufacturing*, Krieger, Malabar, Florida, 1979.

Harrington, Joseph: *Understanding the Manufacturing Process. Key to Successful CAD/CAM Implementation*, Marcel Dekker, New York, 1984.

Hirschhorn, Larry: *Beyond Mechanization: Work and Technology in a Postindustrial Age*, The MIT Press, Cambridge, Mass. - London, 1984.

Odgaard, Irene: *In practise it was worse than expected. Production groups at Aalestrup, Grundfos, Denmark. A case study on new forms of work organization. [in Danish]*, General Workers' Union in Denmark, 1994.

Orlikowski, Wanda J.: "CASE Tools as Organizational Change: Investigating Incremental and Radical Changes in Systems Development," *MIS Quaterly*, no. September 1993, 1993, pp. 309-340.

Patton, M. Q.: *Qualitative Evaluation Methods*, Sage Publications, Beverly Hills, CA, 1980.

Schmidt, Kjeld: "Riding a Tiger, or Computer Supported Cooperative Work," in L. Bannon, M. Robinson, and K. Schmidt (eds.): *ECSCW '91. Proceedings of the Second European Conference on Computer-Supported Cooperative Work*, Kluwer Academic Publishers, Amsterdam, 1991, pp. 1-16.

Schmidt, Kjeld: "Of maps and scripts: The status of formal constructs in cooperative work," *Information and Software Technology*, vol. 41, 1999, pp. 319-329.

Suchman, Lucy A.: *Plans and situated actions. The problem of human-machine communication*, Cambridge University Press, Cambridge, 1987.

Todd, Robert H., Dell K. Allen, and Leo Alting: *Fundamental Principles of Manufacturing Processes*, Industrial Press, New York, 1994a.

Todd, Robert H., Dell K. Allen, and Leo Alting: *Manufacturing Processes Reference Guide*, Industrial Press, New York, 1994b.

Womack, James P., Daniel T. Jones, and Daniel Roos: *The Machine that Changed the World: The Story of Lean Production*, Rawson Associates, New York, 1990.

Yin, Robert K.: *Case Study Research: Design and Methods*, Sage Publications, Beverly Hills, 1989.

7

DEVELOPING A WEB SCHEDULING SYSTEM BASED ON XML MODELING

Leonilde Rocha Varela[1], Joaquim Nunes Aparício[2], and Sílvio Carmo Silva[3]
[1]*University of Minho, School of Engineering, Dept. of Production and Systems*
leonilde@dps.uminho.pt
[2]*New University of Lisbon, Faculty of Science and Technology, Dept. of Computer Science*
jna@di.fct.unl.pt
[3]*University of Minho, School of Engineering, Dept. of Production and Systems*
scarmo@dps.uminho.pt

In manufacturing enterprises, it is important nowadays, as a competitive strategy, to explore and use software applications, now becoming available through the Internet and Intranets, for solving scheduling problems. This work gives a contribution for a better resolution process of scheduling problems, by means of web-based computation. An XML-based specification framework for scheduling is proposed. This specification provides a general model of scheduling problems and related tasks, and consequently a method of describing each particular problem and algorithm, by user information introduction. The main objective of this kind of specification is to make possible flexible communication among different scheduling applications, in a web-based scheduling decision support system.

1. INTRODUCTION

Production Scheduling is an important function strongly contributing to the competitiveness of industrial and service companies. Manufacturing Scheduling may be defined as the activity of allocating tasks to production resources, during a certain period of time.

An effective and efficient resolution of a scheduling problem begins with the identification of suitable scheduling algorithms. When there are some alternative methods and algorithms to solve the problem it is important to make the evaluation of solutions based on the alternatives available and in accordance with the specified criteria or objectives to be reached. We should be able to solve a problem, through the execution of one or more scheduling algorithms and, choose the best solution provided by them. These algorithms can be local or remotely available through the web. Thus, this work intends to be a contribution for a better resolution process of scheduling problems, by means of web-based computation.

It is proposed an XML-based specification framework for manufacturing scheduling concepts modeling. This specification provides a general model of scheduling problems and related tasks, and consequently a method of describing each particular problem and algorithm. This requires identification of such problems, which can be classified by a set of factors, which, in turn, enable specifying a clear and objective problem categorization structure to which real problem instances belong. The existence of a great variety of scheduling problems motivates the utilization of a systematic notation for problems representation that serves as a basis for its classification (Varela, 1999). The nomenclature includes the manufacturing system identification, definition of the performance measure and some constraints that characterize the problem.

According to the notation used for representing scheduling problems, the XML language is used as a specification language for data modeling and processing. The main objective of this kind of specification is to make possible flexible communication among different scheduling applications, in a web-based scheduling decision support system. The specification also contributes to the improvement of the scheduling processes, by allowing an easier selection of several alternative algorithms or methods available for problem solving, as well as an easier maintenance of the knowledge base itself.

This paper is organized as follows. The next section describes the nature of scheduling problems and presents a nomenclature for problem characterization. Some algorithm references to common scheduling problem classes are also presented. Sections 3 and 4 describe the web-based scheduling system main functionalities. Section 4 shows a sample XML specification of scheduling problem classes and other related modeling aspects. The last section presents some concluding remarks and additional discussion points related to the future developments of this work.

2. SCHEDULING PROBLEMS DESCRIPTION

Scheduling problems belong to a much broader class of combinatorial optimization problems, which may either be easy or hard (NP-hard problems) to solve. Detailed information about complexity of scheduling can be found in (Blazewics, 1996), (Brucker, 1995), (Jordan, 1996) and (Pinedo, 1995). In the presence of NP-hard problems we may try to relax some constraints imposed on the original problem and then solve the relaxed problem. The solution of the latter may be a good approximation to the solution of the original one and only polynomial time algorithms are likely to be acceptable to solve complex problems. Fortunately, not all NP-hard problems are equally hard from a practical perspective. Some NP-hard problems can be solved pseudo-polynomially using approximation algorithms that generally provide only feasible solutions, which although normally sub-optimal are within a fixed percentage of the optimum. Examples of this kind of methods are the nowadays widely used local (or neighborhood) search techniques, such as Genetic Algorithms (GA), Simulated Annealing (SA), and Tabu Search (TS), which are also known as extended neighborhood search techniques. All these approaches tend to provide good results in the available time to take decisions, reasons why, in this work, we intend to incorporate them in the web scheduling system we are developing.

Good schedules strongly contribute to the increase companies' success. This is achieved, among other ways, through deadlines satisfaction for the accepted orders, low flow times, few ongoing jobs in the system, low stock levels, high resource utilization and low production costs. All these objectives can be better satisfied through the execution of the most suitable scheduling algorithms available for the resolution of each particular problem.

In order to execute the scheduling process it is necessary to clearly specify the problem to be solved. As mentioned above, scheduling problems have a set of characteristics that must be clearly and unequivocally defined. These characteristics include a class of factors related with the production environment, i.e. system and machines, and other classes that allow defining the characteristics of the jobs and resources and the performance measure or evaluation criterion. The first group of characteristics is related with the environment where the production is carried out. The manufacturing environment specification is denoted by α and includes the production system type definition and, eventually, the indication of the number of machines that exist in that production system. Typical such systems include several types of flow shops usually used in Product Oriented Manufacturing Systems (POMS) (Silva, 2001) and in cellular manufacturing systems. Other characteristics associated with scheduling problems, important and necessary for an adequate characterization of problems, are the constrains imposed to the manufacturing environment and resources (β), e.g. machines and operators, and job processing conditions. Some important processing conditions are, for example, related with the existence of auxiliary resources, like robots and transportation devices and/or the existence of buffers, among others factors. Table 1 shows partial information about the problem classification notation in the form of $\alpha|\beta|\gamma$ (Varela, 1999) that serves as a basis for the XML-based problem specification model underlying to this work. This notation is based on notations proposed by (Blazewics, 1996), (Brucker, 1995) and (Jordan, 1996), as well as on other information presented by (Morton, 1993) and by other authors (Pinedo, 1995), (Artiba, 1997), and (Chrétienne, 1995).

The classification nomenclature includes a wide range of factors, which may be combined in many ways. Some of those factors are related with constraints, such as precedence constraints. In presence of this kind of constraint and under forward scheduling, a job can be started only after all of its predecessor jobs have been completed. Another usual constraint is associated with processing times and affects job start and completion times.

The use of this notation can be illustrated by the example "F||Cmax" which reads as: "Scheduling of non-preemptable and independent tasks of arbitrary processing times (lengths), arriving to the system at time 0, on a (simple) flow shop, in order to minimize schedule length".

Table 1 – A sample of scheduling problems characteristics.

Class	Factor	Description	Value
α	α1	manufacturing system type	0, *P*, *Q*, *R*, *F*, J, O, X, PMPM, ...
	α2	Number of machines	0, *k*
β	β1	Job/operation preemption	0, pmtn
	β2	Precedence constraints	prec, chain, tree, sp-graph, ...
	β3	Ready times	0, r_j
	β4	Restrictions on processing times	p_j=1, p_{ji}=1, p_j=p, $p_{inf} \leq p_j \leq p_{sup}$, ...
	...	...	...
γ	γ	Performance measure	C_{max}, $\sum C_j$, $\sum w_j C_j$, L_{max}, $\sum T_j$, ...

Table 2 shows some typical examples of scheduling problems and algorithms, based on (Bruker, 1995). It is a small sample for makespan flow shop scheduling problems among a vast universe of possible ones. This information is stored in the system knowledge base in order to help the user to identify their problems. The system also helps the user to assign methods to problems. This is further explained in the next section.

Table 2 – A sample of scheduling algorithms attributed to problems.

Problem classes	Algorithm reference	Observations
F2 | | Cmax	Johnson (1954)	Maximal polynomially solvable Without preemption
F2 | rj | Cmax	Lenstra et al (1977)	Minimal NP-hard Without preemption
F2 | rj; no-wait | Cmax	Roeck (1984)	Maximal polynomially solvable With no wait
F3 | pmtn | Cmax	Gonzalez & Sahni (1978) Cho & Sahni (1981)	Maximal polynomially solvable With preemption
F | pji=1; prec | Cmax	Leung et al (1984) Timkovsky (1998)	Minimal NP-hard Without preemption
FMPT | n=3 | Cmax	Kraemer (1995)	Minimal NP-hard With multiprocessor task
FMPM, 3 | | Cmax	Garey et al (1976)	Minimal NP-hard With multipurpose machines
FMPM, m | rj;pji=1| Cmax	Brucker et al (1997)	Maximal polynomially solvable With multipurpose machines

3. SYSTEM FUNCTIONALITIES

Since 1995 great happenings have changed the world of information technology, especially the emergence of new Internet technologies. The eXtensible Markup Language (XML) is one of those new technologies that has been having a wide acceptance and caused great impact on Internet real world applications, since its release by the World Wide Web Consortium (W3C) in 1998 (Ceponkus, 1999). XML enables to describe structures and meanings of data with a simple syntax and is an ideal candidate format for exchanging and processing data through the Internet. Other advantages of an XML based representation are its openness, simplicity and scalability (Abiteboul, 2000). This is one of the main reasons why we have chosen XML to develop our application. For details about XML and related technologies (DTD, XSL, XML Schemas, Namespaces, etc.) see, for example (Ceponkus, 1999), (Abiteboul, 2000) or (Harper, 2001).

Web applications can use XML for local data processing, for showing multiple views of the data and for representing more complex data structures. Therefore, XML may guarantee the future utilization of data formats and the exchange of data structures, so that the web documents and the platforms become more robust for systems integration (Aparício, 2001). XML based data exchange is becoming very popular in global manufacturing, and this will cause connectivity becoming more and more convenient and necessary.

Some XML applications, which are more or less related with this work, are PDML (Product Data Markup Language), RDF (Resource Description Format) and STEPml (Pardi, 1999). Other XML specifications devoted to manufacturing processes are JDF (Job Definition Format), PSL (Process Specification Language), PIX-ML (Product Information Exchange), PIF (Process Interchange Format) and XML-based workflow (Harper, 2001).

As it has been said before, the main purpose of this work consists on trying to improve the resolution of scheduling problems. The system we are developing has a main element that is an interface for introduction, validation, and transformation of manufacturing scheduling data. The interface is mainly controlled by DTD and XSL documents stored in a database on a server. The system allows the execution of either local or remote algorithms. On remote executions, XML data is easily read and processed in every computer system since it is stored and sent as strings.

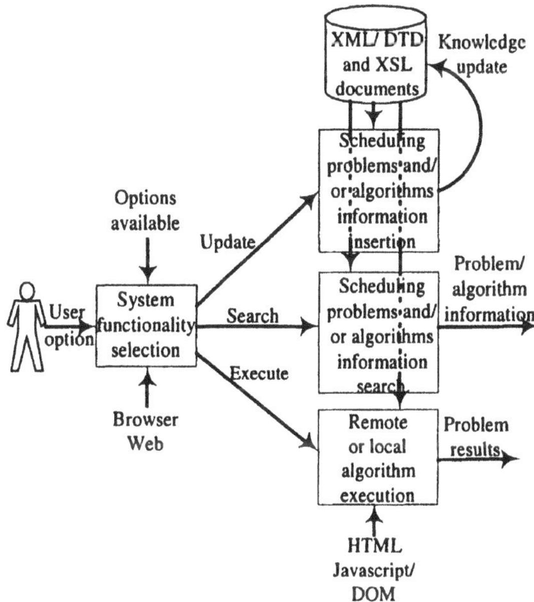

Figure 1 – Web-system functionalities.

The fundamental system functionalities are those related to information modeling, which can be summarized as follows:

- Classification and identification of problems, by using the notation previously presented in section 2.
- Classification and identification of scheduling methods and algorithms.
- Association of scheduling algorithms to scheduling problems.
- Ability to solve scheduling problems, through the selection of one or several algorithms, allowing comparison of results.

The scheduling information is stored in XML documents (e.g. problems.xml, algorithms.xml and implementations.xml, c.f. Figure 2). These documents are validated by corresponding Document Type Definition documents (DTDs), before being put in the XML database. Users can seek for scheduling problem classes, algorithms information and update, algorithms execution and scheduling problem results presentation and storage. The data can be shown in different views, using existing XSL documents, adequate for each specific visualization request.

Figure 2 illustrates the main update options available, underlying to the previously general update option shown in Figure 1.

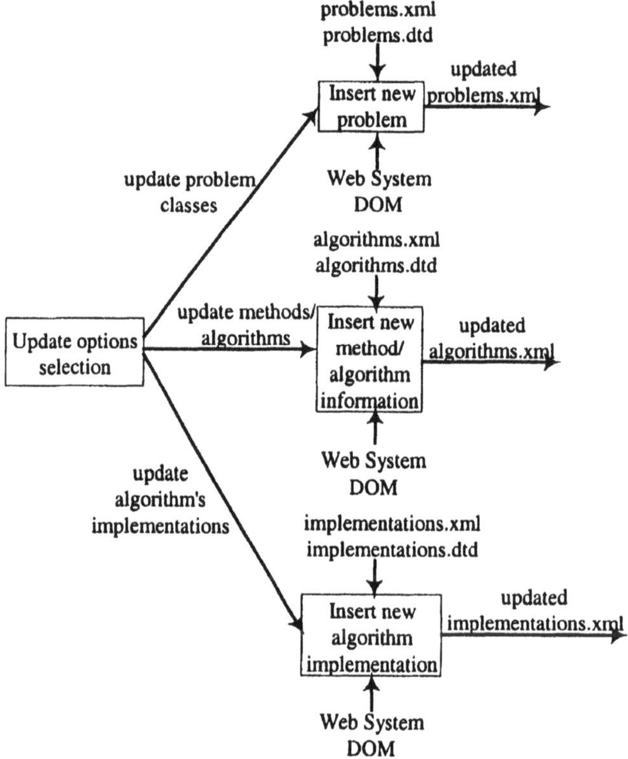

Figure 2 – System's update options.

4. XML SPECIFICATION PRIMITIVES: AN EXAMPLE

This section presents an XML-based specification of scheduling concepts. In a narrow sense, the specification of scheduling concepts gives us syntax of data description for this kind of scheduling problems, but in a broader sense, it can be seen as a general modeling form of such problems. The proposed specification framework provides a general model of scheduling problems and related concepts, and consequently a method of describing each particular problem and algorithm.

With respect to the performance measurement parameters, we think that objectives cannot be put together into one parameter. In other words, the XML specification provides a set of important parameters necessary for the most common kind of scheduling decisions. Then a planner chooses his/her preferences according to the circumstances. However, the XML specification allows users to add their own domain specific performance measures to be considered.

Primitive resource means workstations, machines, equipments, tools, labors, and so on. In these problems a job represents an action that has certain time duration. During that time, the job changes status of inventories of corresponding items, occupying or loading some particular resources. The jobs need some resources and produce some outputs. In XML specification, these objects are referred as items. From the viewpoint of Scheduling Problems, objects in the shop floor can be classified as resource category or as item category. If the target objects are produced or consumed by the job, they are defined as items. Otherwise, if they are renewable after the job being completed, we define them as resources.

In defining job release orders, many attributes have to be considered such as item, quantity, location or destination, due date, processing time, and so on.

One of the most critical success factors for implementation of shop floor scheduling systems is the possibility of dealing with various constraints in each kind of production process, as explained in section 2.

When the designer deals with XML, he/she writes tags hierarchy as elements, and possible attributes. These structures are concerned as a kind of syntax for each application domain. According to that syntax, a XML parser for the particular application translates data for each problem.

Let us now look at a concrete example. Suppose we want to introduce a new problem class. Figure 3 illustrates the system's interface that can be used for the definition of the problem main characteristics. It shows the input data for the problem class FMPM, m| rj, pji=1, n| Cmax, which reads: "Scheduling of non-preemptable and independent tasks with unit processing time lengths, arriving to the system at time rj, on a multipurpose flow shop, with an arbitrary number of machines m, in order to minimize schedule length".

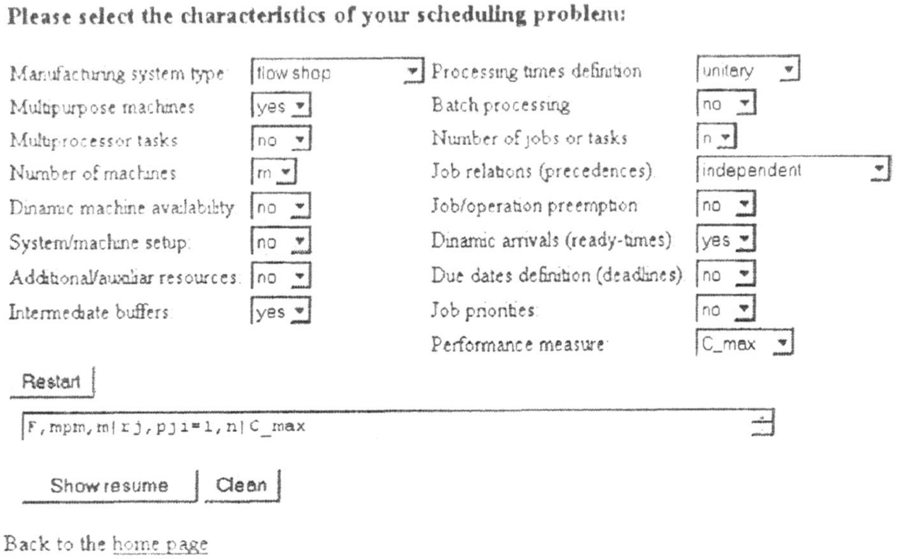

Please select the characteristics of your scheduling problem:

Manufacturing system type: flow shop
Multipurpose machines: yes
Multiprocessor tasks: no
Number of machines: m
Dinamic machine availability: no
System/machine setup: no
Additional/auxiliar resources: no
Intermediate buffers: yes
Processing times definition: unitery
Batch processing: no
Number of jobs or tasks: n
Job relations (precedences): independent
Job/operation preemption: no
Dinamic arrivals (ready-times): yes
Due dates definition (deadlines): no
Job priorities: no
Performance measure: C_max

Restart

F,mpm,m|rj,pji=1,n|C_max

Show resume | Clean

Back to the home page

Figure 3 – A problem characterization.

This interface enables only valid data insertion, accordingly to a DTD (problems.dtd), which enables validating the user data input, allowing only valid data introduction according to the underlying scheduling problem characterization schema used, previously presented in section 2 (c.f. Table 1).

Listing 1 shows the DTD code, which is used for controlling the information related to problem classes identification and insertion in the correspondent XML document.

Listing 1 – Problems.dtd.

```
<!-- Elements and attributes declaration -->
<!ELEMENT problems (problem+)>
<!ELEMENT problem (alpha?, beta?, gamma)>
<!-- Alpha elements -->
<!ELEMENT alpha (alpha1?, alpha2?)>
<!ELEMENT alpha1 EMPTY>
<!ATTLIST alpha1 production_system (0 | P | Q | R | PMPM | ...) "0">
<!ELEMENT alpha2 EMPTY>
<!ATTLIST alpha2 machines (1 | 2 | 3 | m) "1">
<!-- Beta elements -->
<!ELEMENT beta (beta1?, beta2?, beta3?, beta4?, ..., beta12?)>
<!ELEMENT beta1 EMPTY>
<!ATTLIST beta1 interruption (0 | pmtn) "0">
<!ELEMENT beta2 EMPTY>
<!ATTLIST beta2 precedences (0 | prec | chain | tree | sp-graph, ...) "0">
<!ELEMENT beta3 EMPTY>
<!ATTLIST beta3 job_arrivals (0 | rj) "0">
<!ELEMENT beta4 EMPTY>
<!ATTLIST beta4 processing_times (0 | pj=1 | pji=1 | pj=p | pinf≤pj≤psup, ...) "0">
...
<!ELEMENT beta12 EMPTY>
<!ATTLIST beta12 system_setup (0 | setup) "0">
<!-- Gamma element -->
<!ELEMENT gamma EMPTY>
<!ATTLIST gamma measure (Cmax | ...) "0">
```

After having confirmed the problem class, submitted it, and validated it by the system, its information is then added to the correspondent XML document (updated problems.xml), as illustrated in section 3 (c.f. Figure 2). Listing 2 shows a sample of that document, which contains only the information associated to the problem class just added. In that specification the tag <problems> is the root element and can have several <problem> tags as second level tags. These tags, on the other hand, include tags such as <alpha>, <beta> and <gamma> which, in turn, can be further subdivided in other third level tags.

Listing 2 – Problems.xml.

```
<?xml version="1.0"?>
<!DOCTYPE problems SYSTEM "problems.dtd">
<problems>
  <problem>
  <!--FMPM, m | rj; pji=1 | Cmax-->
    <alpha>
      <alpha1 system_type="FMPM"/>
      <alpha2 machines_quantity="m"/>
    </alpha>
    <beta>
      <beta3 ready_times="rj"/>
      <beta4 processing_times="pji=1"/>
    </beta>
    <gamma measure="Cmax"/>
  </problem>
</problems>
```

Listing 1 acts as a model for the description of problem according to Table 1, and Listing 2 acts as the actual repository of that information.

Furthermore, problems.dtd acts as a valuator for information being input to the knowledge base about problems (problems.xml).

For the algorithm execution, of local or remotely registered algorithms, it is still necessary to have DTDs, which describe and control their input and output data. In this case, we also need to have an interface that transforms the problem data, introduced by the user, through the problem identification process, into a valid input data format for the resolution algorithms and this is controlled through the appropriate DTDs. The same happens in the opposite direction, when we need to transform the algorithm results in valid problem results that can be properly processed: visualized and added to the corresponding XML documents.

It is still an open question how the Resource Description Format (Pardi, 1999) can be used for describing resources in our system. It seam that the RDF is too general for our purposes but an adequate subset of the vocabulary may be used in the system.

5. CONCLUSIONS

In manufacturing enterprises, it is important nowadays, as a competitive strategy, to explore and use software applications, now becoming available through the Internet and Intranets, for solving scheduling problems.

This communication proposes an XML-based specification framework for production scheduling concepts modeling, in a web-based production scheduling decision support system. Some of the important functions include the ability to represent scheduling problems and the identification and execution of appropriate available algorithms to solve them.

In order to make possible flexible communication among different scheduling applications, it is used an XML-based data modeling. This specification contributes to the improvement of the scheduling processes, by allowing an easy selection of several alternative available algorithms for problem solving, as well as an easy maintenance of the knowledge base itself. This primarily includes both scheduling problems and algorithms, which are available through the Internet. It is also an adequate specification format for the exchange of data, since it enables to handle with loosely coupled systems and with complex hierarchical data.

With the addition of DTDs, XML can handle much more complex tasks, but the DTDs also have some negative aspects, and their main disadvantages are related to the source code, which is not XML code. Therefore, in terms of future work we aim to transform them into XML Schemas, which are more easily integrated and used in the web system.

The XML based specification can be generated and visualized by computers in appropriate and different ways. An important issue is that the data representation model is general, accommodating a large variety of production scheduling problems.

6. REFERENCES

1. Abiteboul S et al, Data on the web - from relations to semi structured data and XML. USA: Morgan Kaufmann Publishers, 2000.
2. Aparício JN et al, Applications development with XML. Portugal: New University of Lisbon, 2001.
3. Artiba A, Elmaghraby SE, The planning and scheduling of production systems. UK: Chapman & Hall, 1997.
4. Blazewics J et al, Scheduling computer and manufacturing processes. Germany: Springer-Verlag, 1996.
5. Brucker P, Scheduling algorithms. Germany: Springer-Verlag, 1995.
6. Ceponkus A, Hoodbhoy F, Applied XML. USA: Wiley Computer Publishing, 1999.
7. Chrétienne P et al, Scheduling theory and its applications. England: John Wiley & Sons Inc., 1995.
8. Harper F, XML standards and tools. USA: eXcelon Corporation, 2001.
9. Jordan C, Batching and scheduling. Germany: Springer-Verlag, 1996.
10. Morton T, Pentico DW, Heuristic scheduling systems. USA: John Wiley & Sons Inc., 1993.
11. Pardi WJ, XML: Enabling next-generation web applications. USA: Microsoft Press, 1999.
12. Pinedo M, Scheduling theory, algorithms and systems. USA: Prentice-Hall Inc., 1995.
13. Silva SC, Alves AC, SPOP - Sistemas de Produção Orientados ao Produto, TeamWork'2001 Conference, Lisbon, Conference, Lisbon, Portugal, 2001; 1-19.
14. Varela LR, Automatic scheduling algorithms selection. Portugal: Msc. Thesis, University of Minho, 1999.

8

A FLEXIBLE FLOW SHOP MODELLING AS A DISTRIBUTED PRODUCTION SYSTEM

Rui M. Lima and Sílvio do Carmo Silva
Department of Production and Systems
School of Engineering of University of Minho
Campus de Azurém
4800-058 Guimarães – Portugal
rml@dps.uminho.pt / scarmo@dps.uminho.pt

A model of Distributed Production Systems and a formal representation is presented applied to a flexible flow shop. This model is based on recent organizational paradigms like Holonic, Fractal and Bionic production systems. An approach to the problem of resource allocation to production units is developed.

1. INTRODUCTION

All Production organizations are faced with an increased need for change, based on the necessity of reducing the time to market new products, timely delivering customer orders and dealing with increased technological evolution. These needs may be satisfied on the basis of a set of new manufacturing organization paradigms like Fractal (Warnecke, 1993), Holonic and Bionic Manufacturing Systems (Tharumarajah, Wells and Nemes, 1996; Mathews, 1995). These are organization conceptual meta-models based on autonomous production units composed of other similar units.

Nowadays technology is available, based on global communications and distributed data bases and information systems, to allow efficient allocation of globally available resources and services for the production of specific products while demand subsists. This adds up to dynamically putting together distributed resources for designing dedicated and virtual production systems. One concept based on these lines, called OPIM – One Product Integrated Manufacturing, has been put forward in (Putnik and Silva, 1995). Our definition and model of Distributed Production System is closely related with this concept. Furthermore we argue that the underlined characteristics of Distributed Production Systems are the autonomy and distribution of production units or resources and possibility of frequent system reconfiguration, i.e., dynamic reconfiguration, in order to adapt to production changing requirements. In line with this view, in this work, we model a flexible flow shop as a distributed production system. This modelling adapts the flow shop studied in (Azevedo, 1999). The definition, modelling and formal representation of Distributed Production Systems here discussed are oriented for the dynamic design and operation of systems based on the above mentioned organizational and operation paradigms.

2. DISTRIBUTED PRODUCTION SYSTEM MODEL

In our view (Lima, Silva and Martins, 1999) a Distributed Production Systems is composed of a network of autonomous processing units, with the possibility of dynamic reconfiguration of the production system. Three fundamental characteristics are emphasized: distribution, autonomy and reconfiguration.

We can view a system as distributed if there is the need for modelling the distance between units, due to either or both information and physical communication between production units. The problem of distribution may be seen as a problem of system integration as described in (Vernadat, 1996). A platform of integration is needed for the information and physical object communication and a business model with a common semantic reference for mutual understanding of different systems. The integration problem is common to all systems. Traditionally this problem use to be addressed in large design cycles under a homogeneous design and organisational environment. We use the view of production systems integration as a more heterogeneous problem treated in small design cycles, under frequent system reconfigurations.

Autonomy is a relative and not absolute characteristic related to production units. They have the autonomy to use the means of production they choose to manufacture the product as required. The autonomy is constrained by the overall system objectives. In this sense this concept respects the concept established in (Warnecke, 1993) in the Fractal Company, and as been referred in other works, namely in (Mathews, 1995). Ideally, dynamic system reconfiguration should happen instantaneously for optimal adaptation of the production system to some disturbance. In practice, however, this always takes some time which could be used as a measure of system agility.

In our modelling approach, a production unit autonomously able to manufacture a product is called a cell. This is made up from either non-autonomous production units or other cells or both. A cell executes a particular service always delivering a product. This may be delivered to the next cell for further processing, handling or storage. In this sense, any kind of service may be provided by autonomous cells. This approach was initially described in (Lima and Silva, 1998).

In our view, a distributed production system is designed for carrying out production of a product quantity required by some product order and ceases to exist after order completion. Such a system is made of several cells, each one, dedicated to the production of each product, i.e. component, of a product structure (Figure 1). It must be noted, that a component of the product structure is also named product. Our model of a distributed production systems is therefore a particular view of a product oriented manufacturing system (Silva and Alves, 2002), since it is specifically designed for achieving production requirements associated with a single production order of a specific product, including all it's components.

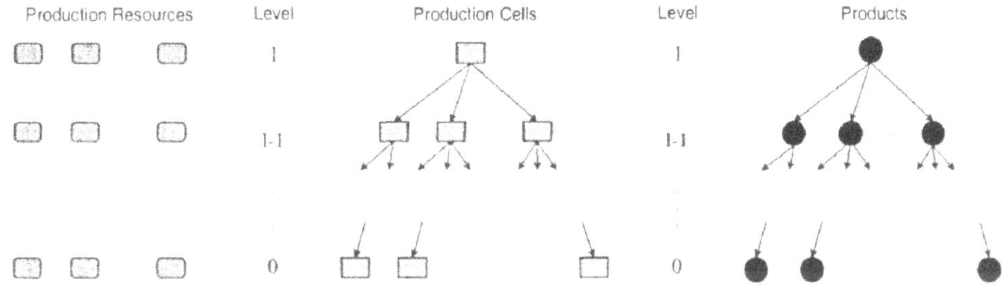

Figure 1: Distributed Production System Levels

3. THE FLEXIBLE FLOW SHOP

In the flow shop problem each job i ($1 \leq i \leq n$) consists of a set of m operations O_{ij} ($1 \leq j \leq m$) with processing times p_{ij}, where each operation must be processed on machine M_j in the exact sequence 1 to m (Brucker, 1995). A flexible flow shop (FFS) is a generalisation of the flow shop with parallel processors at least in one stage of processing (Pinedo and Chao, 1999).

The modelled FFS and alternative choices of production are shown in Figure 2, presenting a view based on production stages. The product oriented modelling view, dependent on product structure, used in this modelling approach is based on the products delivered at each production stage. Additionally we view, in a FFS, a product as the result of processing in "n" production stages, considering that at each stage the input is the result of the previous stage plus, if necessary, one or more raw material or component.

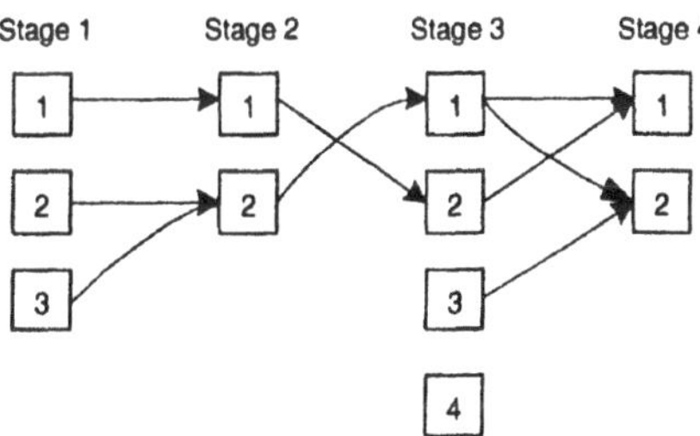

Figure 2: A FFS example (adapted from Azevedo, 1999).

4. ALGEBRAIC REPRESENTATION

Our modelling approach to distributed production systems embeds Holonic and fractal principles of systems design, considering systems inside systems, i.e., systems aggregation, to reach a final system configuration. The Generalised Scheduling work put forward in (Lecompte, Deschamps and Bourrières, 2000), allows the formal representation of distributed production systems modelled as FFS. A formal model of FFS, seen as a distributed production system is developed, representing aggregated systems, the relations between them, and the relation between the candidate resources and the tasks.

4.1 Aggregating/Disaggregating Level Mechanism

In out model a high level cell, executing a task, can aggregate several other cells executing other tasks, in a fractal view of the system, as stated by our model. The product structure is the foundation of the aggregating mechanism, i.e., a cell delivering a product aggregates all services related to the delivering problem of components of that product, in our model also called products. The number of tasks in a level will always be superior to the number of tasks in the upper level, because a set of tasks will be represented in the upper level as one task.

In one level the number of objects will be non-superior to the number in the immediately lower level. At the lowest, more detailed level, all objects / products, are represented and consequently all tasks responsible for delivering those objects. At the highest level, only the representation of the final product delivering service is considered, based on transformation of raw materials. In this modelling process raw materials are all production objects delivered by tasks that we do not want to control or model. Each level down will have the additional representation of the set of tasks responsible for delivering the products immediately lower in the product structure, and it is possible to have the same number of objects between levels if parallel tasks are aggregated. Levels associated with the FFS example will be represented in the forthcoming subsections.

4.2 Lower Level *v=0*

The previous example is represented at the lowest level 0, which is the more detailed level, as the Petri net represented in Figure 3, where each task t_j performed by one cell represents one stage of the FFS (Figure 2) and each object o_i represents one product. Other levels will exist, each one related to the encapsulation of the tasks in one more general task, until the upper task, which is the one that is responsible for delivering the final product.

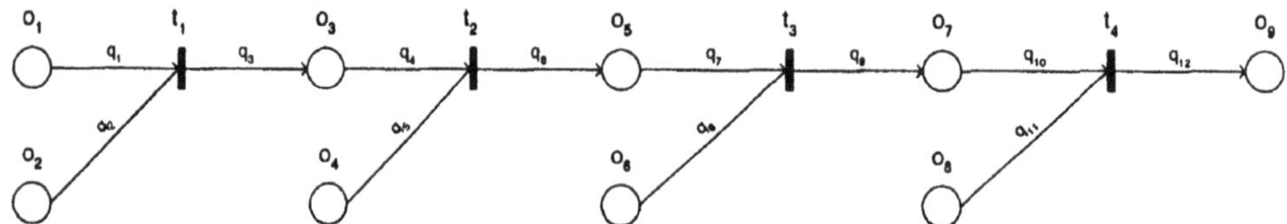

Figure 3: Production System Lowest Level Petri Net

Each Petri Net, as represented in (Lecompte, Deschamps and Bourrières, 2000), can be associated with the transformation matrix **C** (equation (1.1)), with elements C_{ij} representing object quantities consumed or manufactured by t_j task. The upper index of matrices represents the level number. The quantity of work executed in a task consumes or generates objects on the system, in quantities proportional to **C**. So, the change of object quantities is given by the product of the quantity of work by the matrix of objects consumed-generated by the tasks. Tasks on the Petri Net are associated to a quantity of work vector **W**, representing the task effort necessary to deliver a desired quantity of the output objects of each task. A unitary quantity of work delivers q_Q units indicated by the product structure of an object. The product structure is closely related to the level zero Petri Net of the system. In this example $1 \leq Q \leq 12$.

$$\text{Pre}: O \times T \rightarrow \aleph; \quad \text{Post}: O \times T \rightarrow \aleph; \quad \mathbf{C}^0 = \mathbf{Post} - \mathbf{Pre} = \begin{bmatrix} -q_1 & & & \\ -q_2 & & & \\ q_3 & -q_4 & & \\ & -q_5 & & \\ & q_6 & -q_7 & \\ & & -q_8 & \\ & & q_9 & -q_{10} \\ & & & -q_{11} \\ & & & q_{12} \end{bmatrix}; \mathbf{W}^0 = \begin{bmatrix} W_1^0 \\ W_2^0 \\ W_3^0 \\ W_4^0 \end{bmatrix} \qquad \text{Equation (1.1)}$$

4.3 Upper Level $v=l=3$

At the upper level of aggregation of cells one only cell executes a production task, delivering the final product. This final product is the same as o_9 in Figure 3. This upper level can be represented by the Figure 4 Petri Net and respective **C** and **W** matrices.

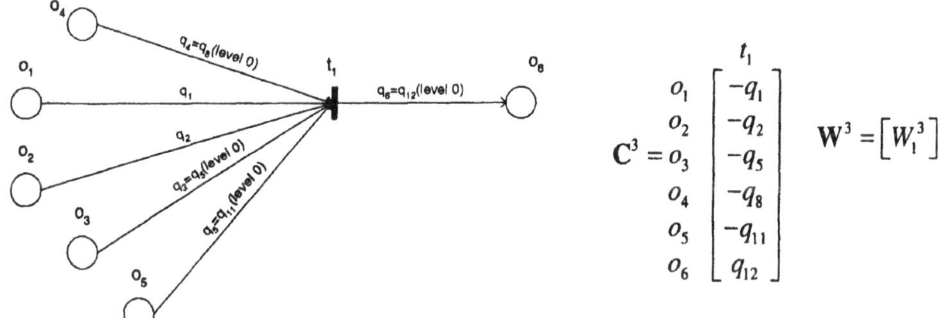

Figure 4: Level $v=l=3$ cell and object representation.

Task t_1 from Figure 4 aggregates all production system tasks, i.e., tasks t_1 to t_4 from Figure 3. Objects o_1 to o_6 from Figure 4 are the same as objects o_1, o_2, o_4, o_6, o_8, o_9 from Figure 3.

4.4 Level $v=l-1=2$

Task t_1 from Figure 5 aggregates tasks t_1 to t_3 from Figure 3 and task t_2 is the same as task t_4 from Figure 3 and the same as task t_1 from Figure 4. Objects o_1 to o_6 from Figure 5 are the same as objects o_1, o_2, o_4, o_6, o_7, o_8, o_9 from Figure 3.

$$\mathbf{C}^2 = \begin{array}{c} o_1 \\ o_2 \\ o_3 \\ o_4 \\ o_5 \\ o_6 \end{array} \begin{bmatrix} -q_1 & \\ -q_2 & \\ -q_5 & \\ -q_8 & \\ q_9 & -q_{10} \\ & -q_{11} \end{bmatrix} \quad \mathbf{W}^2 = \begin{bmatrix} W_1^2 \\ W_2^2 \end{bmatrix}$$

4.5 Level $v=l-2=1$

Task t_1 from Figure 6 aggregates tasks t_1 and t_2 from Figure 3 and tasks t_2 and t_3, not aggregated, are the same as tasks t_3 and t_4 from Figure 3. Objects o_1 to o_8 from Figure 6 are the same as objects o_1, o_2, and o_4 to o_9 from Figure 3.

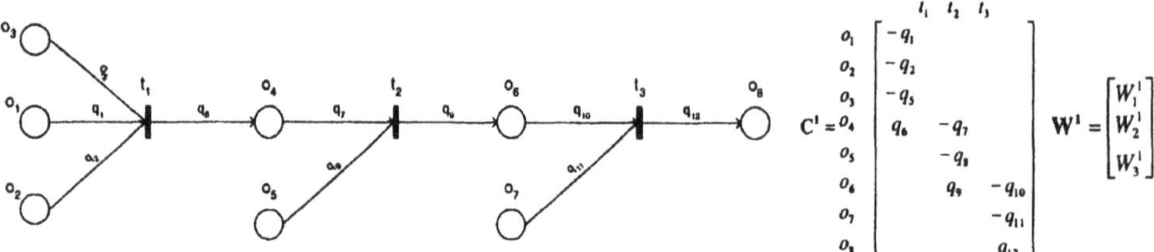

Figure 6: Level $v=l-1=2$ cells and objects representation.

5. RESOURCE ALLOCATION

In the case we are analysing in this work there are 4 tasks that can be executed by some resources for each task. The quantity of work w_{jk} is the task or work of type j ($1 \le j \le n=0$) executed by resource k ($1 \le k \le r$). If some resource does not execute some type of work, than the respective quantity of work is zero. Our problem resides on the assignment of resources to tasks and the assignment problem can be transformed (Hillier and Lieberman, 1989) to the transportation problem. This kind of problems has two fundamental restrictions: supply and demand restrictions.

Demand restriction is related to the satisfaction of ordered quantities, named as covering restrictions in (Lecompte, Deschamps and Bourrières, 2000). The total amount of work done by all resources involved on a task work must be equal to the required amount of work for that task as represented in equation (1.2).

$$\sum_{k=1}^{r} w_{jk} = W_j,\ j=1,\dots,n \Leftrightarrow \begin{cases} w_{11}+\dots+w_{1k}+\dots+w_{1r}=W_1 \\ \dots \\ w_{n1}+\dots+w_{nk}+\dots+w_{nr}=W_n \end{cases} \quad \text{Equation (1.2)}$$

Supply restriction is related to the available resource capacity, i.e., the total amount of work developed by each resource must not exceed his total capacity in all tasks he is involved with (see equation (1.3)). The α_{jk} parameter (Lecompte, Deschamps and Bourrières, 2000) represents the total amount of work that may be accomplished by resource k on type of work j during a period of time.

$$\sum_{j=1}^{n} \frac{w_{jk}}{\alpha_{jk}} \le 1,\ k=1,\dots,r \Leftrightarrow \begin{cases} {}^{w_{11}}\!/_{\alpha_{11}}+\dots+{}^{w_{j1}}\!/_{\alpha_{j1}}+\dots+{}^{w_{n1}}\!/_{\alpha_{n1}} \le 1 \\ \dots \\ {}^{w_{1r}}\!/_{\alpha_{1r}}+\dots+{}^{w_{jr}}\!/_{\alpha_{jr}}+\dots+{}^{w_{nr}}\!/_{\alpha_{nr}} \le 1 \end{cases} \quad \text{Equation (1.3)}$$

Introducing a new parameter c_{jk}, as the time for a resource k to execute one unit of work j, which we call, a unit processing time, and considering the available time of resource k represented by T_k, the relation between α_{jk} and c_{jk} is given by eq. (1.4).

$$\alpha_{jk} = T_k / c_{jk} \quad \text{Equation (1.4)}$$

Decision variables are integers restricted by equation (1.5).

$$w_{jk} \ge 0,\ w_{jk} \text{ are integeres} \quad \text{Equation (1.5)}$$

5.1 Resource Allocation Strategy

The 5 fundamental steps on distributed resource allocation problems referred in (Tharumarajah, 2001) are: 1.Decompose orders into operations; 2. Assign operations; 3. Select machine; 4. Allocate operation; 5. Coordinate allocation & build schedule. In this distributed production system model the 1st step is reduced to the decomposition of one order into tasks associated to each product in the product structure. Problem 2 and 3 referred above is treated as a resource allocation at each level of aggregation and results from the replies that are received from candidate cells. The problem of finding the optimal resource allocation vector for one level of aggregation depends on the used strategy. If we want to minimize the total processing time of all resources in all tasks, than we have the minimization problem represented in equation (1.6), constrained by equations (1.2), (1.3) and (1.5), that can be solved by integer programming.

$$\min \sum_{j=1}^{n}\sum_{k=1}^{r} c_{jk} \cdot w_{jk} \qquad \text{Equation (1.6)}$$

5.1.1 Example

Considering an order of 100 units of object o_9 and random object quantities q_Q (Figure 3) represented at Table 1, with the objective of maintaining the stock of intermediate components it is possible to compute the quantity of work at each task, obtaining: $W_1=300$; $W_2=300$; $W_3=200$; $W_4=100$. This would lead to the following raw materials requirements: o_1 – 600; o_2 – 900; o_4 – 600; o_6 – 800; o_8 – 200. Table 2 represents random available capacities by resource for each task for a period of time.

Table 1: Quantities q_Q consumed and generated by all system tasks.

q_1	q_2	q_3	q_4	q_5	q_6	q_7	q_8	q_9	q_{10}	q_{11}	q_{12}
2	3	1	1	2	2	3	4	1	2	2	1

Table 2: Available capacity by resource and required by task for a period of time.

Task	W_j	Resource	a_{jk}	
1 (t_1)	300	1 ($a_{1,1}$)	210	If
		2 ($a_{1,2}$)	100	$T_k = 1$, for all k
		3 ($a_{1,3}$)	35	Than
2 (t_2)	300	4 ($a_{2,4}$)	240	
		5 ($a_{2,5}$)	150	$c_{jk} = 1/\alpha_{jk}$
3 (t_3)	200	6 ($a_{3,6}$)	55	
		7 ($a_{3,7}$)	100	
		8 ($a_{3,8}$)	120	
		9 ($a_{3,9}$)	10	
4 (t_4)	100	10 ($a_{4,10}$)	40	
		11 ($a_{4,11}$)	90	

The solution presented in Table 3 represents the allocation of resources to tasks by the quantity of work indicated. This is a solution for a particular random example, indicating the applicability of the model, at least, for the particular case.

Table 3: Quantity of work allocated to each resource.

Quantity	$w_{1,1}$	$w_{1,2}$	$w_{1,3}$	$w_{2,4}$	$w_{2,5}$	$w_{3,6}$	$w_{3,7}$	$w_{3,8}$	$w_{3,9}$	$w_{4,10}$	$w_{4,11}$
of work	210	90	0	240	60	0	80	120	0	10	90

6. CONCLUSION

A fundamental problem to be solved in the design and operation of distributed production systems is the allocation of resources to different tasks to be performed. An algebraic model was used for representing a Flexible Flow Shop as a Distributed Production System. The model was applied for solving the resource allocation problem based on a particular strategy of allocation for a case study.

The production system structure is modelled matching the structure of the product to be manufactured, through mechanisms of generation and boundary delimitation of sub-systems.

Future work will address model test and validation using industrial and academic cases under several allocation strategies, associated with order requirements or production system objectives. These strategies may involve aspects such as parallel processing and system loading levels.

7. REFERENCES

1. Azevedo, AL. Apoio à Decisão na Negociação de Encomendas em Redes de Empresas. Dissertação para obtenção do Grau de Doutor em Engenharia Electrotécnica e de Computadores (in portuguese). Faculdade de Engenharia: Universidade do Porto, 1999.
2. Brucker, P. *Scheduling Algorithms*: Springer-Verlag, 1995.
3. Hillier, FS and Lieberman, GJ. *Introduction to Operations Research*: McGraw-Hill, 1989.
4. Lecompte, T, Deschamps, JC and Bourrières, JP. A data model for generalized scheduling for virtual enterprise. *Production Planning & Control*, 2000; **11**(4): 343-348.
5. Lima, RM and Silva, SC. Object Oriented Modelling of Product Oriented Manufacturing Systems, *in Intelligent Systems for Manufacturing: Multi-Agent Systems and Virtual Organization (LM Camarinha-Matos, H Afsarmanesh and V Marik)*. Prague, Czech Republic: Kluwer, 1998: 325-334.
6. Lima, RM, Silva, SC and Martins, PM. Sistemas Distribuídos de Produção, *in 1° Congresso Luso-Moçambicano de Engenharia (JFS Gomes, A Matos and C Afonso)*, Maputo, Moçambique, 1999; B13-B20 (in portuguese).
7. Mathews, J. Organizational Foundations of Intelligent Manufacturing Systems - the Holonic View Point. *Computer Integrated Manufacturing Systems*, 1995; **8**(4): 237-243.
8. Pinedo, M and Chao, X. *Operations Scheduling with Applications in Manufacturing and Services*: McGraw-Hill, 1999.
9. Putnik, GD and Silva, SC. One-Product-Integrated-Manufacturing, *in Balanced Automation Systems: Architectures and Design Methods (LM Camarinha-Matos and H Afsarmanesh)*, 1995.
10. Silva, SC and Alves, A. Design of Product Oriented Manufacturing Systems, *in 5th IEEE / IFIP International Conference on Information Technology for Balanced Automation Systems in Manufacturing and Systems - BASYS'2002*, Cancun, Mexico: Kluwer, 2002.
11. Tharumarajah, A. Survey of resource allocation methods for distributed manufacturing systems. *Production Planning & Control*, 2001; **12**(1): 58-68.
12. Tharumarajah, A, Wells, AJ and Nemes, L. Comparison of the Bionic, Fractal and Holonic Manufacturing System Concepts. *International Journal of Computer Integrated Manufacturing*, 1996; **9**(3): 217-226.
13. Vernadat, F. *Enterprise Modeling and Integration: principles and applications*: Chapman & Hall, 1996.
14. Warnecke, HJ. *The Fractal Company*: Springer-Verlag, 1993.

9

SIMULATION SERVICES FOR TRAINING OF PLANT OPERATORS

Gerhard Schreck
Fraunhofer IPK
Pascalstraße 8-9
10587 Berlin, Germany
Gerhard.Schreck@ipk.fhg.de

This paper presents an approach for machinery and equipment manufacturers to provide qualification services as value-added-services to its customers. A concept for the provision of a virtual training center by cost-effective simulation services via Internet is outlined. The concept has been developed within a project of the Fraunhofer Association e-Industrial Services. Aspects of simulation service implementation and application are illustrated by a realized system demonstrator for the training of operators of water treatment plants.

1. INTRODUCTION

Recently, production systems tend to have shorter life cycles, an increased diversity of variants as well as increased complexity. This development also requires innovations for the training of personnel. Qualification is becoming a competitive factor for producers of production systems, who want to guarantee increased availability and a more efficient operation.

A qualified personnel is an essential prerequisite for the safe and effective utilization of production systems. By applying new mediums and electronic work tools, it is possible to extract the fundamental aspects from the, up until now, rigid learning context of operator training and to flexibly arrange the training in terms of time, duration and place (Qualification on demand). Didactically, this opens up new perspectives since such a learning process is, to a great degree, carried out actively as well as interactively.

Within the framework of the Fraunhofer Association e-Industrial Services, adaptive qualification services are being developed for operation, maintenance and service personnel. Innovative and customer-specific training courses and systems can be provided over network portals. A main focus of development at Fraunhofer IPK is the planning and design of qualification services for operator personnel, especially the implementation of simulation-based training systems for system operators (Bernhardt, 2001).

2. TRAINING OF PLANT OPERATORS

2.1 Developments towards e-Learning

As working systems become more complex, they require higher qualifications of the work personnel. Due to the increasing degree of automation, the workers are becoming more and more removed from the actual process. Increasingly, the production takes place under the control of a central system which results in fewer workers who operate and supervise systems that are constantly becoming more complex. Especially in highly automated systems, the operator's tasks are limited to making sure that a system runs its course smoothly. However, it is necessary that the operator has the capability to manually operate the process control in case of a disturbance. Accordingly, the standards for the operator's qualification, knowledge and skills become greater.

Computer-based Training (CBT), Distance Learning, WEB-based Training, etc. are the current keywords in connection with the new IT-based educational and training concepts. For this, the internet plays an increasingly important role as the standard platform for the providing and calling up of training programs. In the following text, qualification services that are offered on the internet will be referred to as e-Learning.

For the broad market of EDP-standard products (word processing, spread-sheet calculations, etc.) there is already a wide-array of e-Learning course modules offered. Even the major manufacturers of automation components and systems are beginning to organize training for their products on the internet. Such offers, however, are concentrated on individual components or systems (ex. PLC system) and not on entire customer-specific solutions which are usually implemented in the plant engineering and construction as an individual system. The system operator's training is normally carried out by the manufacturer, on-location, during the line-up and start-up phase of the production system.

However, an effective use of the system resources and the guarantee of a safe and reliable operation require qualification measures and services, which would accompany the entire life-cycle of the system. The previously described marginal conditions have supported the employment of online and simulation-based training systems especially in the applications of process engineering (Winter, 2001). The further application of this approach to production systems in general, alongside economical solutions for the implementation of e-Learning services, has very high potential.

2.2 Simulators for the Training of Plant Operators

Training simulators have already been successfully applied for many years to specific industries, such as power stations or large-scale installations of the chemical industry. They represent an important tool for a danger-free and efficient training of the operation personnel. Qualification goals for the use of training simulators are:

- Training of control system operation,
- Training of the initial operation,
- Training of the normal operation,
- Training of the start-up and shut-down procedure,

- Training of exceptional situations,
- Development of execution alternatives,
- Operator support of the operation.

Training simulators enable the training at a real control system albeit in a virtual set-up, i.e. in a simulated system (virtual plant). Through this set-up, work procedures for the normal operation can be practiced as well as rarely occurring work processes, such as start-up and shut-down of plant operation. Additionally, a danger-free training of how to handle usually very risky disturbances (i.e. system breakdown) as well as the necessary measures to be taken by the operator can be executed. Due to costs, the use of training simulators takes places nowadays almost exclusively in processes and systems that are multiply constructed in the same or similar form.

Training simulators are complex systems which require specially trained technicians for its operation. This includes, for example, a system manager for the maintenance of hardware and system software, at least one instructor as well as a process engineer, who has a strong knowledge on process modeling and knows how to handle the engineering tools in order to update the system. Only with such a simulator-operation personnel is the system capable of being fully employed (NAMUR, 1995). Because of this, training simulators are usually operated in training centers and are sought out by plant operator in scheduled courses (Figure 1).

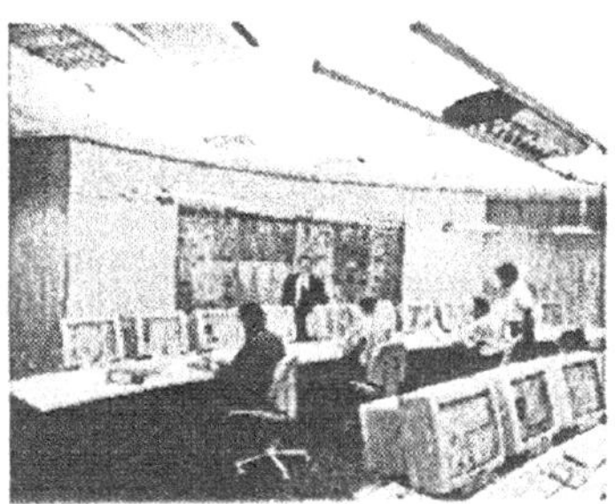

Figure 1 – Training Center for Power Plant Operator
(SimPower Simulator Systems GmbH)

3. SIMULATION SERVICES FOR TRAINING

3.1 Simulation-Based Qualification Services via Internet

High costs for simulator development, as well as for its on-site operation within central training centers, are a barrier for the widespread application of training simulators in production plants in general. Solutions are required, which enable a cost-efficient provision and application of simulation based qualification services for plant operators.

A concept for the provision of a virtual training center by cost-effective simulation services via Internet has been developed within the project e-Industrial services (Hohwieler, 2001). It is based on a client-server architecture, where the training simulator is located at the site of a service provider, e.g. the machinery and equipment manufacturer. The service provider maintains the underlying simulation models of the plant, as well as data bases containing training exercises and profiles of system usage. The operator has access to the training services via an Internet browser. Exercises are offered with reference to his personal qualification profile and training state. Training sessions can be executed self-contained by the operator or, on requested, by support of an human instructor (Figure 2).

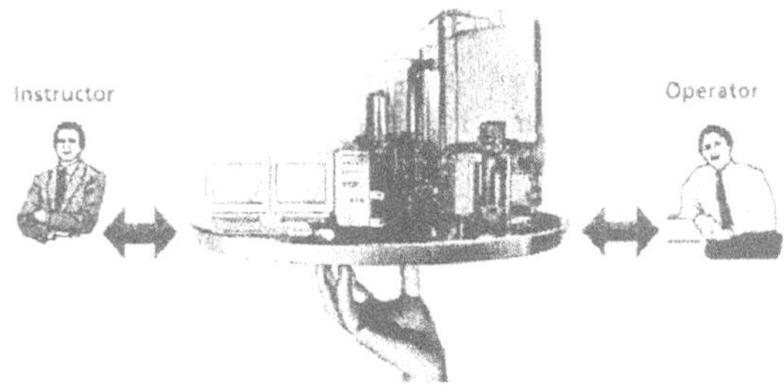

Figure 2 - Access to a Virtual Training Center via the e-IS Service-platform

3.2 Qualification Services as Value-Added-Services of Machinery and Equipment Manufacturers

If the system manufacturer is included in the development, or even the operation, of the qualification services, then the greatest synergy occurs in the aforementioned e-Learning concept. Through the project phases of planning, implementation and line-up of the system, the system manufacturer has the necessary information and models of the customers system. Furthermore, by making this service continuously available, the underlying information model is subjected to adjustments and improvements. This is the basis for a close co-operation between manufacturer and customer, even during the operation phase, and increases customer relation.

The system manufacturer receives valuable information about the application and operation of his product. Through the evaluation of available operational data, it is possible to identify and analyze the user's problems with the system. From this, both specific training courses and training modules can be derived and concrete suggestions for product improvements are generated (Figure 3).

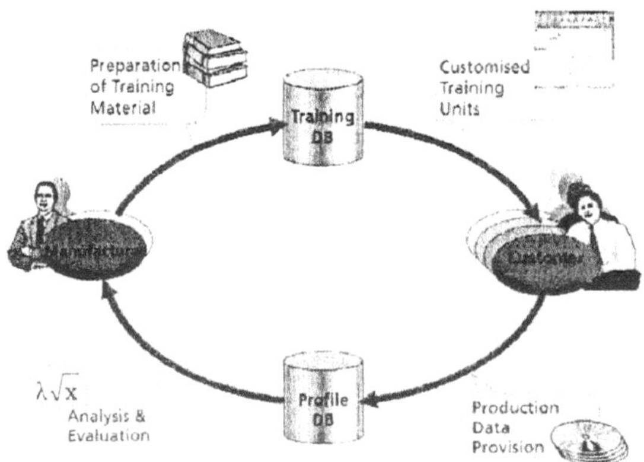

Figure 3 - Manufacturer - Customer Relation

By such an approach, machinery and equipment manufacturers are able to provide qualification services for the complete product life cycle. In this way, the system manufacturer can provide a variety of new services for operator qualification for his implemented system:

- basic education about the product (before the system's delivery),
- system and process related training course,
- specific re-training when the system has been modified.

4. PLATFORM CONCEPT FOR E-INDUSTRIAL SERVICES

With its service platform, the Fraunhofer Association e-Industrial services has created a portal, which will allow both the ordering and execution of e-Services through the Internet. The architecture of the service platform is based on a scalable business model in which the roles of the participants are defined. The model distinguishes between customers, users, retailers and service providers.

The platform includes an application server to authenticate users. The authentication data is sent via an SSL-protected http connection to the application server before being handed over to the service platform using CORBA. Then, the service platform checks the user database to verify the authentication data. The authentication server provides a list of services available to the user and, if applicable, previously interrupted service sessions. Once the user has selected a service, the platform activates the relevant application logic and produces the proper graphic user interface. The user employs this interface to interact with the application logic, which in turn uses other components of the service platform (Figure 4).

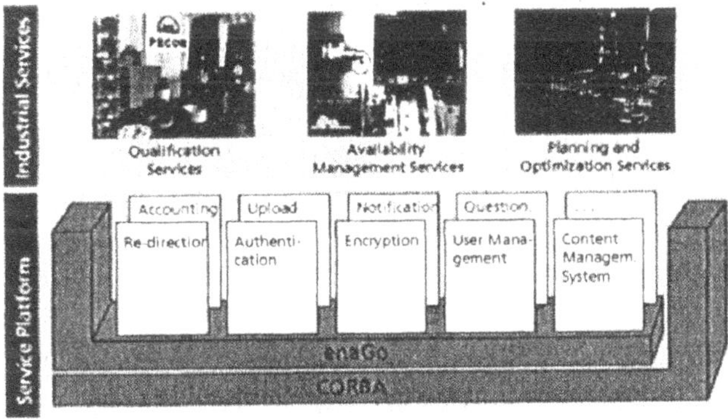

Figure 4 - Service Platform for Implementation and Execution of e-Services

The electronic services integrated in the service platform are offered over an Internet portal operating in a distributed environment. Accordingly, the system architecture makes a clear distinction between application logic and user interface. The application logic is part of the service provider's computer system, whereas the user interface appears on the user's workstations. In order to make the usage of the service as easy as possible while simultaneously enabling the greatest possible platform independence, the service platform relies solely on HTML applications. Only services requiring a great deal of interactivity, such as data evaluation or on-line simulation, are handled through applets or even browser-external applications.

5. APPLICATION EXAMPLE

5.1 Training Operators of Water Treatment Plants

As an example, the previously described e-Learning concept of the simulation-based training was implemented, in cooperation with an automation supplier, for the operation personnel of water treatment plants. Modern water treatment plants are equipped with control technology which allows a safe operation and a continuous monitoring. The pre-set values of the process technician determine the system's operating points which will afterwards be maintained by the supervisory control system. The selection of operating points is dependent on the know-how of the technician. For this, objective criteria of system management (i.e. specific energy consumption, frequency of change-over processes, planning of cleaning procedures and maintenance work) are only rarely taken into consideration.

The main objective of the process management consists of ensuring a proper operation of the system. For this, the following criteria must be fulfilled:

- Allocation of the required quantity of pure water,
- Consideration of the different modes of working and use of resources,
- Compliance with requirements for the quality of water,
- Adherence to a minimal consumption of energy,
- Maintenance of the purification cycle of individual filters,
- A continuous and smooth running of the system,
- Adherence to the prescribed limits of the tanks with a quick reaction to deviations.

Energy tariffs and prognosis of water decline over a given time period (ex. 24 hours) are marginal conditions of the process management which have to be taken into consideration. Such demanding tasks of process management require the appropriate experience of the operator (Lisounkin, 1999).

Through the implementation of the training simulator, it was possible to set up available models of the system with fundamental simulation components. They were supplied for the necessary functions of training purposes and integrated into the service platform. The use of the individual training modules were organized and managed by a training database.

Figure 5 shows the plant operator's control panel. The individual display and operation elements represent those of the real system. The dynamic reaction to the operators entries, however, are realized by the simulator, which is connected to the internet. Besides using the online simulator for the training of operation personnel, the system operator can also use it for trying out alternative ways of running the system.

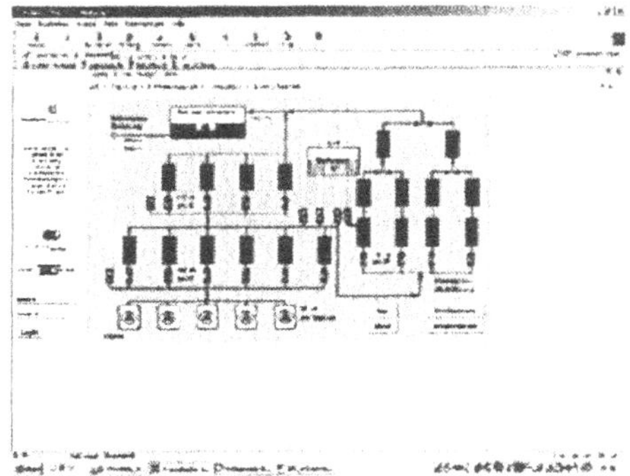

Figure 5 - Example of an Operator Control Panel Screen

5.2 Adaptation of Training Contents to the User's Needs

In order to control and document the dynamic course of events within the water treatment plant, the relevant variables of state are recorded in data archives. This information represents a profile of the system's running and will be used for analysis and assessment. It is possible to evaluate the profile of the training exercise as well as the profile of the actual running of the system. From this, training elements can be constructed that coordinate with specific system situations with the training phase of the operator (adaptive).

In Figure 6, there is an example of plant operation profiles, which shows the relation between water consumption, execution of purification cycles, and water production. When optimizing the operation of the system the scheduling of the purification cycles plays an important role for saving energy costs. Such aspects of operation can be very well trained by simulation exercises and analysis of the used plant operation profiles (Lisounkin, 2002)

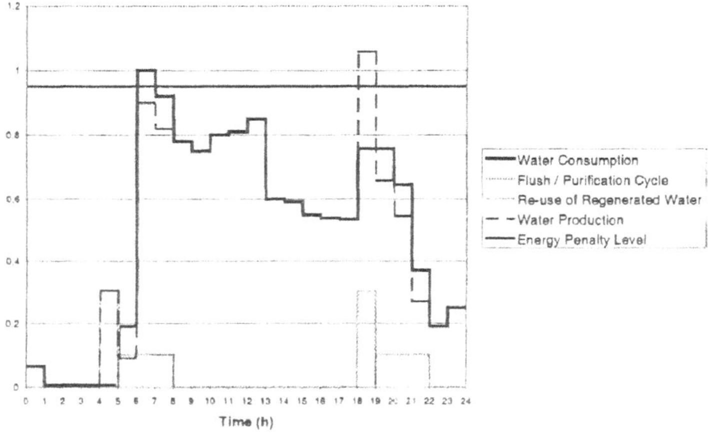

Figure 6 - Example of Plant Operation Profiles

6. CONCLUSIONS AND OUTLOOK

Both manufacturer and user profit from the application of simulation based qualification services through the following advantages:

- Higher availability and optimal use of production systems due to a qualified and trained personnel,
- More effective training through programs that are specifically adjusted to the system and user,
- World wide availability and application possibilities from innovative educational and training programs,
- Possibilities for team training, even when the systems are in different locations.

Within the framework of the developmental environment of the Fraunhofer Association e-Industrial Services, there is a suitable platform for an efficient realization of qualification services via Internet. The prototype training simulator for the operators of water distribution systems serves as a reference point. The available communication and management functions for the handling of services as well as the database structure and models for e-Learning are application-independent and therefore are available for the use of further applications. Plans for the next application include the integration of information modules for qualification of machine tool operators at the shop floor. Further application scenarios will be implemented in cooperation with machine and system producers in order to enable them to offer their customers innovative educational and training services.

7. ACKNOWLEDGMENTS

The basic e-Service infrastructure has been implemented by the partners of the Fraunhofer Association e-Industrial services (Fraunhofer e-IS, 2002). Simulation based qualification services are developments of Fraunhofer IPK. We thank our launching customer Elpro Prozessindustrie und Energieanlagen GmbH, Berlin, for the close co-operation and support in the development of the demonstrator system.

8. REFERENCES

1. Bernhard R, Schreck G. "Teletraining – Simulationsbasierte Schulung von Bedienpersonal". In Futur 1/2001, 12-13.
2. Winter H, Schmidt, F. "Online-Trainingssystem für Bedienerschulung in Unternehmen der verfahrens-technischen Industrie". Düsseldorf: VDI Verlag, 2001 (VDI-Berichte; 1608), S. 457 - 467.
3. NAMUR. "Management von Trainingssimulatorprojekten". NAMUR-Arbeitsblatt NA 60, Version 22.11.95.
4. Hohwieler E, Schreck G, Berger R. "Bereitstellung elektronischer Dienstleistungen für Produktionssysteme". In Proceedings of X. Internationales Produktionstechnisches Kolloquium – PTK, Berlin, 27.-28. September 2001, 107-112.
5. Lisounkin A, Schmidt H.-W. "Modellbasierte Prozessführung in einem Wasserwerk". In Journal Wasser und Boden. Vol. 51, 11, 1999, 44-47.
6. Lisounkin A, Schreck G. "Water Consumption Profile Analysis for Facility Control and Operator Training". To be published in Proceedings of ASM 2002, June 25-28, 2002, Crete, Greece.
7. Fraunhofer e-IS. /www.e-industrial-services.de/

10 SUPPORT FOR B2B E-CONTRACTING – THE PROCESS PERSPECTIVE

Samuil Angelov, Paul Grefen
Computer Science Department
University of Twente
The Netherlands
sangelov@cs.utwente.nl
grefen@cs.utwente.nl

In business-to-business relations, contracts serve both as a protection mechanism of trading partners, as well as a prescription document for activities to be executed by the parties. The processes of contract establishment and its enactment are often expensive and time consuming. E-contracting aims at automation of these processes, making them faster and cheaper. For the design of an information system for support of e-contracting, a clear vision of the e-contracting processes is required. In this paper, we introduce a process model for flexible business-to-business e-contracting. To separate concerns, we distinguish structured function and communication perspectives of e-contracting processes complemented with consistency rules. The proposed approach allows achieving completeness and consistency in building complex contracting processes.

1. INTRODUCTION

Business process modeling and reengineering aims at improving the efficiency and effectiveness of business processes that are executed in a company. Initially, only intra-organizational business processes were considered. Software applications with different levels of complexity are provided for the coordination and automation of intra-organizational processes. After the rapid development of information technology, the possibility for the support of cross-organizational business processes emerged (Grefen, 2000), (Alonso, 1999), (CrossFlow, 2000). Many research institutes and standardization efforts, e.g. ebXML (ebXML, 2001), RosettaNet (RosettaNet, 2001), work on the problem of modeling cross-organizational processes and realization of supporting information systems. Business-to-business contracting is a key example that faces this problem. It governs most business transactions and it comprises a collection of coherent intra- and cross-organizational activities. The choice of the activities to be performed during contracting and the order of execution is context dependent. This adds for the complexity of the process.

Standard paper contracting processes are often slow and require involvement of human actors in all contracting phases. Electronic contracting provides faster and cheaper contract establishment and offers new opportunities to the partners, e.g., micro-contracting (Grefen, 2002). However, implementation of information technology for the support of business-to-business electronic contracting requires a clear vision of the activities that are to be performed by the participating companies. In this paper, we present an approach to achieve this.

We describe a method for process modeling of flexible business-to-business e-contracting. The modeling approach is based on two perspectives of the e-contracting process, i.e., function and communication perspectives. We model the cross-organization activities in a separate view, in order to achieve coherence of communication between parties. Use of process decomposition and process inheritance in the function and communication views respectively, allows achieving a structured and complete model. The two perspectives do not suffice for composing e-contracting processes, as they do not specify sequence, mutual exclusion, etc. of activities. For this reason, we define a set of consistency rules that are used for the specification of the relations between the e-contracting activities. The relation specification facilitates the construction of concrete e-contracting processes.

The combination of function and communication perspectives and the consistency rules provides a tool for the construction of complete and correct concrete e-contracting process specifications. The model can be used for analysis of existing e-contracting process specifications as well. Requirements that are not satisfied or inconsistencies in existing specifications can be discovered. A software architecture is required for realization of e-contracting systems. The elaboration of this software architecture demands clear description of the e-contracting process. The model proposed in this paper is the basis for obtaining requirements for an e-contracting system.

This paper is organised as follows. In Section 2, the approach for the e-contracting process model is described. In Sections 3 and 4, the function and communication perspectives of the model are depicted. Consistency rules that are applied to processes are explained in Section 5. To show the use of the defined model, we use it in Section 6 to construct sample concrete processes. Finally, we draw conclusions on this paper and outline future research issues.

2. MODELLING APPROACH

In this section, we describe our modeling approach and present related work in this field. To provide a complete and consistent model of the e-contracting process, we separate concerns by elaborating different perspectives of the process. To achieve completeness, we depict a function perspective of e-contracting activities. In this view, e-contracting activities are specialized at several levels of abstraction. This perspective provides a complete picture of e-contracting activities to a certain level of specialization. Its hierarchical presentation allows further specialization for the support of specific context requirements. Specific issues of the business domains (such as the insurance domain) can be addressed in this way.

E-contracting is a blend of intra- and cross-organizational activities. An e-contracting model should guarantee coherence of cross-organizational activities as well as coherence between the cross- and intra-organizational activities. To achieve this, next to the function perspective we elaborate a communication perspective. The communication perspective is a specialization tree of the different communication activity types that occur during e-contracting. The communication hierarchy is coupled with internal processes that are associated with the communication activities. This supports modeling of coherent cross- and intra- organizational process. Being a hierarchy, the communication perspective can be further specialized, if specific business situations require this. The leaves in the communication perspective are a subset of the activity leaves in the function perspective. The communication perspective aims at facilitating the process of defining consistent communication activities in the function perspective. It is applied for the construction of the third level of specialization of the function perspective, where concrete communication activities are identified

To model the relations between the e-contracting activities, we define a set of consistency rules. These rules support the proper construction of the e-contracting process from the identified activities. They can be applied at the different levels of abstraction of the function perspective. For some of the rule types, rule inheritance is applicable.

To position our approach, we relate it to other developments in this field. First, we relate our approach to a research project that was carried out at the University of St. Gallen. A number of efforts exist for the standardization of cross-organizational activities (Angelov, 2001b). For this reason, next, we relate our approach to RosettaNet, which is an established standardization effort for cross-organizational activities.

In (Gisler, 2000), three views on the e-contracting process are depicted. The view on e-contracting activities is equivalent to our highest level of abstraction of the function view. However, the authors describe only briefly the phases and the processes that constitute them. In their paper, a document and a legal perspective are aligned to the activities view. The document view shows the documents delivered at the end of each phase. This is not enough to give a clear vision over the communication activities performed by the parties, through which these documents are delivered. In the legal perspective, legal issues are discussed that are not of importance to our approach. The three views are described at a high level of abstraction and only sketch the general characteristics of the e-contracting process. In our work, we describe in greater details the contracting process, reaching level of concrete contracting activities. As already explained, to achieve coherence of communication activities between parties, we distinguish a separate communication view in the model.

RosettaNet is a standardization effort aiming at a description of the cross-organizational business processes. In RosettaNet, a three level hierarchy of the activities of the collaborating parties is used to guarantee completeness of the standard. This hierarchy is built as a specialization of the domain of e-business supply chain activities. In RosettaNet, in contrast to our approach, no attention is paid to the internal business processes and their relation to the cross-organizational processes. As a result, only the e-contracting communication activities can be extracted from this standard. In this paper, we look towards description of the complete e-contracting process.

3. FUNCTION PERSPECTIVE

In this section, the function perspective of the e-contracting process model is described. The perspective is presented as a combination of a subtyping hierarchy and collection relations. We distinguish three levels of abstraction in the hierarchy. Each level is briefly discussed below.

An e-contracting process consists of a number of e-contracting phases. A phase constitutes of activities, specific for a stage of the e-contracting process. These phases are successively executed in the time. We distinguish four phases: information, pre-contractual, contracting and enactment phases (see Figure 1– phase level). In the information phase, general preparations are made, information is provided (for a request or offer of services) and possible partners are identified. In the pre-contracting phase, preparatory contracting processes are performed. In the contracting phase, the contract is negotiated and established. During the enactment phase, the contract is executed and accompanying activities are performed. For a successful e-contracting process, at least the last two phases must take place (Angelov, 2002a) (this requirement can be defined using the consistency rules described in Section 5).

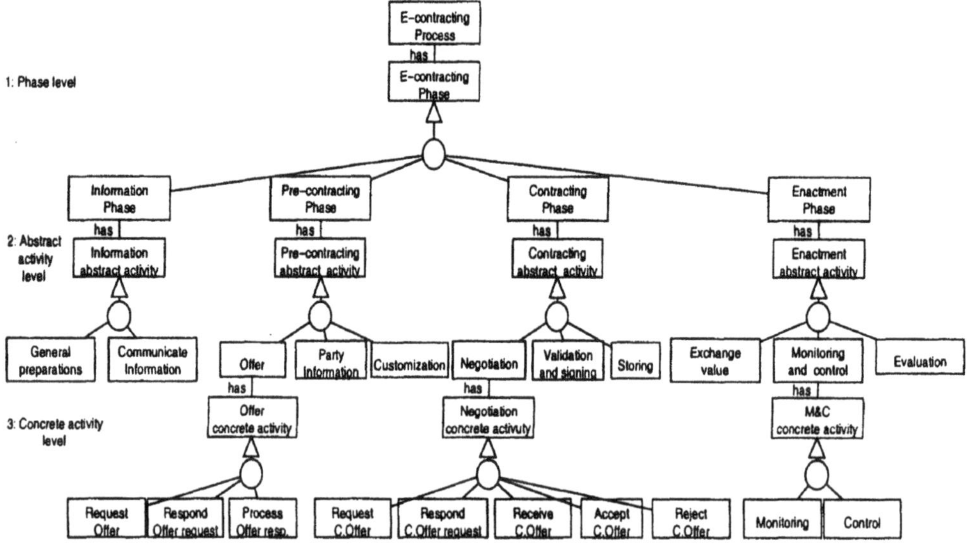

Figure 1 – Function perspective

Each phase contains abstract activities. Abstract activities for each phase are sub-typed to specific abstract activities. They form the second level of abstraction. Abstract activities are a collection of concrete activities that form a logical unit and that in combination deliver a value to the parties. For example, the *offer* activity is a collection of sub-activities that support the exchange of offers between parties (see concrete activity level). Concrete activities form the third level of abstraction of the function perspective. Figure 1 shows a sample specialization of the *offer*, *negotiation,* and *monitoring and control* concrete activities. For reasons of brevity, the other specializations are not depicted. A detailed description is available in (Angelov, 2002b).

The activities identified at the concrete activity level are leaves in the function perspective. This level of specialization is sufficient for modeling standard e-contracting processes. Depending on the business situation, specific activities that are performed during e-contracting might be required. These specific activities can be specialized from the leaf activities in the function perspective. In this way the defined activity tree can be specialized to new levels of detail, e.g., domain level, company level, service level, etc.

In the sequel of the paper, we concentrate on the *offer* abstract activity. The *offer* abstract activity is best used to illustrate the benefits of the proposed approach. It contains the *request offer, respond offer request,* and *process offer response* concrete activities.

4. COMMUNICATION PERSPECTIVE

The function perspective is required to guarantee completeness of the model. At the abstract activity level, the level of specialization allows to distinguish activities as intra- or cross-organizational. Internal activities can vary in their concrete specification, depending on the parties and the business context. However, well-formed communication for the cross-organizational activities, i.e., communication activities between parties, is required to guarantee coherence of the communication activities of parties and thus to guarantee successful exchange of information between parties. Additionally, coherence between the communication activities and the internal activities associated to them must be guaranteed. To specialize cross-organizational activities in the function view and to guarantee their consistency, we need a communication perspective.

In this section, we discuss the communication perspective of the e-contracting process (see Figure 2).

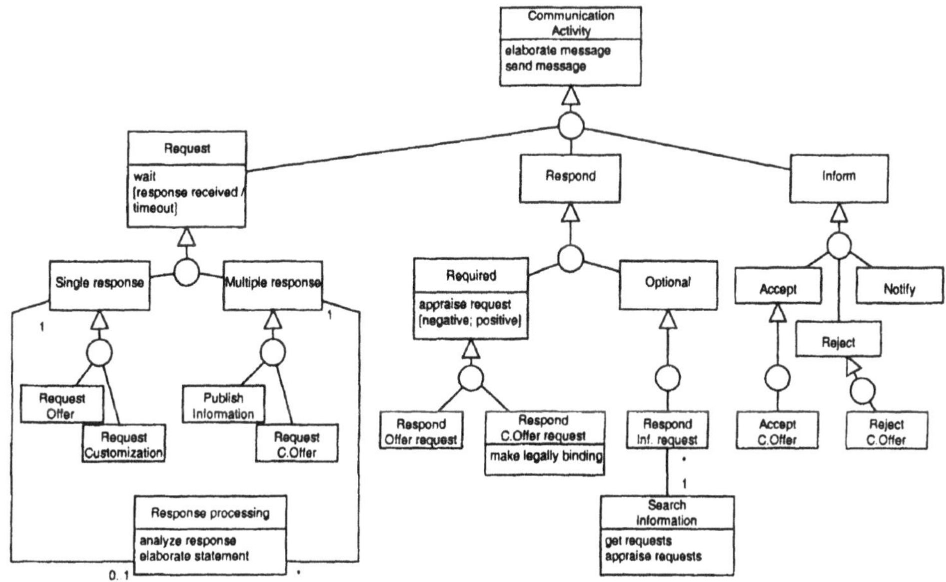

Figure 2 – Communication perspective

Communication processes are sub-typed from a root communication activity. We specialize the communication activity into request, respond and inform activities. This set of activity types covers all aspects of a communication process. The defined communication activity tree, with this level of specialization, suffices to represent the cross-organizational perspective. It defines the communication patterns for the communication activities and thus it guarantees their consistency. All concrete communication activities can be specialized from this last level. However, to achieve coherence between the intra- and cross-organizational activities, we add to this perspective the internal activities that are directly connected to the communication activities. Such activities are, for example, *response processing* (i.e. when a party receives a response from another party resulting from previous request activity) and *search* activities (i.e. when a party searches in a market place to find requests for information from other parties). By adding intra-organizational activities in this view, communication activities and internal activities associated to them are linked to each other. In Figure 2, the internal activities are positioned below the communication hierarchy. Internal activities cause a third level of specialization of communication activities to be defined. We specialize the communication activities according to their relation with the internal activities. A request activity is specialized into requests that expect a single response and requests that expect multiple responses. The internal activity according to which they are specialized is the response processing activity. For example, the request for offer expects only one response, while a request for information, published in a market place, expects many responses from different parties. Analogously, the respond activity is specialized to a required and optional response. Only the response to a request for information (published in a market place) is optional. For all other response activities, the requesting party requires response. For reasons of brevity, only several leaf activities are given in Figure 2 as examples for specialization from the third level. Using the defined communication perspective, we sub-type the cross-organizational abstract activities in the function perspective, e.g., the *offer* abstract activity.

To facilitate the construction of concrete communication activities, we exploit another feature of the constructed hierarchy, i.e., the inheritance of activities. Communication activities consist of tasks. For example, every communication activity consists of at least two tasks, i.e., *elaborate message* and *send message*. We use the communication hierarchy for inheritance of tasks to sub-activities. For example, the *request* activity inherits *elaborate request* and *send request* tasks from the root communication activity. We add a *wait* state and a triggering event (response received or timeout occurs) for the *request* activity, as each request waits for response. This inheritance of tasks throughout the tree requires adding only activity specific tasks to the leaf activities and facilitates construction of concrete activities, as we show in Section 6.

5. CONSISTENCY RULES

In Sections 3 and 4, we have presented two perspectives of the e-contracting process. These two perspectives do not contain information about the temporal and existence relationships between the executed activities. To provide information about these relations, an appropriate notation is required. In this section, a notation that is used to represent this information is described. We define a set of consistency rules that are used to model the activity constraints. A textual notation is used for their definition. There are also graphical notations to represent rules for temporal precedence of activities that can be used as well, e.g. (Jackson, 1997). We define the following relations:

SEQUENCE(A_1,A_2): The relation expresses that the execution of A_1 has to precede that of A_2. For example, SEQUENCE(Offer, Negotiation) shows that the offer exchange activity precedes the negotiation activity.

EXISTENCE(A_1,A_2): The SEQUENCE relation can be strengthened by the EXISTENCE(A_1,A_2) relation, which expresses the requirement that activity A_2 can be executed only when the activity A_1 has been executed. An example would be EXISTENCE(Offer, Customization). A customization activity can be executed only when an offer has been exchanged between the parties.

EXCLUDE(A_1,A_2): This relation shows that both activities are mutually exclusive, e.g., EXCLUDE(Accept contract offer, Reject contract offer).

REQUIRED(A_1): The REQUIRED operator indicates that the activity given as an argument must be executed and is not optional, e.g. REQUIRED(Exchange value).

This set can be extended with other rules, if additional constraints must be imposed.

The hierarchical representation of the function perspective allows rule inheritance for the SEQUENCE and EXCLUDE operators to be applied. Defining SEQUENCE(Contracting phase, Enactment phase), means that all sub-activities of the two phases inherit the defined rule. This rule inheritance is not valid for the EXISTENCE and REQUIRED operators.

6. E-CONTRACTING PROCESS DESIGN

The described model in combination with the defined consistency rules does not define a unique e-contracting process. Business-to-business e-contracting varies in the performed activities depending on the companies and the business context (Angelov, 2001a). The model gives flexibility to construct various concrete e-contracting processes, depending on the business context. By applying consistency rules, a company can define different relations between activities, achieving a correct flexible e-contracting process specification.

In this section, the model is used to construct a fragment of a concrete e-contracting process specification. Activity diagrams are used as a modeling technique (Eriksson, 2000). In the following example, we concentrate on the construction of cross-organizational activities, as they show the application of both perspectives of the model. Concrete specifications for activities that are entirely internal can vary significantly, depending on the specific company. To construct a complete e-contracting process specification, a party starts with identification of the activity leaves that will participate in the process definition. This step might require additional specializations of the activity leaves from the functional perspective. Next, a company uses the consistency rules to define the relations between the identified activities. Then, a process specification for each activity is elaborated.

To demonstrate the use of the defined model, concrete activity diagrams for the *offer* abstract activity are constructed. As the offer activity is a cross-organizational activity, we use both the function and the communication view for the specification construction. First, we identify the activity in the function activity tree. The activity is a sub-activity of the pre-contractual phase. Next step is to select the activity leaves of the *offer* activity.

The offer activity is a request-response activity. It does not involve the third communication category, i.e., inform activity (see Figure 2). Next, the communication perspective is used to identify the leaf activities of the *offer* abstract activity. Usually, the offer activity will start with a request for offer from the consumer in order to get the specifications of the provided service by the supplier. As each offer request is directed to one company, a single response by the supplier is required in return. In this way, the *request offer* and *respond offer request* activities are identified in the request and respond branches respectively of the communication perspective. When received, the response (i.e., the offer) has to be processed by the consumer. As a result, three activity leaves that specialize the offer activity are found, i.e., *request offer, respond offer request* and *process offer response* activities (we use for each of them the abbreviations RqO, RpORq, PrORp respectively, and A_O to denote the set of all three activities). This example shows that the communication perspective facilitates easy definition of communication activities. In the rest of the example, we assume that a company has already identified all the leaf activities that build its e-contracting process.

Next step is to define consistency rules on each of the three activities. We start with using the SEQUENCE operator:

1. We have:
   SEQUENCE (Information phase, Pre-contracting phase), defined in the function perspective.
   From this we infer:
   SEQUENCE (Information phase, A_o)
   Additionally we define:
   SEQUENCE (RqO, RpORq), and
   SEQUENCE (RpORq, PrORp).
2. To strengthen the SEQUENCE operations, we use the EXISTENCE operator:
   EXISTENCE (RpORq, PrORp)
   EXISTENCE (General preparations, RpORq), indicates that general provisions must be available in order to be attached to the offer when the response is elaborated.
3. Finally, the REQUIRED operator gives:
   REQUIRED (RpORq) and
   REQUIRED (PrORp)

Before specifying concrete processes, a start event that triggers the activity and if necessary an end event for it must be defined. In our example, an internal for the company event *offer needed* will trigger the RqO activity. The event *offer request,* generated by the RqO activity or by internal event at the supplier side, will trigger the RpORq activity. Finally, the event *offer received* at the consumer side will trigger the PrORp activity.

Next, activity diagrams can be constructed. First, we construct the *request offer* specification. Using the inheritance of tasks, described in the communication perspective, we see that the offer request contains three basic activities, i.e., elaborate offer request, send offer request, and wait state (see Figure 3).

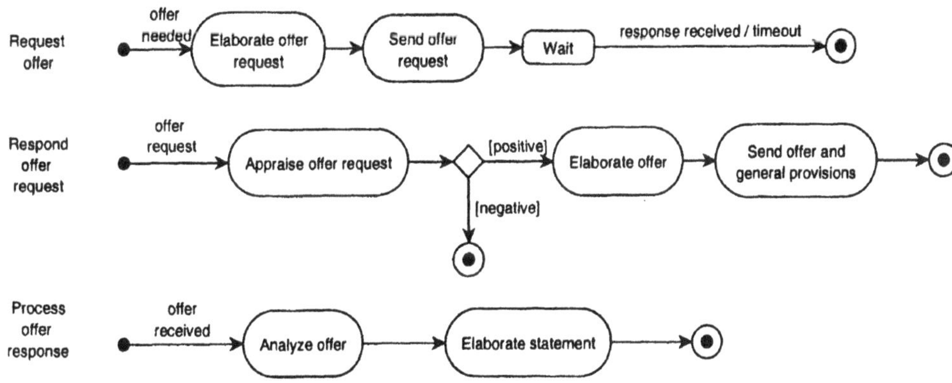

Figure 3 - Offer activity specification

Analogously, using the communication perspective, the *respond offer request* and *process offer response* activity diagrams are constructed. The responding company receives the request for offer and appraises the request. If the request for offer is approved (a positive decision is taken to answer to the request), the company elaborates an offer and sends it. The elaborate message and send message activities are inherited from the root communication activity in the communication perspective and are applied for the respond offer activity context. The offer is sent together with the general provisions prepared during the general preparations activity. The response is received by the requesting party and is analyzed. Based on the analyses, a statement on the received offer is elaborated.

The described specification of concrete activities is based solely on the function and communication perspectives. The example demonstrates that the two perspectives and the consistency rules are a powerful tool that allows consistent and complete e-contracting process specifications to be achieved.

7. CONCLUSION AND FUTURE WORK

In this paper, we have described an e-contracting process model. The model is based on two perspectives, i.e., function and communication. These perspectives, in combination with a set of consistency rules provide for tools to guard completeness and consistency of e-contracting processes. Based on the two perspectives and the set of consistency rules, we define an approach for specification of concrete e-contracting process. The model can be used for the analysis of existing e-contracting process specifications as well. To illustrate the advantages of the proposed modeling approach, the model is used to construct a fragment of a concrete e-contracting process specification.

An information system is required for the partial or full automation of the e-contracting process. However, detailed reference architecture for the support of e-contracting processes does not yet exist. This research work is part of the e-contracting system environment analysis. A data model is required in addition to the process model. More specifically, the e-contract content and its representation are to be researched. The process and data models together allow collecting requirements for an information system that supports an e-contracting process in its four phases. This preliminary work is a step towards the construction of detailed e-contracting reference architecture, which is our research goal.

8. REFERENCES

1. Alonso G, Fiedler U, Hagen C, Lazcano A, Schuldt H, Weiler N. WISE: business to business e-commerce. Procs. 9th International Workshop on Research Issues on Data Engineering: Information Technology for Virtual Enterprises. Australia. 1999.
2. Angelov S, Grefen P. A conceptual framework for B2B electronic contracting. Procs. 3rd IFIP Working Conference on Infrastructures for Virtual Enterprises. Portugal. 2002 (a).
3. Angelov S, Grefen P. An approach for flexible B2B e-contracting process modeling. Twente University: CTIT Technical Report. 2002(b). http://www.ctit.utwente.nl/publications/Tr01/.
4. Angelov S, Grefen P. A framework for the analysis of B2B electronic contracting support. Procs. 4th Edispuut Conference - Multidisciplinary Perspectives on Electronic Commerce. 2001(a).
5. Angelov S, Grefen P. B2B eContract handling - a survey of projects, papers and standards. Twente University: CTIT Technical Report 01-21. 2001(b).
6. CrossFlow project. 2000. http://www.crossflow.org/.
7. ebXML. Technical architecture specification v1.0.4. ebXML. 2001. http://www.ebxml.org.
8. Eriksson H.-E, Penker M. Business modeling with UML: business patterns at work. John Wiley & Sons. New York. 2000.
9. Gisler M, Stanoevska-Slabeva K, Greunz M. Legal aspects of electronic contracts. Infrastructures for Dynamic Business-to-Business Service Outsourcing (IDSO'00). Stockholm. 2000.
10. Grefen P, Angelov S. On τ-, μ-, π-, and ε-Contracting. To appear in Procs. Web Services, e-Business, and the Semantic Web. Canada. 2002.
11. Grefen P, Aberer K, Hoffner Y, Ludwig H. CrossFlow: Cross-organizational workflow management in dynamic virtual enterprises. International Journal of Computer Systems Science & Engineering, Vol. 15, No. 5, pp. 277-290; 2000.
12. Jackson M, Twaddle G. Business process implementation building workflow systems. Addison-Wesley. 1997.
13. RosettaNet. RosettaNet implementation framework: core specification (RNIF 02). RosettaNet. 2001. http://www.rosettanet.org.

11

A SERVICE INTERFACE DEFINITIONS CATALOGUE FOR VIRTUAL ENTERPRISES IN TOURISM

César Garita, Ersin C. Kaletas, Hamideh Afsarmanesh, L.O. Hertzberger
University of Amsterdam, Kruislaan 403, 1098 SJ Amsterdam, The Netherlands
{cesar,kaletas,hamideh,bob}@science.uva.nl

A Virtual Enterprise (VE) in the tourism sector can be defined as a temporary consortium of service provider organizations (e.g. traveling agencies, accommodation providers, etc.), that join their skills and resources in order to offer integrated value-added services. Value-added services are composed of basic services and/or other value-added services that are interconnected to create new higher-level tourism services. In order to support the required level of inter-operability among basic and value-added services offered by different enterprises, it is necessary to define standard semantic models regarding specific service interface definitions and data type structures. These standard service interface definitions can be made available through a common web-based catalogue. This paper focuses on the design and implementation of a Service Interface Definitions Catalogue component aimed at the support of interoperability of value-added services in tourism VEs.

1. INTRODUCTION

With the on-going rise of commercial globalization and market aggressiveness, tourism industries and service providers face the need to strongly collaborate and share their expertise and resources, as well as their costs and risks. In fact, basic collaborations among tourism enterprises based on web information technologies have taken place for several years, since many of them already offer different services through individual or common web sites that allow for instance: gathering of general information about tourism facilities, hotel search and room reservations in a certain geographical area, purchase of plane tickets, selection of organized excursion packages, etc. Typically, the information is presented to end users through static or dynamically generated html pages, which interface with the local or remote company systems using communication mechanisms such as CGI, email, fax, etc. In general, although these services are well established and have a wide acceptance among tourists, the level of integration and interoperability among these services is still quite fragmented and rigid (Afsarmanesh, 2000).

Thus, even though these Web-enabled tourism services are widespread and have substantially broadened the market opportunity horizon for the companies in the tourism sector, there is still a prominent need to support more advanced collaboration scenarios among these companies. The support for *value-added services* (*VASs*) is an example of these advanced collaboration scenarios, through which travel agencies would offer aggregated or *value-added-services* composed of components supplied by a number of different organizations. For instance, a value-added service such as "booking complete journeys", may include booking several means of traveling, arrangement of hotel reservations, leisure tour bookings, etc (see also (Garita, 2001)).

In order to provide *on-line value-added-services* in the tourism sector, both service provider and service requester enterprises must have access to an integrated *federation of services* that are made available for specific purposes (and under specific circumstances) by many different organizations (see Figure 1). This federation of services logically represents a group of distributed and heterogeneous tourism services and resources that are presented to end users through a single infrastructure. This infrastructure would provide an easy and common access to a massive collection of distributed resources and services that would be able to interoperate and be combined in order to build new higher-level value-added services. Clearly, advanced ICT models and mechanisms must be applied in order to standardize and integrate the disparate models and service implementations that are internally used by the tourism enterprises world-wide, and to allow the flexible configuration, execution and follow up of these value-added services involving different enterprises.

Therefore, the concept of Virtual Enterprise (VE) can be applied to the tourism domain in order to support the proper interaction and cooperation of alliances of existing enterprises towards the accomplishment of a common goal (see also (Camarinha-Matos, 2000), (Goranson, 1999)). In particular, a Virtual Enterprise in the tourism sector can be defined as a temporary consortium of different service provider organizations (e.g. traveling agencies, accommodation providers, organizers of leisure programs, public tourism organizations, etc.), that join their skills and resources in order to offer an integrated and aggregated service

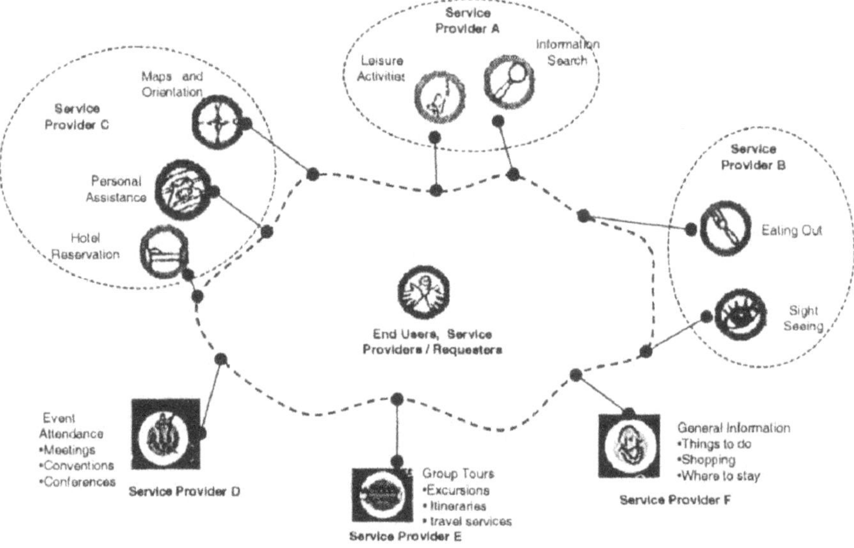

Figure 1 - Federation of heterogeneous and distributed tourism services.

(Afsarmanesh, 2000). In this way, enterprises can offer new tourism services that represent tailored solutions to customers, and they would also be able to participate more actively in certain business scenarios that are currently not well supported by existing information technology infrastructures in the tourism area.

Please notice that to become widely accepted, the design of the common federation layer must follow standardized *semantic models* regarding the service interface definitions and their associated *data type structures*. Namely, the meaning of the service interface definitions and their parameters must be documented and commonly agreed by tourism enterprises in the VE within the target geographical region of the system. Here, the use of already existing *ontologies* and *data types definitions* in the tourism areas is strongly needed. The standard service interface definitions can be made available through a common *Service Interface Definition Catalogue*, which could be accessed via web interfaces. The data type structures needed by the service interfaces, could also be made available through this catalogue.

In this context, this paper focuses on the internal system design and final implementation of a Service Interface Definitions Catalogue (SERV-CAT) for the support of VE in tourism. Part of the system described in this paper was implemented within the European 5FP project FETISH. In short, the FETISH project aims at the integration of the fragmented tourism information systems and their IT-based services into a federation of distributed resources that are presented through a single infrastructure to end users and other service provider enterprises.

The rest of this paper is organized as follows. Section 2 describes a reference structure of a support infrastructure for VEs in tourism. Section 3 presents the detailed design and implementation of the SERV-CAT system as one of the main components of this reference infrastructure. Finally, Section 4 summarizes the achieved results after the implementation of the SERV-CAT component.

2. A SUPPORT INFRASTRUCTURE FOR TOURISM VES

It is clear that the support for complex VE collaborations involves the application of advanced information models and technologies, including distributed business processes, workflow management, ontology definitions, standard data models, Internet facilities, middleware components, multi-agent approaches, and advanced distributed information management techniques among others (Garita, 2002). In this section, a proposed structure for a VE support platform in tourism incorporating some of these technologies is presented.

The diagram presented in Figure 2 depicts the main structural components of the proposed system. The system architecture presented here is internally based on Java/Jini technologies. In short, the Jini architecture has been specifically designed for deploying and using generic services in a distributed network (Edwards, 1999), (Freeman, 1999), (Arnold, 1999). In this way, services can be plugged/unplugged into network directories, and specific lookup mechanisms allow the retrieval of services to be used and executed by client applications or end users. In the Jini approach, a service proxy must be defined for each actual tourism service (which can be already implemented in heterogeneous hardware/software platforms). A

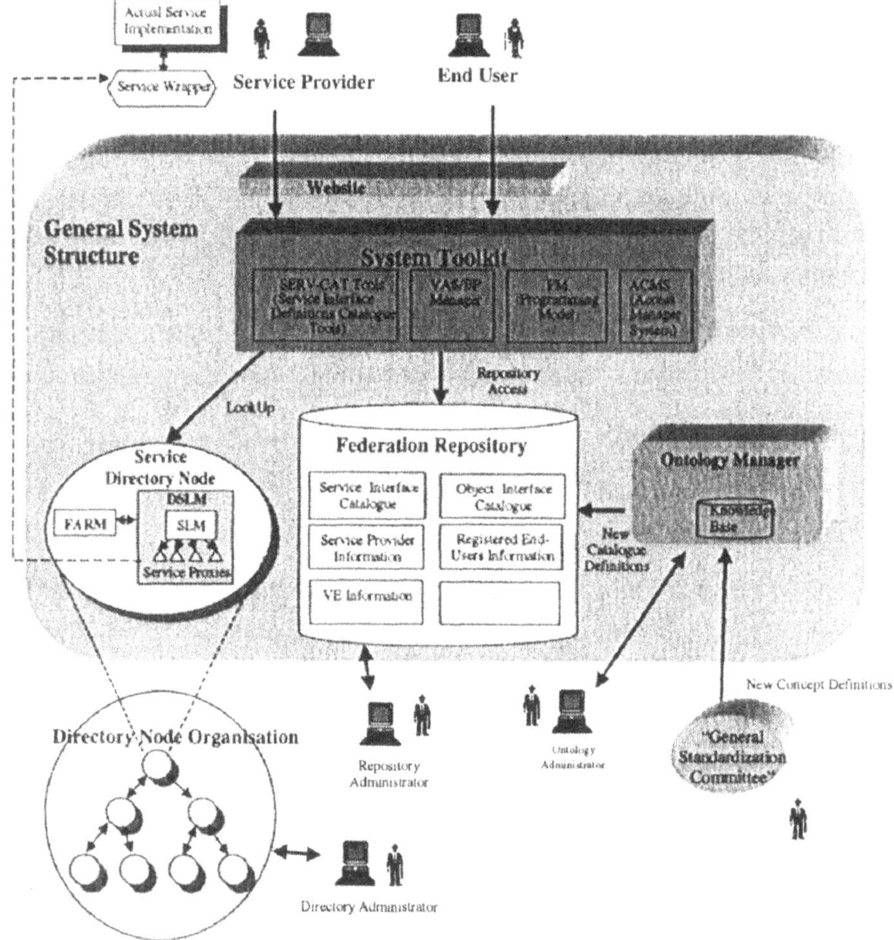

Figure 2 -General architecture components for a VE platform for tourism sector.

proxy represents a pointer or a remote reference to an actual service (or a wrapper to it), and acts as a front-end for other systems or applications that ultimately need to access the tourism service implementation. Thus, service requesters must be able to retrieve these proxies and integrate them into their own systems. In other words, the actual tourism services will be accessed and executed through proxies located in other enterprises.

Each major component of Figure 2 is briefly described in the paragraphs below.

First of all, please notice that the end users and service providers have access to several system toolkit components, which can be downloaded via a web site. Namely, the system toolkit includes all the tools and applications that are made available to service providers and end-users in order to facilitate their access to services and/or adaptation of the basic services (and value-added-services) that they provide in compliance with the global federation specifications. The tools and applications in the system toolkit include four main components:

- The *Service Interface Definitions Catalogue* (SERV-CAT) tools. The main objective of the SERV-CAT tools is to allow service requesters and providers to access the precise service and object definitions for the tourism services that are handled within the federation.

- The *VAS Process Management System* (VAS/BP Manager). This system allows the definition and execution of business processes (BPs) representing value-added services in the context of Virtual Enterprises. In the remaining of this paper we refer to this toolkit component as PROMAN (Camarinha-Matos, 2001).
- *Programming Model* (PM). This component represents a set of APIs and documents that can assist service providers that wish to extend their service implementations with wrappers and proxies to be plugged into the global service federation. For instance, this "model" can include templates to facilitate the generation of service wrappers and proxies complying with the JINI technology.
- *Access Manager System* (ACMS). This module serves as the entry gateway for the end users and service providers to the system, and supports interaction scenarios in which some kind of "human intervention" may be required.

Furthermore, the set of service proxies that are available within the federation are organized and managed within "Service Directory Nodes" of the system architecture. The main components of this node are described below:

- *Distributed Service Lookup Manager* - DSLM. The DSLM component represents an advanced look-up service manager facility that extends the basic JINI look-up mechanism in order to allow the distributed access and management of service proxies, that are physically distributed and located at different nodes. The management of local proxies at each node is carried out by the SLM (Service Lookup Manager) component using built-in JINI look-up services. In general, the directory nodes are logically inter-linked following an acyclic graph or a hierarchical tree-like organization, which represents the distributed service directory of the global service federation.
- *Federated Access Rights Manager* (FARM). This module allows the definition and validation of access rights to services defined at the level of service proxy in the general context of the global federation, as well as services defined within the Virtual Enterprises. For instance, service providers can specify that their given service proxies can be available for lookup only to certain specific sets of service requesters or only to specific VE members. Such access rights provision is extremely important for the support of VE infrastructures.

Besides the system toolkit, DSLM node and FARM components, there are two other important elements addressing different aspects of the data and meta-data that need to be managed in order to support the operation of the tourism VE infrastructure that are described below:

- *Ontology Manager*. This component basically represents the knowledge base repository in which the definition of all concepts belonging to the tourism specific domain are represented and stored. New service / object catalogue definitions that are generated here, are pushed into the federation repository
- *Federation Repository*. The Federation Repository represents a database containing all the information that is required to support the operation of the global service federation, and that needs to be accessed by different modules and end users. The main components of the repository contain the data related to: service interface catalogue, object interface catalogue, service providers' information, registered end-users information, and VE-related information.

Finally, the General Standardization Committee represents a group of people who must decide if a new tourism service-interface definition is accepted to become a part of the interface definition specifications for generic federation services.

Based on the system structure defined in Figure 2, it is possible to illustrate different use-case scenarios, such as the procedures for definition of a new federation service, registration of a basic service in the federation, distributed service look-up, and user access to an existing service. Furthermore, the system structure can also support more complicated cases, such as the definition, registration, and access to value-added services within the global federation. Some of these scenarios and functionalitites have been addressed in previous publications (Afsarmanesh, 2000),(Camarinha-Matos, 2001). In the next section, the internal design and implementation of the SERV-CAT component of the presented reference infrastructure is described in details.

3. SERV-CAT DESIGN AND DEVELOPMENT

As mentioned previously, SERV-CAT applications allow end users to access the Service Interface Definitions Catalogue. The SERV-CAT architecture embodies a catalogue database (part of the Federation Repository) containing the service interface definitions, software components to access the catalogue, application servers to manage different information management requests, and several graphical and programming interfaces for end users and applications.

The end-users of the service federation should be able to browse service interface definitions information via for instance, a web interface. This information also needs to be accessed by other internal components of the tourism infrastructure to perform some validation actions that may be necessary for instance, when defining a business process for a value-added service.

In the following subsections, the SERV-CAT architecture and its components are described in details.

3.1 General SERV-CAT Architecture

In general, multi-threaded web-based applications can be defined and modeled by a three-tier architecture, also called client-agent-server architecture. In this architecture the clients are only concerned with presentation services, such as the user interface design specificities. As such, the agent, referred to as application server in this paper, processes the application logic for the client, hiding the underlying implementation and access details of the server tier, and adding higher-level support functionalities for the client. The SERV-CAT architecture has been designed following such a multi-tier approach (see Figure 3). By making a clear separation between the client and application server tiers, the client components are designed as relatively light processes, which are mostly concerned with user-interface details, and representation and formatting of the data. The functionality itself is supported in the middle tier (Application Server), which in turn gets relieved of all the specific details of the end-user and module interfaces.

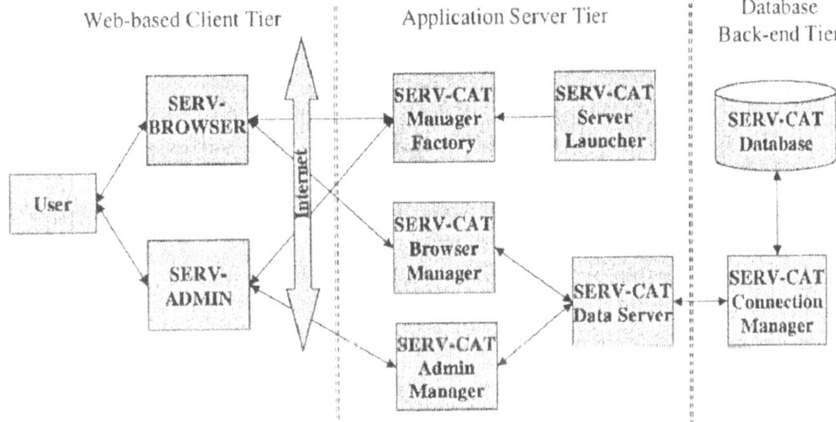

Figure 3 - General SERV-CAT 3-tier architecture.

Following this approach, the tiers in the SERV-CAT architecture and the components in each tier are described in the next sub-sections.

3.2 SERV-CAT Client Tier

The client tier of SERV-CAT architecture contains the components that directly interact either with the end users or with other system components e.g. PROMAN system. From a general point of view, the SERV-CAT Client Tier is composed of two types of interfaces: graphical interfaces for end-users, and programming interfaces for other system components.

The graphical interfaces support functionalities required by ordinary end users and administrator users. Currently, there is one main client interface for ordinary end users: the Service Interface Definitions Catalogue Browser (SERV-BROWSER). SERV-BROWSER allows a regular user, which can be a service provider, a travel agency, etc., to access the contents of the Service Interface Definitions Catalogue. The functionalities provided by the SERV-BROWSER to end users include:

- Downloading a jar file (Java archive file containing compiled Java code), which contains the compiled Java codes of the data types in SERV-CAT.
- Viewing the service packages in the catalogue and displaying their corresponding descriptions. Service interface definitions in SERV-CAT are logically grouped into packages, which correspond to packages in Java.
- Viewing the types in each package. Service interfaces in SERV-CAT are represented as types in Java programming language, which can be either a Java class or a Java interface. Detailed descriptions of each type can be obtained via SERV-BROWSER, including: name of the type, super classes, package name, access modifiers of this type, textual description, and a mark indicating whether this type is representing a value-added service.
- Viewing the members of each type. The activities or events associated to a service are represented as the members of a type in the Java programming language. A member can be either a field or a method. The detailed description of each member can also be obtained, including for instance: name of the

member, type of a field or return type of a method, access and other modifiers of this member, and the parameter list if the member is a method. Details of the type definitions (i.e. type of a field, return type of a method, or parameter types of a method) can be displayed in a separate window. Using this window, users can both browse and download the Java source code if the type is a complex type, or the XML description if the type is a primitive type.

Please notice that ordinary users can only view the catalogue contents; they are not allowed to modify the contents of the catalogue.

A snapshot of the browsing interface is shown in Figure 4. As can be seen in this figure, the interface that allows the user to browse the service catalogue information is divided in three main areas. In the first area (left), the user can browse the service packages that are available. In the second area (middle), the user can see the service types e.g. Java classes and interfaces, that are defined within a given package. Finally, for a given type, the user can see which methods and field members are defined (right area). When the user double-clicks on a selected item, the detailed information associated with that specific item is displayed. For instance, in the case of the methods, the user can see the parameters, modifiers, return type, etc. that are defined according to a given method (see Figure 4).

The SERV-BROWSER is a Web-enabled application. It can run both as a stand-alone Java application and as a Java applet within a Web browser. It communicates with the middle tier of SERV-CAT via RMI.

Besides the regular end-user SERV-BROWSER tool, the client tier of the SERV-CAT application also includes a specific component for system administrators, namely the SERV-ADMIN. This administrator graphical interface supports the extended functionality required by administrator users. In addition to providing all of the SERV-BROWSER functionalities, SERV-ADMIN allows the administrators to modify the contents of the SERV-CAT; e.g. to insert new service interface definitions to SERV-CAT, or edit an already existing service interface definition.

Finally, the SERV-CAT client tier also includes lower-level application programmers interfaces (APIs). These interfaces represent high-level information management functions specifically developed to support other system components, such as PROMAN. Currently, PROMAN and SERV-CAT are integrated through the SERV-CAT programming interfaces. PROMAN uses the SERV-CAT functions to access the Service Interface Definitions Catalogue in order to obtain the available service interface definitions during the definition of a value added service.

3.3 SERV-CAT Application Server Tier

The middle tier of SERV-CAT contains specific application servers, which encapsulate the application logic for the SERV-CAT Client Tier components. Currently, there are four server tier components: SERV-CAT Manager Factory, SERV-CAT Browser Manager, SERV-CAT Admin Manager, and SERV-CAT Data Server, as described below (see also Figure 3):

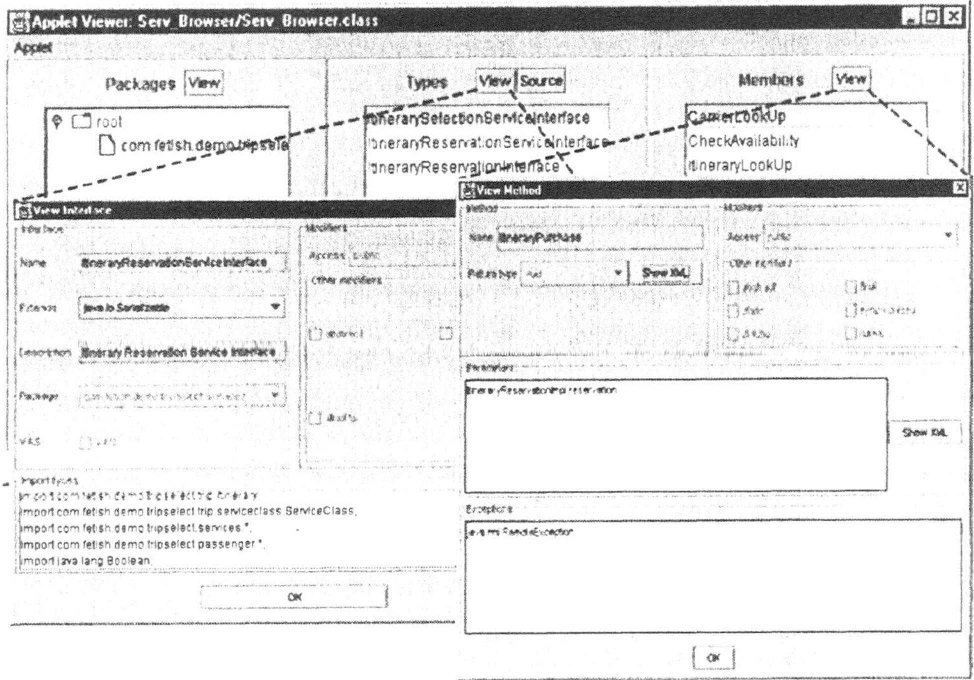

Figure 4 - End user interface for Service Interface Browser.

- SERV-CAT Manager Factory. The application server tier is internally designed following the factory pattern (Gamma, 1995),(Sun-Microsystems, 2001). In this context, the SERV-CAT Manager Factory is a server, to which client applications (SERV-BROWSER and SERV-ADMIN) connect via RMI, and request a manager instance to access the SERV-CAT. The Manager Factory creates a new manager instance for each request coming from the client application; i.e. a Browser Manager for a request from a SERV-BROWSER instance or an Admin Manager for a request from a SERV-ADMIN instance. The remote reference to the newly created manager instance is passed to the client application, and from this point on the manager handles the communication between the client application and the catalogue.
- SERV-CAT Browser Manager. The SERV-CAT Browser Manager provides the functionality to support the client applications being executed by ordinary users (such as SERV-BROWSER). The Browser Manager application server allows read-only access to the catalogue. The information retrieval functions are encapsulated in methods, each retrieving a specific piece of information from the catalogue. Below, some of the methods available to client applications are given as examples:
  - getInterface: to retrieve a specific interface or all interfaces.
  - getTypeMembers: to retrieve the members (methods and fields) in a given type.
  - getParameter: to retrieve a set of parameters in a given method.
  - getInterfaceSourceCode: to retrieve the Java source code for a given interface.
- SERV-CAT Admin Manager. The SERV-CAT Admin Manager provides the functionality to support the administrative components of the client tier (e.g.

SERV-ADMIN). Please notice that besides all SERV-CAT Browser Manager functionality, the SERV-CAT administrator provides the functionality to modify the contents of the SERV-CAT database. The SERV-CAT Admin Manager is password protected.

- SERV-CAT Data Server. The SERV-CAT Data Server handles all database-related operations for the Service Interface Definitions Catalogue. The data server is the only component directly accessing the catalogue database. Requests to the remote SERV-CAT Browser/Admin Manager are forwarded to the underlying data server. The database operations are performed using a connection object obtained from the connection pool in the back-end tier. The Data Server provides the functionality to support all of the client tools, such as SERV-BROWSER and SERV-ADMIN.

Besides the application servers described above, the application server tier of SERV-CAT contains an extra component (server launcher) and a Java package, which are used to support the proper operation of the application servers and to provide some miscellaneous functionalities. In particular, the SERV-CAT Server Launcher is a Java program that starts up the SERV-CAT application by initializing and launching a new SERV-CAT Manager Factory. Furthermore, based on the data structures defined for the Service Interface Definitions Catalogue (the catalogue database model), a Java package was created, which contains a set of Java classes that exactly correspond with the data structures defined in the catalogue database model. Other system components that need to interact with SERV-CAT use this package in order to exchange Service Interface Definitions Catalogue information in the common format of Java objects.

3.4 SERV-CAT Database Back-end Tier

The database back-end tier of the SERV-CAT architecture corresponds to the SERV-CAT DB containing the data repositories and the SERV-CAT Connection Manager handling the connections to the database. The Oracle DBMS is currently used for the SERV-CAT DB. Since the DB is accessed exclusively through JDBC, any other JDBC-compliant database engine can be easily used instead of Oracle, if necessary.

The SERV-CAT DB contains the definitions of the service interfaces available in the system. In the catalogue database, the service interfaces are basically modeled following the syntax of the Java programming language. Thus, the catalogue database model describes packages of service interfaces, fields and methods of each interface, types of fields, parameters and return types of methods, and exceptions thrown by the methods.

The relational database model of the SERV-CAT DB is given in Figure 5. A detailed description of this diagram is outside the aim of this paper; instead, a short characterization of each entity is described below. In brief, the entity TFET_TYPES represents a root class for the main data types that are handled in the current system. The entity TFET_FET_TYPES is a generalization of the concepts of both Java classes (TFET_CLASSES) and interfaces (TFET_INTERFACES). Please notice that both classes and interfaces can be defined recursively in terms of other types, and that they are encapsulated in packages (TFET_PACKAGES). Furthermore,

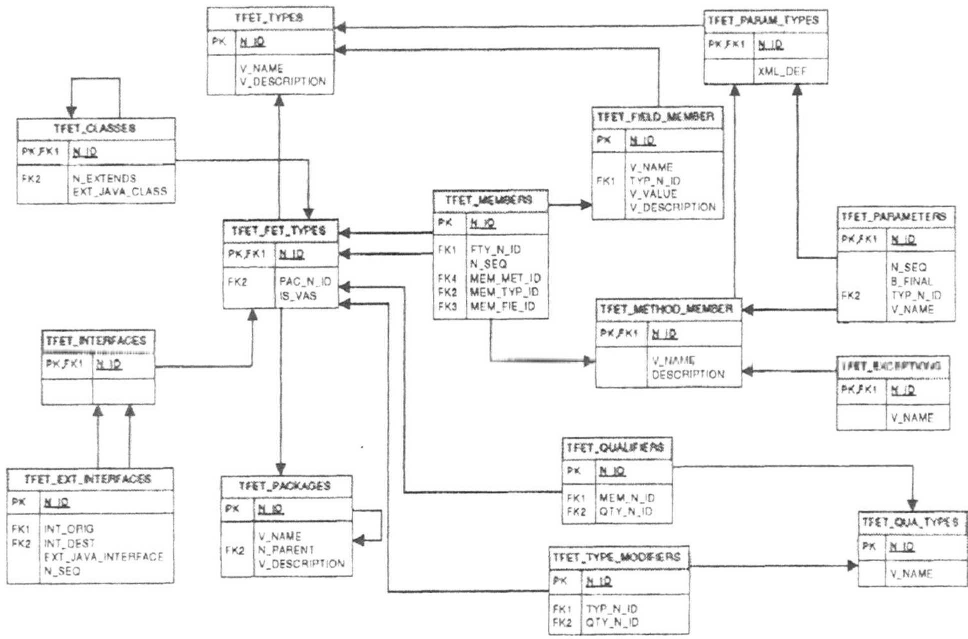

Figure 5 -Entity Relationship Diagram for Service Interface Catalogue Definitions.

both classes and interfaces are associated with class members (TFET_MEMBERS), which in turn can be either methods (TFET_METHOD_MEMBER) or fields (TFET_FIELD_MEMBER). In general, type members can be associated (through TFET_QUALIFIERS) with zero or more specific qualifier types (TFET_QUA_TYPES). The qualifiers types represent for instance private, public and protected declarations of type members. The method members are also associated with certain parameters (TFET_PARAMETERS) of a given type.

Besides the catalogue database, a second component is involved in the back-end tier: the SERV-CAT Connection Manager. The Connection Manager handles the connections to the database by using a connection pooling mechanism.

Finally, the SERV-CAT system functionality has also been extensively documented using UML Use Case Diagrams and Use Case Models (Fowler, 1999),(Larman, 1998).

4. CONCLUSIONS AND FUTURE WORK

The Virtual Enterprise paradigm can be applied to the tourism sector in order to support the provision of integrated value-added services as a composition of services provided in turn by different independent organizations. In this context, a reference model for web-based tourism infrastructure to support VE collaborations was proposed and described. One of the main components of the proposed VE infrastructure is the Service Interface Definitions Catalogue (SERV-CAT), through which standard service interfaces and data type can be formally specified.

Therefore, this paper focused on the description of the internal system design and implementation of the SERV-CAT three-tier architecture, which properly supports the requirements identified for different kinds of end-users and client applications. The SERV-CAT tools provide the necessary facilities for browsing, downloading, and maintaining the common interface specifications. All these functionalities aim at the support of value-added service definition and interoperability within a VE framework.

Finally, future extensions that can be considered for the SERV-CAT architecture described in this paper include: a link with ontology system, manipulation of VE configuration topology and VE members information, application of WSDL, and incorporation of searching capabilities for the SERV-CAT applications.

5. REFERENCES

1. Afsarmanesh, H., and Camarinha-Matos, L. M. "Future Smart-Organisations: a Virtual Tourism Enterprise." *1st International Conference on Web Information System Engineering - WISE'2000*, Hong Kong, China, 2000.
2. Arnold, K., O'Sullivan, B., Scheifler, R., Waldo, J., and Wollrath, A. *The Jini Specification*, Addison-Wesley, 1999.
3. Camarinha-Matos, L., Afsarmanesh, H., Kaletas, E. C., and Cardoso, T. "Service Federation in Virtual Organizations." *11th International PROLAMAT Conference on Digital Enterprise - New Challenges*, Budapest, Hungary, 2001, 305-324.
4. Camarinha-Matos, L. M., Afsarmanesh, H., and Rabelo, R. "E-Business and Virtual Enterprises - Managing Business-to-Business Cooperation.",, Kluwer Academic Publishers, Boston, 2000, 552.
5. Edwards, W. K. *Core Jini*, Prentice Hall, 1999.
6. Fowler, M., and Scott, K. *UML Distilled: Applying the Standard Object Modeling Language*, Addison Wesley, 1999.
7. Freeman, E., Hupfer, S., and Arnold, K. *JavaSpaces Principles, Patterns and Practice*, Addison Wesley, 1999.
8. Gamma, E., Helm, R., Johnson, R., and Vlissides, J. *Design Patterns: Elements of Reusable Object-oriented Software*, Addison-Wesley, 1995.
9. Garita, C. "Federated Information Management for Virtual Enterprises," Doctoral Thesis, University of Amsterdam, Amsterdam, The Netherlands, 2001.
10. Garita, C., Afsarmanesh, H., and Hertzberger, L. O. "A Survey of Distributed Information Management Approaches for Virtual Enterprise Infrastructures." Managing Virtual Web Organizations in the 21st Century: Issues and Challenges, U. J. Franke, ed., Idea Group Publishing, 2002, 164-183.
11. Goranson, H. T. *The Agile Virtual Enterprise: Cases, Metrics, Tools*, Greenwood Publishing Group, Inc., 1999.
12. Larman, C. *Applying UML and Patterns*, Prentice Hall, 1998.
13. Sun-Microsystems. "Factory Pattern", http://java.sun.com/j2se/1.3/docs/guide/rmi/Factory.html, 2001.

PART 2

NETWORKED ENTERPRISING

12

DYNAMIC VIRTUAL ORGANIZATIONS, OR NOT SO DYNAMIC?

L. M. Camarinha-Matos[1], H. Afsarmanesh[2]
[1]*New University of Lisbon, Faculty of Sciences and Technology*
Quinta da Torre, 2829-516 Monte Caparica, PORTUGAL, cam@uninova.pt
[2] *University of Amsterdam, Faculty of Science*
Kruislaan 403, 1098 SJ Amsterdam, THE NETHERLANDS, hamideh@science.uva.nl

Expectations created by the early rapid developments in virtual organizations, hoping to resolve the main challenges in the area and continuous emergence of new related facilities are still far from full materialization. Being a multi-disciplinary area that requires the participation of experts in ICT, theory of organizations, sociology, economy, law, etc., there is primarily a need for further developments in terms of modeling and better understanding of concepts, as well as supporting infrastructures and tools. Harmonization of the current approaches and establishment of common reference models and practices is also a pre-requisite. In this context a brief characterization of the state of the art is made and several open research issues are introduced.

1. INTRODUCTION

1.1 Collaborative Organizations

Collaborative and networked organizations have gained momentum during the last years changing the way that commercial, industrial, cultural and social activities are organized. In addition to the rapid evolution of traditional supply chains and outsourcing environments, a growing trend nowadays consists of tasks performed by autonomous teams set up as independent contractors and linked by a network. These teams usually come together, some times in temporary combinations, to tackle various projects, and may dissolve once the work is done. Consider the wide variety of recent radical outsourcing in design for manufacturing, printing industry, software development, or the film industry: in almost every case, in one way or another "Smart Organizations", "Virtual Organizations" or "Networked Organizations" represent a collaborative configuration.

The proliferation and variety of terms applied to forthcoming business structures, such as blurring borders in organizations, alliances, partnerships, aggregations, value constellations, business webs, and business ecosystems, show only the surface of a fast changing paradigm. During the last decade, and in parallel with the development and spreading of Internet technologies, traditional collaboration networks have found new leveraging tools and new collaborative business forms have emerged. New technologies, business processes, and organizational life forms supported by networking tools "invade" all traditional businesses and organizations what requires thinking in terms of whole systems, i.e. seeing each business as part of a wider economic ecosystem and environment. The new collaborative paradigm needs to be better understood and properly supported, not only in terms of the needed technologies, but also through the development of adequate skills, tools & mechanisms, culture and regulations. Complementarily, there is the emergence of new value systems for provided products and services that need to be understood, embedded in the new business practices and supported by new tools.

In the current market scenario, recent trends in industry are also emphasizing the relevance of *agility*, understood as the ability to recognize and rapidly react and cope with the unpredictable changes in the environment [8], with a smooth adaptation of its entire structure to the new / current reality. The idea of highly dynamic organizations, that form themselves and acquire shape according to the needs and opportunities of the market and remain operational as long as these opportunities persist, suggests a number of benefits, among which the following can be emphasized:

- *Agility*: being the capability to recognize, rapidly react and cope with the unpredictable changes in the environment in order to achieve better responses to opportunities, shorter time-to-market, and higher quality with less investment.
- *Complementary roles*: enterprises seek for complementarities (creation of synergies) that allow them to participate in competitive business opportunities and new markets.
- *Achieving dimension*: especially in the case of SMEs, being in partnerships with others allow them to achieve critical mass and appear in the market with a larger "visible" size.
- *Competitiveness*: achieving the cost effectiveness, by proper division of subtasks among cooperating organizations.
- *Resource optimization*: smaller organizations sharing infrastructures, knowledge, and business risks.
- *Innovation*: being in a network opens the opportunities for the exchange and confrontation of ideas, the basis for innovation.

Considerable investments have been made, namely in Europe and the USA, in a large number of research projects applying new organizational forms, which have produced an abundant variety of specific solutions and broad awareness for the necessary organizational changes. Particularly in the case of Europe, given both its cultural background in business and the current emerging development investments, Europe is placed in a key leading position for the development of the organizational forms fit for the digital age. However, the research in many of these cases is highly fragmented being each project focused on solving specific problems and applying IT to partially design and develop a minimal B2B interaction mechanism to support its basic needs. As such, there is no effective consolidation/harmonization among them in order to have an effective impact. How to integrate all these fragmented research contributions and how to empower enterprises in both their regional and global competitiveness are open questions.

On the other hand proliferation of fast changing short-life non-interoperable technologies is a major obstacle for SMEs entering collaborative partnerships. The crash of many unrealistic "dot-com" ventures also slowed down some investments by the industry, but the well-founded research towards the development of adequate support infrastructures based on realistic business models has seen a continuous progress. In fact, while the basic networking infrastructures and the virtual organization (VO) / virtual enterprise (VE) paradigm are spreading, new forms of collaborative virtual communities / virtual communities of practice (VCP), i.e. stronger human-oriented organizations, are emerging. However, the wide variety of terms and concepts, most overlapping and without precise definitions, show the fundamental need to establish a clear baseline. In order to be efficient and competitive in their operation, the VOs and other collaborative organizations of the future have to rely on solid bases and strong methodological approaches.

1.2 Technology Trends

The availability of a large number of contributing elements (technologies, paradigms, best practices and models) constitutes a set of enabling factors for the opportunity of materializing concepts that although not new, were waiting for the enabling factors. Examples are:

- On VE / VO: Significant developments in support infrastructures, various experiments in regional clustering / networking, and various pilot cases of IT supported clusters.
- On spreading, widening, and acceptance of the concept of "sharing": Computational resource sharing through GRID, collaborative engineering, Virtual Laboratories (VL), P2P-ERP/PDM Systems for dynamic SMEs, contracts and negotiation models (acquaintance models, auctions, etc.).
- On new organizational design, including structure and processes, and interactions with the environment.
- On the information and communication technology research advances: Web technology, standards and tools, communication security, federated information management, coordination theory and systems, component-based system design and developments, MAS technology and software mobility, GRID technology, mobile computing.
- Advances in knowledge representation, with particular focus on shared ontologies and imprecise knowledge representation / soft-computing.
- Basic technologies and tools for "traditional" Virtual Communities, still limited and not considering communities of practice under social contracts.

However, most of these technologies and concepts are in their infancy and under development, mostly fragmented and non-interoperable, requiring considerable effort to implement and configure comprehensive VO support infrastructures and operational methods. Even the most advanced infrastructures coming out of leading R&D projects require complex configuration and customization processes hardly manageable by SMEs. There is a lack of common reference models, interoperable infrastructures, and general business support functionalities that constitute major obstacles to resources and information sharing.

1.3 The Way Ahead

There is a growing awareness that the VO developments should be based on contributions of multidisciplinary nature, namely from the Information and Communication Technologies, socio-economic, cognitive aspects, operations research, organizational, business management, legal, social security, and ethical areas. Some trends in this direction are:

- New behavioral forms, which include new ways of work and even new moral and ethical attitudes;
- New cooperation agreements and social contracts;
- New liability agreements and risk negotiation practices;

- New ways of generating value for common developments;
- Correspondingly, new challenges on IPR and ownership identification; and
- Definition of legal frameworks affecting /addressing VOs.

Furthermore there is a need for mechanisms to empower human relationships as a way to induce creativity, to strengthen cohesion and sustainability and to reach responsiveness to market turbulence. However the developments in this area are still **mostly technology-driven** and achieved independently of each other and at different projects, thus repeatedly providing only very primitive *interaction infrastructure* among the organizations involved in the VO.

Understanding the emerging behavior and trends (how and why) is a challenge, requiring further developments in modeling, support mechanisms and tools, coordination principles and leadership, and establishment of collaboration support (virtual) institutions (e.g. e-notary, e-dispute-solving).

Similarly there is a need for planning and establishing new **integrated** metrics. Dynamic evaluation of the fractional value of processes (e.g. value features, rewarding principles, creation of enterprise-wide appreciation of new value features, trust arbitrators, auditability), need to be part of a comprehensive research and development initiative.

This paper summarizes some ideas under discussion in the framework of two international initiatives: IST THINKcreative and IFIP COVE. THINKcreative is an EC funded network of experts that aims at identifying and characterizing emerging organizational collaborative forms and their required infrastructures, modeling and application tools, and socio-organizational needs for the next 5, 10 and 20 years. COVE started as a project aiming to contribute to the harmonization and knowledge dissemination of world-wide research results on virtual organizations, and to foster needed collaborative developments. More recently COVE evolved to a permanent Working Group of the IFIP Technical Committee 5, the WG5.5.

Following sections discuss major aspects in VO: infrastructures, cluster management and VO creation, VO operation, evolution and dissolution, virtual laboratories and virtual communities. For each of these topics, a brief overview of the state of the art and major trends is presented, followed by a list of suggested key topics for further research.

2. INFRASTRUCTURES FOR VIRTUAL ORGANIZATIONS

Although the potential advantages of the Virtual Organizations are well known at the conceptual level [3], [7], their practical implantation is still far from the expectations. In order to leverage the potential benefits of the agile VE/VO paradigm, there is a need for flexible and generic **infrastructures** to support the full life cycle of the VO/VE, i.e. creation, operation, evolution and dissolution. Achieving such infrastructures is still a major challenge. The lack of a common and widely accepted **reference model** and infrastructure is still forcing every vertical development project to design and implement its own mini-infrastructures, deviating some resources from its main focus, while generating something only applicable to that project.

In fact, even the most advanced infrastructures coming out of leading R&D projects still require complex configuration and customization processes, which are hardly manageable by SMEs. Infrastructures combining heterogeneous components from different vendors are also potentially unstable being difficult to determine which component (or tool provider) is responsible when something goes wrong with such complex systems. In spite of the fast growing technological developments, lack of proper interoperability mechanisms among enterprise applications is a major obstacle to agile VO/VEs. As complex organizations, formed by heterogeneous and autonomous entities, VOs need to deal with a combination of **different technologies** and a **variety of application sources.**

Although it is not a new subject but rather the central question in systems integration, **interoperability** remains as a critical topic in the agenda of VO/VE supporting infrastructures. In fact, effective cooperation in a VO/VE requires interoperation among the enterprise applications at two levels: (i) Intra-enterprise interoperability – comprising systems integration at the level of enterprise applications; and (ii) Inter-enterprise interoperability – comprising systems integration at the level of virtual organization (requiring that similar reference models are adopted). Furthermore, when discussing the interoperability approaches we need to carefully address the "**life cycle**" aspects as different enterprise technologies have quite different life cycles (e.g. ICT, manufacturing technology, products, services) and the components to be integrated may be at different stages of their life cycles.

Some of the main trends in the attempt to develop generic VO infrastructures include:

- Layer-based frameworks, which add a *cooperation layer* to the existing ICT platforms of the enterprises. Inter-enterprise cooperation is then performed via the interaction through these layers. Examples of this approach are early efforts in VE infrastructures, as represented by the NIIIP [11], PRODNET [3], [7], or VEGA [18] projects, that aimed at designing open platforms to support the basic information exchange and coordination needs in industrial virtual enterprises.

- Agent-based frameworks, including those approaches that represent enterprises as *agents* and the inter-enterprise cooperation as interactions in a distributed multi-agent system. Although less-developed than the layer-based approaches, various examples focusing the creation and operation of VOs can be found:
  - Agents in VE creation - A growing number of works are being published on the application of multi-agent systems and market-oriented negotiation mechanisms for the VE formation [5], [10], [14].
  - Agents in VE operation – Various projects have been addressing the dynamic scheduling and execution of distributed business processes [2], [12].

- Service-federation / service-market frameworks - According to this model, enterprises should be able to plug/unplug their services to/from service directories [4]. By means of proper "standard" service interface, the interoperability with other (requesting) enterprises, regardless of the heterogeneity associated with the actual implementation of the services themselves, is supported. This means that no matter how the service is actually implemented, in terms of the computer platform, operating system, programming language, internal modules, etc., there is a ***client service interface*** that can be managed by a lookup service and made available to other enterprises that may request it. The underlying concepts of the JINI architecture [15] show how to support, in a transparent way, a **federation of service functions** offered by different service suppliers and running on different nodes of a network. Although

JINI may contribute, in theory, to facilitate the interoperability among services offered by different enterprises, its use in VO environments requires its extension to properly work in wide area networks and the development of additional support functionalities. For instance, the matter of access rights and enterprises information visibility is a very important issue, and therefore when searching and accessing a specific service type it is also relevant to determine both the supplier of the service and the requesting client, in order to check such visibility rights. It is also necessary to define the rules for both service specification/definition and service registration through the service interface. Furthermore, the general acceptance of the service interface by the service providers for developing services compliant with such rules is of great importance. Latest developments such as WSDL / SOAP represent a positive step in this direction.

Suggested research topics. Setting up an infrastructure for VO/VE still requires a large engineering effort, which represents a major obstacle for the implantation of this new organizational paradigm. Furthermore, it shall be noted that the fast evolution of the information technologies often presents a disturbing factor for non-IT companies. Therefore, further research effort is necessary towards the establishment of generic and interoperable infrastructures. Some open research issues include:

- Advanced federated information management, supporting the authorized information exchange, information integration mechanism, and collaborative work among organizations.
- Consideration of new assumptions in interoperability: (i) Interoperability is a continuous process as new technologies are emerging every day! (ii) Interoperability should become a "design principle" in software systems. (iii) Diversity / heterogeneity / autonomy of components must be accepted (not avoided). (iv) Co-existence of components with different life cycles and in different stages of their life cycles must be assumed.
- Progress towards an invisible, pervasive, and safe support infrastructure.
- Inter-domain transactions and recovery mechanisms.
- Effective integration of legacy systems.
- Tracking and auditing support services. Also self-identification (of products), allowing traceability and closing the gap between the physical world and the logical world.

3. CLUSTER MANAGEMENT AND VO CREATION

Although not well understood earlier, it is now clear that the formation of **dynamic VO/VE** requires an appropriate "breeding" or "nesting" environment (e.g. regional **industry cluster**) in order to guarantee basic requirements such as:

- Trust building ("trusting your partner" is a long-term process),
- Common infrastructures and agreed upon business practices (requiring substantial engineering / re-engineering effort),
- A sense of community and some sense of stability.

Industry clusters do not correspond to a new concept as a large number of related initiatives have emerged during the last decades, namely in Europe and the USA. But the advances in information and communication technologies now bring new opportunities to leverage the potential of this concept, namely by providing the adequate environment for the rapid formation of agile virtual organizations.

It is important to notice that there is a potential conflict between fast innovation and the stability requirements that are both part of the human nature. It is necessary to find harmonic solutions to conciliate the dynamism of the new business ecosystems and the needs for stability of individuals (and their families).

If long-term collaborative environments or business ecosystems are in place, it is viable to establish **dynamic VO/VE** as a rapid and optimized response to business opportunities and threats.

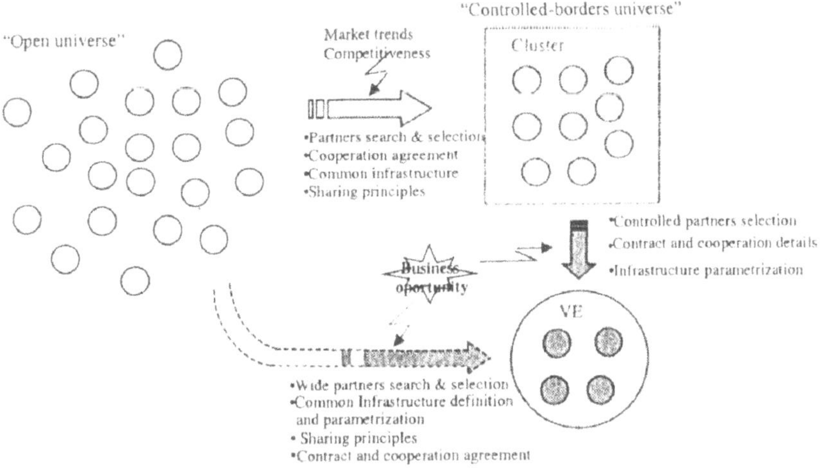

Figure 1 - Two approaches for VE formation

The Brazilian VIRTEC the ALFA COSME-VE, COWORK, and MASSYVE [13] are examples of early initiatives that have addressed specific aspects of creation and management of clusters of enterprises. Some of the aspects that have been subject of more attention are: Brokerage, partners search and selection (e-procurement), definition of cooperation rules (negotiation and contracting), etc.

One of the problems in partners search for VO creation is the availability of directories of companies / organizations where their profile (skills, resources, performance history, etc.) are represented in a standard format. The unavailability of a standard to represent these profiles has been a major obstacle. Recent developments (UDDI, WSDL, SOAP) represent promising steps in this direction. Nevertheless if the catalog is confined to a cluster it is easier to reach a common representation of profiles.

Some ***open research topics*** include:

- Management and configuration of local/regional clusters operating on specific vertical markets with specific business processes requirements.
- The full VO/VE creation framework.
- E-notary and certification services for networked organizations with special services such as: black lists, past performance, credentials, and best practices.
- Modeling and management of cooperation contracts and agreements.
- Methodologies for transforming existing organizations into VO-ready organizations.

4. VO OPERATION

Coordination of distributed business processes (DBP) and activities is an important element in the VO operation. Most of the early approaches took a workflow-based approach, starting with the WfMC reference architecture [17] and experimenting with extensions for supervision of distributed processes (cross-organizational workflow) including some preliminary but very limited works on exception handling, multi-level coordination and its relationship to coordination roles of the VO members, and flexible workflow models to support less structured processes.

In terms of DBP planning and modeling some graphical languages have been suggested but a standard is still necessary in order to allow effective distribution / sharing of business processes. Proposals like PIF and PSL have been discussed but there is still more work to do. A recent European initiative, the UEML network, might contribute to some harmonization in the modeling area.

In terms of business support functions, most of the projects have addressed application specific cases. ERP vendors have been extending their monolithic single-enterprise-centric systems in order to comply with more dynamic supply chains and networks, but this is an area requiring more investment on generic functionalities.

Some ***open research topics***:

- Coordination, administration and management of highly distributed activities, tasks, processes, and roles. Planning and supervision of distributed processes (including complex services).
- Risk management / assessment tools.
- Design, development, provision and management of value-added services provided in the context of VE/VOs.
- Dynamic evaluation of revenues, rights and liabilities of every VE relationships, and dynamic selection of new partners in order to make the VE network more effective.
- Clarify / re-define notions of value in a society of relationships, focusing on the added-value contribution (how to measure it?) of each node and how to reward it in order to preserve the business ecosystem (dynamic sustainability concept). What is valuable, where does the value reside, who generates value? Cooperation adds an overhead that has to be compensated by the added-value and agility.
- Soft-modeling and reasoning with special decision support mechanisms for supply chain management, selection of partners or efficiency of VE relationships.
- E-contract management and adaptation to the legal frameworks.
- Advanced simulation models and tools for networked collaborative organizations.
- New business support functions and better integration with enterprise applications.
- New user interfaces, seeking an entertainment facet as a way to overcome cultural barriers.

5. VO EVOLUTION AND DISSOLUTION

During the life cycle of a VO it is natural that some partner leaves the consortium and be replaced by a new organization. The termination of this collaboration process or even the ending of a VO, are subjects not properly addressed yet.

The consequences of the operation of a VO/VE cannot be simply discarded when the VO/VE dissolves. Most of these consequences are of a legal nature and shall be regulated by the cooperation agreements. That is the case, for instance, of the responsibility of customer support / product maintenance during the life cycle of the product / service generated by a VO/VE. Environment regulations are also forcing companies to plan provisions regarding the product disposal and recycling after its end of life.

Recent regulations in some countries also state that the liabilities regarding each component of a product may ultimately lie with the component's supplier. In the case of a network chain type of manufacturing this forces each node in the chain to keep track of the history of each component/sub-product that "passed by" this node. This is a functionality that is properly supported by most of the more advanced ERP systems, but not by most of the scheduling systems, for instance.

There are, however, several other less "material" issues which are more difficult to handle. One of these issues is the Intellectual Property Rights (IPRs) policy, namely for the post-dissolution phase and its consequences in terms of information accesses by the VE members. In some cases there is also the possibility that the VE evolves into a more permanent organization, a joint venture enterprise created by the VE members, to exploit the intellectual and industrial property results developed in cooperation. There is also considerable knowledge that can be elicited from the ending cooperation experience, namely the knowledge about what went right, what went wrong, partners performance / reliability, jointly defined business process templates, etc. Defining the ownership and access rights to this knowledge is not an easy task and requires further investigation.

Therefore, some important ***research topics*** include:

- Definition of a legal and organizational framework for the termination of a cooperation process.
- Creation of mechanisms for handling post-cooperation IPRs and liabilities.
- Management functionalities to support the post-VO access to common resources and information.
- Mechanisms to support extensive traceability.

6. VIRTUAL LABORATORIES

A Virtual Laboratory (VL) is another form of collaborative network, representing a heterogeneous, distributed problem solving environment that enables a group of researchers located in different geographical places to work together, sharing resources (equipments, tools, experimental data, etc.), i.e. a specialized form of VO.

In some domains requiring expensive equipment and a large critical mass of researchers, e.g. bio-informatics, there is a pressing need to assist researchers with enhanced environments in conducting their complex scientific experiments.

Another application scenario for VL requiring specific support tools is remote education (e-learning).

VL can benefit from the integration of results and approaches from related areas such as tele-operation / tele-supervision federated information management, and collaborative spaces, and involves:

- Interaction between people, instruments, and information:
  - Collaboration tools: Teleconferencing, chat, shared e-whiteboard, notepad, etc.;
  - Scientific instruments connected to the network;
  - Sharing and authorized exchange of information among collaborators;
  - Large scale simulations;
  - Data filtering and reduction facilities;
  - Visualization tools and devices.
- Remote experiment execution and control.
- Access to information from the distributed public and proprietary sources.
- User-friendly interfaces.
- The basic necessary functionality and tools.
- Integration/fusion of distributed and diverse meta-data, data, and results.
- High-performance, secure, distributed and collaborative experimentation.
- Semi-intelligent assistance to define/perform experiments.

Tele-robotics and tele-supervision applications which make use of the Internet have been progressively increasing for a wide domain of applications (remotely operated robots and telescopes, manufacturing systems, virtual laboratories, etc.). The traditional approaches taken in this area assume a set of pre-defined services which a user can activate on simple machine and sensorial remote environments. However, if complex machinery or sensorial environments are considered to be remotely operated with maximum flexibility, a set of pre-defined services and simple monitoring/recovering procedures are not sufficient. Also, for large or variable time-delays and low availability of the communication channels, remote low level closed loop control is impractical and higher levels of control (such as supervisory control, for example) and autonomy are required. So, more sophisticated and more reliable solutions have to be found leading to an increase of the autonomy of the equipment being operated, yet preserving a high degree of flexibility. One promising approach consists of applying intelligent mobile agents [16]. Adaptable agents, carrying high level missions, can adapt themselves to the available resources in the visited places, allowing for a higher autonomy namely in the case of a temporary unavailability of network connections. Agents can also provide a facility to implement assistance mechanisms and to support asynchronous cooperation.

Recent advances in networking, high performance computing and resource management have introduced new possibilities for secure communication and computation intensive resource management [1], [9]. The GRID is a world-wide effort in this area, which takes advantage of improvements in the overall network bandwidth, and adds a new dimension to the distributed computing. Through the GRID environment, a large number of Unix-based workstations and supercomputers can be connected in an efficient way, offering users a vast amount of computational power. However, the development of communication infrastructures such as the GRID architecture and the supporting GRID middle-ware (e.g. the GLOBUS toolkit), are on going world-wide efforts which will not be completed any time soon. Therefore, although GRID is promising as a foundation for networked organizations, still many of its facilities are under development, and in specific at its current state, GRID falls short of supporting the necessary base for collaboration among autonomous business-oriented organizations. Unlike the pure scientific research, many organizations are keen about their autonomy and their rights to both their proprietary data and local resources, as it is also required in most applications within the VE/VO paradigm. Therefore, GRID is so far mostly being used as a partial infrastructure, on top of which, depending on the application, other functionality is developed.

Some important ***open research topics*** in VL include:

- Integration of component technologies into a coherent platform.
- Coordinated and dynamic resource sharing for collaborative problem solving - Direct access to hardware, software, data, etc.
- High-performance data integration for scientific collaboration - Identification of the best path for exchange of large data sets among VO members based on the on-line monitoring of distributed resources.
- Tele-supervision and tele-operation assisted by intelligent mobile agents.
- Facilities for dynamic definition of information (and services) access rights / different visibility levels for different VL community members - Encouraging the joint developments while preserving rights, responsibilities, and liabilities.
- Definition of adequate representation languages for Cooperation formalization - *Cooperation* agreement / contracts, liability and risks negotiation, credit assignment (based on contributions), value and ownership of common developments, intangible entities (IPR, services).
- Social aspects and remote collaboration (lack of "silent language" of body motions and spatial positions).
- Asynchronous cooperation and delegation. Further developments in coordination approaches for diverse, autonomous, semi-cooperative, semi-reliable, heterogeneous, and evolving organizations.
- Improved mechanisms for specification of access rights and separation of virtual spaces / experiments.
- Extended error recovery mechanisms.
- Training methodologies based on VL for manufacturing professionals.

7. VIRTUAL COMMUNITIES SUPPORT

When a proper cooperation nesting or breeding environment (e.g. cluster or long term network) is in place, **virtual communities of practice (VCP)** / virtual teams may emerge within such environment, constituting a fundamental element of value creation and sustainability. Virtual Communities and Communities of Practice are not new concepts but they acquire specific characteristics and increased importance when considered in the context of the collaborative networks of organizations. These communities, although spontaneously created, are bound to certain social rules resulting from the commitment of their members to the underlying organizations (new concept of social-bound VCPs) (Fig. 2).

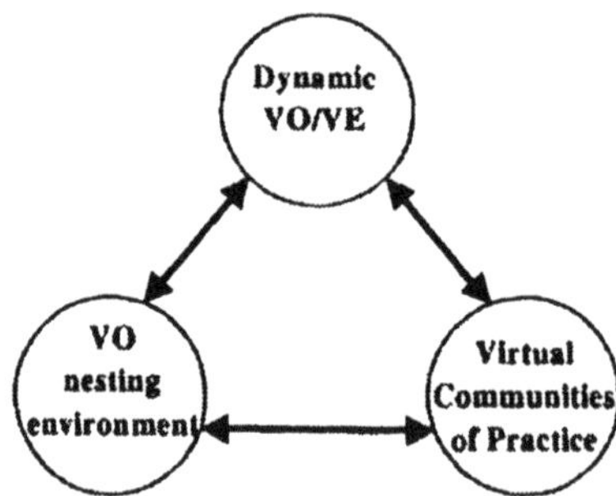

Figure 2 – VCPs in the context of VOs and cooperation nesting environments

This is the case, for instance, in *concurrent* or *collaborative engineering* where teams of engineers, possibly located in different enterprises, cooperate in a joint project such as the co-design of a new product. A large number of computer supported cooperative tools are becoming widely available for synchronous cooperation. Some examples are teleconference, and chat tools combined with application sharing mechanisms. Considering the geographical distribution, the autonomy of the VE members, the local corporate cultures, and also the individual working preferences of the team members, it is likely that most of the activities will be carried out in an asynchronous way.

In terms of coordination, several approaches to develop *flexible workflow* systems have been proposed. In the case of processes mainly executed by humans, rigid forms of procedural control are not adequate. People like to keep their freedom regarding the way they work. Product design, like any other creative process evolves according to a kind of "arbitrary" flow. It is therefore necessary to also support *loosely constrained* sets of *business processes*.

The trend is followed by other communities of professionals (e.g. consultants) that share the body of knowledge of their professions such as similar working cultures, problem perceptions, problem-solving techniques, professional values, and behavior.

Another special area of application, as for instance represented by the TeleCARE project [6], is the creation of virtual communities for providing care services to elderly. These communities involve organizations and people such as care providers, health care professionals, relatives of elderly, and the elderly.

Some open ***research topics***:

- Development and management of shared, smart spaces for geographically distributed teams of the same or different organizations, which develop complex engineering products.
- Provision of adequate visibility and access rights definition and management.
- Understand and model multi-level relationships among VC members.
- Coordination of (asynchronous) activities performed in different places by different actors; flexible coordination models.
- Frameworks for collaboration in mobile contexts.
- Tools for community management, leadership, and creation of incentives.
- Provision of notification mechanisms regarding major events in the design / planning process (e.g. conclusion of a step by one actor).
- Mechanisms to handle Intellectual Property in VCP under social contracts.

8. OTHER ISSUES

Although VOs should be addressed by multi-disciplinary teams, some early developments have been tackled separately either by the ICT community or by the organizations and management community. In particular in the European context, most of the early Esprit and IST projects were technology-driven. A few recent projects put more emphasis on the management and organizational issues (with a corresponding decrease on the ICT infrastructure) but a balanced integration between the "ICT" and the "Management and Organizational" communities still seems to be missing. One exception is present at the EC-funded THINKcreative network that involves a balanced composition of experts from these two main areas.

In addition to the mentioned aspects, there are other important factors to be considered in VO, such as the social, ethical, and educational issues. The barriers for implantation of VOs are more of a socio-organizational and command logic than of technological nature. One of the early attempts to combine a "sociology" component with the technology development was represented in the Esprit PRODNET II [3].

Although there is a growing awareness for the advantages of taking a multi-disciplinary approach, it is important to not under-estimate the difficulties of putting together communities with different backgrounds, different language and culture, and different approaches to problem solving. Even within the engineering area it is not always easy to reach a common language and understanding. For instance, many of the European projects on VO, although ICT-based, are mostly developed by industrial-, mechanical-, or electrical-engineers, where there is, in many cases, a "divorce" between this community and the software engineering community. The difficulties are much bigger when other non-engineering communities are put together with engineers.

There is therefore a need for an integrated multi-disciplinary approach leading to truly joint work (mutual understanding and mutual respect for the other areas!) among: Theoreticians, System engineers and ICT developers, Social & organizational experts, Economists, Standardization bodies, and the Application Domain experts. In order to make this possible, there is also a need for further investment in formal languages – a must in order to ensure mutual understanding in a complex multi-disciplinary domain.

Furthermore, there is a need to elaborate new individual (social) protection mechanisms – agility in partnering and establishment of relationships cannot be adopted, without adequate protection mechanisms for the involved individual. Namely, mechanisms must be introduced to guarantee some long-term stability to individuals and their families in the context of highly dynamic market changes.

9. CONCLUSIONS

The area of virtual organizations and networked collaborative organizations in general correspond to a very dynamic domain, where new concepts, mechanisms, infrastructures and tools are emerging at a fast pace.

There is however the need for a more systematic and comprehensive understanding of the area, namely in terms of the emerging collaborative organizations that will likely play an important role in the next 5, 10, 15 years, as well as in terms of developing appropriate support infrastructures and tools. In parallel with such developments it is mandatory to reach some harmonization of models and approaches in order to reach inter-operability and reduce the engineering efforts still required to launch an operative VO.

Such developments shall necessarily be undertaken by teams with a multi-disciplinary composition, for which the difficulties of communication / understanding among different communities should not be under-estimated.

10. ACKNOWLEDGMENTS

The authors acknowledge partial support to this work from the European Commission (IST THINKcreative project) and IFIP (COVE / WG 5.5) and thank other partners of these projects for their valuable contribution to the discussion of some of the topics reported here.

11. REFERENCES

1. Afsarmanesh, H.; Kaletas, E.C.; Hertzberger, L.O. – A Reference Architecture for Scientific Virtual Laboratories, Future Generation Computer Systems, vol. 17, 2001.
2. Broos, R.; Dillenseger, B.; Guther, A.; Leith, M. – MIAMI: Mobile intelligent agents for managing the information infrastructure, www.infowin.org/ ACTS/ANALYSYS/PRODUCTS/THEMATIC/AGENTS/ch3/miami.htm, 2000.
3. Camarinha-Matos, L.M.; Afsarmanesh, H. – Infrastructures for Virtual Enterprises - Networking Industrial Enterprises, Kluwer Academic Publishers, ISBN 0-7923-8639-6, Oct 1999.
4. Camarinha-Matos, L. M.; Afsarmanesh, H. - Service Federation in Virtual Organizations, Proceedings of PROLAMAT'01, 7-10 Nov 2001, Budapest, Hungary.
5. Camarinha-Matos, L. M. and Afsarmanesh, H. - Virtual Enterprise Modeling and Support Infrastructures: Applying Multi-Agent Systems Approaches, in *Multi-Agent Systems and Applications*, M. Luck, V. Marik, O. Stpankova, R. Trappl (eds.), Lecture Notes in Artificial Intelligence LNAI 2086, Springer, ISBN 3-540-42312-5, July 2001.
6. Camarinha-Matos, L.M.; Afsarmanesh, H. – Design of a virtual community infrastructure for elderly care, in *Collaborative Business Ecosystems and Virtual Enterprises, Kluwer Academic Publishers, May 2002.*
7. Camarinha-Matos, L.M.; Afsarmanesh, H.; Rabelo, J. – Infrastructure developments for agile virtual enterprises, to appear in *J. Computer Integrated Manufacturing*, 2002.
8. Goranson, H.T., 1999 – The Agile Virtual Enterprise – Cases, metrics, tools. Quorum Books, ISBN 1-56720-264-0.
9. Kaletas, E. C.; Afsarmanesh, H. ; Hertzberger, L. O. – Virtual Laboratories and Virtual Organizations supporting biosciences, in *Collaborative Business Ecosystems and Virtual Enterprises, Kluwer Academic Publishers, May 2002.*
10. Li, Y.; Huang, B.; Liu, W.; Wu, C.; Gou, H.– Multi-agent system for partner selection of virtual enterprise, Proceedings of the World Computer Congress 2000, Track on Information Technology for Business Management, R. Gan (Ed.), Publishing House of Electronics Industry, ISBN 3-901882-05-7, Beijing, China, 21-25 Aug.*2000.*
11. NIIIP. www.niiip.org.
12. Rabelo, R.; Afsarmanesh, H.; Camarinha-Matos, L.M. - Federated multi-agent scheduling in virtual enterprises, in *E-business and Virtual Enterprises, Kluwer Academic Publishers,* Oct *2000.*
13. Rabelo, R.; Camarinha-Matos, L.M.; Vallejos, R. - Agent-based brokerage for virtual enterprise creation in the moulds industry, *in* E-business and Virtual Enterprises, Kluwer Academic Publishers, ISBN 0-7923-7205-0, pp.281-290, Oct 2000.
14. Rocha, A.; Oliveira, E. – An electronic market architecture for the formation of virtual enterprises, in [3], 1999.
15. SUN - JINI Technology Architectural Overview, www.sun.com/jini/whitepapers/architecture.html, Jan 1999.
16. Vieira, W.; Camarinha-Matos, L.M. - Adaptive mobile agents: Enhanced flexibility in Internet-based remote operation, *in Advances in Networked Enterprises, Kluwer Academic Publishers,* ISBN 0-7923-7958-6, Sept 2000.
17. WfMC - Workflow Management Coalition, 1994 - The Workflow Reference Model - Document Nr. TC00 - 1003, Issue 1.1, Brussels Nov 29.
18. Zarli, A.; Poyet, P. – A framework for distributed information management in the virtual enterprise: The VEGA project, in [3], 1999.

13

CONSIDERATIONS ON SECURE FIPA COMPLIANT AGENT ARCHITECTURE

Tomáš Vlček[1], Jan Zach[2]
[1] *Czech Technical University in Prague, Czech Republic; vlcek@labe.felk.cvut.cz*
[2] *CertiCon a.s., CAK, Prague, Czech Republic; zach@certicon.cz*

This paper is intended to support security instruments for FIPA (http://www.fipa.org) compliant architectures. These security instruments, should increase trust and confidentiality within and among agent communities/technology and provide security mechanisms, as encryption, authentication, message integrity services, etc., employing cryptography algorithms.

1. INTRODUCTION

In the paper proposed secure architecture is FIPA compliant in the sense that every common FIPA compliant agent should be able to interact with agents having this extended architecture even not knowing the security mechanisms. On the other hand, agents demanding for security can, of course, refuse plain, non secured communication with non authenticated agents, etc.

The security mechanisms can utilize existing agent platform mediators such as the Agent Management System (AMS), Directory Facilitator (DF), or Agent Communication Channel (ACC), e.g. for authentication purposes[1]. But these new tasks enforce to make requirements for these mediators much more thoroughness, as FIPA specifies them too loosely[2] for these purposes (FIPA 1998, FIPA 2000). Other approaches could be found in (Wulf 1995, Wong 1998).

This paper is aimed mainly to "static", i.e. non-mobile, agents, but it should be possible to extend the architecture by mobility support easily[3].

2. ARCHITECTURE DESCRIPTION

All the requirements defined as a data items for architecture design are grouped into General Requirements – see Table 1, and Security Requirements – see Table 2, and are labeled by Requirement Identifier (RID) for future reference.

The specification uses common abbreviations as well as the terminology of FIPA standards (FIPA 1998, FIPA 2000); definitions of basic terms used, e.g. Agent Platform (AP), Home Agent Platform (HAP), directory Facilitator (DF) etc. can be found in (FIPA, 1998).

Table 1 summarizes explicit general requirements imposed on the architecture design from the point of view of its compliancy with the FIPA system standards, transparency, legacy systems compatibility, reliability and optimal performance.

Table 1 – Requirement Specification – General Requirements

ID		Requirement
G1		The resulting architecture should fit into the FIPA compliant system standard [1]
	G1.1	Security services should be transparent whether within or outside an Agent Platform (AP).
	G1.2	An agent residing on an insecure platform (i.e. with enabled secure mechanisms) should be able to receive insecure messages, e.g., from outside of the AP. Whether the agent is willing to respond in an insecure way or at all depends on the agent itself.
	G1.3	Messages should consist of a FIPA compliant, non encrypted envelope[4] extended by encryption information as well as of a plain or encrypted content of the message. Furthermore, authenticity of the envelope should be easily verifiable as well.
G2		The resulting architecture should be vendor, patent, proprietary algorithm independent.
G3		The resulting architecture should be available and reliable.
G4		All the necessary security infrastructure should be accessible within an AP. If any security service requires an inter-platform communication, this should be transparently provided by trusted AP's mediators.
G5		For performance and maintenance reasons, the resulting architecture should enable security based on trusted relationships and thus request/service delegation. E.g., an agent authenticated in his Home Agent Platform (HAP) is trusted in an adjacent AP which shares the trusted relationship with this HAP.
G6		All the security services should be transparent to an agent.
G7		The security architecture should be easily applicable to and integrable with any legacy system.
G8		The architecture should support administrative domains in order to avoid administration troubles.
	G8.1	It should be possible to settle administrative domains in a hierarchical way so that one can be immersed to another.
	G8.2	In any domain it should be possible to specify groups and roles assignable to agents belonging to that domain.

Table 2 defines the basic set of security services related to the platform and agent security, security threads resistance, security polices and authentication mechanisms. Dependencies among particular architectural security services are depicted in Fig. 1.

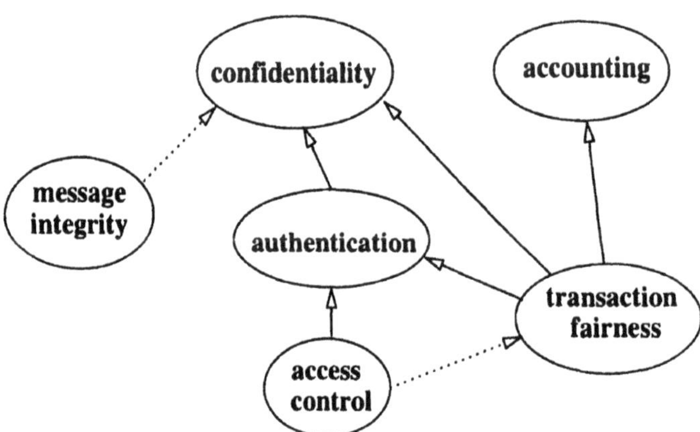

Figure 1 – Service Dependencies

Table 2 – Requirement Specification – Security Requirements

ID			Requirement
S1			The architecture should support at least the following security services
	S1.1		**Authentication Service**, i.e., an arbitrary agent should be able to prove its identity.
	S1.2		**Confidentiality Service**. This service should protect communication against passive attacks as eavesdropping or traffic analysis.
	S1.3		**Access Control Service** should support access control to agents' particular resources and alleviate agents' burden associated with it.
		S1.3.1	The architecture should support access control to resources based on **roles** and **groups** assigned to a particular agent.
		S1.3.2	Roles and groups should be unique within a domain and all its subdomains.
		S1.3.3	An agent could have assigned an arbitrary number of roles and groups.
	S1.4		**Transaction Fairness Service** should provide protection of a particular transaction against repudiation or an attempt not to fulfill obligations, etc. In addition, it should serve as a trusted third party, i.e. as an arbitrator or transaction mediator, and support accountability and fairness within an agent community.
	S1.5		**Accounting Service** should support logs and their analysis, monitoring, intrusion detection, etc. Besides it is required by the Transaction Fairness Service, it should improve availability and reliability of the system as a whole.
	S1.6		**Message Integrity and Protection Service** should provide message protection against modification, alternation, errors, etc. This protection includes not only the content of a message but even its plain envelope. Easy detection of the message integrity should be possible.
S2			The resulting architecture should be as much as possible resistant at least against the following security threads:
	S2.1		Eavesdropping.
	S2.2		Masquerading.
	S2.3		Reply attack.
	S2.4		Message alternation.
	S2.5		Denial of service (DoS) and interruption.
S3			An AP should be able to set up its security policy dependent on which **environment** it operates:
	S3.1		**Secure.** The security is switched off.
	S3.2		**Unsecure.** All security mechanisms are switched on.
	S3.3		**Security Debugging.** Extensive logging is switched on.
S4			An agent should be able to use at least the following security services:
	S4.1		**Authentication Service.** All counterparts of communication should be able to prove their identity. If an unauthenticated message is received, the agent can throw it away or respond with an authentification request/failure.[5]
	S4.2		**Access Control Service.** The service demander should prove its identity and rights to the service.
	S4.3		**Message Integrity and Protection Service.** Messages should be protected against modification or other corruption during their transport. This option does not imply that the messages are encrypted.
	S4.4		**Confidentiality Service.** All messages should be encrypted to prohibit their unauthorized access.
	S4.5		**Transaction Fairness Service.** This service can be employed for assuring fairness during particular transactions.
	S4.6		**Filtering.** This policy enables to filter incoming messages according to the source address, authentication, etc. Filtering should be performed within agents.
S5			Resulting security level should be derived from security requirements of an agent and its HAP.
S6			An AP should be able to force its agents to start using a security mechanism.

S7	The architecture should be open for additional security services as availability, accounting, accountability, etc. These services are too sophisticated to be included into the basic security model but it should be possible to add them easily.
S8	There should be specified interfaces supporting both a symmetric, i.e. a private key, and an asymmetric, i.e. a public-key, encryption.
S9	An agent, accessing a service, should prove its identity, if its HAP is insecure, the service is not public, and/or the authentication is just required.
S10	Every agent should be able to authenticate at least in its HAP.
S11	Every service provider, including the public one, i.e. a mediator, running on an insecure AP and providing data should authenticate to its client.
S12	Identity of an agent should be proved by a time limited certificate issued by an authorization authority as the AMS or the PKI maintainer.

3. DESIGN DECISIONS

It seems reasonable to suppose an agent platform to be either secure or insecure. The decision about platform security (and security policy) is up to the platform owner. If an agent within a platform requires some security mechanisms (authentication, confidentiality, message protection, etc.) and its home platform does not support it, an error message is returned.

The inter- and intra- platform security should be distinguished because of considerable inherent differences: The inter-platform security concerns larger agent communities, e.g., the Internet, whereas the intra-platform security will be used in smaller communities, e.g., on a factory floor. It is apparent there are a bit different requirements in both cases concerning performance[6] and features they provide, e.g., agents on a factory floor can be supposed to provide much more prolific repertoire of services than their open-community counterparts, they could require the control access support for their particular services (not for the agent as a whole), etc.

There will be both the symmetric (shared secret key) and the asymmetric (public key) crypto algorithms employed depending on wether we deal with the inter-platform or the intra-platform security.

Inter-platform security will be provided by two means: trusted platforms and the public-key cryptography.

The term trusted platforms means that AMS's of both AP's share a secret key and they mutually trust in provided authentication information, i.e. certificates. This technique is available, e.g., within an enterprise, it is simple and does not require the sophisticated PKI infrastructure. Some potential issues can stem from the trust intransitivity. In addition, every platform or a trusted group of platforms can have its own public key which authenticates it within the agent universe.

In an open environment, e.g., the Internet, the public-key cryptography is much more applicable. The main advantage is the possibility of hierarchical certification, the main drawback[7] is the complexity of maintaining (and assuring security of) such hierarchical certificates. Of course, it is possible for a single agent to have its own public key, if necessary.

Intra-platform security requires the same security mechanisms as in the case of the inter-platform security but, in addition, some mechanism, e.g., the single service access control, should be provided. This can be done in a Kerberos-like manner. All security mechanisms should be implemented using the symmetric key encryption.

3.1 Trust Relation

To reason about trust within and among AP's we introduce the trust relation by the following definition:

Definition: As the **trust** it is meant a binary relation defined as

$Agent \times Agent \rightarrow \{true, false\}$

expressing that the first agent trusts or mistrusts the second agent. The symmetric trust will be denoted as $\Leftrightarrow_T$, the asymmetric one as $\Rightarrow_T$. The trust $Agent_1 \Rightarrow_T Agent_2$ can be established after the $Agent_2$ proves its identity, i.e. authenticates, to the $Agent_1$. This relation is not commutative.

In principle, the authentication can proceed in two manners as outlined in the following schema:

(i) The agent A and agent B share a secret key $K_{A,B}$, the authentication protocol then can look as follows:

1. $A \rightarrow B : E_{K_{A,B}}[nonce_A]$
2. $B \rightarrow A : E_{K_{A,B}}[nonce_A + 1, nonce_B]$
3. $A \Rightarrow_T B$

The protocol can further continue in the following way:

4. $A \rightarrow B : E_{K_{A,B}}[nonce_B + 1]$
5. $B \Rightarrow_T A, A \Leftrightarrow_T B$

(ii) The agent A holds its own, by a 3rd authority certified, public key:

1. $A \rightarrow B : nonce_A, Sgn_A[data\_verifiable\_by\_B]$
2. $B \Rightarrow_T A$

This protocol can continue:

3. $B \rightarrow A : Sgn_A[nonce_A]$
4. $A \Rightarrow_T B, A \Leftrightarrow_T B$

By a *nonce*, in the context of the protocols, it is denoted an arbitrary piece of data, the only condition that has to hold is that both the agents know the transformation *nonce+1* so that the agent which generated that nonce knows which value to expect after the transformation. The main reason for introducing a nonce is the countermeasure against the reply attack and a proof that the counterpart understands the message.

3.2 Authentication

Identity of an agent will be proved for other agents by a certificate issued by a **trusted authority** (TA). If the identified agent does not possess its public key, the certification authority will be its home TA, otherwise the certificate can be issued by any AP. The issued certificate will be valid within the authorizing TA's AP only. Part of the certificate will be a secret session key used for the consecutive session.

The following prepositions are assumed to be valid:

1. A TA trusts an agent if the agent proves its identity by a secret key (sometimes called the master key) shared between the agent and the TA.

The TA then attests this trust by issuing a **certificate**. After the certificate delivery, the proposition $agent@HAP \Leftrightarrow_T TA@HAP$ is valid. This type of certification will be possible only within the agent's HAP.

2. A TA trusts an agent if the agent proves its identity by its public key which is certified by the PKI authority. The TA then assets this trust by issuing a **certificate** and it holds $agent@HAP \Leftrightarrow_T TA@HAP$. This type of authorization is possible even across APs.
3. A certificate issued by a TA is issued for one specific agent. If the agent being authenticated needs to be authenticated to another agent, it needs a new certificate issued for that another agent.
4. An agent *a@HAP* trusts another agent *b@HAP* if that agent possesses a valid certificate issued by its home TA agent *ams@HAP*.
5. The trusted AP relationship means that the trusted APs share secret keys which allows their mutual authentication.
6. The shared secret key for AP's trust will be held by TAs of the trusted APs.
7. Trust is not transitive in general, transitivity, i.e.
   $(TA@AP_1 \Rightarrow_T a@AP_1) \wedge (TA@AP_2 \Rightarrow_T TA@AP_1) \wedge (b@AP_2 \Rightarrow_T TA@AP_2) \rightarrow$
   $\rightarrow (b@AP_2 \Rightarrow_T a@AP_1)$
   holds within the trusted platforms only, i.e. where $(TA@AP_1 \Rightarrow_T TA@A_2)$

In principle, we can distinguish the following authentication cases:

- **Authentication within an AP without a Public Key.** This is the most common generic way to authenticate within an AP, see Fig. 2(1). The TA issues a certificate to the agent *A*, authenticating *A* to *B*, as TA proved its identity by acquaintance of the shared secret key. The certificate contains a session key which identifies the agent *A* to *B*.
- **Authentication within an AP with a Public Key.** See Fig. 2(2). This method works as in the case 1, but the public key is used for authentication. Communication 2 and 3 serves for acquiring the valid public key to verify the agent's identity.
- **Authentication in a trusted AP without a Public Key.** See Fig. 2(3a). In this case, the scenario is: 1. *A* acquires an authentication certificate issued by the home AMS and 2. In virtue of the certificate, *A* acquires another certificate valid in the adjacent trusted platform AP_2.
- **Authentication in a trusted AP with a Public Key.** See Fig. 2(2), or 2(3b).
- **Authentication in a non-trusted AP with a Public Key.** See Fig. 2(2). This is the most general way to get the certificate.

In all the mentioned cases, the result is a valid authentication certificate usable in the destination platform. A direct authentication with a public key, i.e., without any mediation with an AMS it is not prohibited but it is not recommended.

3.3 Access control

The access control (i.e. authorization) to agent's resources will be provided by the following means:

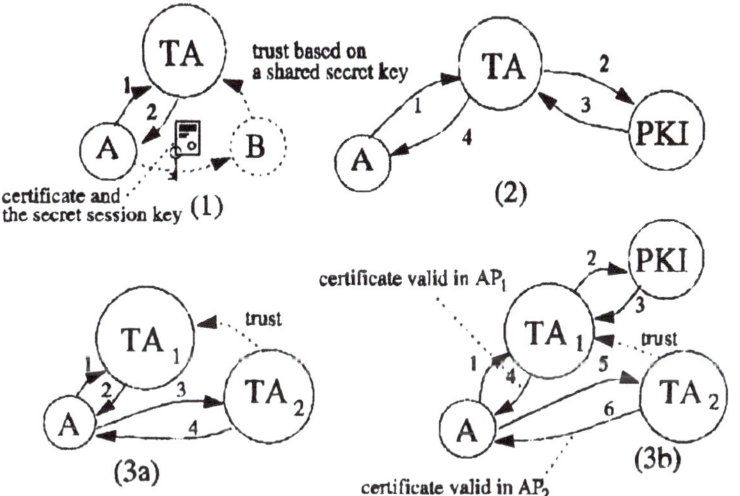

Figure 2 – Authentication Cases

a) An agent will be responsible for the access control to its resources by itself. This implies that the service providing agent has to maintain a list of authorized agents, i.e. their AID's, and operations granted to them.
b) An access to particular resources will be granted by a voucher issued either by a TA, e.g. the DF, or the service providing agent. Access to the requested resource/service will be granted in exchange for that voucher[8].
c) Access is based on mapping domain access rights appertaining to an accessing agent the rights of the local system. For the rights mapping, the resource providing agent will be responsible. Such a mapping makes the system interoperable with legacy systems with its own access control mechanism.

The approach ad a) can be denoted as a traditional approach, well known from the client/server applications. It is feasible for resources with few accessing agents as the overhead caused by the access control list maintenance increases with the number of accessing agents. The approaches ad b) and c) move the access control responsibilities to a central location, thus those methods are feasible for environments having large number of agents. Utilization of AID for decision making on access rights to services implies that the very first authentication should proceed as early as during agent's registration to an AMS.

The architecture relies on three types of vouchers:

- Time limited voucher granting access to the service for all time of its validity and bound to its holder it was issued for. This type of the vouchers will be issued by the DF according to the AP's access control policy.
- Voucher application limited, negotiable, and by the Transaction Fairness Service registered. Every application has to be mediated by the Transaction Fairness Service. This type of voucher can be issued by the service provider.
- Portable and platform independent voucher digitaly signed by a TA.

As a part of the voucher information on administrative domains, roles, and groups assigned to the agent will be included. Administrative domains are introduced to maintain the access control lists easily and are proposed to be settled hierarchically above the FIPA agent platforms.

4. CONCLUSIONS

Basic efforts aimed at achievement of FIPA agent security, which are currently being implemented within our multiagent infrastructure, are discussed in the paper. To be honest, there are additional requirements concerning the FIPA standard augmentation to support the proposed architecture - namely introduction of public-key infrastructure agent and accounting and trusted arbiter agent - which were not discussed and depart beyond the limited extent of the paper.

5. ACKNOWLEDGMENTS

This work was partially supported by the Ministry of Education of the Czech Republic under the Project LN00B096.

6. REFERENCES

1. The Foundation for Intelligent Physical Agents (FIPA). http://www.fipa.org.
2. FIPA Agent Management. Part 1 - document number FIPA00002. Foundation for Intelligent Physical Agents, 1998.
3. FIPA Agent Security Management. Part 10, Version 1.0. Foundation for Intelligent Physical Agents, 1998.
4. FIPA Agent Management Specification - document number XC00023H. Foundation for Intelligent Physical Agents, 2000.
5. FIPA Agent Message Transport Service - document number XC00067D. Foundation for Intelligent Physical Agents 2000.
4. Schneier, Bruce. Applied Cryptography. New York: John Willey & Sons, 1996.
5. Stallings, William: Cryptography and Network Security. Principles and Practice. Prentice Hall, 1999.
6. Wong, H. Chi and Sycara, Katia: Adding Security and Trust to Multi-Agent Systems. Carnegie Mellon University, Pennsilvania:1998
7. Wulf, Wm A., Wang, Chenxi, Kienzle, Darrell: A New Model of Security for Distributed Systems. Computer Science Technical Report CS-95-34, University of Virginia, Virginia: 1995.

---

[1] The reason to extend the FIPA mediator functionality instead of adding new mediators stems from the fact that the new mediators would essentially double functionality of the existing ones. The only exception is introducing of a new security agent responsible, e.g., for the PKI infrastructure maintenance.

[2] E.g. in (FIPA, 2000): "... it (DF) must strive to maintain an accurate, complete and timely list of agents ...", in the next paragraph one can read: "... the DF cannot guarantee the validity or accuracy of the information that has been registered with it ...". Some of these problems are evidently caused by lack of built-in security elements as authentication, etc.

[3] If we view a mobile agent as a service extension of the host machine (agent) and the host agent is responsible for it, i.e. the mobile agent is authenticated, trusted, etc., i.e. the mobile agent delegates its responsibility to the host agent, then everything should fit in with the paper well.

[4] It enables processing and forwarding of the message even by agents not knowing the security mechanisms.

[5] An authentication in connection with the Transaction Fairness Service, e.g., a signed message digest, can serve as an evidence about transactions, etc.

[6] In (Schneier, 1996), it is stated that symmetric algorithms are generally at least 1000 times faster than the public-key algorithms.

[7] Moreover, there are some safety reasons predestinating the public-key cryptography mainly for identity proofs and secret key exchanges, e.g., see (Schneier, 1996) and (Stallings, 1998).

[8] The voucher figures here as a digital cash.

14

A REVIEW ON ENVIRONMENTS SUPPORTING VIRTUAL ENTERPRISE INTEGRATION

Maria Manuela Cunha
Instituto Politécnico do Cávado e do Ave, Portugal, mcunha@ipca.pt
Goran D. Putnik
Universidade do Minho, Portugal, putnikgd@dps.uminho.pt
José Dinis Carvalho
Universidade do Minho, Portugal, jdac@dps.uminho.pt
Paulo Ávila
Instituto Politécnico do Porto, Portugal, pavila@dem.isep.ipp.pt

Since the mid nineties, a considerable effort have been undertaken to develop environments to support the Virtual Enterprise life cycle. This effort includes the development of technologies and the development of applications either at the academia or at industrial level to facilitate supply chain management and virtual enterprise integration and its reconfigurability dynamics.
In the paper we intend to present those main contributions, viewing the creation of an environment for the effective and efficient integration of virtual enterprises. We also present the model of the Market of Resources, proposed by the authors, as an electronic brokerage service, designed with this purpose, and discuss its benefits face to other developments.

1. INTRODUCTION

The goal of the enterprise is to fulfil the customer requirements. Traditionally, the enterprise uses the set of resources existing inside its walls. As this selection domain is relatively limited and of small size, it cannot, in general, provide the desired competitive performances, the enterprise searches for cooperation with other enterprises, corresponding to a shift from "self-centred closed-enterprises" to "global open-enterprises" (Browne & Zhang, 1999).

Several factors determine the competitiveness of the enterprise, being the most important requirements for competitiveness, the fast adaptability or fast reconfigurability to environmental change (Cunha, Putnik, & Gunasekaran, 2002). The paradigms satisfying those requisites are the Agile and the Virtual Enterprise ones, which, in the context of the present work, will be designated as the Agile/Virtual Enterprise model (A/V E), corresponding to the Virtual Enterprise model offering the characteristics of the Agile Enterprise.

The requirements of fast adaptability or reconfigurability implies the ability of (1) flexible and almost instantaneous access to the optimal resources to integrate in the enterprise; (2) design, negotiation, business management and manufacturing management functions independently from the physical barrier of space; and (3) minimisation of the reconfiguration time (Putnik, 2000).

We can identify several phases on the life cycle of an A/V E namely: (1) Creation, involving search and selection of partners, and its integration, (2) Operation, (3) Reconfiguration and (4) Dissolution. Reconfiguration happens during A/V E operation and implies a redesign of the A/V E, with search and selection of new partners and integration of the same in a new A/V E instantiation. Fast reconfigurability means that an A/V E can have as many instantiations as required in order to keep permanent alignment with the market requirements, and that these reconfigurations happen with a low reconfiguration time and cost (Cunha & Putnik, 2002). Dissolution is seen as a special case of reconfigurability.

In our work, when referring the A/V E integration, we will implicitly include the upstream phase of search and selecting the partners to integrate. Although much research is being undertaken around the several steps of A/V E integration, its management and co-ordination, insufficient attention has been devoted to the necessity of creating the environment where those processes take place, i.e., the environment to enable an efficient and effective integration, offering strategies for dynamically align the virtual enterprise with business.

This paper reviews some of the most significant contributions towards A/V E integration, namely tools and environments for electronic brokerage, negotiation and integration. Section 2 introduces the main concepts and supporting technologies and techniques. The main contributions towards environments for A/V E integration are addressed in section 3 and section 4 presents the Market of Resources as an environment for A/V E integration. Section 5 concludes the paper, with a simple relationship between techniques/environments and A/V E organisational models.

2. TECHNOLOGIES AND TECHNIQUES SUPPORTING ENVIRONMENTS FOR VIRTUAL ENTERPRISES INTEGRATION

Information and Communication Technologies and Internet-based Agent technology are the main technologies for implementation of techniques supporting or contributing to the integration of A/V E[1]. These techniques or applications include electronic negotiation, electronic marketplaces and market brokerage. In this section we briefly present the main aspects of Agent technology and of the mentioned techniques. Other fundamental technologies for A/V E operation are workflow management systems, collaborative design, virtual product, concurrent engineering.

2.1 Agent Technologies

According to a commonly used definition proposed by (Wooldridge, 1997), agents are software systems capable of flexible, autonomous action in some environment in order to meet its design objectives. Agents consists on software than can travel over networks, activate and control remote programs, interrogating host Web sites, interacting with other agents and return to source with information.

Some specific domains where, according to (Oliveira, 1999), the agent-based solution proved to be appropriate include[2]:

- *Softbots*, (software robots) are agents living in virtual environments, having access to multiple heterogeneous and geographically distributed information sources as Internet, to perform active searches for relevant information, like Web pages containing information considered important for its user.
- *Virtual Organizations*, in Internet-based marketplaces and in the integration virtual enterprises, agents can search for partners to integrate a supply chain or a virtual organisation, negotiate, organise auctions and manage bids.
- *Electronic Commerce*, where agents can search for products /services, negotiate and manage the transaction, and organise bids, in an electronic marketplace.

Other applications could be referred, but are out of our scope of interest.

2.2 Electronic Automated Negotiation (e-Negotiation)

(Beam & Segev, 1997) define electronic automated negotiation as the process by which two or more parties multilaterally bargain resources for mutual intended gain, using the tools and techniques of electronic commerce in networked computers. Automated negotiation is difficult, namely because of: (1) the need for an ontology for categorizing objects, such that they are semantically meaningful to a software agent, and (2) the need for a algorithmic negotiation strategy.

The most basic form of e-Negotiation is no negotiation at al, i.e., fixed-price sale, where the seller offers the goods or services through a catalogue at take-it-or-leave-it prices. Other styles of negotiation are auctions, bilateral bargaining (which involves making proposals and counter-proposals until agreement is reached), combinatory auctions or direct negotiation within a small set of eligible resource providers (bilateral bargaining within a smaller domain manually performed).

Agent technology plays an important role in the automation of e-Negotiation.

2.3 Electronic Marketplaces (e-Marketplaces)

Firms exist to reduce the costs of negotiating, monitoring and executing transactions that are necessary to produce or acquire goods and services on the market. Market is the mechanism that allows buyers and sellers to change things. Its main characteristic is to link buyers and sellers to define prices and quantities. An Electronic Marketplace is an Internet-based environment where participants (buyers and sellers) can meet to exchange goods and services or to cooperate in order to achieve a common business goal. The economic benefits to firms are participation and value creation in wider market-like relationships organised electronically while reducing costs through automation of a higher volume of transactions.

Compared with other electronic procurement solutions, e-Marketplaces represent a relatively neutral position between buyer and seller, providing services to both sides of a transaction (Segev, Gebauer, & Beam, 1998). In a multiagent supported e-Marketplaces, where agents can meet to exchange services or trade with a variety of merchandise, the agents can represent various organisations and companies. A negotiation on price and quantity and a contract between two agents can be set up and the transaction carried out within minutes or even seconds.

2.4 Market Brokerage

The concept of broker, capable of acting on behalf of a customer in guiding the selection of the most suitable product, has long been well known and the extension of this concept to the electronic marketplace is a natural progression.

Market brokerage is a core concept to overcome the current limitations of e-Marketplaces, namely the problems of semantic matching and the coordination of the selection of resources to integrate in an A/V E (Cunha, Putnik, & Ávila, 2000). Appropriate brokerage services should support new market-led relationships between producers and consumers, where the large number of suppliers and customers are geographically separated, where there are many comparable products or when prices and product features or models change rapidly. A purpose of electronic brokerage is the reduction of costs of search and discovery mediated by a third party (the broker) for buyers and sellers of physical or logical goods and services within an e-marketplace (Bichler, 1998). Market brokerage can be performed with different degrees of automation, from manual or fully automated using intelligent agent technology. The importance of brokerage is discussed in the Reference Model proposed by (Putnik, 2000), and a detailed broker functions taxonomy can be found in (Ávila, Putnik, & Cunha, 2002).

3. ENVIRONMENTS TOWARDS VIRTUAL ENTERPRISE

We refer in this section some relevant environments contributing for A/V E integration, supporting any or all of the following functions: A/VE design, selection, negotiation and integration of resources into A/V E enterprises, and coordination functions. Examples include electronic marketplaces and agent-based brokerage.

3.1 Electronic Marketplaces

Recent years have seen a dramatic emerging of e-marketplaces for business opportunities and Internet-based online auctions. There exist several Electronic markets operating in a variety of industries, from industrial metals, chemicals, construction, textile and many others, distinguished by factors such as main focus or scope, revenue strategies, restriction to entry or openness (limitation on number of participants), contents in databases or references (degree of distributiveness of catalogues), degree of automation in negotiation, support to transactions, etc.

A valuable example is *Covisint* (http://www.covisint.com), an e-marketplace consisting on a Virtual Supplier Network (a service encompassing the complete interaction between suppliers or suppliers and their customers, using network technology) specifically created for the automotive industry. The service is projected to be a one-stop-shop, supporting procurement transactions, pre-production collaborative engineering and exchange of information during production or for supply chain management. *Covisint* was officially announced in December 2000 as an independent company, created by Ford, Chrysler, General Motors, Renault and Nissan and a number of development partners.

3.2 Agent-based Brokerage and Marketplaces

Agent-based approaches have been already applied for enterprise integration, manufacturing production planning, scheduling and process control, material handling for one decade. Several researchers have proposed the organisation of the supply chain as a network of cooperating, intelligent agents, just to mention:

- (Sauter & Parunak, 1999) proposed the Agent Network for Task Scheduling (ANTS) architecture with techniques inspired by both human institutions and insect colonies, in which large populations of simple agents support scheduling in supply chains;
- The project MetaMorph II (Shen & Norrie, 1998) proposed the use of hybrid agent-based architecture for manufacturing enterprise integration and supply chain management, i.e., a mediator-centric architecture to integrate partners, suppliers and customers dynamically with the main enterprise through their respective mediators within a supply chain network via the Internet.
- (Shen, Ulieru, Norrie, & Kremer, 1999) presented a case study of supply chain management for a large manufacturing enterprise, CASA, based on Collaborative Agent System Architecture;

The implementation of marketplaces based on Agents is also usual. Several projects have been found, such as:

- The experiment at BT Laboratories intends to build a broker-less marketplace based on agents (Collis & Lee, 1998a, 1998b). In this scenario, each agent will have the ability to contact every other agent and negotiate to buy and sell directly; this means there is no role for intermediary agents such as brokers.
- The OFFER Project (Object Framework for Electronic Requisitioning) (Bichler, Beam, & Segev, 1998) is an object framework for business-to-business electronic commerce that contains a CORBA-based electronic broker who assists the user in two ways during a market transaction: first, it helps search in many, often unknown electronic catalogs of suppliers; second, it provides auction mechanisms to support price negotiation between buyers and sellers.
- The Global Electronic Marketplace (GEM) (Rachlevsky-Reich & Ben-Shaul, 1999) is an electronic commerce platform containing a complex and distributed structure of trading facilities based on brokers and a central market server. GEM simulates a trading floor by bringing together and bids collected by the brokers.
- MAGMA (Minnesota Agent Marketplace Architecture) is an architecture for Agent-based virtual marketplace, providing all services essential to agent-based commercial activities, available through an open-standard messaging API, which allows use of a heterogeneous set of agents independently of platform and language (Tsvetovatyy, Gini, Mobaster, & Wieckowski, 1997).
- In the model for negotiation in virtual organisations formation proposed by (Oliveira & Rocha, 2000), when a specific consumer's need is identified, it is created a new agent that will formulate an announcement for goal satisfaction in the electronic marketplace, will receive and evaluate bids from potential suppliers of the product and negotiate in order to integrate the partnership.

However it was not possible to find many applications of this technology covering the whole process of enterprise selection, negotiation, integration, and coordination of integration.

4. MARKET OF RESOURCES AS A VIRTUAL ENTERPRISE INTEGRATION ENVIRONMENT

Three relevant requisites are identified in relation with the process of A/V E design or integration: (1) Flexible and almost instantaneous access to the independent candidate resources to integrate a virtual enterprise, negotiation process between them, selection of the optimal combination and its integration; (2) Design, negotiation, business management and manufacturing management functions independently from the physical barrier of space; and (3) Minimisation of the reconfiguration and integration time and cost. These requisites imply the existence of a market of independent candidate resources for integrating a virtual enterprise, able: (1) to provide the environment and technology for efficient access to resources, efficient negotiation between them and its efficient integration; and (2) to provide a domain for selection of participant resources in a virtual enterprise, large enough to assure a good combination of resources.

The concept of Market of Resources was introduced by the authors in (Cunha et al., 2000), as an electronic and virtual market, mediating offer and demand of resources to dynamically integrate in an A/V E. Enterprises (resources providers) subscribing the Market of Resources, make their resources available as potential servers /partners for A/V E integration. The Market of Resources supports the A/V E model proposed in the Virtual Enterprise Reference Model (BM-VEARM) by (Putnik, 2000).

The service provided by the Market of Resources is supported by (1) a knowledge base of resources and results of the integration of resources in previous A/V E, (2) a normalised representation of information and (3) intelligent agent and algorithms, (4) a brokerage service and (5) regulation, i.e. management of negotiation and integration processes. It is able to offer (1) knowledge for A/V E selection of resources, negotiation and its integration, (2) specific functions of A/V E operation management, and (3) contracts and formalising procedures to assure the accomplishment of commitments, responsibility, trust and deontological aspects, envisaging that the integrated A/V E accomplishes its objectives of answering to a market opportunity. The environment supports not only the ***integration*** process, but, what is most important when the fast and proficient reaction to change is a key element, is able to effectively support ***dynamic integration***, which is the main reason for the concept of Market of Resources as an institution.

5. CONCLUSIONS

Although it was not possible an exhaustive review, we tried to present the main developments and contributions towards the creation of environments able to support the processes of A/V E (design and) integration. We were able to conclude that all the required technologies and techniques already exist, most of them dispersedly developed, as well as many valuable applications are already in operation, however there is missing what we designate as an adequate ***environment*** to support the inherent need of dynamics required by the emerging paradigm of

A/V E. Market of Resources was conceived precisely to "boost" the dynamics as well as to support the high dynamics of the A/V E reconfiguration and integration[3].

The table bellow summarises the contribution of each technology/technique and of each environment on the main Virtual Enterprise models: Electronic Commerce, Supply Chain, Extended Enterprise, BM_VEARM and OPIM (One Product Integrated Manufacturing), (Putnik, Guimarães, & Silva, 1996). It is also referred the importance of reconfigurability dynamics for each VE model.

The Market of Resources is proposed as an ideal environment to support the requirement of fast adaptability of the most dynamic VE models life cycle (BM_VEARM and OPIM), while the other environments are designed to cope only VE models that do not require a high reconfigurability dynamics.

		Technologies / Techniques				**Environments**			Importance of reconfig. dynamics
		Agents Technol	*Electr. Negot.*	*Market places*	*Market Broker.*	*Electron. Marketp.*	*Agent Broker.*	*Market Resour.*	
VE Models	e-commerce		x	x		x	x		low
	Supply chain	x	x	x		x	x		medium
	Extended Enterprise	x	x	x	x	x	x		medium
	BM_VEARM	x	x	x	x			x	high
	OPIM	x	x	x	x			x	high
Ability to support fast reconfigurability						low	low/med	high	

6. REFERENCES

1. Ávila, P., Putnik, G. D., & Cunha, M. M. (2002). Brokerage Function in Agile/Virtual Enterprise Integration - A Literature Review. In L. M. Camarinha-Matos (Ed.), *Collaborative Business Ecosystems and Virtual Enterprises*: Kluwer Academic Publishers.
2. Beam, C., & Segev, A. (1997). *Automated Negotiations: A Survey of the State of the Art.* Retrieved, June 2001, from the World Wide Web: http://www.haas.berkeley.edu/~citm/nego-proj.html/
3. Bichler, M. (1998). An Electronic Broker to Business-to-Business Electronic Commerce on the Internet. *International Journal of Cooperative Information Systems, 7*(4).
4. Bichler, M., Beam, C., & Segev, A. (1998). OFFER: A Broker-Centered Object Framework for Electronic Requisitioning, *Proceedings of IFIP Conference: Trends in Electronic Commerce*. Hamburg, Germany.
5. Browne, J., & Zhang, J. (1999). Extended and Virtual Enterprises: similarities and differences. *International Journal of Agile Management Systems, 1/1*, 30-36.
6. Collis, J. C., & Lee, L. C. (1998a, May 1998). *Building Electronic Marketplaces with the Zeus Agent Toolkit.* Paper presented at the Workshop of the Agents'98 2nd International Conference on Autonomous Agents, Minneapolis, USA.
7. Collis, J. C., & Lee, L. C. (1998b). *Building Electronic Marketplaces with the Zeus Agent Toolkit.* Suffolk, UK: Intelligent Systems Research Unit, BT Laboratories.
8. Cunha, M. M., & Putnik, G. D. (2002). Discussion on Requirements for Agile/Virtual Enterprises Reconfigurability Dynamics: The Example of the Automotive Industry. In L. M. Camarinha-Matos (Ed.), *Collaborative Business Ecosystems and Virtual Enterprises*: Kluwer Academic Publishers.
9. Cunha, M. M., Putnik, G. D., & Ávila, P. (2000). Towards Focused Markets of Resources for Agile / Virtual Enterprise Integration. In H. Afsarmanesh (Ed.), *Proceedings of the 4th IEEE/IFIP International Conference on Information Technology for Balanced Automation Systems in Manufacturing and Transportation*. Berlin: Kluwer Academic Publishers.

10. Cunha, M. M., Putnik, G. D., & Gunasekaran, A. (2002). Market of Resources as an Environment for Agile / Virtual Enterprise Dynamic Integration and Business Alignment. In A. Gunasekaran (Ed.), *Knowledge and Information Technology Management in the 21st Century Organisations: Human and Social Perspectives*. London: Idea Group Publishing.
11. Jennings, N. R., Farantin, P., Johnson, M. J., O'Brien, P., & Wiegand, M. E. (1996). Agent-based Business Process Management. *International Journal of Cooperative Information Systems, 5*(2-3), 105-130.
12. Jennings, N. R., & Wooldridge, M. (1998). Applications of Intelligent Agents. In M. Wooldrodge (Ed.), *Agent Technology: Foundations, Applications and Markets*: Springer-Verlag.
13. MIT_Media_Lab. (2001, May 2001). *Projects*. Software Agents Group, Massachusetts Institute of Technology. Retrieved December 2001, from the World Wide Web:
14. Oliveira, E. (1999). *Applications of Intelligent Agent-Based Systems*. Paper presented at the 4° Simpósio Brasileiro de Automação Inteligente, SBAI, São Paulo, SP.
15. Oliveira, E., & Rocha, A. P. (2000). Agents advanced features for negotiation in Electronic Commerce and Virtual Organisations formation process. In C. Sierra (Ed.), *Agent Mediated Electronic Commerce, the European AgentLink Perspective, Lectures Notes in Artificial Intelligence* (Vol. 1991, pp. 77-96): Springer-Verlag.
16. Putnik, G. (2000). BM_Virtual Enterprise Architecture Reference Model. In A. Gunasekaran (Ed.), *Agile Manufacturing: 21st Century Manufacturing Strategy* (pp. 73-93). UK: Elsevier Science Publ.
17. Putnik, G. D., Guimarães, P. F., & Silva, S. d. C. (1996). Virtual Enterprise / OPIM Concepts: an institutionalization framework. In H. Afsarmanesk (Ed.), *Proceedings of the 2nd IEEE/ECLA/IFIP International Conference on Architectures and Design Methods for Balanced Automation Systems* (pp. 391-400). Portugal: Chapman & Hall.
18. Rachlevsky-Reich, B., & Ben-Shaul, I. (1999). GEM: A Global Electronic Market System. *Information Systems, 24*(6), 495-518.
19. Sauter, J. A., & Parunak, R. (1999, May 1999). *ANTS in the Supply Chain*. Paper presented at the Agent's 99 Workshop on Agent-Based Decision Support for Managing the Internet-Enabled Supply Chain, Seattle.
20. Segev, A., Gebauer, J., & Beam, C. (1998). *Procurement in the Internet Age - Current Practices and Emerging Trends (Results from a field study)* (CMIT Working Paper 98-WP-1033). Berkeley, CA: Fisher Center for Management and Information Technology, University of California at Berkeley.
21. Shen, W., & Norrie, D. H. (1998). An Agent-Based Approach for Manufacturing Enterprise Integration and Supply Chain Management. In G. J. e. al (Ed.), *Globalization of Manufacturing in Digital Communications Era of the 21st Century: Innovation, Agility and the Virtual Enterprise* (pp. 579-590): Kluwer Academic Publishers.
22. Shen, W., Ulieru, M., Norrie, D. H., & Kremer, R. (1999, May 1999). *Implementing the Internet-Enabled Supply Chain Through a Collaborative Agent System*. Paper presented at the Agent's 99 Workshop on Agent-Based Decision Support for Managing the Internet-Enabled Supply Chain, Seattle.
23. Tsvetovatyy, M., Gini, M., Mobaster, B., & Wieckowski, Z. (1997). MAGMA: An Agent-based Virtual Market for Electronic Commerce. *Journal of Applied Artificial Intelligence, 11*(Special Issue on Intelligent Agents).
24. Wooldridge, M. (1997). Agent-based Software Engineering. *IEE Proc. Software Engineering, 144*, 26-37.
25. Wooldridge, M., & Jennings, N. R. (1995). Agent Theories, Architectures and Languages: A Survey. In N. R. Jennings (Ed.), *Intelligent Agents: Theories, Architectures and Languages* (Vol. LNAI Vol 890, pp. 1-39). Heidelberg, Germany: Springer-Verlag.

---

[1] Understanding A/V E integration as including the processes of selection and negotiation between candidate resources and the integration of the selected resources.

[2] For detailed descriptions of agents theory, architectures and languages we suggest (Wooldridge & Jennings, 1995) and for agents applications, (Jennings, Farantin, Johnson, O'Brien, & Wiegand, 1996; Jennings & Wooldridge, 1998; Oliveira, 1999), among many other valuable sources of information. The MIT Media Lab site provides interesting and valuable information on underway research projects at MIT's Software Agents Research Group (MIT_Media_Lab, 2001).

[3] We did not address the issues of emerging standards for interoperability and information interchange, Internet protocols and other essential infrastructures, as we were concerned, in the present work, with the technologies and environments supporting A/V E integration.

15

E-SERVICES FOR VIRTUAL ENTERPRISE BROKERAGE

Ricardo Mejía, Joaquín Aca, Eunice García, Arturo Molina
CSIM-ITESM
Ave. Eugenio Garza Sada 2501 Sur
Monterrey, N.L. 64849 Mexico
rmejia@tamayo.mty.itesm.mx, jaca@tamayo.mty.itesm.mx
iegarcia@tamayo.mty.itesm.mx, armolina@campus.mty.itesm.mx

Nowadays the global competitive environment has special impact on Virtual Business development. A special issue related to the exploitation of global business opportunities is the role played by Information Technologies in Virtual Enterprises. There have been several e-application developments to support key processes of a Virtual Enterprise Broker (VEB). However, it is important to design and develop not only e-applications, but also e-Services that are easy to implement and have an impact in the performance of VEB activities. This paper describes a methodology to evaluate, structure and implement e-Services in order to assure that these applications will improve the operations of the VE. These e-services will demonstrate how their implementation improve the performance of the VEB activities in the creation of Integrated Supply Chains between Small and Medium Enterprises (members of Virtual Industry Clusters) to OEMs (Original Equipment Manufacturers).

1. INTRODUCTION

In the actual global competitive environment, big companies are taking more care about their sourcing strategies and they are demanding quality and shorter cycle times at the best price. Therefore, the Virtual Enterprise Broker (VEB) must improve its process of business opportunities exploitation, in order to take advantage of the huge amount of opportunities that global sourcing might offer. These aspects are very important not only for mass production but also for special projects or product outsourcing to potential suppliers. Large firms like, OEM and Maquiladoras[1] offer to the VEB the challenge to explore new strategies and redefine how new business can be exploited.

A VEB must use available resources from partners to form a business entity by means of network communication technology. The Information Technology enlarges the working space to globalization and sets up a new type of enterprise through Internet. The change of organization form requires the corresponding

[1] Maquiladoras are international manufacturing companies established in other countries with special taxes agreements.

management technology, thus it should seek a new management model and technology to fit the implementation of Virtual Enterprises (VE).

The supportive role of Information Technology for handling information is particularly important because nothing else (people, parts, products, machines) can act if information is not accessible to make decisions. To the extent that information should be handled in a efficient and effective manner in order to allow the flows of inputs into, through and out of manufacturing systems be improved (Gunasekaran and McGaughey, 2002). Information Technologies can optimize and support the core processes carried out by the VEB in order to fulfill customer needs through the creation of Virtual Enterprises. VE will be the efficient organization form in the future, due to the rapid development of computer techniques and information technology (Xu et. al., 2002).

2. VIRTUAL ENTERPRISE BROKER CORE PROCESS

The Virtual Enterprise Broker (VEB) performs an important role in virtual enterprises development, being the entity responsible of create, manage and dissolve a VE in order to exploit global business opportunities. The activities carried out by the VEB through its Core Processes are very important for the fulfillment of customer requirements. Therefore, the creation of new tools to support VEB activities is an important area of research in order to improve the VE performance. Four core processes have been defined to support VEB activities (Mejía and Molina, 2002): Analysis of Market Requirements, Project Planning, Project execution and Customer Service (Follow-up). The main tasks carried out by the VEB can be analyzed through the Virtual Enterprise Life Cycle that is divided into five main phases: Identification, Formation, Design, Operation and Dissolution (Kanet et. al., 1999). The broker in a VE is foremost a member of the enterprise. It acts as an information broker, an initiator of business by recognizing new opportunities and exploiting them through searching and choosing appropriate, competent and complementary partners. It is the coordinator of the VE and moderator during the execution/operation of the VE's mission and is the primary point of contact for customers of the VE. Information Technologies are necessary to support key activities related to the VEB processes. Furthermore, the process of creating VE's is composed of tasks that can be facilitated by specific computer applications in order to achieve the automation of some of the VEB core processes.

In the Virtual Industry Clusters (VIC, 2001) there have been several e-application developments to support the activities carried out by the Virtual Enterprise Broker (VEB). Those e-applications support VEB activities in order to have the right information, at the right moment, in the right place. Some applications are: Enterprise Core Competence Database, Enterprise Capability Broker Matrix and Broker Capacity Planning Tool (Mejía and Molina, 2002). All these applications are computer based tools, but are not e-services, as shown in figure 1. In our research, an e-service is the integration of e-applications to offer a brokerage service by the VEB.

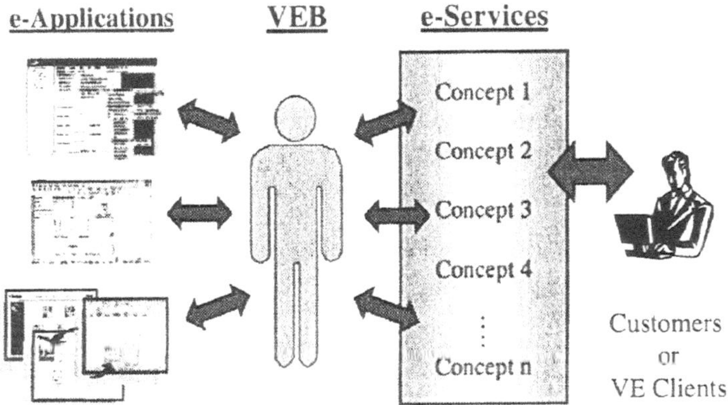

Figure 1 – e-Applications and e–Services concepts

3. METHODOLOGY

The methodology described here allows the VEB to evaluate and design different e-services in a systematic form, in order to implement those e-services with high potential to improve VE performance.

3.1 Conceptualization

This phase is focused on Brainstorming for potential e-services, where concepts generated at this stage must be classified in five categories:

a) *Information*. It implies information, as laws, news, technological innovations, etc. Its implementation is very easy with a low business impact. It is a time depending tool, requiring actualization over the time.
b) *Community*. It implies interaction with experts or lead users of different industries in order to share experiences to take advantage in productive process. It is easy to implement and medium impact in the business.
c) *Directories*. It implies access to manufacturers and providers databases. It is medium difficulty implementation and impact business.
d) *Collaboration*. It implies the dynamic interaction between parties of the project in order to manage it. It is difficult to implement and it has medium to high impact in the business.
e) *Process facilitation*. It implies the automation of key activities using a specific technological tool. This is very difficult to implement, but it has high impact.

It is necessary to decide which concepts are going to continue through the evaluation process. Depending on the actual organization needs, the broker use two main criteria to decide which idea is going to be the most feasible: "*Easy implementation*" and "*business impact*", based on the Cisco Methodology "Net Ready" (Hartman and Sifonis, 2000).

3.2 Evaluation

All brainstormed e-services within a chosen category are evaluated individually through the Cisco Methodology again at this stage. The results should be reflected in a graph like in Figure 2. In this case Concept 4 is considered as "quick wins" and

Concept 5 is considered as "hanging fruit". A concept is selected and the next step is evaluating the concept regard two variables:

- *Process issues*: Cost effects, Optimize channel structure, National coverage, Channel fragmentation reduction and Partner integration.
- *Economical issues*: Superior service, Business support, Time reduction cycle and Knowledge / cluster intelligence.

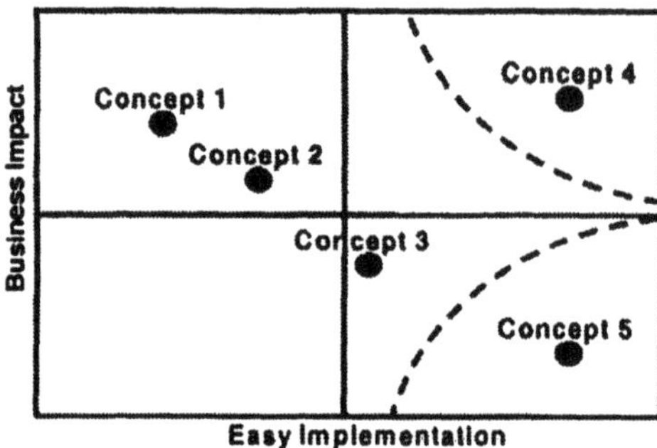

Figure 2 – Evaluation graph for e–services concepts

3.3 Process Modeling

An e-service is the automation of a given methodology or process. Depending on the level of detail, the modeling of the process is going to be more complex, and is important for the application developer to achieve the necessary level in order to design an effective e-service. In our research the VEB processes are structured but not detailed. The experts are in charge of modeling and structuring VEB processes in order to design an automated application. The process modeling has two levels: a) first level defines the activities, deliverables and resources of the process, the result is a list process; b) second level is the flow diagram for each process (see Figure 3).

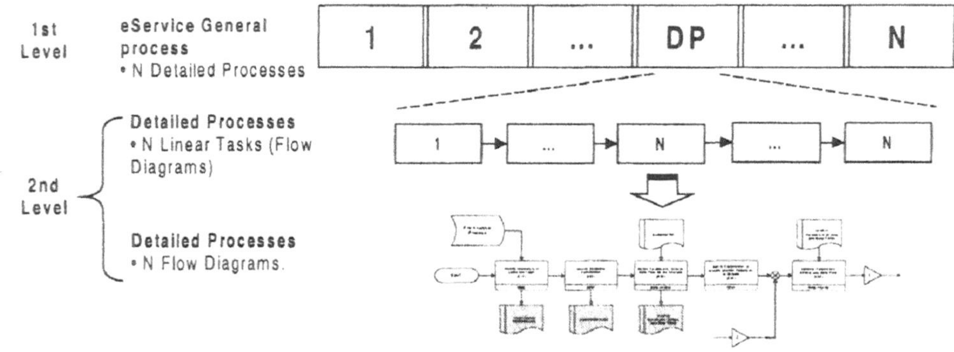

Figure 3 – e-service process modeling

3.4 Applications Selection

This stage is the identification, evaluation and selection of e-application vendors. The application must be represented in functional structure in order to evaluate performance functionality for each vendor. The valuation matrix and valuation symbols are show in Figure 4.

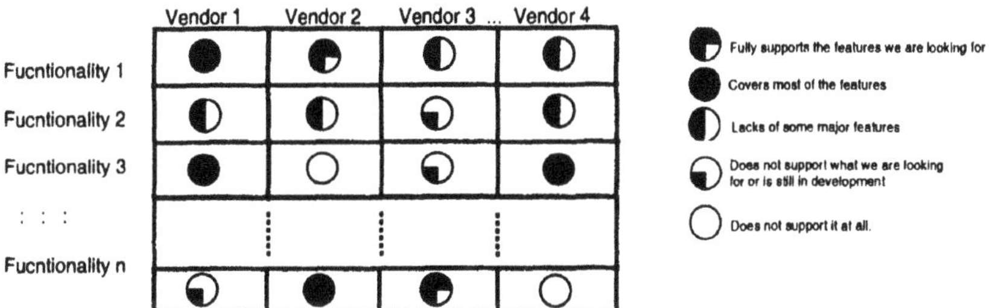

Figure 4 – Matrix valuation and valuation symbols

3.5 Infrastructure Design

Detailed descriptions of the technological requirements of the e-application are selected at this stage. The technical and economical feasibility is checked until technical diagrams are done. The infrastructure design is the architecture definition, and some metrics for the environment must be considered:

- *Technology*: Supports latest standards?, is a proven solution?, differentiates the product from other vendors?, is it robust?, allows fail-over, redundancy?, supports major OS platforms?
- *Integration*: Supports open standards?, is an integrated solution?, can the product be easily connected with other systems?, is it easy to migrate? Has the product support from middleware vendors?, can we easily connect it with other modules of the architecture?
- *Scalability*: Is the product designed for a scalable scenario?, does it support clustering?, has a record of proven scalable solutions?, is it recognized in the market as a scalable solution?
- *Support of package applications*: Is it easy to integrate new packaged applications?, do major vendors support the product?, has a proven record of incorporating packaged applications?
- *Development Tools, time to market (TTM)*: Has development tools designed specially for the product?, is it easy to develop new applications with the product using the existing tools?, development cycle reduces time to market?, requires high technical skills?, are the development tools integrated among them?, and with the product?

3.6 Roadmap Implementation

The last stage of the methodology is the implementation of the e-application. The tasks covered in this process are:

- *Verification Test:* Stand-alone installation verification and the Interfaces installation must be done.
- *Users Acceptance Test:* LAB installation and verification, Building all possible scenarios and running by key users.
- *Beta Test (Soft launch):* Some enterprises are selected for Beta Test mode. The employees are trained and ran a pilot event. Logistic arrangements are made and the last step is the invitation to all enterprises.
- *Go-Live:* Intensive technical support at the first weeks, Extensive technical support during the next weeks, continuous remote and physical assistance per request, performance management tracking & report.

4. CASE STUDY

Using the methodology described above, a list of new concepts and ideas was generated in order to select those e-services with high potential into the VE environment considering the Mexican SME characteristics. However, the time for implementation depends on the complexity of the applications to be developed and if it is systems configuration or new development. From that list, four e-services were selected through the proposed methodology in order to be designed and implemented for the brokerage activities in the Virtual Industry Cluster. Two e-services were related to "Process facilitation e-services": e-RFQ and e-selection; and two for "Collaboration e-services": e-inspection and e-fax communication.

4.1 e-RFQ (Electronic Request for Quotation):

Time and accuracy can define a new business opportunity, needing an application that reduces quotation time through automated quotation services over a web-based tool. These tools reduce administrative time spent on creating and issuing manual RFQ´s and negotiating with suppliers using phone calls, faxes and face-to-face meetings.

Quotation knowledge automation is needed, allowing customers to fill standard RFQ or specially products or process RFQ. That process is shown in Figure 5, where the standard RFQ goes trough a module specially designed in order to receive an automated quotation. The special products RFQ must go through the VEB, and then distributed among evaluated and selected cluster members. Then, the VEB send the quotation to the client. However the Client-Broker communication is still optimized.

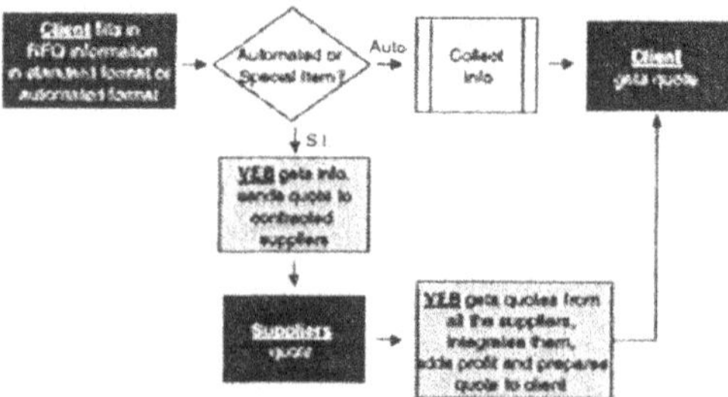

Figure 5 – e-RFQ Process Map

4.2 e-Selection:

One of the most important activities carried out by the VEB is the *partner selection*. The companies involved in the project execution are the direct responsible of the product manufacture obligating the VEB to consider, from the first stages of its Core Process, the potential players to be evaluated in order to satisfy customer requirements.

Thereby the VEB needs a technological enabler with the capability to identify, select, communicate and establish a formal agreement among the partners involved in a specific project. Also allow partners ranking for future players selections based on previous performance. Four main processes were defined for the players selection service, as shown in Figure 6.

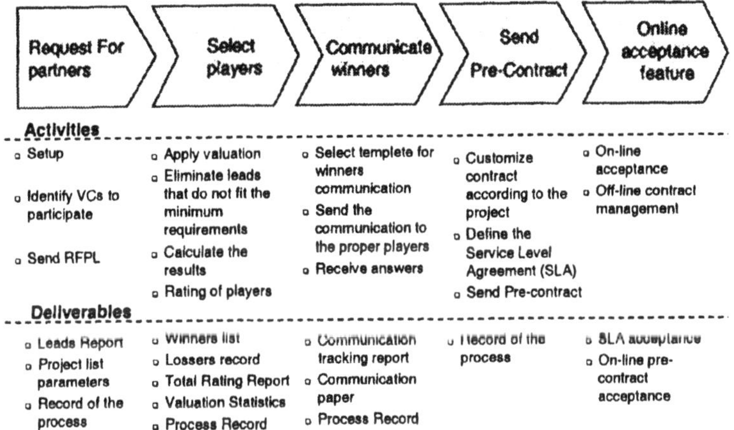

Figure 6 – e-Selection main processes

4.3 e-Inspection:

It is common to have foreign customers, where the auditing costs are high because the travel expenses. To allow customers to follow-up their products, a web-based service is proposed trough a video camera to visually inspect products, as they are being created and tested in the supplier's factory.

Virtual Inspection will be available to customers through a web interface providing virtual auditing sessions with a Web-cam based tool. The remote interviewing between customers and Mexican Small and Medium companies (SME´s) provides: A) Customer experience related to inspection, B) Customer travel time & expenses decreasing and C) Reduction in customer notification period (Cycle time reducing)

4.4 e-Fax Communication:

One of the most common problems for Virtual Industry Clusters Management is the lack of Internet culture. The micro and small industries are tended to conventional communication services for doing business, as face-to-Face, Telephone and Fax.

The proposed service will act like a bridge between the "online" and the "traditional telephony" worlds, by allowing the conversion of web-generated information requests into faxes. This application will promote the e-culture in the SME´s working as a warning that an important e-mail arrives, due to the fact that SME´s owners will receive simultaneously a Fax with the information on the e-mail.

This e-service is easy to implement because it is a low cost communication solution by assembling "off the shelf" existing web services to be paid depending on usage. It will be accomplished by "assembling" different functionalities provided by different and remote ASP (Application Service Providers). In this scenario each company will provide a value that is complementary to reach the final required service: Web-Form Application and Email Translation and Fax Forwarding as shown in Figure 7.

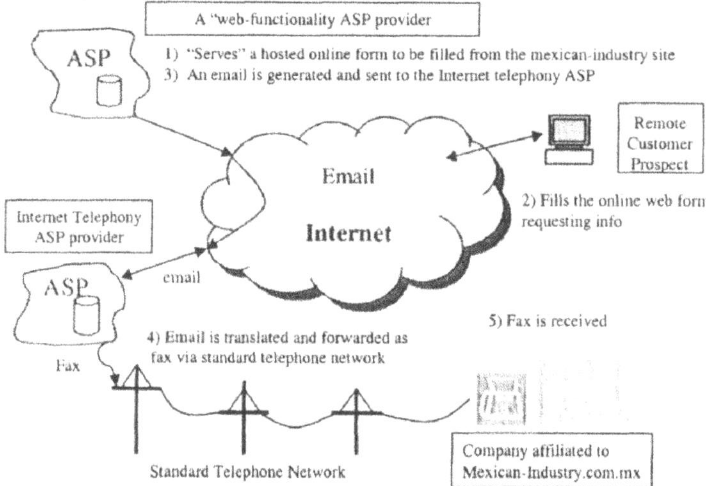

Figure 7 – "Off the shelf" e-Fax communication

5. CONCLUSION

Information technologies can support the development of e-services that support brokerage processes in Virtual Enterprises. In this paper a systematic methodology has been defined in order to develop e-services, which have major impacts on the VEB operations. These e-services also must offer a value added to customers that are looking for brokerage services. The proposed methodology allows VEBs, not only to identify new services concepts, but also to design and implement potential ideas into automated services. Four examples of e-services are described that are the results of applying the methodology and assuring that they will impact the performance of the VEB services.

6. ACKNOWLEDGMENTS

The authors gratefully acknowledge the contribution to this work of the Masters students on Global e-Management (GEM) at the EGADE business school, from the Monterrey Institute of Technology (ITESM).

7. REFERENCES

1. Hartman and Sifonis. "Net ready: Strategies for success in e-conomy", McGraw Hill. N.Y., 2000.
2. Gunasekaran A. and McGaughey R. "Information technology/information systems in 21st century manufacturing", International Journal of Productions Economics, 2002. pp. 1-6.
3. Kanet J., Faisst W. and Mertens P. "Application of information technology to a virtual enterprise broker: The case of Bill Epstein". International Journal of Production Economics, 1999. pp. 23-32.
4. Mejia R. and Molina A. "Virtual Enterprise Broker: Process, Methods and Tools", 3rd IFIP Working Conference on Infrastructures for Virtual Enterprises (PRO-VE'02), Portugal, 2002. pp. 81-90.
5. Xu W., Wei Y. and Fan Y. "Virtual Enterprise and its intelligence management", Institute of Policy and Management, Chinese Academy of Sciences, Computers & Industrial Engineering, 2002. pp. 199-205
6. VIC Web Site (2001), (http://www.mexican-industry.com)

16

COMPETITOR BASED STRATEGIC NETWORKS OF SME

Michel Pouly[*], Rémy Glardon[**], Charles Huber[***]
[*] *MTO Network / Swiss Federal Institute of Technology, Lausanne*
michel.pouly@epfl.ch
[**] *MTO Network / Swiss Federal Institute of Technology, Lausanne*
remy.glardon@epfl.ch
[***] *MTO Network / ZPA, Fachhochschule Aargau*
ch.huber@fh-aargau.ch

Small subcontracting companies have difficulty getting in touch with large customers which drastically reduce the number of their suppliers to those able to provide a complete service. Setting up strategic networks is a new way of doing business where companies which are normally competitors can successfully cooperate to address new markets they will never be able to address alone. This paper presents a methodology for creating competitor based strategic networks as well as a case study showing how this methodology has been applied to set up Swiss Microtech, the first network in the screw machining domain.

1. INTRODUCTION

Networks of enterprises can be set up for different reasons. Some of the most frequently used models are (Brütsch, 1999) :

- *virtual factories*, aiming to optimise the load of the production resources of its members to enhance their overall competitivity
- *vertical networks* built around companies working in the same domain but at different stages of a product
- *virtual enterprises* built around complementary companies wishing to cooperate to develop and manufacture new products
- *strategic networks* built around competitors wishing to cooperate to enter new markets they would not be able to address alone

The main difference between strategic networks and the other forms of alliances is the fact that the future partners see each other as competitors, at least at the beginning of the project. Thus, the main challenge is to build up enough trust to share the information required to run the network. A certain amount of transparency concerning the current and future workload as well as pricing data is a prerequisite, but such information is normally kept confidential.

This paper presents a methodology for creating a competitor based strategic network of SME. A real case study will illustrate the developed concepts.

2. ELEMENTS OF A COMPETITOR BASED STRATEGIC NETWORK

Two basic elements are required to create such a network (see figure 1) :

- the industrial cluster
- the virtual enterprises

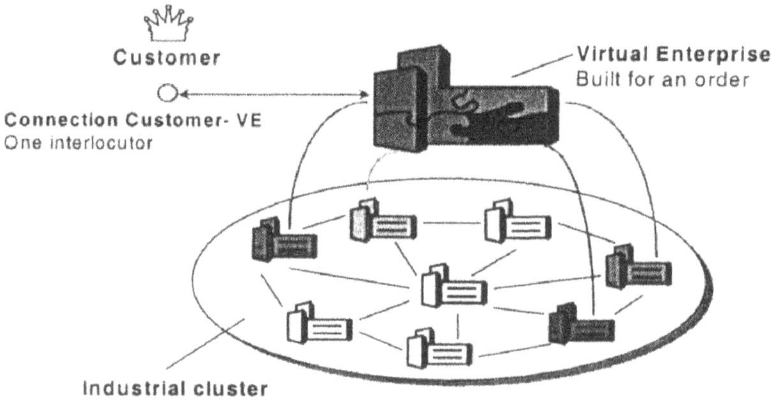

Figure 1 – Elements of a competitor based strategic network

2.1 The Industrial Cluster

The industrial cluster is the backbone of a strategic network. The cluster members are independent enterprises which are and will remain competitors within their own markets but will also be partners to enter new markets they will not be able to address alone (for instance because they are too small or too far away from these markets).

Selecting the members of the initial cluster is a key process during the creation of such a network (Flores et. al, 2000).

These members should :

- bring a certain amount of complementarities at the technical (machine park, technological know-how etc.) and economical (markets, products etc.) levels; the alliance is then better suited to fulfil the customer needs than any individual partner alone
- have a similar level of quality, for instance an ISO 9000 certification
- share a common approach of doing business with customers, suppliers, partners and competitors (common business ethic)
- be deeply convinced that an alliance is really a solution for the future and be ready to give something before receiving

Other enterprises bringing complementary competencies will also join the cluster to be able to provide a complete solution to the customers.

2.2 Virtual Enterprises Based on the Cluster

Virtual enterprises will be set up around cluster members to fulfil a customer need in an optimal way. The best-suited enterprises will join together to realize an order for the lowest costs and within the required delay. Once the order is delivered, the corresponding virtual enterprise may be dissolved or take other new orders.

3. METHODOLOGY TO CREATE A COMPETITOR BASED STRATEGIC NETWORK

The proposed methodology is based on the four following modules :

- strategy
- structure and roles
- business processes and rules
- business plan

3.1 The Strategy

As the cluster members are and will also remain competitors within their own markets, a clear strategy must be defined. This module must give an answer to the following questions :

- definition of the expectations of the customers : this is a key issue as the network, like any other business, will only succeed if it meets the needs of the potential customers and brings significant advantages ! These can be lower costs, shorter delays, complete heterogeneous orders, engineering services and so on
- definition of the market/product segments to be addressed by the network and those remaining in the competition area
- definition of the industrial cluster as defined here above

3.2 Structure and Roles

Even a light construction like a network needs a minimal structure to work. The proposed structure is based on *roles* (Katzy et. al, 1996, Schuh et. al, 1998). A role is a function, which must be fulfilled by one or more persons. Four main roles have been identified (see figure 2) :

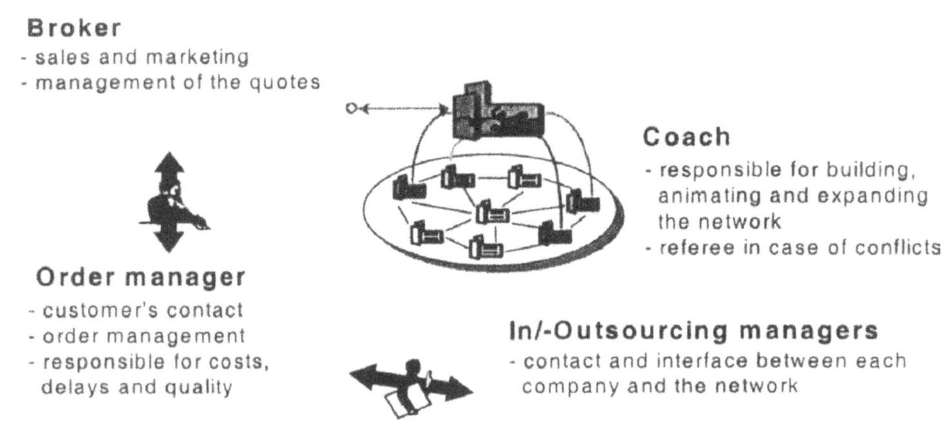

Figure 2 – Roles within the virtual enterprise

1. In-/Outsourcing Managers

Each enterprise belonging to the cluster must appoint an In-/Outsourcing Manager responsible for the contacts within the network. The I/O manager receives the requests for quotation from the brokers and prepares the bids in case of interest.

As reaction time is important for a customer, he is responsible for a timely answer. He is also the contact person for the order manager within a virtual enterprise his company is participating in. Finally, he represents his company within the cluster.

2. The Coach

The responsibility of the coach is the animation of the network. He will prospect and evaluate new possible cluster members, organize the information and knowledge transfer and also be the referee in case of problems between cluster members or within a virtual enterprise.

3. The Order Manager

Once a quote is transformed into an order, the Order Manager will take over the responsibility up to the delivery and beyond. He will be the unique business partner for the customer and must set up and pilot the virtual enterprise built for this particular job. He is responsible for the delays, costs and quality of the order as well as for the commercial part (internal and external invoices).

Someone working for the company having the biggest share of the order will normally take the role of the Order Manager.

4. The Broker

The broker « sells » the network to the potential customers and manages the requests for quotations. He will select the enterprises able to realize the possible order in the most economical way (best suited machines, know-how, remaining free capacity and so on) and ask for bids. He is also responsible for preparing and following the quotations until transformation into a possible order.

5. The work groups

Work groups can also be created to address particular problems in a smaller circle and propose solutions for the cluster. Possible work groups are : common purchases, IT solutions and so on.

3.3 Business Processes and Rules

Once the roles have been determined, it is necessary to define the main business processes (Schönsleben, 1998) as well as the corresponding responsibilities :

- incoming requests for quotation : acceptance or not
- transmission of the accepted requests for quotation : distribution and reception of the internal bids
- preparation of a quotation and follow-up
- incoming order : order confirmation and set up of the corresponding virtual enterprise
- order follow up : engineering, production, delivery, invoicing and repartition of the payment
- after sales service and warranty
- dissolution of the virtual enterprise

The rules of the game must also be defined for the cluster :

- membership (acceptance, begin, end, exclusion)
- rights and duties of the members (chart)
- fees and other contributions of the members
- juridical form of the cluster, corporate identity
- treatment of conflicts

3.4 Business Plan

A business plan for the first 2-3 years must be prepared using for instance three scenarios :

- limited success
- probable success
- important success

4. CASE STUDY : SWISS MICROTECH, SCREW MACHINING STRATEGIC NETWORK

Originally, the screw machining industry in the Swiss Jura region was a supplier of parts for the clock and watch industry. Many family based very small and small enterprises (from 10 to 100 employees) produced parts for just a couple of customers. The industrial culture was based on individualism and mistrust; the competition was for them the neighbour workshop. A survey executed in 1998 (Bigoni et. al, 1998) showed the difficulties faced by this branch :

- these small companies were unable to get in touch with large customers of the automobile, electronics and medical branches which drastically reduced the number of their suppliers to those able to provide a complete delivery including engineering, machining, thermal treatments and assembly
- these SME were technically up to date, but their commercial services were lacking
- their delivery schedules were too long and not very reliable

Following the recommendations of this survey, 10 enterprises belonging to the same professional association decided to join an applied research project aiming to develop a competitor based strategic network.

4.1 Towards the Creation of the Network

The first step was the definition of the strategy : the expectations of potential customers were gathered by the way of a questionnaire-based survey followed by interviews with selected potential customers. Following results emerged :

- 70% of the potential customers just needed classical subcontracting relationships. They expected a better price, shorter but over all more reliable delays and the ability to deliver large heterogeneous orders (all kind of materials, lengths and diameters) combined with further machining (drilling, threading etc.) and thermal treatments. They further demanded a unique interlocutor responsible for the whole order
- 30% of the potential customers wished to develop a closer partnership with their subcontractors by delegating the industrialization of parts. For them, using the production know-how of the suppliers is a good way of reducing their costs. It is very interesting for a supplier to penetrate deeper into the value added chain of

its customers as it is a way to bind them and as services often yields more revenues than pure fabrication operations

- a large majority of the potential customers would have no problems in doing business with a virtual enterprise they considered as an interesting model for the future
- even if classical communication methods (phone, fax, letters) stayed at the top, e-mails ranked close behind

The definition of the product and market segments to be addressed by the network was directly derived from these results. Even if e-market places are still rare in the segment of special mechanical parts, the project showed that something is still going on in this domain. The 10 enterprises members of the project group naturally formed the initial industrial cluster.

The structure, roles and business processes were defined as explained here above and have been tested by simulation during 4 months. The role of broker was split between the salesmen and representatives of each participating member and the coach who is responsible for all direct inquiries as well as e-market places activities. Finally, the rules of the game were summarized in a chart to be signed by every partner.

4.2 The Crisis

After one year, when the time had arrived to formally create the network, half of the initial cluster members decided to leave the project. Mistrust and fears were stronger then the desire of collaboration. The four most committed members decided to continue until the creation of Swiss Microtech Enterprise Network, which was officially announced at the end of June 2001. The last activities within the frame of the project were :

- Definition of the legal form (statutes, bodies, registration of the name)
- Corporate identity (logo, website : http://www.swissmicrotech.ch
- Communication (press, professional journals etc.)

4.3 First Experience

During the first six months of existence, 10 enterprises applied for membership. The first most important success was reached when 3 partners decided to buy together new washing machines and received a very interesting quantity rebate, enough to cover the project costs.

5. CONCLUSIONS

The main objectives of this research project were to develop a methodology that can be used to create competitor based strategic networks and to apply this methodology to create a first network for the screw machining industry. Such networks can really help SME to address important markets they would never be able to address alone as the trend towards further reduction of suppliers to those able to provide complete deliveries will certainly continue (Guide européen des alliances, 1998). These networks can also reduce the production costs through common grouped purchases of raw material, tools, machines and services. Adding services like development and industrialization of parts allows a deeper penetration into the value added chain of the customers, a way to becoming an important partner instead of remaining just a supplier.

The creation of a competitor based strategic network must be initiated by the future members themselves, they must fully support the project and share a common business ethic. Members participating only to get some advantage in the case of success really jeopardize the project as mutual trust and readiness to share confidential information quickly disappear. The chosen strategy must represent a "win-win" situation for each member; no doubts or second thoughts should be left. Conflicts of interests must be thoroughly discussed and an acceptable consensus must be reached before going on. Technical issues like the structure of the network, the roles, the business processes and the necessary IT tools are easier to define. It is also important for the motivation to quickly reach an initial success like a first order or an interesting common purchase. Building trust between the future partners requires important personal contacts that can be established during meetings, workshops and reciprocal company visits.

The creation of Swiss Microtech Enterprise Network is an important step for the screw machining industry in the Swiss Jura region. It shows that it is better to share opportunities than to stay in a splendid isolation and finally disappear.

6. ACKNOWLEDGMENTS

The authors would like to thank the ten enterprises members of the project group and their professional association for their commitment and support. The authors would also like to thank the CTDT (Centre Technique du Décolletage et Taillage) for its outstanding technical support as well as the Commission for Technology and Innovation of the Swiss Federal Government, which funded this research.

7. REFERENCES

1.Bigoni P, Glardon R, Pouly M, Décolletage dans l'arc jurassien, Rappport final CTI, 1998
2.Brütsch, David, Virtuelle Unternehmen, v/d/f Hochschulverlag an der ETH Zürich, 1999
3.Flores M, Molina A, Virtual Industry Clusters : Foundation to create virtual enterprises, in Advances in Networked Enterprises, pp 111-120, edited by L. Camarinha, H. Afsarmanesh, H Erbe, Kluwer Academics Publishers, 2000
4.Katzy B, Schuh G, Millarg K, Die virtuelle Fabrik – Produzieren im Netwerk – neue Märkte erschliessen durch dynamische Netzwerke, in Technische Rundschau 43/1996, pp 30-34
5.Schönsleben, Paul, Integrales Logistikmanagement : Planung und Steuerung von umfassenden Geschäftsprozessen, Springer, Berlin, 1998
6.Schuh G, Millarg K, Göransson A, Virtuelle Fabrik, neue Marktchancen durch dynamische Netwerke, Carl Huber Verlag, Munich, 1998
7.Guide européen des alliances entre PME de la sous-traitance, Office des Publications des Communautés Européennes, Luxembourg, 1998

17

RELATIONSHIP MANAGEMENT IN ENTERPRISE NETWORKS

Arian Zwegers, Herbert Wubben
Baan, azwegers@baan.com, hwubben@baan.com
Ingo Hartel
Swiss Federal Institute of Technology Zurich
Center for Enterprise Sciences (ETHZ-BWI), Ingo.Hartel@ethz.ch

Enterprises cooperate more extensively with other enterprises in various forms. To enable the cooperation of multiple organizations in supply chains or virtual enterprises, configuration and set-up tools need to define the relations between partnering enterprises. In the one-of-a-kind industry, enterprises collaborate within a Virtual Enterprise (VE). For the definition of relationships among partners in a VE, standard project management 'tools' can be used. EXtended Relationship Management (XRM) services define the relationships among partners in a VE. These services need to support a network view, viral effects, many-to-many relations, and 'configuration' of the integration infrastructure.

1. INTRODUCTION

One of the trends in the global market is the increasing cooperation among enterprises during the entire product life cycle. This is related to business drivers, such as the need for cost reduction, flexibility, focus on core competencies, and so on. The result is anything from a rather stable alliance between partners as in a supply chain to a more transitory cooperation as in a virtual enterprise.

To enable the cooperation of multiple organizations in supply chains or virtual enterprises, the relations between these partners need to be defined. Configuration and set-up tools are needed to define inter-enterprise relationships, in addition to applications for monitoring, management, and optimization of inter-enterprise business processes. Before processes within a supply chain or virtual enterprise can be executed, the relations between the various partners have to be defined by means of tools for the set-up of these cooperation forms. These so-called eXtended Relationship Management (XRM) services can be used to configure a whole supply chain or virtual enterprise (Radjou *et al.*, 2001; Forrester, 2002)*. Changing

* Please note that this paper adopts a slightly different interpretation of the term 'XRM' than Forrester in (Radjou *et al.*, 2001). According to Forrester's definition, XRM applications manage, monitor, and/or optimize inter-enterprise business processes. Here, we restrict ourselves to the services that allow an enterprise to define relations between enterprises. In Forrester's definition, this is only part of XRM applications. This functionality is in fact quite interesting for all collaborative applications, and should be made available to these applications as specialized services.

configurations of partners in a virtual enterprise necessitate dynamic configurations of both inter-enterprise business processes and the integrations with partners' enterprise applications. Both should be easily modified. XRM tools aim to provide this easy and effective reconfiguration of cooperating partners.

The objective of this paper is to define how relationship management services should support the set-up and reconfiguration of a virtual enterprise out of an enterprise network. The focus is on the decomposition of an inter-enterprise project in order to obtain a more accurate picture of the distribution of work. Only then, it will be clear with what partners enterprises share specifications, on what basis they report progress, when they can start certain parts of the work, and so on. Irrespective of collaborative (project management) applications, the basis of collaboration is found in such a "cooperation structure".

The next section provides some background about 'collaborative commerce', virtual enterprises, and collaborative project management. They are respectively the business model, the organizational structure, and one of the most obvious applications in which XRM plays a role. In section 3, the characteristics of XRM services are defined, and its place in an integration infrastructure is outlined. A case of a virtual enterprise in practice is presented in section 4. The paper gives a first glance of how the relations between the partners in that virtual enterprise can be modeled. A discussion closes this paper. The research has been carried out as part of the IMS project 'GLOBEMEN – Global Engineering and Manufacturing in Enterprise Networks' (IMS 99004, EC project IST-1999-60002).

2. BACKGROUND

2.1 Trend Toward "Collaborative Commerce"

Nowadays, three major movements put additional requirements to enterprises: globalization, outsourcing, and customization. Organizations expand their scope to become really global, and differentiate their patterns of cooperation to encompass collaborative activities. Outsourcing and a focus on core competencies requires better collaboration, synchronization of processes, and appropriate handling of time and distance constraints. Customization demands make-to-order manufacturing, better demand visibility, and more flexibility in general in order to execute faster and more efficiently. Closer collaboration with partners is required by globalization, outsourcing, and customization.

However, the trend towards closer collaboration is hindered by a number of factors. Current applications focus on single-tier environments, and provide limited support for complex partner relationships. Popular solutions which are available in the market today, such as Supply Chain Management applications, typically address cooperation within 'paired relationships'. The latter means that companies are inclined to optimize the relationships with their closest suppliers and customers in a one-to-one fashion. Only the cooperation between an enterprise and its closest suppliers or customers is considered. The supplier's suppliers and the customer's customers are not taken into consideration. Although the logistics management of an enterprise towards its direct partners might be optimized, the overall supply chain is far from optimal.

Nevertheless, it is apparent that enterprises will have to adopt approaches such as "collaborative commerce" (or "c-commerce") to remain competitive in most industry segments (Forrester, 2002; Gartner, 2002). Gartner defines c-commerce as follows:

> "C-commerce is the collaborative, electronically enabled business interaction among an enterprise's internal personnel, business partners, and customers throughout a trading community. This trading community can be an industry, industry segment, supply chain or supply chain segment." (Gartner, 2002)*

Perhaps the most essential element of c-commerce is the extension of an enterprise's knowledge assets to include those outside the enterprise. When intellectual capital is leveraged across enterprises, the benefits of c-commerce can be realized. Sharing intellectual capital and combining core competencies with partners are the major ingredients of collaboration.

C-commerce should be considered as a business model rather than a solution that can be offered by vendors. It benefits an enterprise by extending the enterprise's visibility and cooperation throughout the value chain, thereby contributing to the realization of virtual enterprises.

2.2 Virtual Enterprises

Virtual Enterprises (VEs) are examples of implementations of the c-commerce business model. They are 'set up' from Enterprise Networks (see Figure 1). Such a network is a cooperative alliance of enterprises established to jointly exploit business opportunities through setting up virtual enterprises. The main purpose of a network is to prepare and manage the life cycle of VEs. It establishes mutual agreements among its members on issues such as common standards, procedures, intellectual property rights, and ICT, so that these time-consuming preparations can be significantly shortened when a customer request arises, and a VE is put in place. The network should be seen as a potential from which different VEs can be established in order to satisfy diverse customer demands. The network will seek out and await customer demands, and when a specific customer demand is identified the business potential is realized by forming a VE. Accordingly, compared to a virtual enterprise, a network can be perceived as a relatively long-term cooperation since it typically sets up multiple VEs. Conversely, the VEs have a more temporary nature.

A network is principally created based on core competencies and capabilities assigned from different cooperating enterprises. The network can therefore be characterized as a portfolio of core competencies that are available to realize VEs and products. This competence portfolio is dynamic in the sense that competencies can leave and join the network. In addition, a network can be characterized as a product-oriented network focusing on the strategically important, value adding partner competencies in the potential VEs, while typically excluding off-the-shelf suppliers (Van den Berg *et al.*, 2000).

A Virtual Enterprise is a temporary alliance of enterprises that come together to share skills or core competencies and resources in order to better respond to a business opportunity, and whose cooperation is supported by ICT (derived from

---

* See Eschenbächer and Zwegers (2002) for a discussion on different interpretations of the term 'c-commerce'.

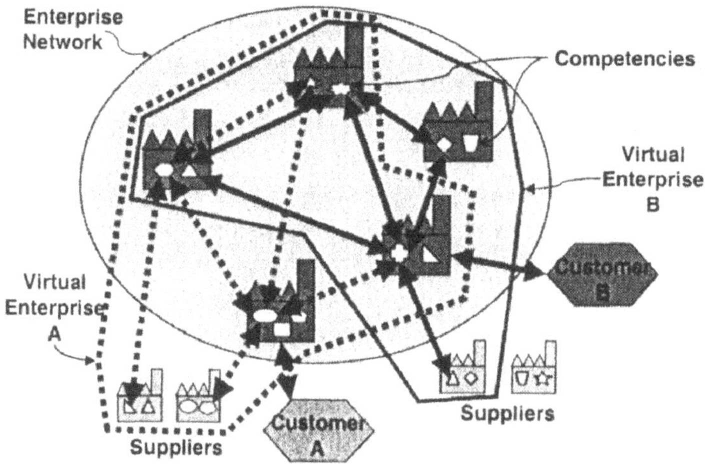

Figure 1 – Enterprise Network and Virtual Enterprises

(Camarinha-Matos, 2000)). Formation of the VE materializes through configuration of the core competencies and capabilities available in the network and possibly through inclusion of additional, required competencies provided by non-network participants, cf. Figure 1. Though being comprised by competencies from various partners, the VE performs as one, unified, and attuned enterprise. Hence its virtual nature. Accordingly, the business processes are not carried out by a single enterprise, but every enterprise is a node in the VE that adds some value to the product chain.

Please note that in the set-up of a VE from an enterprise network, the rather 'loose' relations that exist among enterprises in a network become 'solid' in a VE. In a network, there is no notion of a specific product or project. On the other hand, the VE is set up with a specific purpose in mind, i.e. a specific project delivering a specific product for a known customer. The configuration of the VE comprises the definition of the tasks/roles of individual enterprises and the relations between them. Concrete agreements are made regarding deliverables, schedules, payments, and so on, which are detailed in contracts and project plans.

2.3 Collaborative Project Management

This paper focuses on the one-of-a-kind industry. In this industry, enterprises participate in complex projects with significant durations and resource usages. These projects are split into many activities, deliverables, and milestones. They take place in a distributed environment within a temporary, product driven, inter-enterprise structure (the virtual enterprise) and usually with geographically distributed sites (plants, construction sites, and so on).

Due to these difficulties, collaborating enterprises are looking for more reliable project plans with a shared model of project activities and requirements. That way, they can monitor the project through on-line access to activity progress, with real-time notification of events and 'alert' conditions and impact evaluation for deviations based on changes of downstream activities. This will enable enterprises to diminish risks, since unexpected events or plan deviations are reduced and there is clear visibility between all activities. In addition, it will allow enterprises obtaining a higher level of flexibility and efficiency, responding faster to customer change requests, exploiting partner competencies from the network potential in a better way, and accelerating and controlling the flow of information during the project life cycle.

3. EXTENDED RELATIONSHIP MANAGEMENT (XRM)

3.1 Definition of Relationships Among Partners in a VE

For the definition of relationships among partners in a VE, rather standard project management 'tools' should be used. These 'tools' are:

- *Work Breakdown Structure*, i.e. a deliverable-oriented grouping of project elements that organizes and defines the total work scope of the project. Each descending level represents an increasingly detailed definition of the project work (PMBOK, 2000).
- *Organization Breakdown Structure*, i.e. a depiction of the project organization in which work packages are related to organizational units (PMBOK, 2000).
- *Project Network Diagram*, i.e. a schematic display of the logical relationships of project activities, which is always drawn from left to right to reflect project chronology. It is often referred to as a PERT chart (PMBOK, 2000).
- *Bill of Material*, i.e. a diagram presenting a hierarchical view of the physical assemblies, subassemblies, and components needed to fabricate a manufactured product. It contains the products that are required and must be produced, installed, assembled, and described in a hierarchical way.

The key point is the combination of these structures. A Work Breakdown Structure can be decomposed into more detailed activity structures, which eventually drill down to normal Bills of Material. The components in such a Bill of Material are provided by suppliers according to normal supply chain relationships. Tools are available to support these supply chain relationships. In addition, some project management tools support multi-enterprise Work Breakdown Structures. However, the combination is still unique.

3.2 Characteristics of XRM Services

XRM services defining the relationships among partners in a virtual enterprise need to exhibit certain characteristics, namely they need to support a network view, viral effects, many-to-many relations, and 'configuration' of the integration infrastructure.

XRM services need to provide a *network point of view*. Enterprise applications such as ERP and SCM typically consider an enterprise or an enterprise plus its direct suppliers and customers. They adopt an enterprise view and an 'enterprise + tier 1' view respectively. However, XRM must go beyond the paired relationships and must create transparency across multi-tier boundaries. They take the whole supply chain or virtual enterprise and thereby supplier's suppliers and the customer's customers into consideration. In addition, each individual virtual enterprise member has visibility into its position in the virtual enterprise, possibly restricted to one tier only, depending on the authorities it was given.

XRM services need to support *viral effects*, so that partners can introduce their own suppliers and customers. While XRM services are sponsored and hosted by a single firm (usually a main contractor or dedicated service provider), partners can pay to extend the services to their other partners and customers. The whole virtual enterprise can be set up more efficiently this way (Radjou *et al.*, 2001).

XRM services need to support *many-to-many relationships*. Especially in supply chains with rather standard products, a component manufacturer supplying to multiple OEMs, wants to give access to its production schedules to all OEMs. However, a building contractor hosting XRM services and collaborative project management applications does not want its subcontracted engineering firms to set up virtual enterprises with other, competing building contractors.

XRM services need to *'configure' the integration infrastructure*, i.e. regardless of where a partner is located in the virtual enterprise, it will be able to set security, encryption, alerts, permission and data access to enterprises further up or complementary in the value chain. This way, information flows can be orchestrated.

3.3 XRM in the Integration Infrastructure

XRM is seen as one of the services provided by an integration infrastructure. Collaborative applications are positioned on top of the infrastructure. Van Busschbach *et al.* (2002) describe the capability stack of services needed for the complete integration backbone. It consists of four functional layers (from bottom to top):

- *Connectivity Layer*, linking applications in different programming languages, databases, middleware, protocols, and other technologies.
- *Transformation Layer*, reconciling differences in data and functions on a functional level.
- *Routing Layer*, providing dynamic behavior based on the contents of a message, to be configured by a business analyst.
- *Process Management Layer*, allowing the end user to dynamically trigger, execute and monitor business processes.

XRM services reside in the Process Management Layer. They use "yellow pages" about the enterprise network, which includes for example information about competences of potential partners. In addition, documents such as general agreements, procedures, and so on, can be stored for later use during the setup and operation of a VE. XRM models enterprises and their relationships in one or more projects based on Work Breakdown Structures, Activity Structures, and Bills of Material. These models form the basis for monitoring and management of the business processes in virtual enterprises by collaborative project management applications. The business processes managed in the Process Management Layer dictate the flow of information between applications and other data sources. Perhaps the ultimate goal of this layer is to provide inter-enterprise workflow management services that support multiple dynamic workflows crossing organizational boundaries.

4. AN INDUSTRIAL CASE STUDY

Within the context of IMS project 'GLOBEMEN', XRM services have been developed. Though these services do not entirely implement the ideas as presented above, the basic principles behind the XRM services and especially their characteristics are identical. The services have been developed with the following reasoning in mind: enterprises close contracts; contracts contain obligations; obligations are linked to deliverables; deliverables can be organized in a project; every deliverable is related to a matched deliverable if this deliverable is subcontracted; and every planned deliverable is related to an actual deliverable.

The case is that of a paper mill producer (PMP), its customer (C), and one of its subcontractors (SC). C is customer of PMP. Both enterprises agreed on the delivery of (a part of) a paper machine by PMP to C. As a customer, C requests to be reported on the progress of the part of the paper machine that is developed by PMP.

PMP organizes the delivery of that paper machine as a project, and decomposes the paper machine in three parts (Conveyor, Wrapper, and Rolls) for internal project management and subcontracting of one part. The Rolls will be constructed by another company (SC) and it is agreed that SC will report progress on the total and on three deliverables/activities for the Rolls: design, build and installation. For all deliverables, progress is being registered on actual deliverables that realize planned deliverables. Figure 2 shows the accompanying 'cooperation structure'. Note that this picture seamlessly integrates a Work Breakdown Structure with a sales order for a deliverable and a purchase order with one deliverable and three sub-deliverables.

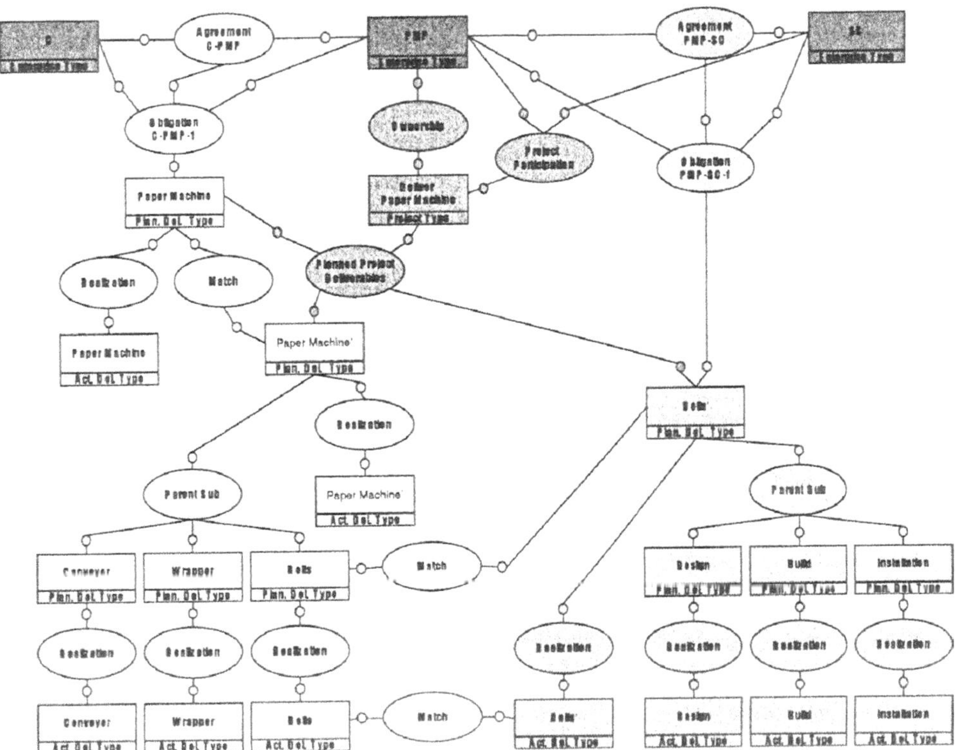

Figure 2 – Cooperation structure

SC reports the progress on the deliverables Design, Build, and Installation, and Rolls'. These instances are also in the scope of PMP, since PMP and SC have agreed on the deliverables and their structure. Therefore, it is possible for PMP to track the progress. Note that SC does not (yet) organize the delivery of the Rolls as a project. SC could define the parts of Rolls which are subcontracted again, thanks to the viral capabilities of the XRM services.*

PMP is able to track progress on a subcontracted part of the Paper Machine': Rolls'. PMP also tracks and reports progress on Paper Machine' and its sub-deliverables internally, and is able to report progress on the Paper Machine to customer C.

5. DISCUSSION

XRM services can be found in various forms in collaborative applications. After all, a cooperation can only be defined and detailed with XRM-like services. The cooperation structures and XRM characteristics mentioned in this paper are mostly based on experiences with collaborative project management applications in the one-of-a-kind industry. Other applications, e.g. focused on short-lived VEs such as virtual service enterprises, which fulfill services like maintenance, inspection or repair collaboratively, might need simpler cooperation structures (Hartel, 2001).

This paper presents the first results obtained with XRM services within the IMS project 'GLOBEMEN'. Further research will focus on the genericity of the identified structures within the one-of-a-kind industry and on the genericity of the characteristics in XRM services. A prototype of an integration infrastructure realizing the desired XRM characteristics is also planned.

6. REFERENCES

1. Berg R. van den, Hannus M, Pedersen JD, Tølle M, and Zwegers A. "Evaluation of state of the art technologies". Globemen EU (IST-1999-60002) deliverable D411, 2000.
2. Busschbach E van, Pieterse B, Zwegers A. "Support of Virtual Enterprises by an Integration Infrastructure". In Collaborative Business Ecosystems and Virtual Enterprises (L.M. Camarinha-Matos (ed.)), pp. 311-326. Kluwer, Boston, 2002.
3. Camarinha-Matos LM. "Trends in virtual enterprise infrastructures". In Proceedings of WCC2000/ITBM 2000 - IFIP World Computer Congress/International Conference on Information Technology for Business Management. Beijing, China, 21-25 Aug 2000.
4. Eschenbächer J, Zwegers A. "Collaboration in value creating networks: the concept of collaborative commerce". In Proceedings of APMS 2002, Eindhoven, Netherlands (to be published), 2002.
5. Forrester. Various documents on URL: http://www.forrester.com, 2002.
6. Gartner. Various documents on URL: http://www.gartner.com, 2002.
7. Hartel I, Burger G. "Virtual Service Enterprise - A Model for virtual collaboration in after-sales service in the one-of-a-kind industry" In Proceedings of the IMS Forum, Ascona, Switzerland, 2001.
8. PMBOK. A guide to the Project Management Body of Knowledge (PMBOK® guide). Project Management Institute, Newtown Square, 2000.
9. Radjou N, Orlov LM, Child M. "Apps For Dynamic Collaboration". The Forrester Report. Cambridge, MA: Forrester Research, 2001.

* The quotation mark is used to make a difference between two representations of the Rolls deliverable. The representation without quotation mark is the representation that both C and PMP agree on. The representation with quotation mark is the representation that both PMP and SC agree on.

18

EVALUATION OF ORGANIZATIONAL STRUCTURE IN EMERGENCY FROM THE VIEWPOINT OF COMMUNICATION

S. Nishida, M. Nakatani, Y. Hijikata, and T. Koiso

Department of Systems and Human Science, Graduate School of Engineering Science
Osaka University, Toyonaka, Osaka, 560-8531 JAPAN
nishida@sys.es.osaka-u.ac.jp

This paper focuses on evaluation of organizational structure in emergency from the communication viewpoint. The communication process in emergency is analyzed first, and the problems caused in the process are discussed. Then a communication model is proposed, in which human related factors such as "competence", "duty", "responsibility" and "knowledge" are considered. Then a system to evaluate organizational structure in emergency from the viewpoint of communication is designed on the basis of the model. Finally, a prototype system with GUI is developed and its evaluation results are discussed.

1. INTRODUCTION

It is frequently observed in the emergent situation that important information does not reach to an appropriate person or department in the organization because of the confusion after the emergency or in some case because of lack of knowledge on contact address. This phenomenon happens especially when the size of organization becomes large, and we believe it is very important to predict communication problems in advance and improve the organizational structure from the viewpoint of communication.

Several types of communication models have been studied in the field of CSCW (Computer-Supported Cooperative Work). For example, conversation model based on the Speech Act Theory was developed (Winograd, 1988) and it is used for a support system which deals with E-mail processing. The IBIS (Issue Based Information System) model was proposed (Conklin, et al., 1988) and it is used for a support system to enhance software productivity. Furthermore, trouble communication model in software development project was studied (Nakatani, et al., 1992)

In this research, we first investigate in the important factors in emergent situations and propose a communication model in emergent situation in which human related factors such as "competence", "duty", "responsibility" and "knowledge" are focused. Then a system to evaluate organizational structure in emergency from the viewpoint of communication is proposed based on the model.

Finally, a prototype system with GUI is developed and its evaluation results are discussed.

2. ANALYSIS OF DECISION MAKING IN EMERGENCY

Recently, "commandware" is recognized to be very important in the field of crisis management. (Kawata, 1995) "Commandware" is regarded as the chain of commands to manage emergent situations. Commandware is closely related to the structure of organization. Hierarchical structures are usually adopted for the large scale system such as fire department, police system, management system for large scale chemical plants, and so on. In the hierarchical structure, problem solving is conducted by mutual communication among the nodes in the hierarchy.

Here we made interviews to the people who manage large scale plants such as power plant etc. to investigate how decisions or judgments are conducted and what types of communications occur in emergent situations. Concretely, we asked what type of communications occurred, and what was the objective of the communication. By summarizing these data, we reached to the conclusions that many communications, which were observed in plant management, are caused by the following factors.

(1) Who is the person that has competence to execute the operation?
(2) Who is the person that must execute the operation?
(3) Who is the person that takes responsibility for assuring some results on the troubled situation?
(4) Who is the person that has knowledge on the current situation or on the actions to be taken?

The above factors are called as "human related factors" , and it is thought that they play a very important role in selecting proper actions in the judgment process. The human related factors are the causes of communications between each node in the hierarchy, and the destination or the quantity of the communication depends on the human related factors. Though little attention has been given to the communication caused by these factors so far, we recognized the importance of the human related factors through the analysis of the interviews to the fire department.

3. COMMUNICATION MODEL IN EMERGENT SITUATION

In this section, a communication model is introduced in which human related factors are considered. The following four types of the communications generated at each node of the hierarchical organization are considered here.

(1) Communication generated by competence
It is defined as the communication to get permission of executing some operation, since the person has no competence, that is, no right to execute the operation.

(2) Communication generated by duty
It is defined as the communication to contact to the other person who has the duty to execute some operation under a given situation, since current situation is thought to need the operation and the person has no duty of executing it.

(3) Communication generated by responsibility
It is defined as the communication to contact to the other person who has the responsibility to execute some operation for assuring some results, since the person has no responsibility on it. Here responsibility means to assure the results by taking any means.

(4) Communication generated by knowledge
It is defined as the communication to contact to the other person who knows the situation or the operation very well, since the person does not know it well.

Our communication model in emergent situations consists of the above four types of basic communications, and the model is composed of both "physical structure" of the large scale system and "human related factors" in it. Figure 1 shows the concrete components of physical structure and human related factors. Physical structure is decided by the structure of artifacts. Physical structure is divided into four sub- structures as follows:

(a) Plant Structure (PS): PS shows names, location of each part.
(b) Sensor Structure (SS): SS shows sensor name, location, measurement and values.
(c) Actuator Structure (AS): AS shows actuator name, location and type of actuator.
(d) Trouble Operation Structure (TOS): TOS shows the relation between trouble situation, action to be taken and result of the action.

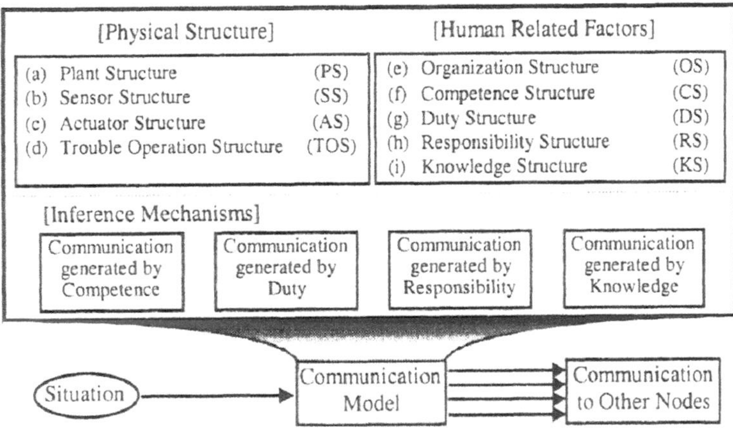

Figure 1 Communication Model

These sub-structures are determined by the physical factors of the system, and it is independent of the human related factors. On the other hand, the human related factors are concerned with competence, duty, responsibility and knowledge. The factors are determined by the formation of organization, bylaw related to persons, each person's knowledge and so on. The human related factors are expressed by the following five sub-structures:

(e) Organization Structure (OS): OS shows names of each person in the organization and location of hierarchical organization.
(f) Competence Structure (CS): CS indicates persons who can execute some actions to be taken.
(g) Duty Structure (DS): DS indicates persons who must execute some action to be taken in the trouble situation.
(h) Responsibility Structure (RS): RS indicates persons who assure some results for the trouble situation.
(i) Knowledge Structure (KS) : KS indicates persons who know the part of physical structure well.

Adding these structural data, the model has inference mechanism to predict "who has the competence on the operation?" "Who has the duty on the given troubled situation?" and so on. When some situation is given as an input, the destination of each type of communication mentioned before is determined by the following inference mechanisms based on the physical structure and the human related factors.

(1) Communications generated by competence
Some appropriate actions to be taken under a given situation are selected from TOS. Then persons who have competence for the selected actions are predicted from CS, and the destination of communication generated by competence is decided.

(2) Communications generated by duty
Some appropriate actions to be taken for the given situation is selected from TOS. Then persons who have duty on the trouble situation and the selected actions are calculated from DS. The derived persons correspond to the destination of communication generated by duty.

(3) Communications generated by responsibility
Some appropriate actions to be taken and results of the action under the given situation are selected from TOS. Then persons who have responsibility for the trouble situation and assumptive results are predicted from RS. The derived persons correspond to the destination of communication generated by responsibility.

(4) Communications generated by knowledge
Some parts of the plant concerned with given situation are selected from SS, or some appropriate actions to be taken under the given situation are selected from TOS. Persons who have information on the part selected by SS are calculated from KS. Moreover, persons who have information on the selected actions are also

calculated from KS. The destination of communication generated by knowledge is decided in this way.

As a total, the communication model in emergent situations can predict the destination of four types of basic communications by symbol processing using the data of both physical structure and the human related factors, when the situation of the system is given as an input.

4. A PROTOTYPE SYSTEM TO EVALUATE ORGANIZATIONAL STRUCTURE FROM THE VIEWPOINT OF COMMUNICATION

A prototype system to evaluate organizational structure in emergency is developed based on the above communication model.

The system can deal with four types of communications, that is, communication generated by competence, communication generated by duty, communication generated by responsibility and communication generated by knowledge. Figure 2 shows an example data for the prototype system. The structure of organization is assumed to be two layer hierarchy. The member which corresponds to root node is "C" and the two members which correspond to leaf nodes are "A" and "B". The physical plant consists of two plants, "Pa" and "Pb". Pa is composed of four parts and has seven sensors and four actuators. Pb is composed of two parts and has three sensors and two actuators.

(a) organization structure

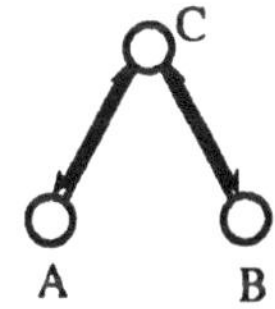

(b) plant structure

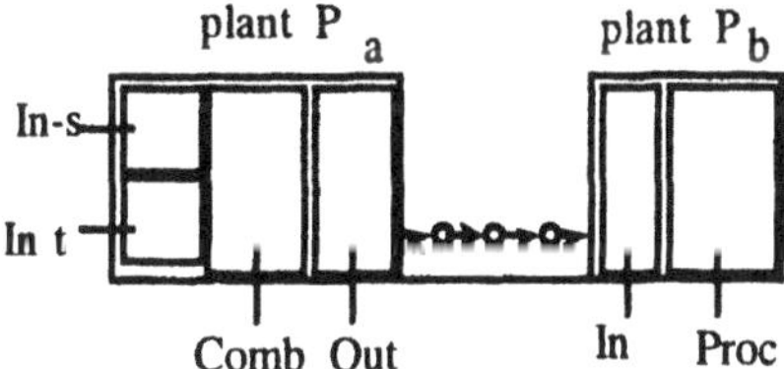

Figure 2 An Example Data

Parameters of sensors take values of "H(igh)", "M(iddle)" and "L(ow)". Parameters of actuators take values of "U(p)" and "D(own)".The data of the prototype system are managed by the frame-type data. For example, Plant Structure (PS) data "pnm, 1, Pa, In-s" means that the part "In-s " in the plant "Pa" is defined as "No.1" Plant Structure data. By using these nine types of data, destination of each kind of communication, which is generated from competence, duty, responsibility and knowledge, is determined by the mechanism mentioned in the section of communication model.

By using this system, we can find communication problems for the current organization structure, and also we can search improved organizational structure from the viewpoint of communication. The following functions are provided in the prototype system.

(1)Visualization of communication frequency distribution
By using the communication model in emergency, we can calculate the frequency of communications caused by some accidents in the physical system. If the probability of each accident is given in advance, then the communication frequency in the organization is calculated and it is visualized in the system.

(2)Detection of communication bottlenecks
The "communication bottlenecks", which have high possibility to receive many communications in emergency, can be predicted in the system. Furthermore, by changing human related factor data, we can find a new improved organizational structure.

(3)Comparison of different organizational structures
If the different organizational structures are given to the system, we can compare the structures from the viewpoints of communication and evaluate which structure is better. For example, hierarchical structure and flat structure can be compared quantitatively from the communication viewpoint.

The prototype system is developed on the PC using JAVA language. Figure 3 shows the comparison between hierarchical structure S1 and flat structure S2. In S1, communications are concentrated on E and F, however, in S2, there is no concentration. On the other hand, S1 has higher extension index value than S2, which means that S2 is more distributed organization than S1.

5. CONCLUSIONS

In this paper, decision-making in emergent situations is analyzed, and the important factors are investigated from the viewpoint of communication. Then communication model which considers human related factors such as "competence", "duty", "responsibility" and "knowledge", is introduced and a prototype system to evaluate organizational structure in emergency is developed based on the communication model.

We plan to try more complex examples in the next stage, and to improve the function of the evaluation system.

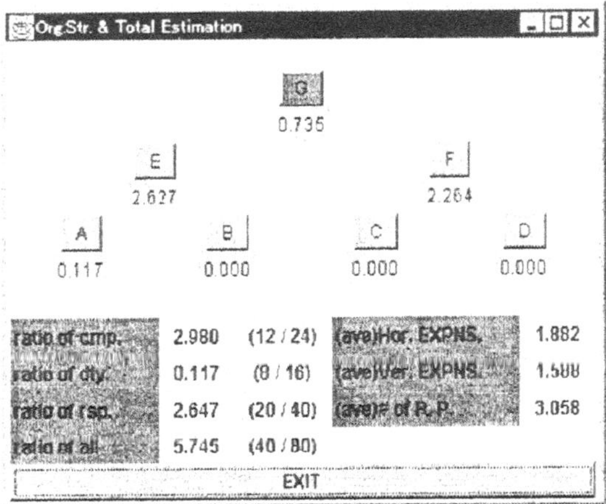

(a) Hierarchical Structure S1

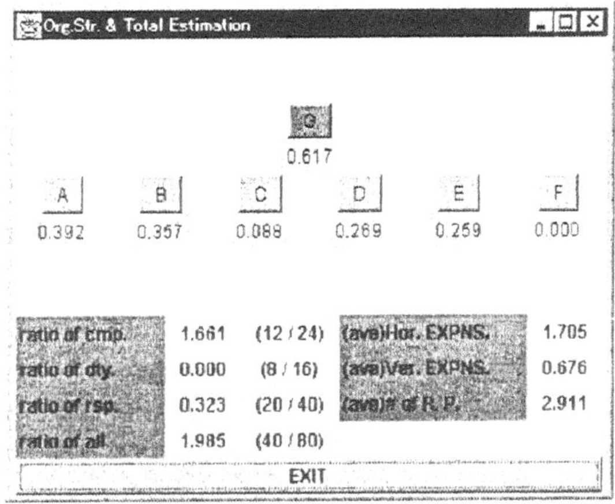

(b) Flat Structure S2

Figure 3 Evaluation Results

6. ACKNOWLEDGEMENTS

This work was partially supported by the Japan Society for the Promotion of Science under Grant-in- Aid for Creative Scientific Research (Project No. 13S0018)

7. REFERENCES

1. Koiso, T. and Nishida, S: Communication Support System for Operators in Emergency of Large Scale Plant, Proceedings of INCOM'98, pp.491-496. 1998.
2. Kawata, Y.: " Catastrophic Urban Disasters", Kinmirai-sha (in Japanese), 1995.
3. Nakatani, M. and Nishida, S.: " Trouble Communication Model in a Software Development Project", IEICE Trans. Fundamentals, Vol.75-A No.2, pp.196-206, 1992.
4. Nunamaker, J..F.: editor, Special issue on GDSS, Decision Support Systems, 5(2).1989.
5. Conklin, J. and Begeman, M.L.:" gIBIS : A Hypertext Tool for Exploratory Policy Discussion", Proceedings of CSCW'88, pp.140-152, 1988.
6. Winograd, T.: "A Language Perspective on the Design of Cooperative Work.", Proceedings of CSCW'88. pp203-220, 1988.
7. Malone, T.W. "Modeling coordination in organizations and markets, Management Science", 33(10), pp.1317-1332, 1987.

19 WORKFLOW HISTORY MANAGEMENT IN VIRTUAL HEALTHCARE ENTERPRISE

Tauqir Amin, Pung Hung Keng
Department of Computer Science, National University of Singapore
{amin,pung}@comp.nus.edu.sg

There are various applications of workflow history information maintained by Workflow Management System in the organizations. Most of such applications are also relevant and required in the context of a Virtual Enterprise. To make these applications of workflow history information feasible, sharing of geographically distributed history information among participating organizations of a virtual enterprise is vital. Such sharing requires a common systematic way of identification of history information. As a part of development of research project HISFlow, we develop a simple and generic scheme to identify history information of workflows across a Virtual Healthcare Enterprise. This scheme provides a robust foundation for more sophisticated Workflow History Management of a Virtual Enterprise. The scheme also caters the concept of partial view of a virtual process i.e. a view of virtual process seen by a participating organization. We use an example to demonstrate the working of the scheme for the identification of workflow history information.

1. INTRODUCTION

An integrated health care service built upon partnerships, alliances, and relationships with physicians, polyclinics, laboratories, pharmacies, hospitals and payers is emerging as the operating model for health care organizations (Horsch, 1999). The concept of a Virtual Enterprise is the solution to establish such integrated health care. As defined in the literature, virtual enterprise is a consortium of autonomous, diverse, geographically dispersed organizations that accumulates resources to achieve common objectives efficiently. The interaction of processes of the participating organizations is essential to build such a Virtual Healthcare Enterprise.

Workflow Management System has been widely conceived as principal supporting technology for automation of business processes and interaction with other organizations. Consequently, it provides a basic framework for the Virtual Enterprise paradigm. As mentioned in (Amin, 2002), such a framework is a set of WfMSs that are collaborating in a loosely coupled way to achieve automation of business processes of the Virtual Healthcare Enterprises. As the workflow technology is approaching first level of maturity, new strengths of it have been discovered. One of them is exploitation of history of workflow processes for various different purposes.

The rest of this section presents background and the problem to be solved in the paper. Section 2 elaborates the identification scheme for history information and also proposes two models to conceptualize the history information space. The Section 3 presents an example to demonstrate the working of proposed scheme. Section 4 talks about different workflow history applications and their relevance to a Virtual Enterprise. Conclusion is given in the Section 5.

1.1 Background

From WFMS viewpoint (Amin, 2002), a Virtual Enterprise is defined as an enterprise whose processes are virtual in the sense that they consist of geographically distributed processes. In other words, a Virtual Process is a set of processes that are connected with each other to fulfill a bigger goal of the Virtual Enterprise. Each of such processes runs on different autonomous WfMSs of respective organizations. As these processes are executed locally, the history information of the processes is stored in and maintained by the respective WfMSs. Such history information of the local process is only accessible to local WfMS and hence it can only be used by the respective organization. As the local process is part of the virtual process, related portion of the history of the process should also be shared with relevant organizations. Such sharing of history of local processes with the other participating organizations produce three complex problems. Firstly, we need a systematic mechanism to let the organization identify interested history information residing on other organizations. (Tagg, 2001) also raises the same problem and names it the workflow case identifier problem. Secondly, not all the history information is meant to be shared with or accessed by other organizations and this accessibility varies from organization to organization. So we need a way to abstract history information for sake of sharing. Thirdly, we need to have an application level communication protocol for WfMSs to communicate history information among the participating organizations. In this paper we only discuss first problem.

1.2 Problem Statement

A Workflow Management System of a participating organization handles its own process instances and instance related data autonomously. Hence every WfMS has its own identification of its workflow history information. Such identification is only valid inside the organization. But for different applications of history information, one organization has to refer to the workflow history information of peer organizations. Therefore, to let the organization identify workflow history information of a peer organization is the problem that has to be solved for making use of workflow history information of a Virtual Enterprise.

To further explain the problem, suppose two clinical processes X and Y are part of one Virtual Process but running on different hospitals. In the definition of X, we want to have a workflow branching condition based on the history of instances of Y. We have to put this as an expression in the definition of X so that when an instance of X is running, this expression is resolved to get the data of required instances of Y.

Such expressions require two things: identification of workflow history information and some operators. The operators are beyond the scope of this paper. We only propose the identification scheme. This scheme would provide a base not only for such expressions, but also for different kinds of analysis and monitoring.

2. STRUCTURE OF HISTORY INFORMATION

2.1 Instance Identification Scheme

Both Workflow Relevant Data and Workflow Internal Data are tied to the process instances. Once the process instance is identified, all the information attached to it can be obtained. So the first step of identification of history information is identification of process instances. Taking this observation into consideration, we define a process instance the first basic unit of workflow history information of a Virtual Enterprise. In this paper, we only propose the identification scheme of process instances across the organizations. This scheme needs to be further enhanced to have workable identification of workflow history information.

There are two levels of identification scheme: definition level and instance level. Definition level identification involves only process definitions of participating organizations. It is a step towards achieving instance level identification which involves process instances of the participating organizations. The approach of instance level identification scheme is based on the fact that a virtual process instance is a logical container that contains process instances of participating organizations. Being participants of such a logical container, process instances belonging to different organizations have same context. This same context along with definition level identification provides necessary information to identify the process instances of the peer organizations. In the following part of the paper, we develop this identification scheme by using Set theory and mathematical notations.

The participating organizations of the given Virtual Enterprise VE can be presented as

$O(VE) = \{o_1, o_2, o_3, ...o_i\}$ Where $o_1, o_2, o_3, ...o_i$ stand for the identification of organizations. And i is the total number of organizations in the Virtual Enterprise

Definition: Following the modeling approach of (Amin, 2002), Virtual Process is defined by two things: participating process definitions and peer to peer link among them. Hence, Definition of Virtual Process VP can be represented as

$VP = \{P(VP), \|(VP)\}$ Where $P(VP)$ means all the process definitions participating in Virtual Process Definition VP and $\|(VP)$ means all the peer to peer relations of the participating process definitions of VP.

All the process definitions belonging to organization O_1 are represented as

$P(O_1) = \{p_1, p_2, p_3, ...p_{k_1}\}$ Where $p_1, p_2, p_3, ...p_{k_1}$ are identifiers of process definitions of organization O_1 which are unique within the organization. And k_1 is the total number of process definitions in organization O_1.

Please note that $P(O_1)$ should be read as P of O_1 meaning the processes of O_1.

Similarly for organization O_i, its process definitions can be represented as

$P(O_i) = \{p_1, p_2, p_3 .....p_{k_i}\}$ Where $p_1, p_2, p_3 .....p_{k_i}$ are identifiers of process definitions of organization O_i which are unique within the organization. And k_i is the total number of process definitions in organization O_i.

The participating organizations of Virtual Process Definition VP can be represented as

$O(VP) = \{o_1, o_2, o_3, ...o_j\}$ Where $O(VP) \subseteq O(VE)$ and j is the total number of organizations participating in Virtual Process Definition VP.

A process definition can uniquely and globally be identified with the combination of two identifiers: the locally unique process definition identifier and its organization identifier, provided the organization identifier is globally unique. For example process definition $p_{(a,b)}$ is globally unique, where 'a' stands for process definition identifier and 'b' stands for organization identifier. For sake of simplicity we assume that only one process definition of the organization participates in the Virtual Process Definition VP. In terms of globally unique identifiers, the participating process definitions in Virtual Process Definition VP can be represented as

$$P(VP) = \{p_{(m_1,o_1)}, p_{(m_2,o_2)}, p_{(m_3,o_3)}, ...p_{(m_j,o_j)}\}$$

Where $m_1, m_2, m_3, ...m_j \in P(O_1), P(O_2), P(O_3), ...P(O_j)$ respectively and $o_1, o_2, o_3, ...o_j \in O(VP)$

For nth Virtual Process Definition

$$P(VP_n) = \{p_{(m_j^n,o_j)}\} \quad .... \text{(A)}$$

We represent peer to peer relations of processes definition p_1 with other process definitions, say p_2 and p_3, as $p_1 \| (p_2, p_3)$.

Therefore all the peer to peer relations of $P(VP)$ in the Virtual Process Definition VP can be represented as

$$\|(VP) = \{p_{(m_1,o_1)} \| (p_{(r_1,q_1)}), p_{(m_2,o_2)} \| (p_{(r_2,q_2)}), ...p_{(m_j,o_j)} \| (p_{(r_j,q_j)})\} ..... \text{(B)}$$

Where $q_j \subseteq O(VP)$ and $m_j \not\subseteq r_j$ and

$$(r_j, q_j) = \{(\Phi_1, \lambda_1), (\Phi_2, \lambda_2), (\Phi_3, \lambda_3), \ldots\ldots (\Phi_h, \lambda_h)\}$$

Where $h = card(q_j)$ and $\lambda_h \in q_j$ and $\Phi_h \in P(\lambda_h)$

and $\lambda_a \neq \lambda_b$ if $a = b$

After having expressions (A) and (B), we apply above identification scheme on the Partial View concept of (Amin, 2002).

Definition: As defined in (Amin, 2002), a Virtual Process Definition is a set of Partial Views seen by individual participating organizations.

$$VP = \{PV_1VP, PV_2VP, PV_3VP, \ldots\ldots PV_jVP\}$$

Where PV_1VP, PV_2VP, PV_3VP and PV_jVP are Partial Views of VP seen by the organizations o_1, o_2, o_3 and o_j respectively.

Definition: To an organization, Partial View of a Virtual Process Definition is a set of its local process definition and peer to peer relations with other participating process definitions of the same Virtual Process Definition.

Following above definition of Partial View, PV_1VP can be represented as

$$PV_1VP = \{(p_{(m_1,o_1)}), (p_{(m_1,o_1)} \| p_{(r_1,q_1)})\}$$

Similarly

$$PV_jVP = \{(p_{(m_j,o_j)}), (p_{(m_j,o_j)} \| p_{(r_j,q_j)})\}$$

For jth Partial View of nth VP

$$PV_jVP_n = \{(p_{(m_j^n,j)}), (p_{(m_j^n,j)} \| p_{(r_j^n,q_j^n)})\} \ldots\ldots\ldots\ldots (C)$$

With the help of above expression definition of local process and its relations can be identified. Please note that Proxy Process of Meta Model of Partial View given in (Amin, 2002) is just a way of implementation of relation of local process with other processes.

As mentioned above, notion of Virtual Process Instance provides a context that logically connects all the participating process instances belonging to different organizations. All the instances of Virtual Processes Definition VP can be represented as

$I(VP) = \{I_1VP, I_2VP, I_3VP, \ldots\ldots I_gVP\}$ Where I_gVP is the identifier of gth instance of Virtual Process Definition VP.

Following the expression (A)

$I_gVP = \{I_g p_{(m_j,o_j)}\}$ Where $I_g p_{(m_j,o_j)}$ are all the process instances of participating organizations that belong to Virtual Process Instance I_gVP.

Similarly, for the gth instance of Partial View PV_jVP of Virtual Process Definition VP can be represented as

$$I_g PV_j VP = \{I_g p_{(m_j,j)}, I_g (p_{(m_j,j)} \| p_{(r_j,q_j)})\} \quad \text{.........} \quad \text{(D)}$$

Where $I_g (p_{(m_j,j)} \| p_{(r_j,q_j)})$ is the *gth* instance of relations between local process definition $p_{(m_j,j)}$ and $p_{(r_j,q_j)}$. Remember $p_{(r_j,q_j)}$ are process definitions of peer organizations with which local process definition is connected.

The semantic of instance of relation, say $I_a(p_b \| p_c)$, is one complete interaction between two process instances $I_a p_b$ and $I_a p_c$. Where $I_a p_b$ and $I_a p_c$ are *ath* instances of process definitions p_b and p_c respectively. Process instance $I_a p_b$ is a local process instance and $I_a p_c$ is a process instance of a peer organization. The expression (D) let the organization know which process instances of peer organizations are interacting with which local process instances. In simpler words, the relationship of local process instances and process instances of peer organizations is captured in expression (D). And this relationship helps the organization identify process instances of peer organizations.

2.2 Workflow History Space

2.2.1 *Process/Place/Time Model*

We conceptualize Workflow History Information as three co-ordinate space, axes of which are Process, Place and Time. "Process" and "Place" symbolize Virtual Process Definition and Organization respectively. A single point in this space is a set of instances of a process definition belonging to an organization. For example, a point (VP_1, O_2, T_6) shown in "Figure 1 (a)" gives us a set of all instance identifiers of a local process definition $p_{(m_2^1,O_2)}$ that exist at time T_6. And as we know from expression (A), $p_{(m_2^1,O_2)}$ is a participating process definition of VP_1 and belongs to the organization O_2. This set of instances includes both the instances that are currently active and the instances that have been executed by the time T_6. In this view of the workflow history information space, we only consider to identify the instances, not the internal details of the instances.

2.2.2 *Instance/Place/Time Model*

This model gives another view of the workflow history that can be used to have internal detail of a process instance. Axes of this space are Instance, Place and Time. The "Instance" symbolizes a Virtual Process Instance. A single point in this space is a snap shot of a local process instance belonging to an organization at given time. For example, a point (I_3VP_1, O_1, T_4) shown in "Figure 1 (b)" gives a snap shot of a local process instance $I_3p_{(m_1^1, O_1)}$ of organization O_1 at time T_4 that belongs to I_3VP_1. By snap shot we mean the values of all kind of data attached to the process instance at given point of time. This includes the data and the states of both finished and active activities, the relevant data, and the instance internal run-time data.

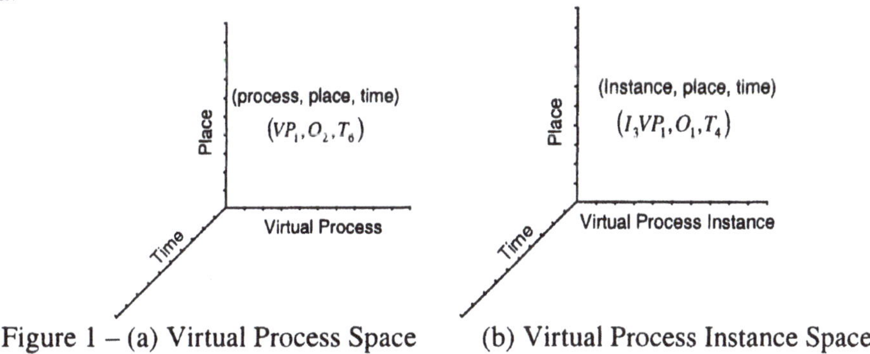

Figure 1 – (a) Virtual Process Space (b) Virtual Process Instance Space

3. APPLICATION OF INSTANCE IDENTIFICATION SCHEME

A simplified form of the example given in (Amin, 2002) is used to demonstrate the application of proposed instance identification scheme. We ignore the internal details of the process definitions as we are not concerned with it. We also add few extra process definitions into picture to make it more suitable for the current purpose. Four organizations, the Police, the Community Pediatrics, the Examination Room Provider and the Post AFE Care Provider, are collaborating to form a Virtual Enterprise. A child rape case is reported to the Police and it asks the Community Pediatrics to do AFE examination. The Community Pediatrics requires an examination room from nearby hospital, the Examination Room Provider. After the initial AFE examination, the patient is admitted to the Post AFE Care Provider for further treatment. All the four participating organizations have their own processes that interact with each other to form a Virtual Process to achieve the bigger goal.

As shown in the "Figure 2", the process definition P2 of The Police is participating in the Virtual Process Definition VP_1, and linked with one of the process definition P3 of The Community Pediatrics. Similarly process definition P3 of Community Pediatrics is further interacting with process definitions P1 and P4 of Post AFE Provider and Room Provider respectively.

Suppose VP_1 denotes the virtual process given in the example. By using equation (A), all the participating process definitions of VP_1 are presented in terms of globally unique identifiers as

$$P(VP_1) = \{p_{(p_2,o_1)}, p_{(p_4,o_2)}, p_{(p_1,o_3)}, p_{(p_3,o_4)}\}$$

By using equation (B), all the relations among the local process definitions of VP_1 are presented as

$$\|(VP_1) = \left\{ \begin{matrix} p_{(p_2,o_1)} \|(p_{(p_4,o_2)}), p_{(p_4,o_2)} \|(p_{(p_2,o_1)}, p_{(p_1,o_3)}, p_{(p_3,o_4)}), \\ p_{(p_1,o_3)} \|(p_{(p_4,o_2)}), p_{(p_3,o_4)} \|(p_{(p_4,o_2)}) \end{matrix} \right\}$$

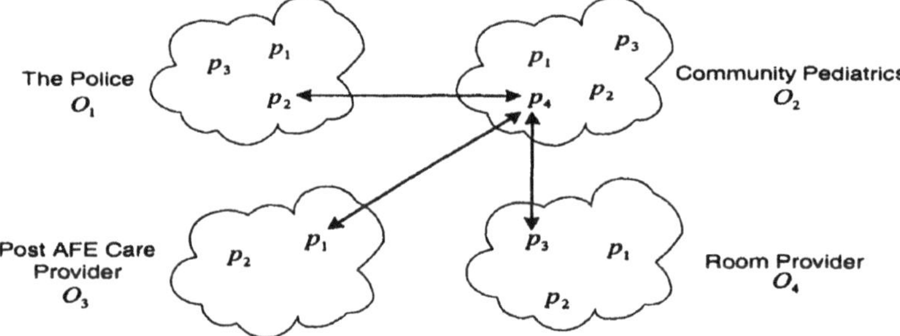

Figure 2 – Interaction of participating processes of a Virtual Process

For the Partial View of VP_1 seen by the Police in terms of global identifiers can be represented as

$$PV_1VP_1 = \{(p_{(p_2,o_1)}), (p_{(p_2,o_1)} \|(p_{(p_4,o_2)}))\}$$

Similarly for the Partial View seen by Community Pediatrics

$$PV_2VP_1 = \{(p_{(p_4,o_2)}), (p_{(p_4,o_2)} \|(p_{(p_2,o_1)}, p_{(p_1,o_3)}, p_{(p_3,o_4)}))\}$$

For the Partial View seen by Post AFE Care Provider

$$PV_3VP_1 = \{(p_{(p_1,o_3)}), (p_{(p_1,o_3)} \|(p_{(p_4,o_2)}))\}$$

For the Partial View seen by Room Provider

$$PV_4VP_1 = \{(p_{(p_3,o_4)}), (p_{(p_3,o_4)} \|(p_{(p_4,o_2)}))\}$$

Now lets take an example of one instance of the partial view seen by Community Pediatrics, say $I_3PV_2VP_1$. Following expression (D), Community Pediatrics can identify process instance $I_3 p_{(p_2,o_1)}$ belonging to the police. Similarly other process instances can also be identified.

4. APPLICATIONS OF WORKFLOW HISTORY IN A VIRTUAL ENTERPRISE

We have observed that the applications of workflow history information is generally scattered in the literature. Every work tries to focus on one or a few applications of workflow history information. As a part of the contribution of this paper, we first consolidate all the applications of workflow history information and then discuss their relevance in a Virtual Enterprise.

The applications of workflow history are generally divided into two broad categories: Monitoring and Controlling. Monitoring deals with the history of currently running process instances. Controlling deals with the history of already finished process instances over a longer period of time. (Muehlen, 2000) and (Muehlen, 2001) further categorize monitoring into two categories based on the purposes of the monitoring. There are two types of purposes: technical and business oriented. As the framework of a Virtual Enterprise is a set of loosely-coupled WfMS, the technical monitoring is less relevant for the virtual enterprises. For example, an organization is not concerned with the system load, response time and license management of the WfMSs of its peer organizations. But it is very much concerned to know the business states of the process instances of the peer organizations.

As one of the facets of controlling, an important application of workflow history is to do analysis of it over a very long period of time for business process re-engineering. Workflow history is analyzed to improve accuracy, efficiency and timeliness of the processes. Beate in (List, 2000) proposes a separate read-only analytical repository of history information for this purpose. This kind of analysis has new aspects in the case of Virtual Enterprise. The analysis can help the organizations to refine the current arrangements of the virtual enterprise. It can also set the guidelines for creating new virtual enterprises.

Application of the history information for sake of History-dependant Authorization (Casati, 1999) has larger scope in a Virtual Enterprise. The criteria of authorization of tasks to the users could be based on the workflow history of current instance or past instances of the peer organizations. For example, whenever user 'Y' of the peer organization executes some activity 'A', only user 'X' of this organization will execute the particular activity 'B'. Similarly workflow branching logic can also be based on the workflow history of the peer organization. In some domains like medical, workflow history serves for legal purposes as well. Future of an instance can be predicted based on the projection of the workflow history. Other applications of workflow history information include finding of workflow exception patterns to have guidelines for handling them (Sadiq, 2000) and helping the organizations maintain an Organizational Memory discussed in (Kaathoven, 1999) and (Wargetitsch, 1997). Knowledge Management is another emerging area where benefits of workflow history are yet to be discovered fully. (Zhao, 1998) and (List, 2001) bring some of such benefits to light.

In short, not many published works talk about Workflow History Management. Even fewer touch this issue in the context of Inter-organizational Workflows or Virtual Enterprises. Peter in (Muth, 1999) discusses it as part of research project Mentor, but the focus is on architectural aspects of it. Querying of History Information and its optimization are the main topics of (Koksal, Mar 1998) and (Koksal, Oct 1998).

5. CONCLUSION

Although we refer to some particular process model, in this paper we try to keep our discussion and solution at abstract level and independent of details of any process model. This makes the approach equally useful for any process model. But on the other hand, because of being primitive, the solution is not complete enough to be practical unless it is enhanced to cover detailed data of process instances The main focus is to solve the problem of identification and linking of the processes of a Virtual Enterprise for sake of history information. We believe that the approach can be useful in any form of process automation that involves geographically distributed processes.

6. REFERENCES

1. Amin T., Keng P. H.: Inter-organizational Workflow Management System for Virtual Healthcare Enterprise (To be appear), 3rd IFIP Working Conference on Infrastructures for Virtual Enterprises PRO-VE'02, Portugal, May 1-3, 2002.
2. Casati, F., Castano, S., Fugini, M. G.: Managing Workflow Authorization Constraints Through Active Database Technology", Information Systems Frontiers, 3(3). 1999.
3. Horsch, A., Balbach T.: Telemedical Information Systems IEEE Transactions on information technology in biomedicine, Vol. 3, No. 3, September, 1999
4. Kaathoven, R. V., Manfred, A., Martin, S., Ulrich, R.: Organizational Memory Supported Workflow Management, Organizational Memory supported Workflow Management. In Proc. 4th Intl. Conference Wirtschaftsinformatik (WI'99), Saarbrücken, Germany, March 3-5, 1999
5. Koksal, P., Arpinar, S., Dogac, A.: Workflow history management ACM SIGMOD Record March 1998 Volume 27 Issue 1
6. Koksal, P., Arpinar, S., Dogac, A.: History Management in Workflow Systems, international Symposium on Computer and Information Sciences (ISCIS XII), Antalya, Turkey, October 1998
7. List, B., Schiefer, J., Tjoa, A.: Customer Driven E-business Process Improvement with Process Warehouse, IFIP2000, Peking
8. List, B., Schiefer, J., Robert, M.: Measuring Knowledge with Workflow Management Systems, DEXA'01, IEEE Computer Society Press, pp. 467-471, Munich, Germany, September 2001
9. Muehlen, M. Z., Rosemann, M.: Workflow-based Process Monitoring and Controlling Technical and Organizational Iusses, HICSS 2000
10. Muehlen, M. Z.: Process-driven Management Information Systems-Combining Data Warehouses and Workflow Technology, International Conference on electronic commerce research (ICECR-4), Dallas, Nov. 8-11, 2001, pp. 550-566
11. Muth, P., Weissenfels, J., Gillmann, M., Weikum, G: Workflow History Management in Virtual Enterprise using a Light-Weight Workflow Management Systems, Proc. of 9th International Workshop on Research Issues in Data Engineering (RIDE), Australia, March 1999
12. Sadiq, S. W., Maria, E. Orlowska: On Capturing Workflow Exceptions in Workflow Process Models, In Proceedings of the 4th International Conference on Business Information Systems. Poznan, Poland. Springer-Verlag. April 12 -13 2000
13. Tagg, R.: Workflow in Different Styles of Virtual Enterprise, Workshop on Information Technology for Virtual Enterprises, ITVE 2001, Queensland
14. Wargitsch, C., Wewers, T., Theisinger, F.: Workbrain: Merging Organizational Memory and Workflow Management System, University of Erlangen-Nuremberg, FORWISS, 1997.
15. Zhao, J. L.: Knowledge Management and Organizational Learning in Workflow Systems, Proceedings of the AIS Americas Conference on Information Systems, Baltimore, Maryland, August 14-16, 1998

20

CONFIGURING OF SUPPLY CHAIN NETWORKS BASED ON CONSTRAINT SATISFACTION, GENETIC AND FUZZY GAME THEORETIC APPROACHES

Alexander V. Smirnov[1], Leonid B. Sheremetov[2,3], Nikolai Chilov[1]
Jose Romero Cortes[2]
[1]*St.Petersburg Institute for Informatics and Automation of the Russian Academy of Sciences*
SPIIRAS, 39, 14th Line, St.Petersburg, 199178, Russia
smir@.iias.spb.su
[2] *Computer Science Research Center of National Technical University (CIC-IPN),*
Av. Juan de Dios Batiz esq. Othon de Mendizabal s/n Col. Nueva Industrial Vallejo,
México, D.F., C.P. 07738, Mexico
sher@cic.ipn.mx
[3] *Mexican Oil Institute,*
Av. Lazaro Cardenas, 152, Col.san Bartolo Atepehuacan, México, D.F., CP 07730 ,

In this article, the problem of the supply chain network (SCN) generation as a dynamic, flexible and agile system with dynamic configurations is considered. The proposed method consists in the product and SCN configurations with resource allocation in multi-agent environment. For this purpose an application of different techniques is examined. Object oriented constraint networks are used for solving SCN configuration and resource allocation tasks using constraint satisfaction methodology. The second approach permits to find sub-optimal solution applying the theory of games with fuzzy coalitions. FIPA compliant agent platform and a CASE tool for SCN development, modeling and simulation are used to provide the experiments. The above techniques are compared and the simulation results are discussed.

1. INTRODUCTION

Supply-chain network (SCN) is a philosophy for enterprise integration based on a society formed by autonomous agents by bonding together to solve a common

This paper presents several solutions to the problem of configuration of a SCN considered as a problem of task allocation among groups of autonomous agents. These groups are called coalitions. Important properties of the techniques and algorithms solving the task allocation problem are: (i) avoiding central authority, (ii) a low computational complexity, and (iii) increasing both individual utility and the overall outcome of the system (Shehory, 1999). There are two different approaches to the coalition formation problem, the former is based on the optimisation and combinatorial methods and the later on the game-theoretic approach (Axelrod, 1997; Jennings, 2001; Mares, 2000).

The paper considers the case when each task is attached to a group of agents (better to say, they try to form a coalition to perform this task) because they cannot be performed by a single agent, a single agent cannot perform them efficiently or cannot meet system's constraints. Earlier, the approach of forming fuzzy coalitions with full involvement was considered, when each agent may be a member of only one coalition and each task can be fulfilled by only one agent (Romero & Sheremetov, 2001). In this paper an approach when capacity constraints are added to the problem statement is presented. Techniques of the first type are based on the conventional optimization approaches. Object oriented constraint networks are used for solving SCN configuration and resource allocation tasks using constraint satisfaction methodology (Smirnov and Chilov, 1999). The second approach permits to find sub-optimal solution applying the theory of games with fuzzy coalitions. The above techniques are compared and the simulation results are discussed.

2. A CASE STUDY DESCRIPTION

For the demonstration purposes a rather simple example of an automobile SCN was considered. The case study deals with production of a hypothetic vehicle (a *Car*). The price of the car is *$20,000*. The production process (fig. 1) consists of the following two phases: *Component Production* and *Car Assembly*. *Component Production* consists of three parallel operations: *Body Production*, *Motor Production*, and *Transmission Production* (Bokma, 2001).

Demand is represented by a uniform distribution around the linear trend:

$d_t = a + b \cdot t + \mu \cdot \sigma$, where

t – time instant

d – demand (d_t corresponds to time interval $[t-1, t]$)

a – basis value ($a = 100$)

b – trend component (0 for demand without trend)

μ – random noise uniformly distributed within $[0{:}1]$

σ – distribution amplitude

For simplicity, an example without trend and with low noise ($\sigma = 5$) is considered. In this case the technique of Single Moving Average for the demand forecasting can be used:

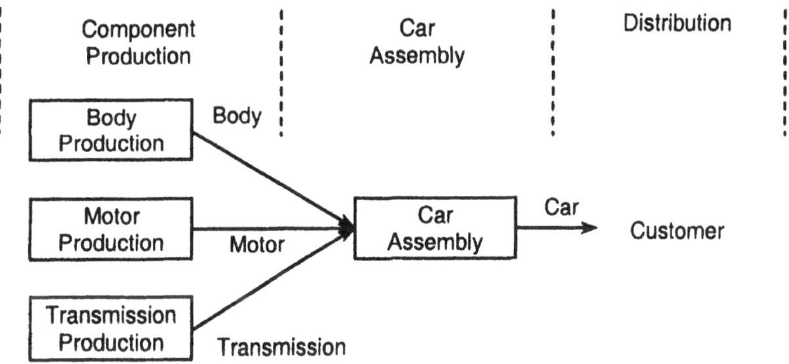

Figure 1 – Structure of the Production Process

$$f_{t+2} = f_{t+1} = \frac{\sum_{i=t-n+1}^{t} d_i}{n}, \text{ where}$$

f – forecasted data (forecast)
n – forecast base ($n = 5$);

Car Assembly can be performed by one unit (*car assembler* or Unit 7) with the following parameters:

- *Capacity = 105.* A case without fixed capacity (no changes) is considered.
- Stocks are *unlimited*
- Stocking costs are *$750* per car/week, *$300* per body/week, *$200* per motor/week, *$100* per transmission/week.
- Assembly costs are *$1500* per car

Component Production can be performed by 6 units, each with different facilities (see Table). The stocks are considered unlimited. Payoffs for Component Production are *$7000* per body, *$5000* per motor, and *$4000* per transmission. Penalties for backorders are *$1500* per car/week (paid by the car assembler to the customer), *$400* per body/week, *$300* per motor/week, *$250* per transmission/week (paid by the component producers to the car assembler).

Table 1. Data for the production units (potential supply chain members)

Unit	Capacity	Facility	Production Costs	Stocking
Unit 1	*100*	Body Production	*$4500* per body	*$250* per body/week
Unit 2	*100*	Motor Production	*$3500* per body	*$150* per body/week
Unit 3	*100*	Transmission Production	*$2500* per transmission	*$50* per transmission/week
Unit 4	*303*	Body Production	*$4900* per body	*$300* per body/week
		Motor Production	*$3800* per body	*$200* per body/week
		Transmission Production	*$2700* per transmission	*$80* per transmission/week
Unit 5	*100*	Motor Production	*$3600* per body	*$170* per body/week
		Transmission Production	*$2600* per transmission	*$60* per transmission/week
Unit 6	*200*	Body Production	*$4700* per body	*$270* per body/week
		Motor Production	*$3600* per body	*$170* per body/week

3. DESCRIPTION OF SOLUTION METHODS

3.1 Constraint Satisfaction Approach to Configuration and Resource Allocation of the SCN

Generally a task of a resource optimization can be described as follows: it is necessary to define efficient allocation (where is situated) and schedule (when is available) of a given resource components and when and which of the components should be used. As a criterion such indices as costs of the resource acquiring and/or delivery or required for this purpose time, can be used. It is necessary to take into account relationships existing between resources and resource components (for instance, a resource may consist of some other resources). The fact of existence of these relationships allow considering the task of resource optimization as a constraint satisfaction problem (Smirnov and Chilov, 1999).

A constraint satisfaction problem is defined as (X, D, C). It consists of n variables $X = \{x_1, x_2, ..., x_n\}$, whose values are taken from finite, discrete domains $D = \{D_1, D_2, ..., D_n\}$, and a set of constraints on their values $C = \{c_1, c_2, \ldots c_m\}$. A constraint is defined by a predicate. That is, the constraint $c_k(x_{k1}, ..., x_{kj})$ is a predicate that is defined on the Cartesian product $D_{k1} \times \ldots \times D_{kj}$. This predicate is true if the value assignment of these variables satisfies this constraint. Solving a constraint satisfaction problem assumes finding an assignment of values to all variables such that all constraints are satisfied. In other words, a constraint satisfaction problem is a task of finding a consistent assignment of values to variables (Mackworth, 1992; Yokoo, and Hirayama 2000). A simple example of such task is given in (fig. 2).

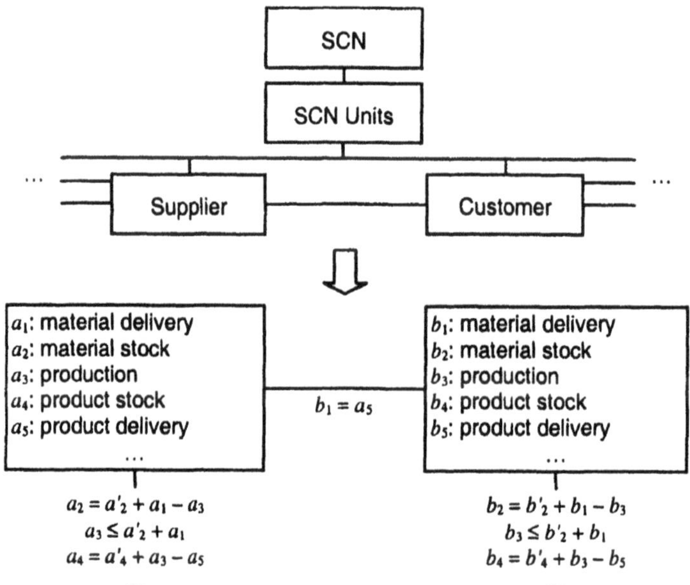

Figure 2 – Example constraint network

Regarding to the considered here task, the components of the task have the following notations:

x_{ijt} – the quantity of the j component to be produced by unit i at a time interval $[t-1, t]$;

D_{ijt} – the sets of integer positive numbers (I^+);

C – the constraints responsible for synchronization and consistency of the considered SCN system. The following groups of constraints were selected: capacity-based constraints, constraints on materials availability, delivery or synchronization constraints.

3.2 Game Theoretic Approach with Fuzzy Coalitions to SCN Configuring

Another approach developed in this article is based on fuzzy coalition game of players with full involvement (Mares, 2000; Romero and Sheremetov, 2002). Each player corresponds to the node of the SCN. According to (Mares, 2000), the core (the set of solutions) C_F of the game (I, w) (where I is the set of players and w is the characteristic function associated with fuzzy payoffs) is defined as follows:

$$C_F = \{\sum_{i\in I} x_i \le w(I), \sum_{i\in K} x_i \le w(K) : K \subset I\} \tag{1}$$

The core has the following membership function associated with it:

$$\gamma_c(x) = \min_{K\subset I}(\nu_{\succ=}(w(I), \sum_{i\in I} x_i), \nu_{\prec=}(\sum_{i\in K} x_i, w(K))) \tag{2}$$

where: $\nu \succ= (w(I), \langle \sum_{i\in I} x_i \rangle)$, with the preference $\succ=$ as a weak order fuzzy relation with membership function $\nu \succ=: R\times R \to [0,1]$.

The expressions (1) and (2) correspond to the game-theoretic model with fuzzy coalitions and contain only the terms relative to the fuzzy payments. For the purposes of this article the fuzzy core was changed to include the capacities of each agent and the tasks to fulfill defined by the demand, product bill and specified in the problem domain ontology. The new core definition follows (without lacking of generality, for simplicity this model doesn't include the fluctuations caused by inventories):

$$C = \{2500x_{11t} + 2100x_{41t} + 2300x_{61t} + 1500x_{22t} + 1200x_{42t} + 1400x_{52t} + 1400x_{62t} +$$
$$1500x_{33t} + 2500x_{74t} + 1300x_{43t} + 1400x_{53t} \ge (100 + 5t + \mu 5)w(I),$$
$$2500x_{11t} + 2100x_{41t} + 2300x_{61t} \le (100 + 5t + \mu 5)w(k_1)$$
$$1500x_{22t} + 1200x_{42t} + 1400x_{52t} + 1400x_{62t} \le (100 + 5t + \mu 5)w(k_2)$$
$$1500x_{33t} + 1300x_{43t} + 1400x_{53t} \le (100 + 5t + \mu 5)w(k_3)$$
$$2500x_{74t} \le (100 + 5t + \mu 5)w(k_4)$$

$$\begin{aligned} x_{11t} + x_{41t} + x_{61t} &= 100 + 5t + 5\mu \\ x_{22t} + x_{42t} + x_{52t} + x_{62t} &= 100 + 5t + 5\mu \\ x_{33t} + x_{43t} + x_{53t} &= 100 + 5t + 5\mu \end{aligned} \tag{3}$$

$x_{74t} = 100 + 5t + 5\mu$

$x_{11t} \leq 100$ $\quad x_{41t} \leq 302.5$ $\quad x_{61t} \leq 200$

$x_{22t} \leq 100$ $\quad x_{42t} \leq 302.5$ $\quad x_{52t} \leq 100$ $\quad x_{62t} \leq 200$

$x_{33t} \leq 100$ $\quad x_{43t} \leq 302.5$ $\quad x_{53t} \leq 100$

$x_{74t} \leq 102.5$

$x_{ijt} \in R^+,\ i = 1,\dots,7;\ \ j = 1,\dots,4\ \ t = 1,\dots,5\}$

where:

x_{ijt} = the quantity of the j component to be produced by agent i in time t.

$w(I)$ = fuzzy payoff per unit for car production.

$w(k_1)$ = fuzzy payoff per unit for Body Production.

$w(k_2)$ = fuzzy payoff per unit for Motor Production.

$w(k_3)$ = fuzzy payoff per unit for Transmission Production.

$w(k_4)$ = fuzzy payoff per unit for car assembly.

μ = uniform random variable in [0,1].

The forecasting model for the demand is the following:

$100 + 5t + 5\mu,\ for\ t = 1,\dots,5$ and μ is uniform in [0,1] (4)

Two solution techniques were studied. First, the Excel solver was used. Next, genetic algorithms were used and Evolver software. Testbed implementation details and simulation results are discussed in the following section.

4. IMPLEMENTATION DETAILS AND OBTAINED RESULTS

4.1 A Multiagent Testbed

To implement the prototype and provide the experiments with the proposed methods, a multiagent testbed has been developed. For the implementation of the testbed, Zeus v1.2.1 software (JRE v1.3.1.02) was used as FIPA compliant agent platform (Nwana et all., 1999).

Each domain agent associated with a node of the SCN was equipped with the contract net negotiation protocol (CNP). The SCN Head agent (called Assembly in the presented case study) was the one who decided the final configuration based on the computations performed by the solvers. Problem solving methods (PSM) are implemented as external legacy software modules. Genetic algorithms are implemented using the Evolver software (Evolver, 2001), accessed through the Excel Wrapper agent. Constraint solver is implemented using ILOG Configurator constraint programming engine (ILOG, 2001) and accessed by means of another Wrapper agent implemented in C++. Agents were running on the agent platform and PSM software on another computer.

Some scalability problems were detected while running the simulations. First, an execution of the batch files generated in a predetermined way: run1.bat (executing Agent Name Server - ANS), run2.bat (domain agents) and run3.bat (visualizer and Directory Facilitator - DF), was tried. The problem of this approach is that each agent is executed in his own virtual machine consuming many computer resources. As a result, it was impossible to execute more then 10 agents in a single-host fashion. To handle this problem, the utility (Zsh) that allows to execute several agents in the same virtual machine was used. The second parameter of this utility <param2> is a number representing the time period that any DF agent started will wait between querying the agent system for their capacities to be properly recognized by the rest of the system, which can affect the system performance. This way it was possible to reach the following configuration: 10 Tail Agents, Assembler Agent, ANS, Visualizer Agent, and DF Agent. The agents were running on a Compaq Presario 5473 (Celeron 550 Mhz, 128 MB RAM) computer. Using this computer, the case study SCN shown in the figure 3 has been simulated.

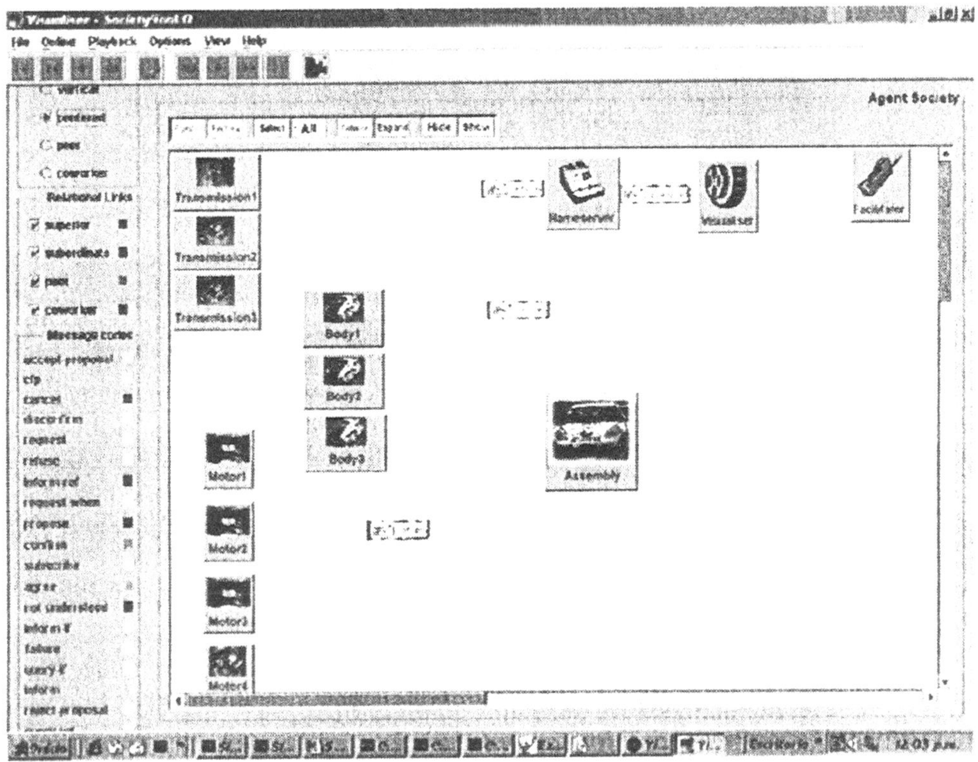

Figure 3 – A screenshot of the Visualizer with an example configuration (Society Viewer's window).

As it shown in fig.3, the case study consisted in eleven domain agents (one for each facility and an assembly one) and three utility agents of the platform. Each domain agent had an access to a DB where it's capacity, production cost and stocking data was stored. In the case of a fuzzy game, domain agents were also equipped with the interface windows to capture the parameters of the individual membership functions. Special purpose Coalition Agents have been generated for each component every time a new demand occurred. Additional software accessed by these agents has been developed to calculate coalition membership functions. Assembly Agent served as a SCN coordinator initiating negotiation protocols. CNP was used to collect the biddings for the demand.

4.2 Results of Constraint Satisfaction Approach

As it was mentioned above to solve considered here task the engine of ILOG Configurator was used. It represents constraint network to be processed in an object-oriented form. The system supports the following two types of relations: (i) "is a" between classes and objects, and (ii) "is connected to" between objects. In turn relations "is connected to" can be of the following two subtypes: (i) "has part" or "part of" and (ii) "uses". The objects own attributes whose values belong to defined domains and are controlled by constraints existing in the problem domain. This representation allows rapid and convenient model creation and maintenance. On the other hand an advanced ILOG Solver performs the task solving process in an efficient way. Obtained results for 5 time intervals are given in table 2.

Table 2. Production levels per unit for five time intervals

t	x_{11t}	x_{22t}	x_{33t}	x_{41t}	x_{42t}	x_{43t}	x_{52t}	x_{53t}	x_{61t}	x_{62t}	x_{74t}
1	100	100	100	0	0	0	0	5	5	5	105
2	100	100	100	0	0	0	0	12	12	12	112
3	100	100	100	0	0	0	0	15	15	15	115
4	100	100	100	0	0	0	0	24	24	24	124
5	100	100	100	0	0	0	0	28	28	28	128

The common network payoffs per car obtained for each time interval are equal 9,480.95; 9,457.14; 9,447.83; 9,422.58; 9,412.50 respectively. The payoffs (p) of the participating units per car/component are as follows: $p_{unit\ 1} = 2{,}500$; $p_{unit\ 2} = 1{,}500$; $p_{unit\ 3} = 1{,}500$; $p_{unit\ 4} = 0$; $p_{unit\ 5} = 1{,}400$; $p_{unit\ 6} = 1{,}850$; $p_{unit\ 7} = 2{,}500$.

Utilizing combination of constraint-based technique allowing obtaining a global optimal solution, and ILOG Solver engine allowing utilizing both linear and non-linear constraints, makes it possible to solve large tasks with complicated dependencies between their components.

4.3 Results of Game Theoretic Approach with Fuzzy Coalitions

For the case study, positive ramp membership functions were selected: payoff per car - [7,100, 8,000]; gross payoffs for body - [6,500, 7,000]; motor - [4,500, 5,000]; transmission - [3,800, 4,000]; and assembly - [2,000, 4,000] respectively. Two solvers were used to find the solution. The first one, the Excel solver was able only to approximate the integer solution (table 3). Table 3 shows the imputations for each time interval, the last column shows the number of cars to be assembled according to the forecasting defined by (4).

Table 3. Production levels per unit for five time intervals

t	x_{11t}	x_{22t}	x_{33t}	x_{41t}	x_{42t}	x_{43t}	x_{52t}	x_{53t}	x_{61t}	x_{62t}	x_{74t}
1	100	100	100	0	0	0	5.299	5.3	5.3	.001	105.3
2	100	100	100	0	0	0	8.399	11.5	11.5	3.101	111.5
3	100	100	100	0	0	0	10.25	15.2	15.2	4.95	115.2
4	100	100	100	0	0	0	14.50	23.7	23.7	9.20	123.7
5	100	100	100	0	0	0	16.75	28.2	28.2	11.45	128.2

The second solution method used was that of genetic algorithms. The solution converged within several seconds (though communications between agents took considerable time). The rates of mutation and crossover in the typical values of 6 and 50% respectively, with a size of population of 50 organisms were fixed. Time convergence parameters and number of iterations was also fixed (Romero and Sheremetov, 2001).

The common network payoffs per car obtained for each time interval are equal to 7,578.46, 7,578.22, 7,578.22, 7,577.84, 7,577.84 respectively. The payoffs (p) of the participating units per car/component are as follows: $p_{unit\ 1}$ = 2,500; $p_{unit\ 2}$ = 1,500; $p_{unit\ 3}$ = 1,500; $p_{unit\ 4}$ = 0; $p_{unit\ 5}$ = 1,400; $p_{unit\ 6}$ = 1,400; $p_{unit\ 7}$ = 2,500. The same gross payoffs per unit were obtained for each time interval for each component: $w(I)$ = 20,000; $w(k_1)$ = 7,000; $w(k_2)$ =5,000; $w(k_3)$ =4,000 $w(k_4)$ =4,000. The possibility of the fuzzy game $\gamma_c(I,w)$ = 1.00 (because of the simplicity of the case study), though the imputation obtained took into account the subjective estimations of the players defined by their fuzzy payments.

5. DISCUSSION AND CONCLUSIONS

Different problem statements and solution techniques have been discussed in this article. The problem statement defined in section 3.2 permits to consider non-lineal membership functions, integer variables, multi-objective functions and non-lineal constraints. But only the use of heuristic and soft-computing techniques such as genetic algorithms as it was shown in (Romero and Sheremetov, 2001), permit to find the best converged imputation in a reasonable time for real world applications. The use of genetic algorithms has the following benefits: they allow to find a semi-optimal solution in the case when an optimal solution can't be found analytically because of the problem's complexity, they allow to find a local optimal solution in the cases when the optimal solution even doesn't exist (when the game is not convex), and also they can be used to find solutions for the mixed approaches similar to the discussed in this paper when a game-theoretic approach is combined with the combinatorial one.

The constraint-based approach assumes *complete* information sharing while the game theoretic approach assumes *minimal* or *no* information sharing. Since in real-world situations the both cases as well as some intermediate ones are possible, the application of presented here techniques in a combined way is preferable. The subsequent research efforts are planned to be devoted to investigation of combined techniques for tasks representing more realistic situations according to the following:

1) wider range of parameters to optimise,
2) more complicated strategies of the units (e.g., including safety stocks forming),
3) more complicated demand patterns and forecasting techniques,
4) non-lineal relationships in the model.

FIPA compliant agent platform and a CASE tool for SCN development, modeling and simulation are used to provide the experiments. The use of this platform not only ensures interoperability among the agents and reusable components for the future enterprise-based applications, but also allows taking advantage of agent-based, as well as component-based services offered by the SCN units that can be used and customized as needed.

The presented methodology of the coalition formation implies implicit negotiations (vague, imprecise, open), which are guided to maximize the benefits or viabilities (i) of each individual agent of the SCN, (ii) of agents' coalition and even (iii) of a great coalition that contains all the agents of the system. The structure of a virtual company formed this way, has the distinctive point and the advantage in that it takes into account the convenience for the companies to participate in groups (virtual companies), it allows quick adaptations that respond to changes of the environmental dynamics.

6. ACKNOWLEDGMENTS

Partial support for this research work has been provided by the CONACyT, Mexico within the project 31851-A Models and Tools for Agent Interaction in Cooperative MAS and by the National Technical University, Mexico, within the program CGEPI 18.01. The paper is also due to the research carried out as a part of the project # 4.4 of the research program # 18 "Intelligent Computer Systems" of the Russian Academy of Sciences, and grant # 02-01-00284 of the Russian Foundation for Basic Research. Some examples were developed using software granted by ILOG Inc.

7. REFERENCES

1. Axelrod, R. (1997). The complexity of cooperation: agent based models of competition and collaboration. Princeton University Press.
2. Bokma, A. (2001). CogNet: Integrated Information and Knowledge Management and its Use in Virtual Organisations. In E-Business and Virtual Enterprises, Managing Business-to-Business Cooperation. L.M.Camarinha-Matos, H.Afsarmanesh, R.J.Rabelo, ed. Kluwer Academic Publishers, Boston, 361-370.
3. Evolver (2001). Release 4.01. Palisade.
4. Jennings, N.R., Faratin, P., Lomuscio, A.R., Parsons, S., Sierra, C and Wooldridge, M., (2001). Automated negotiation: prospects, methods and challenges. Int. J. of Group Decision and Negotiation 10(2): 199-215.
5. ILOG (2001). Corporate website, URL: http://www.ilog.com.
6. Mackworth, A. (1992). Constraint Satisfaction. In: S.C. Shapiro (ed.): Encyclopedia of Artificial Intelligence. New York: Wiley-Interscience Publication, 285-293.
7. Mares, M. (2000). Fuzzy coalition structures. Fuzzy sets and systems. Elsevier Sciences. 114: 23-33.
8. Nwana, H. S., Ndumu, D. T., Lee, L. C., and Collis, J. C. (1999), ZEUS: A Toolkit for Building Distributed Multi-Agent Systems, Applied Artificial Intelligence Journal 13 (1/2): 129-185.
9. Romero, J. & Sheremetov, L. (2002). Model of Cooperation in Multi Agent Systems with Fuzzy Coalitions. In B. Dunin-Keplicz, E. Nawarecki (Eds.): From Theory to Practice in Multi-Agent Systems. Lecture Notes in Artificial Intelligence, Springer Verlag, 2296: 263-272.
10. Shehory, O. and Kraus, S. (1999). Feasible Formation of Coalitions Among Autonomous Agents in Non-Super-Additive Environments, Computational Intelligence, Vol. 15(3): 218-251.
11. Smirnov, A. (1999). Virtual Enterprise Configuration Management. In: Proceedings of the 14th IFAC World Congress (IFAC'99), Beijing, China, Pergamon Press, vol. A, 337-342.
12. Smirnov, A. and Chilov, N. (1999). Management Decision Making Models and Tools for Estimating Strategic Objectives of Virtual Enterprise Participants. In: Proceedings of the International Conference on Life Cycle Approaches to Production Systems: Management, Control, Supervision (ASI'99), Leuven, Belgium, 5.10 – 5.11.
13. Yokoo, M. and Hirayama, K. (2000). Algorithms for Distributed Constraint Satisfaction: A Review. Autonomous Agents and Multi-Agent Systems, Vol. 3(2): 198-212.

21

QUANTITATIVE INTEGRATION OF THE ANALYTICAL HIERARCHICAL PROCESS AND VIRTUAL ENTERPRISE MODEL TO SUPPORT MANAGER DECISIONS

Giuseppe Confessore
Istituto di Tecnologie Industriali e Automazione – Sezione di Roma
Consiglio Nazionale delle Ricerche
c/o DISP. Via del Politecnico 1, 00133 Roma, Italy
g.confessore@itia.mi.cnr.it

Livio Cricelli
Università di Cassino. Dipartimento di Meccanica, Strutture, Ambiente e Territorio
Via G. Di Biasio 43, 03043 Cassino (Fr) Italy
cricelli@unicas.it

Paolo Mancuso
Università di Roma "Tor Vergata". Dipartimento di Informatica, Sistemi e Produzione
Via del Politecnico 1, 00133 Roma, Italy
mancuso@disp.uniroma2.it

In measuring the global performance of a production system two problems are relevant. The first one is represented by the individuation of a meaningful set of indicators and the second one by the choice of the connected weights system. In this paper, we highlights the advantages of the integration of the Analytical Hierarchical Process and the use of a simulation tool of a production system. The procedure of such integration is explained with more considerations given to its possible dual application, by top managers and systems' designers, to firstly predict the possible changes of production system and then take reasonable courses of action to individuate the best configuration. Moreover, we have tested the proposed methodology for an Italian firm.

1. INTRODUCTION

One of the most relevant topics in production management is the development of integrated systems which are able to co-ordinate different technologies and applications; aiming at making the whole process of production efficient. In a competitive environment, industrial enterprises must continuously improve their productivity to sustain long term growth and profitability. To increase efficiency, without absorbing further resources, productivity measurement and analysis can therefore play an important role in the strategic planning and competitive analysis (Lowlor, 1985, Sudit, 1995).

In many industrial sectors, models of business management that are based on the maximisation of the short run profits are often inadequate to guarantee success in front of changes in the world competitive markets. The problems faced today by each firm have reached high level of unforeseeably and complexity, and so, as a result, the decisions that the managers must take result in hard determination. For a long time management has turned their own attention toward two different directions:

1. to the inside, where the purpose is to improve the processes of production to adjust them to the mutable situations of market and new technologies and to modify the organisational structures, policies and the techniques of management;
2. to the outside, where they try to modify the market, arouse new needs or modify those existing to exploit the action of the competitors and the behavior of the institutions.

To develop their own activity effectively management needs continuous information on the whole economic system and on their own operational units. Difficulties that it meets to effect the correct choices are highly correlated to the quantity and the quality of available information (Avai et al, 2001). It appears therefore evident that the presence of a rational and efficient information system is essential for the existence and the survival of the firm.

The purpose of the information system is therefore to develop a continuous function of control both on the inside environment, constituted by varied business activities, and on the outside environment, represented by the competitors, the institutions and the consumers. The core of the system is represented by the performance measurement system that assumes therefore a fundamental importance in the optimal management of the firm and for its existence and survival.

The term performance has recently entered in the common political and managerial language, to indicate the achieved result obtained by any activities. More precisely, with performance, it is the intended result of management of the activities of an organization in a certain period of time (Lucertini et al, 1995, Hatry, 1980). This interpretation doesn't allow the deepest meaning that the performance assumes in business circles; it is not a simple numerical value. Having performance implicates to have success, to be competitive, to be able to react opportunely to the changes of the external environment and individualizing and improving those activities which are able to provide value to the firm. The performance of a firm today is the key to economic success.

In this sense, the concept of performance is deeply linked to management. In fact, Lebas (1995) shows that performance doesn't refer to the results provided in the past, but rather is projected toward those obtainable in the future, introducing in this way the concept of performance management. Management must, in practice, individualize the causes of performance and to pursue continuous improvement, supported by the measures of the same performance. In fact, the comprehension of the processes of performance generation not only facilitates the identification of these measures and therefore the possible corrective actions, but it allows a clear utilization of strategies to each level of responsibility.

The performance management precedes and follows the performance measurement in a repetitive loop, creating at the same time the environment for the measures. A system of effective performance management must be supported by measures that (Lebas, 1995):
a) give autonomy to managers;
b) reflect relationships of cause and effect;
c) create the bases for the discussion, so supporting continuous improvement;
d) help managers in making their decisions.
The performance management and the measurement of performance can not be separated; if we focus only on the measurements, without understanding that the measures are the consequences of the decisions, we loose the opportunity to reach the control on the processes of performance creation and success for the firm (Prokopenko, 1992). The measurement concept is considered an essential prerequisite getting efficient results and continuously improving business performances. The concept of performance evaluation has always existed; traditionally the measurements were based on historical data, almost never on competitive bases or through the use of financial indicators. These last ones are able to be drawn only after the editing of budgets and therefore they are not able to signal opportunely the presence of problems. The actual market conditions and the firms global competition make these indicators insufficient to obtain a measure of efficiency and we must move attention toward the search for new indexes to measure business performances. The individuation of the proper criterions to evaluate the results really obtained by the firm is still object of researchers discussion. In the literature, in fact, a unique reference model doesn't exist. In general, it depends on the particular considered context and from the specific sector of application. The most diffused and used criterions for performance evaluation (indexes, variations, ratios, etc.) fall into the categories of effectiveness, productive efficiency, and profitability. The significance of this paper can be seen in the definition of framework to evaluate the operative, tactical and strategic decisions of the management. We propose to use the analytical hierarchical process (Saaty, 1977, Saaty and Khouja, 1977, Saaty and Varga, 1979) to evaluate the decisions where the weights of the decision tree are computed by using a simulation model of the production system. To do this, we introduce the concept of virtual enterprise (or virtual factory - VF) as the simulation model of the physical enterprise (or physical factory - PF).

2. THE MODEL

To allow the management to decide which are the best decisions, at operative, tactical and strategic level, we introduce a model in which an analytical hierarchical process tool is integrate with a simulation model representing the physical enterprise (see Figure 1).
In particular, in the simulation model (or virtual enterprise) we simulate the different scenarios originated from different decisions of the management (the different choices that the decision tool has to evaluate) for computing the weights necessary to order the choices by decision tool. The virtual enterprise is a virtual copy of the physical enterprise. The physical and informative flows that are involved in the

physical enterprise are represented in the virtual enterprise by entity flow in the simulation model.

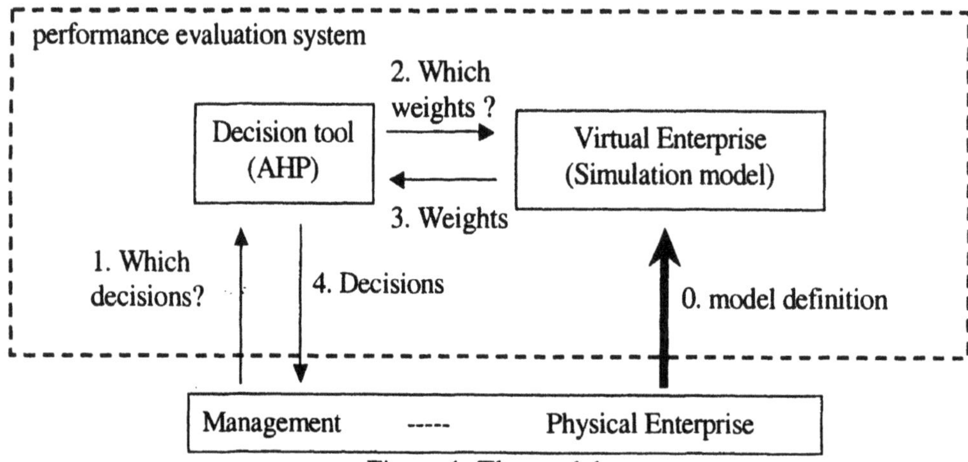

Figure 1. The model.

When a decision has to be make, different choice are make in the simulation model. Then, it is possible to set the weights of the decision tree in order to choice the best decision. The decision could be strategic, tactical or operative, even in the same time.

3. A CASE STUDY

The theoretical model defined in section 2 has been applied at one of the most important Italian industry, at world-wide level of domestic appliances. We have considered three productive plants employed for the production of electric compressors for refrigerators. The three plants are located in different part of the North East of Italy. The first plant located near Pordenone produces copper and cast-iron for electric motors and compressors. The second plant in Rovigo assembles electric motors. Finally, the last plant near Belluno assembles the compressors.
At this point our analysis has been focussed on Rovigo plant characterised by a job-shop productive configuration. In particular we have considered two manufacturing departments in which stators and rotors are produced respectively. Then the performance indicators and their relative weights have been obtained through interviews with plant managers and using the AHP methodology (Chankong and Haimes, 1983, Mesarovich et al., 1970) implemented by Expert Choices® 2000 software (see Table 1).
Performance indicators specification for each nodes level is reported below (note that the numbers 1 and 2 are referred at the two manufacturing departments).

- First level nodes: Pr = Productivity, Production Environment =PE, CS = Customer Satisfaction, Lo = Logistic
- Second level nodes: LP = Labour Productivity, MP = Machinery Productvity, Fl = Flexibility, Ma = Maintenance, TO =Time to Order, LT= Production Lead Time, MLT = Mean Lead Time stock-out, MDT = Mean Delivery Time.

- Third level nodes: LE = Labour Efficiency (total amount of actually worked hour/total amount of paid hours), LPE= Labour Performance (produced volume/total amount of effective worked hours), ME = Machinery Efficiency (actually production hours/scheduled production hours machines), MPE = Machines Performance (produced volume/(actually production hours), PN= Number of different products, MST = Mean Set-up Time, MTBF = Mean Time Between Failure, MTM = Mean Time to Maintenance, PLT = Production Lead Time, TLT = Transport Lead Time, WLT = Waiting Lead Time
- Fourth level nodes: MSTS = Mean Set-up Time between the production of items belonging to the same products typology, MSTD = Mean Set-up Time between the production of items belonging to different products typology.

The second step in our analysis has been the individuation of the strategic scenarios to compare. The base scenario has been obtained starting from the production data collected during the 2000 year. The production level reached in this year has been about 3 millions of compressors. Moreover, in order to consider the existence of seasonality the production period has been divided into two sub-periods: November to April and May to October. The total amount of compressors produced has been of 1.200.000 in the first period and 1.800.000 in the second one. The collected data have been normalised and reported in Table 2.

Table 1. Performance indicators and weights.

First level nodes	Second level nodes	Third level nodes	Fourth level nodes	Fifth level nodes
Pr 0.25	LP 0.33	LE 0.5	LE1 0.545	
			LE2 0.455	
		LPE 0.5	LPE1 0.545	
			LPE2 0.455	
	MP 0.66	ME 0.5	ME1 0.6	
			ME2 0.4	
		MPE 0.5	MPE1 0.6	
			MPE2 0.4	
PE 0.25	Fl 0.389	PN 0.469		
		MST 0.531	MSTS 0.525	MSTS1 0.545
				MSTS2 0.455
			MSTD 0.475	MSTD1 0.545
				MSTD2 0.455
	Ma 0.611	MTBF 0.434	MTBF1 0.5	
			MTBF2 0.5	
		MTM 0.566	MTM1 0.566	
			MTM2 0.434	
CS 0.25	TO 0.524	PLT 0.723		
		TLT 0.277		
	LT 0.476	WLT 0.146		
		PLT 0.61		
		TLT 0.244		
Lo 0.25	MLT0.12			
	MDT 0.88			

Table 2. Performance indicators values

Performance indicators	First period	Second Period
LE1	0.958	0.958
LE2	0.958	0.958
LPE1	0.28	0.563
LPE2	0.28	0.564
ME1	0.937	0.937
ME2	0.917	0.917
MPE1	0.388	0.643
MPE2	0.409	0.669
PN	0.25	0.25
MSTS1	0.545	0.5
MSTS2	0.455	0.625
MSTD1	0.545	0.3
MSTD2	0.455	0.3
MTBF1	0.475	0.475
MTBF2	0.5	0.5
MTM1	0.333	0.333
MTM2	0.25	0.25
PLT	0.45	0.75
TLT	0.5	0.5
WLT	0.6	0.6
MLT	0.45	0.75
MDT	0.6	0.6

The alternative scenarios are four and they are characterised by different assumption on firm's strategic objective, obtained using the virtual enterprise simulated through the discrete simulation software tool ARENA®. In the first scenario, the performance indicators modified respect to the base scenario are relative to Productivity (Pr) and Production Environment (PE); in the second Customer Satisfaction (CS); in the third Customer Satisfaction (CS) and Logistic (L) and in the last one, only the change in the Production Environment (PE) has been examined. The modified values of the indicators under the different scenario, computed by the simulation tool, are shown below:

First Scenario:

Performance indicators	First period	Second Period
LPE1	0.35	0.7
LPE2	0.35	0.7
MPE1	0.45	0.8
MPE2	0.45	0.8
MSTS1	0.8	0.8
MSTS2	0.8	0.8
MTM1	0.5	0.5
MTM2	0.4	0.4

Second Scenario:

Performance indicators	First period	Second Period
PLT	0.75	0.9

Third Scenario:

Performance indicators	First period	Second Period
PLT	0.5	0.8
TLT	0.7	0.7
WLT	0.65	0.65
MLT	0.5	0.8
MDT	0.65	0.65

Fourth Scenario:

Performance indicators	First period	Second Period
PN	0.5	0.5
MSTS1	0.6	0.6
MSTS2	0.6	0.6
MSTD1	0.6	0.6
MSTD2	0.6	0.6
MTBF1	0.6	0.6
MTBF2	0.6	0.6
MTM1	0.5	0.5
MTM2	0.4	0.4

The global alternatives priority computed by the Software Expert Choices® 2000 in the two production periods are summarised in Table 3.

Table 3: Global alternatives priority

Alternatives	First Period	Second Period
Base Alternative	0.183	0.188
Alternative 1	0.197	0.203
Alternative 2	0.222	0.203
Alternative 3	0.195	0.199
Alternative 4	0.203	0.207

The model results for the first production period are shown in Figure 2. The best alternative is the second one, that is proposed to improve exclusively the production lead time. Also differing from the actual situation only for an indicator (PLT), the obtained improvement in the global performance is very high (about 21%). In fact, the production lead time influences in decisive way the internal logistic and also the customer satisfaction. With the aim to evaluate the importance of the first level weights, a sensitivity analysis is performed. As it is shown in Figure 3, for a value of productivity weight equal to 70% the alternatives are equivalents. Therefore, if this objective can become such strategically important in near future, it would be necessary to proceed to a more detailed analysis in order to estimate better which alternative to follow. Moreover variations in all strategic objectives weights within a enough wide range do not involve appreciable differences in the choice of the best alternative.

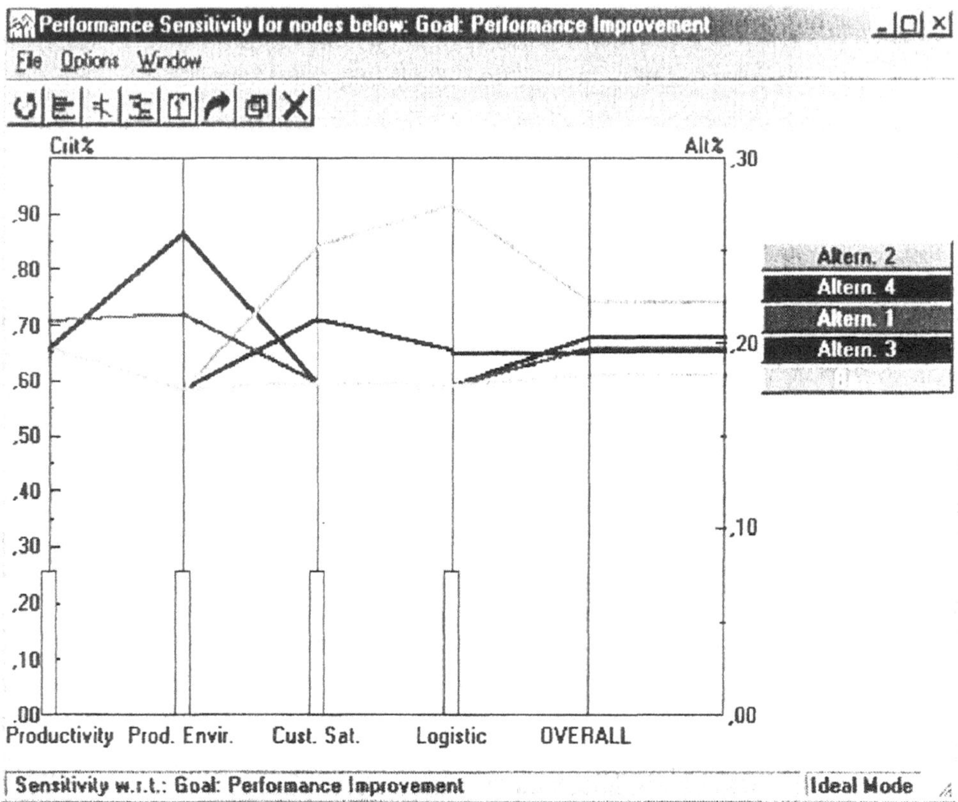

Figure 2: Performance Graph for the first production period.

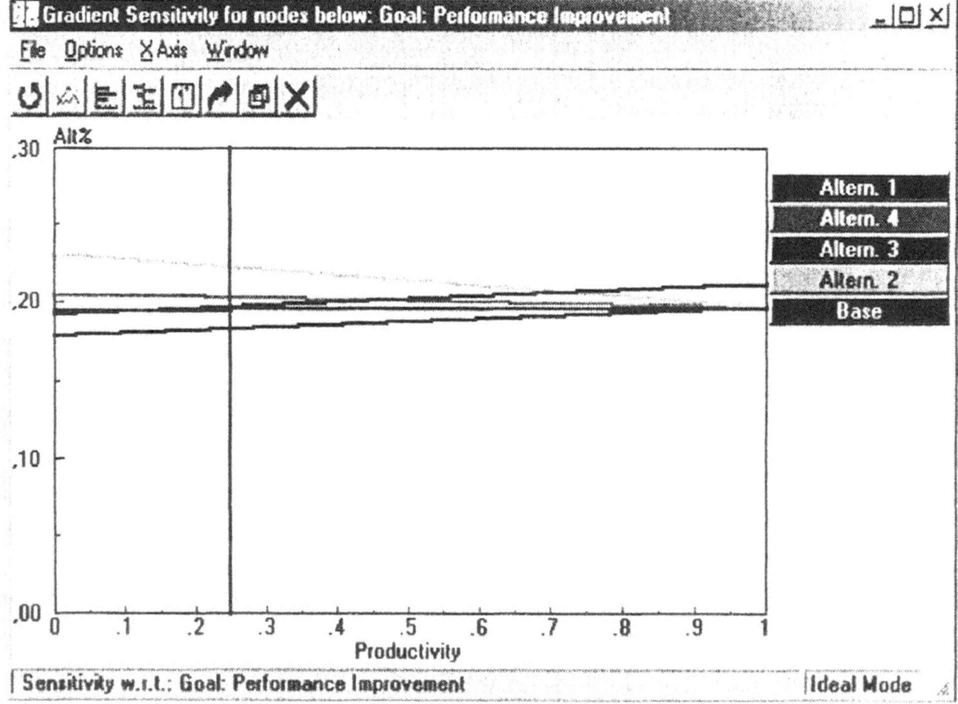

Figure 3: Sensitivity Analysis Graph for productivity

In the second period (see Figure 4), characterized from a large volume of production, the examined alternatives cause not very high improvements in the global performance respect the actual situation.

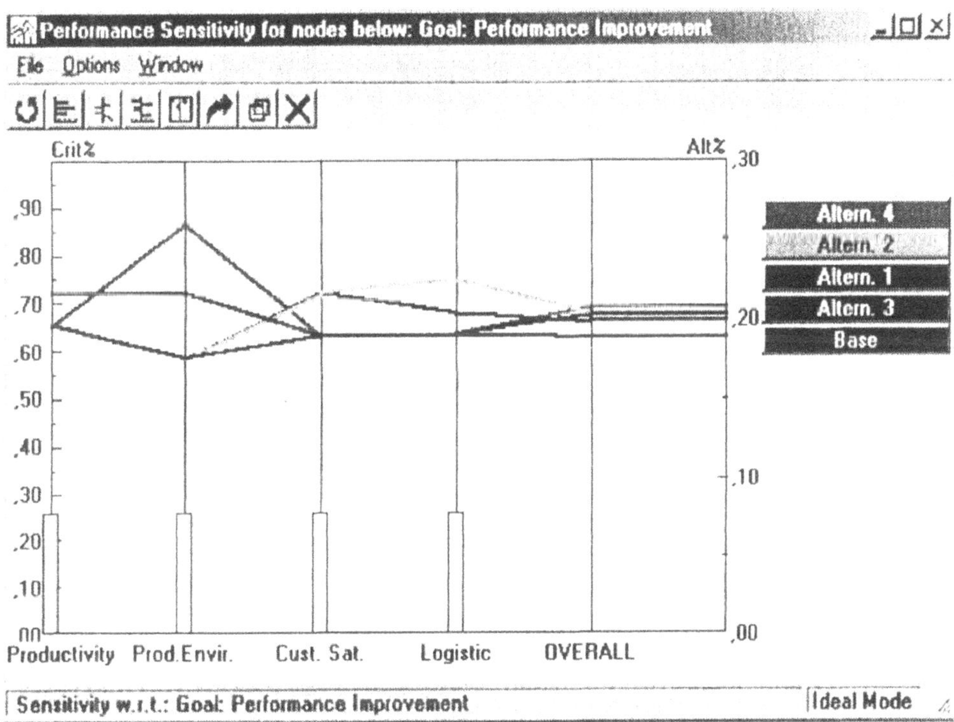

Figure 4: Performance Graph for the second production period.

4. CONCLUSIONS

In this paper we have introduced an integrated procedure based on the analytical hierarchical process methodology and the discrete simulation software in order to allows the management to take decisions. In particular, we have introduced an operational framework to evaluate the operative, tactical and strategic decisions of the management. So, after the simulation model of a plant has been designed, we have generated four scenarios characterized by different assumptions on firm's strategies. Then for each scenario the performance indicators have been computed in the simulation environment and, finally, the best scenario has been individuated through AHP methodology.

Preliminary results related to a plant of an Italian firm shown that our approach is useful when different decisions at different levels are taken in the same time. The next steps will be the following:

to improve the simulation model of the production system in order to obtain a better definition of the performance indicators ;

to extend the proposed analysis to the whole supply chain of the domestic appliances.

5. REFERENCES

1. Avai A., Boer C. R., Carotenuto P., Confessore G., Fornasiero R., "A Performance Indicators Model for the Supply Chain", in Pawar and Muffatto Eds. Logitics and the Digital Economy, University of Nottingham, pp. 315-320, 2001.
2. Chankong V. and Haimes Y.Y. "Multiobjective decision making. Theory and methodology" North-Holland, 1983.
3. Hatry H. P. "Performance measurement principles and techniques: an overview for local government", Public Productivity Review, 4, 312-339, 1980.
4. Lebas M.J., "Performance Measurement and Performance Management", International Journal of Production Economics, 23-35, 1995.
5. Lowlor A., "Productivity Improvement Manaul", Gower Publ., 1985.
6. Lucertini M. , Nicolò F. and Telmon D., "Integration of Benchmarking and Benchmarking of Integration", International Journal of Production Economics, 38, 58-71, 1995.
7. Mesarovich M.D., Macko D. and Takayama Y. "Theory of Hierarchical, Multilevel Systems", Academic Press, New York, 1970.
8. Prokopenko J., "La gestione della Produttività", Franco Angeli/Azienda Moderna Ed., 1992.
9. Saaty T.L., "Scaling method for priorities in hierarchical Structures", Journal of Mathematical Psychology, 15, n. 3, 1977.
10. Saaty T.L. and Khouja M.A., "A measure of world influence", Peace Science, 1977.
11. Saaty T.L. and Varga L.G. "Estimating technological coefficients by the analytic hierarchy process", Socio-Econ. Plan. Sci., 13, pp. 333-336, 1979.
12. Sudit E.F. "Productivity measurement in industrial operations", Invited review, European Journal of Operational Research, 85, 435-453, 1995.

22

PERFORMANCE MEASUREMENT IN VIRTUAL ORGANIZATIONS

Ralf Hieber[1], Ingo Hartel[1], Yoichi Kamio[2]
[1]*Swiss Federal Institute of Technology Zurich – Center for Enterprise Sciences (ETHZ-BWI), Ralf.Hieber@ethz.ch, Ingo.Hartel@ethz.ch*
[2]*Toyo Engineering Corporation, kamio@ims.toyo-eng.co.jp*

The paper gives an overview of a new integral model for performance measurement in virtual organizations. With the focus on the one-of-a-kind production environment, different type of virtual enterprises can be distinguished depending on the deliverables. The paper will focus on the virtual service enterprise, which delivers services such as maintenance, repair, or operation support to customers. By providing generic and aggregated performance indicators an integral and balanced model to measure the performance of a service network as well as virtual service enterprises, which are formed by selected network members, will be provided. A case study has proven the applicability and potential benefits of a collaborative performance measurement in service networks.

1. INTRODUCTION

For over a decade, there has been a growing interest in the concept of virtual organizations to enlarge own business offerings and solutions, not only in production but also in the field of services, in order to gain additional market shares as well as increase customer satisfaction. Thus, by integrating the core competences of each business partner, companies have realized that the efficiency of their own business success is heavily dependent on the performance of the entire production and service network because of the more and more complex linked value adding processes. Hence, collaborative performance measurement of virtual organizations for determining the network organization success is one of the most critical success factors. Based on the common business strategy and goals, the organization has to evaluate common performance as well as to direct management attention to areas for network improvements.

2. VIRTUAL ORGANIZATION

In the search for organization forms for the twenty-first century, the virtual organization concept is beginning to make headway as a dynamic structural pattern. Under this model, organizational units (also called as virtual enterprises) are created, restricted to the primary business purposes and thus, this structural simplicity allows maximum economic efficiency. A virtual enterprise can briefly be characterized as a short-term inter-enterprise cooperation where individual enterprises join core competencies in order to establish a value chain configured exactly to meet a specific customer demand. When the customer demand has been fulfilled, the virtual enterprise is decommissioned. With the focus on the one-of-a-kind production different type of virtual enterprises can be distinguished depending on the deliverables (Hartel, 2002). During the use of the one-of-a-kind product (e.g. chemical production facility) the virtual service enterprise offers services such as maintenance, repair, or operation support to the plant owner.

2.1 The Model of the Virtual Service Organization

The model of the virtual service organization consists of three main elements - the service network with the network members, the resulting virtual service enterprises (VSE) and the service products. To provide a structural arrangement and to capture the characteristics of these entities the Virtual Enterprise Reference Architecture (VERA) is currently being developed in the IMS GLOBEMEN project. VERA is based upon the GERA modeling framework of GERAM (GERAM, 1999).

Figure 1 shows that the network in its operational phase creates VSEs and a VSE carries out some service product life cycle phases (indicated by the double arrows).

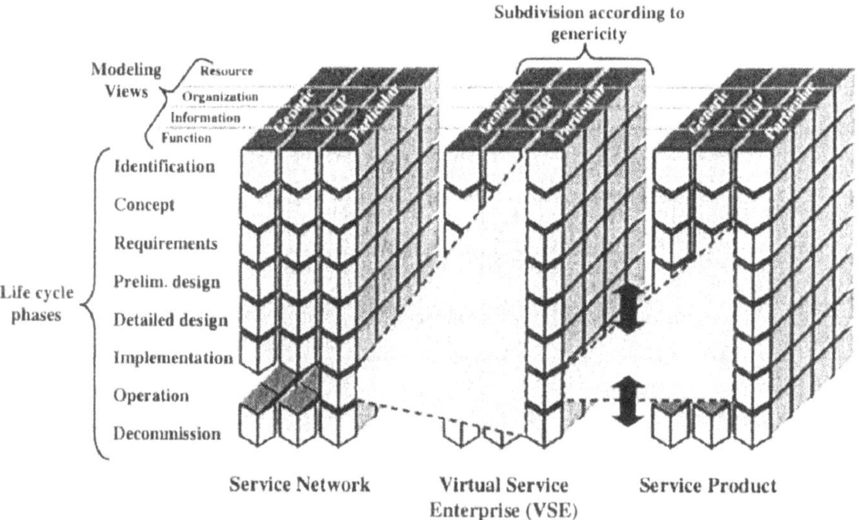

Figure 1 – Virtual Enterprise Reference Architecture (GLOBEMEN, 2000)

The *virtual service enterprise* is formed of selected network members. Together the network members can fulfill the specified service product. The service product is divided into different tasks. Each network member in the VSE is responsible for performing a part of these tasks in accordance with its competencies and available technical aids and ICT. A *service network* in the operation phase has an array of service products, which they can offer to the customers. A *service product* consists of one or several service modules, which through its single or their combined characteristics target distinct customer needs (Hartel, 2002).

3. PERFORMANCE MEASUREMENT APPROACHES AND KEY REQUIREMENTS

The described virtual service organization concept fundamentally changes the nature of organizations, which are nowadays established in this phase of the product life cycle. The service planning and fulfillment is no longer based on own direct ownership and control, but rather on collaboration and coordination across company boundaries as well as interfaces between different departments and different functions, which also finally affects the performance measurement approaches in place. Thus, innovative ways of collaborative performance measurement for virtual service organizations must be developed and new performance dimensions must be taken into consideration that go beyond the traditional dimensions like cost, time and quality. In the following section, the requirements for a new collaborative performance measurement system for a virtual service organization will be derived.

Single network objective-oriented: network members pursue different objectives when participating in a service network. Some members can strive for enhancing and complement core competencies, others for significant know-how increase and further members for developing new markets. As soon as several organizations with different corporate objectives and interests are included, the new challenge is to integrate them in a collaborative way towards a common network objective.

Partnership-oriented: From a collaboration point of view, the partnership orientation in the service network and virtual service enterprise is the most important. The results of numerous studies investigating critical success indicators in the area of supply chain management, have shown put stress on the prerequisite of a win-win partnership for successful network organization. Accordingly, the extent of the partnership that exists between the entities in the network must be evaluated and improved as well.

Balanced-oriented: Many companies have realized the importance of financial as well as non-financial performance measures, but mostly failed to understand them in a balanced framework. According to Kaplan and Norton (Kaplan, 1992), while some managers and researchers have concentrated on financial performance measures, others have concentrated on operational measures. Such an inequality does not lead to metrics that can present a clear and integrated picture of organizational performance.

Model-oriented: On the strength of a systematic approach (e.g. EFQM-model, Malcom Baldrige Award), the performance measurement for service networks and virtual service enterprises should be supported by a generic framework to give guidelines on how to implement and use the recommended performance measures.

Scope-oriented: With respect to the level of detail, the service network and virtual service enterprise performance measurement system should contain any desired eligible elements, thus each network resp. virtual enterprise can tailor its specific scope and objectives after deriving them from overall set of targets and strategies.

Most of the above-described principles for a performance measurement approach are already more or less quite familiar and accepted on a company internal level, however, not from a network perspective as yet, which results by offering joint services towards a common customer (Hieber, 2002). Thus, most of the above principles are nowadays included in recently developed performance measurement approaches and, it seems reasonable to include them in a service network context. However, regardless of the performance approach selected on a corporate level, the primary focus must be on supporting a network perspective as a result of a virtual service organization structure.

4. INTEGRAL MODEL FOR PERFORMANCE MEASUREMENT IN VIRTUAL SERVICE ORGANIZATION

Most of the current approaches for performance measurement are not designed to strive for and contribute to the global optimum of industrial service network organization including independent one-of-a-kind producers, service companies, suppliers or sub-contractors. Thus, a new model will be introduced, which should overcome these deficiencies and provide a framework for measuring performance in service networks and virtual service enterprises.

4.1 Generic Performance Target Areas of Virtual Service Organization

Nowadays, efficient service management has a significant influence on companies performance, especially in the one-of-a-kind industry, in the target areas of quality, costs, and delivery. As a matter of fact, most of the current performance measurement approaches are focusing on these three performance target areas. However, service management in virtual organization enlarges the perspective from a single company's point of view towards a network system's orientation. According to our research, the following three new high-level enabling network and virtual enterprise performance target areas can be identified and are defined as follows:

Service collaboration: The ability to work together by offering joint services and act collaboratively in a win-win partnership to fulfill (final) customer service demand. All service activities should be oriented towards the global optimum of the network.

Service coordination: The ability of service network members to coordinate and communicate efficiently in daily operations. That means that organizations, people, and systems all have access to relevant service information regardless of time, location or company.

Service product configuration: The ability to achieve a high substantial potential of flexibility in (re)configuration of service products between the members in the network by means of practicing and sharing service know-how, capabilities, routines, and skills as well as leveraging ideas and visions.

These performance target areas are dedicated to the overall optimum of a service network and in addition, finally contribute to a very large extent to improvements in inter-company as well as corporate service performance with respect to quality, costs, and delivery.

Thus, these new identified performance target areas of service networks and virtual service enterprises enlarge the current perspective towards a more integral view and hence, will be best reported and measured by common generic network performance indicators. To enable this performance measurement for service networks and virtual service enterprises, the following integral model with the respective assigned performance indicators will be now proposed.

4.2 Integral Model for Performance Measurement in Virtual Service Organization

The integral model is based on the common practices and processes in service management of the participating network entities who are willing to start a joint performance measurement approach. Therefore, the integral model consists of generic as well as aggregated performance indicators of the participating companies in order to (self)assess the performance of the entire service network and virtual service enterprises. However, as figure proposes, a two-phase approach will be recommended.

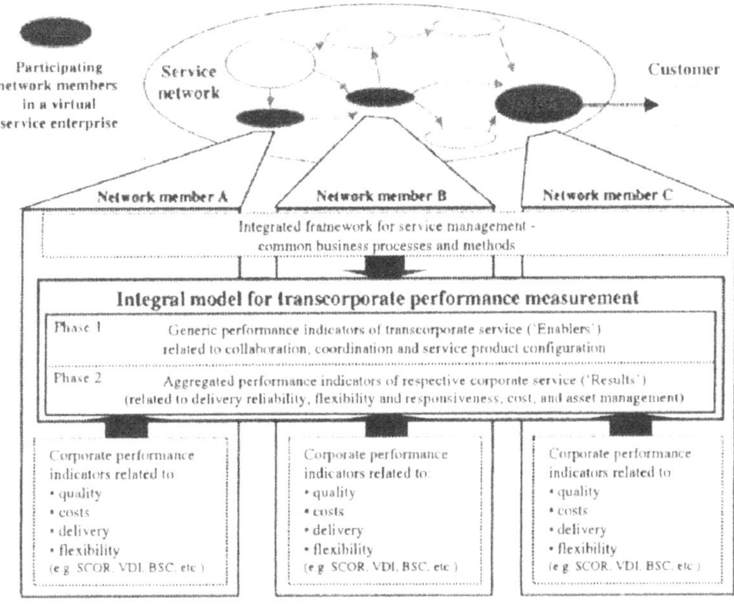

Figure 2 – Integral model for performance measurement

In phase one, generic high-level transcorporate service performance indicators are of main concern (Enablers). These are metrics that mainly address the service collaboration, service coordination, and service product configuration performance target areas of the virtual service organization and record how well the service network and virtual service enterprises are operating. Especially at this early stage of implementing a common performance measurement system, it is very sensitive to already capture and exchange metrics related to internal service cost information or internal service levels. As studies have revealed (Hieber, 2000), network members may be reluctant to share information on service costs or internal service levels, and in addition, the need to release sensitive and confidential information may compound this hesitation. Hence, at the beginning, the performance indicators will first operate on a high-level perspective, rather than on the prevalent result-oriented financial and operational perspective.

In phase two, by building trust and openness and setting up efficient lines of communication during the common operations in the network and virtual enterprises, including monitoring of the generic performance indicators, the integral model can be then enlarged step-by-step with elements of current performance measurement approaches with the respective internal corporate service performance target areas of quality, costs, and delivery by aggregating and transforming those on a network and virtual enterprise level (Results).

4.3 Generic Performance Indicators in Virtual Service Organizations

To meet these new requirements and to overcome the existing identified shortfalls in service network and virtual service enterprise performance measurement, the next table introduces a new set of high-level generic performance indicators on the inter-company level.

Table 1 – Generic performance indicators: Service 'Enablers'

Performance target area	Definition	Generic transcorporate performance indicator
Service collaboration efficiency	The ability to work together by offering joint services and act collaboratively in a win-win partnership to fulfill (final) customer service demand. All service activities should be oriented towards the global optimum of the network.	• Strategic service alignment • Service planning collaboration • Service execution collaboration
Service coordination efficiency	The ability of service network partners to coordinate and communicate efficiently in daily operations. That means that organizations, people, and systems all have access to relevant service information regardless of time, location or company.	• Information availability • Communication efficiency • Information and communication technology (ICT) support
Service product configuration flexibility	The ability to achieve a high substantial potential of flexibility in (re)configuration of service products between the members in the network by means of practicing and sharing service know-how, capabilities, routines, and skills as well as leveraging ideas and visions.	• Service product know-how • Service product skill sharing • Service product (re)configuration flexibility

It is also important to mention, that these performance target areas and assigned performance indicators are the most difficult to record in a quantitative manner. As a consequence, the main interest is not the total score, but more the difference to previous benchmarks. In addition, this proposed set of generic performance indicators should be considered as a starting point for a collaborative performance measurement, rather than a fixed set of predefined indicators. New ones can be added and existing ones can be abandoned, depending on the specific needs of a virtual service organization.

5. CASE STUDY

A Japanese one-of-a-kind producer ("OKP1"), member of the IMS GLOBEMEN project develops and sells large chemical installations. For the manufacture of these installations, it has a large network of suppliers and sub-contractors. Worldwide there are 100 of these installations in operation by customers. In the past, OKP1 developed service components, such as a remote plant monitoring system and a training simulation system, to support after-sales services. However, OKP1 does not have its own team of service technicians. A customer ("C1") operates several installations in Asia and has its own teams for inspection and maintenance. Another large European one-of-a-kind producer ("OKP2"), which is not a direct competitor of OKP1 but works at the same level in the value chain, has a number of its own external service stations in Asia. OKP2 receives support from various service companies if there are capacity bottlenecks or if time is critical. The service network is made up of OKP1 with selected suppliers and sub-contractors, OKP2 with its service stations and service companies in Asia, and C1's service teams. As only OKP1 customers receive the after-sales services, OKP1 takes on the role of hosting provider, who is responsible for network operation and customer contacts.

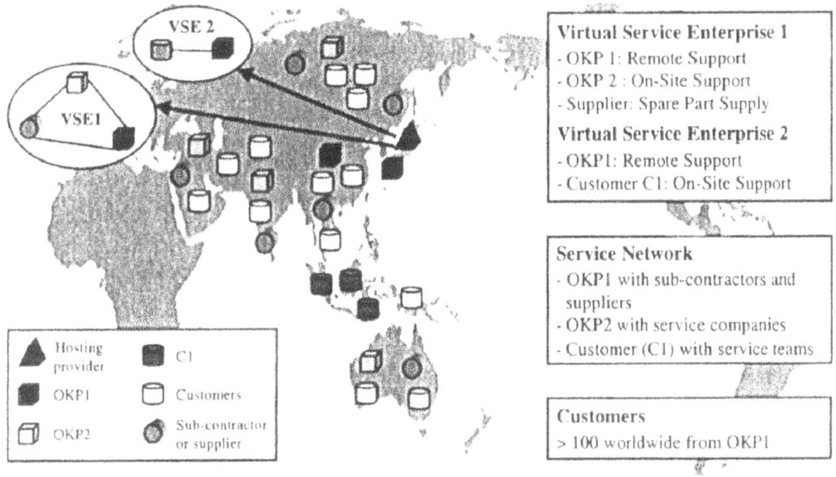

Figure 3 – Structure of the service network

The operating service network is able to provide a wide range of service products, which are configured from available service modules. The service modules are mainly based on the service components, which have already been established at OPK1. For example, if a customer requires maintenance on a reactor and replacement of spare parts of the supply pipes, a virtual service enterprise ("VSE1") could take the following configuration: A service technician from OKP2, who has reactor training, goes on-site to the customer. At the same time, a supplier delivers to the customer the pipes it has manufactured or drawn from inventory. During the repair procedures, the service technician receives additional required information from a developer at OKP1.This form of cooperation described above allows OKP1 to actively offer after-sales services. Through implementing its various service components, OKP1 can gather new experience and data during the operation of the installation. In addition, technicians from C1 will benefit from enlarged experience through service work at other companies. They can apply this experience knowledge within their own company.

By applying the integral model for performance measurement with the assigned service network enabler KPIs, it was possible to detect areas for improvements in a collaborative way. For example, a collaborative service execution in the area of maintenance results in a reduction of the total required service time and cost. Gathered operation data were remotely monitored and analyzed by OKP1 using a data acquisition and simulation system. Regarding the determined plant operation condition a maintenance can then better be planed and scheduled. The execution of the maintenance will be done by C1 or OKP2 supported by remote consulting from OKP1. To further improve the service coordination OKP1 has installed a document management system. This system contains all relevant information from the previous life-cycle phases of the operating plants. All members of an established virtual service enterprise have access via the Internet to the stored data. With the described sharing of skills and the access to relevant service information the overall maintenance efficiency can be enhanced and improvements can be monitored by the newly provided key performance indicators.

6. CONCLUSION

The newly proposed generic key performance indicators (Enablers) can be a useful instrument to discern clearly the strengths and areas in which improvements in service management can be made. Moreover, this set of generic performance indicators should be common to the general service performance target areas of almost every service network. Furthermore, these performance indicators can be further broken down in one of the specific performance target areas as applied in the case study in order to fine-tune the specific service network and virtual service enterprise needs.

In general, this set of performance indicators gives a clear picture of what a service network does **(network enabler)**, which will finally lead towards a more result-oriented financial picture of what a service network achieves by setting up virtual service enterprises **(network results)**.

7. REFERENCES

1. GERAM. Generalized Enterprise Reference Architecture and Methodology. ISO/DIS15704, IFAC/IFIP Task Force on Architectures for Enterprise Integration, 1999.
2. GLOBEMEN. Global Engineering and Manufacturing in Enterprise Networks. IMS 99004 / IST-1999-60002, http://globemen.vtt.fi, 2000 - 2003.
3. Hartel I, Burger G, Billinger S, Kamio Y. Virtual organization of after-sales service in the one-of-a-kind industry. In Luis M. Camarinha-Matos: Collaborative Business Ecosystems and Virtual Enterprises, pp. 405-420, Kluwer Academic Publishers, Boston (USA), 2002, 631 pages.
4. Hieber R. Supply Chain Management - A Collaborative Performance Measurement Approach. vdf Hochschulverlag AG at ETH Zurich, www.vdf.ethz.ch, Zurich (CH), 2002.
5. Hieber R, Windischer A, Alard R, Fischer D. Survey "Successful cooperation in supply chains –trends and practices". Center for Enterprise Sciences (ETHZ-BWI), Zurich (CH), 2000, 24 pages.
6. Kaplan R, Norton D. The Balanced Scorecard – Measures that Drive Performance. In Havard Business Review, January/February 1992, pp. 71-79.

23

AN ANALYSIS ON GAME THEORETIC NEGOTIATION DYNAMISM BASED ON MULTI-AGENT PARADIGM IN VIRTUAL ENTERPRISE

Toshiya Kaihara[1] and Susumu Fujii[2]
[1] *Kobe University, Graduate School of Science and Technology*
[2] *Kobe University, Department of Computer and Systems Engineering*
{kaihara,fujii}@ms.cs.kobe-u.ac.jp

In this paper, we focus on negotiation process in VE formulation as a basic research to clarify its effective management. Each enterprise in VE is defined as agent in multi-utilities and a framework of multi-agent programming with game theoretic approach is newly proposed as negotiation algorithm amongst the agents. Each unit is defined as agent in our VE model, and their decision makings are formulated as a game theoretic methodology. We adopt CNP (Contract Net Protocol) as the coordination and negotiation mechanism amongst the units. CNP models transfer of control in a distributed system with the metaphor of negotiation among autonomous intelligent beings. CNP consists of a set of nodes that negotiate with one another through a set of message. Nodes generally represent the distributed computing resources to be managed, correspond to "enterprises" in this paper. We develop a computer simulation model to form VE through multiple negotiations amongst several potential members in the negotiation domain, and finally clarify the formulation dynamism with the negotiation process.

1. INTRODUCTION

Nowadays, Virtual Enterprise (VE) is a crucial paradigm of business management in agile environment. VE exists in both service and manufacturing organizations, although the complexity of the each enterprise in VE may vary greatly from industry to industry. Realistic VE handles multiple end products with shared components, facilities and capacities (Camarinha-Matos, 1999). Since the flow of materials in VE is not always along an arborescent network, various modes of transportation may be considered, and the bill of materials for the end items may be both deep and large.

Traditionally, marketing, distribution, planning, manufacturing, and the purchasing organizations operated independently. These organizations have their own objectives and these are often conflicting. Marketing's objective of high customer service and maximum sales conflict with manufacturing and distribution goals. Many manufacturing operations are designed to maximize throughput and lower costs with little consideration for the impact on inventory levels and distribution capabilities. Purchasing contracts are often negotiated with very little information beyond historical buying patterns. The result of these factors is that there is not a single, integrated plan for the organization - there were as many plans as businesses. Clearly, there is a need for a mechanism through which these different functions can be integrated together. Although cooperation is the fundamental characteristic of VE concept, due to its distributed environment and the autonomous and heterogeneous nature of the VE members, cooperation can only be succeed if a proper management of dependencies between activities is in place just like Supply Chain Management (Fisher, 1994) (Goldratt, 1983).

In this paper, we focus on negotiation process in VE formulation as a basic research to clarify its effective management. Each enterprise in VE is defined as agent with multi-utilities and a framework of multi-agent programming with game theoretic approach (Von Neumann, 1947) is newly proposed as negotiation algorithm amongst the agents. Each unit is defined as agent in our VE model, and their decision makings are formulated as a game theoretic methodology. We adopt CNP (Contract Net Protocol) (Smith, 1980) (Durfee, 1987) as the coordination and negotiation mechanism amongst the units. CNP models transfer of control in a distributed system with the metaphor of negotiation among autonomous intelligent beings. CNP consists of a set of nodes that negotiate with one another through a set of message (Kaihara, 2002a, 2002b). Nodes generally represent the distributed computing resources to be managed, correspond to "enterprises" in this paper. We develop a computer simulation model to form VE through multiple negotiations amongst several potential members in the negotiation domain, and finally clarify the formulation dynamism with the negotiation process.

2. ENTERPRISE AGENT

2.1 Virtual Enterprise Model

A large number of diversified networked organisations of enterprises fall under the general definition of VE. We assumed our VE model in the possible simplest definition as a basic research, as follows:

i) Duration: Single business

An alliance of the enterprises is established towards a single business opportunity, and is dissolved at the end of such process.

ii) Topology: Fixed structure

There exist established supply chains with an almost fixed structure.

iii) Participation: Single alliance

All the enterprises are participating into only a single alliance at the same time.

iv) Coordination: Democratic alliance

A different organisation can be found in some supply chains without a dominant company. All the enterprises cooperate on an equal basis, preserving their autonomy.

v) Visibility scope: Single level

All the enterprises in VE communicate only to its direct neighbours in its architecture (figure 1). That is the case observed in most supply chains.

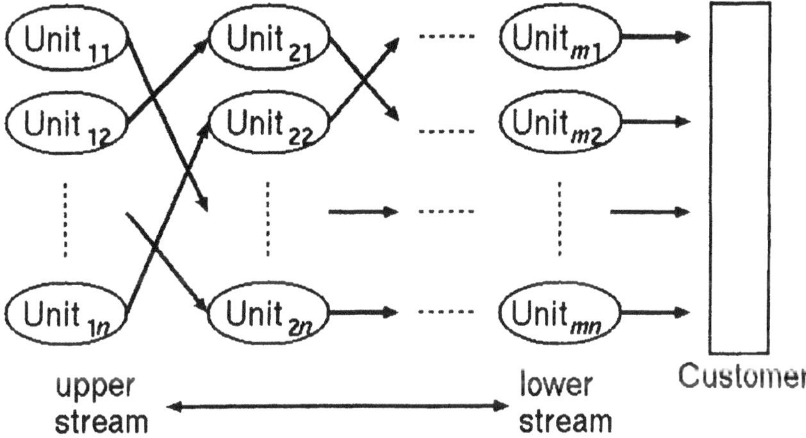

Figure 1 VE model

Figure 1 shows the assumed VE model in this paper. We call an enterprise as *unit*, and there exist m layers, which have m_n units in the VE model. The lowest level corresponds to consumers who can create original task requests to the VE. As the layer number, m, increases, we describe it 'lower' based on the product flow order in this paper.

At first, the customer dispatches new order to all the units in layer m, and then several units, which are satisfied with the order, responds and circulates the order toward upper units in the VE model. Finally a VE with single supply chain will be established for the order as a consequence of their negotiations through all the layers.

2.2 Unit Structure

Each unit is defined as agent in our VE model, and its structure is described in figure 2. We adopt CNP as the coordination and negotiation mechanism amongst the units. CNP models transfer of control in a distributed system with the metaphor of negotiation among autonomous intelligent beings. CNP consists of a set of nodes that negotiate with one another through a set of message. Nodes generally represent the distributed computing resources to be managed, correspond to "units" in this paper.

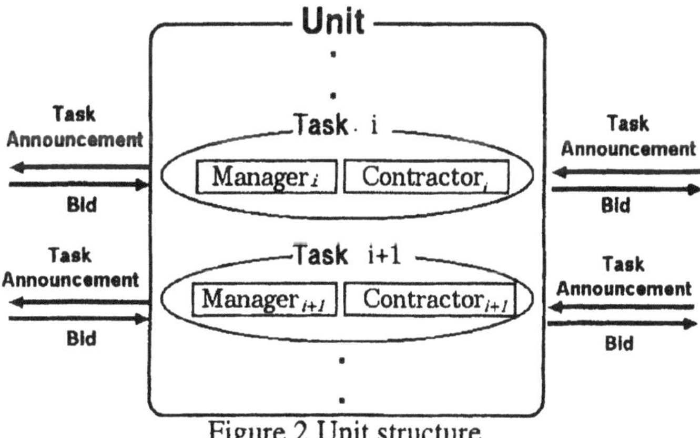

Figure 2 Unit structure

An agent (=unit) can act both as a manager and a contractor of a delivery sets. When a unit receives new order (= task announcement) *i*, it creates a contractor / manager set (Manager *i* / Contractor *i*) for the task inside. Manager *i* creates a new order towards the lower units to secure the contract with the upper layer.

2.3 Basic Assumptions

There exist several situations in partnering amongst enterprise agents. In this paper it is assumed that the product demand is predictable in the negotiation under multipurpose criterion. That means order patterns are previously given and the negotiations start after the order reached to each enterprise agent. They should prepare robust solutions with maximum utilities against the order. We propose agent behaviours based on game theoretic approach according to this assumption.

2.4 Negotiation Algorithm

Negotiation steps according to agent roles are described as follows:

Manager

Step M1: Create a new task based on the received bid information.
Step M2: Task announcement (TA) to the lower units.
Step M3: After the bidding period expired, check all the acquired bids according to its standard. If there exists no bid to select, go to M4. Otherwise go to M5.
Step M4: Modify the task and go to M2.
Step M5: Select the task and send reward (Reward) to the corresponding unit.

Contractor

Step C1: Create an estimated bid.
Step C2: Send the bid.
Step C3: Request task announcement to the manager.

2.5 Agent Behaviour

In this model, all the orders are clearly given before the negotiations. Agent behaviours are described in each negotiation step.

- Bidding (Step C2)

Each contractor (U_{ij}) has three attributes, such as cost, lead time and quality, in their bid for order k defined as follows:

$$Cost_{ij}^{k} = E_{ij}^{k} + D_{ij}^{k} + P_{ij}^{k} \quad (1)$$

$$Leadtime_{ij}^{k} = \lambda_{ij}^{k} / E_{ij}^{k} \quad (2)$$

$$Quality_{ij}^{k} = \mu_{ij}^{k} D_{ij}^{k} (1 - \exp^{-v_{ij}^{k} P_{ij}^{k}}) \quad (3)$$

where

$Cost_{ij}^{k}$: total cost for U_{ij} to process order k

$Leadtime_{ij}^{k}$: lead time for U_{ij} to process order k

$Quality_{ij}^{k}$: product quality for U_{ij} to process order k

$E_{ij}^{k}, D_{ij}^{k}, P_{ij}^{k}$: equipment / development / personnel cost

λ_{ij}^{k} : coefficient of leadtime

$\mu_{ij}^{k}, \nu_{ij}^{k}$: coefficients of quality

Cost vs. lead time, and cost vs. quality, are in trade off relationship in those equations with reality.

- Reward (Step M5)

After the bidding by contractors, managers compute following pay-off matrix according to their utilities against all the bids.

$$\begin{array}{c} \\ Unit_{i1} \\ Unit_{i2} \\ \cdots \\ Unit_{ij} \\ \cdots \\ Unit_{in} \end{array} \begin{array}{c} \begin{array}{ccc} C & L & Q \end{array} \\ \begin{bmatrix} C_{i1}^{k} & L_{i1}^{k} & Q_{i1}^{k} \\ C_{i2}^{k} & L_{i2}^{k} & Q_{i2}^{k} \\ \cdots & \cdots & \cdots \\ C_{ij}^{k} & L_{ij}^{k} & Q_{ij}^{k} \\ \cdots & \cdots & \cdots \\ C_{in}^{k} & L_{im}^{k} & Q_{im}^{k} \end{bmatrix} \end{array} \tag{4}$$

where

$$C_{ij}^{k} = (\overline{c_i^{k}} - Cost_{ij}^{k}) / s_{c_i^k} \tag{5}$$

$$L_{ij}^{k} = (\overline{l_i^{k}} - Leadtime_{ij}^{k}) / s_{l_i^k} \tag{6}$$

$$Q_{ij}^{k} = (Quality_{ij}^{k} - \overline{q_i^{k}}) / s_{q_i^k} \tag{7}$$

C_{ij}^{k} : utility on cost for U_{ij} to process order k

L_{ij}^{k} : utility on lead time for U_{ij} to process order k

Q_{ij}^{k} : utility on quality for U_{ij} to process order k

$\overline{c_i^{k}}, \overline{l_i^{k}}, \overline{q_i^{k}}$: average utility of all the bid on cost, lead time, quality

$s_{c_i^k}, s_{l_i^k}, s_{q_i^k}$: standard deviation of all the bid on cost, lead time, quality

Five strategies are defined as selection mechanism using the payoff matrix in (4).
- method 1: cost minimisation

$$\max_{j=1,2,\dots,n} = C_{ij}^{k} \tag{8}$$

- method 2: lead time minimisation

$$\max_{j=1,2,\ldots,n} = L_{ij}^{k} \tag{9}$$

- method 3: quality maximisation

$$\max_{j=1,2,\ldots,n} = Q_{ij}^{k} \tag{10}$$

- method 4: total utility maximisation

$$\max_{j=1,2,\ldots,n} = C_{ij}^{k} + L_{ij}^{k} + Q_{ij}^{k} \tag{11}$$

- method 5: max-min strategy

$$\max_{j=1,2,\ldots,n} \min\{ C_{ij}^{k}, L_{ij}^{k}, Q_{ij}^{k} \} \tag{12}$$

Method 5 is so called " max-min strategy" in game theory, which has been proved to conduct Nash equilibrium solution by min-max theorem, if the game is in zero-sum situation like our formulation shown in (4).

3. EXPERIMENTAL RESULTS

3.1 Simulation Model

A 3-layered VE model for computer simulation was developed to clarify VE formulation dynamism with the proposed negotiation mechanism. Each layer consists of 5 enterprises in this simulation model described in Figure 1.

Simulation parameters are shown in Table 1. All the results are the average of 500 trials in each simulation scenario.

Table 1 Simulation parameters

m	n	N	E	D	P	λ	μ	ν
3	5	1	5-15*	5-15*	5-15*	300	5	0.1

* followed by uniformed random distribution

Table 2 Simulation results (Negotiation attributes)

	Method 1		Method 2		Method 3		Method 4		Method 5	
	Ave.	St. Dev.	Ave.	St. Dev.	Ave.	St. Dev.	Ave.	St. Dev.	Ave.	St. Dev.
Cost	72.87	5.08	99.89	7.47	104.17	6.61	98.96	8.79	91.19	5.54
LTime	119.53	18.47	68.32	4.84	90.21	18.06	80.72	11.04	91.04	12.24
Quality	65.10	10.58	92.59	18.05	132.34	12.44	106.84	20.22	93.23	12.97

Table 3 Simulation results (Utilities)

	Method 1	Method 2	Method 3	Method 4	Method 5
E_{ij}^{k}	8.13	13.35	9.96	11.68	10.38
D_{ij}^{k}	8.13	10.11	12.84	11.47	10.61
P_{ij}^{k}	8.03	9.84	11.92	9.83	9.41

Simulation results in terms of negotiation attributes and utilities are shown in Table 2, 3, respectively. All the results are shown in the average (AVE.) and the standard distribution (St. Dev.) in Table 2. Figure 3 also illustrates the average of each negotiation attribute to compare the proposed methods.

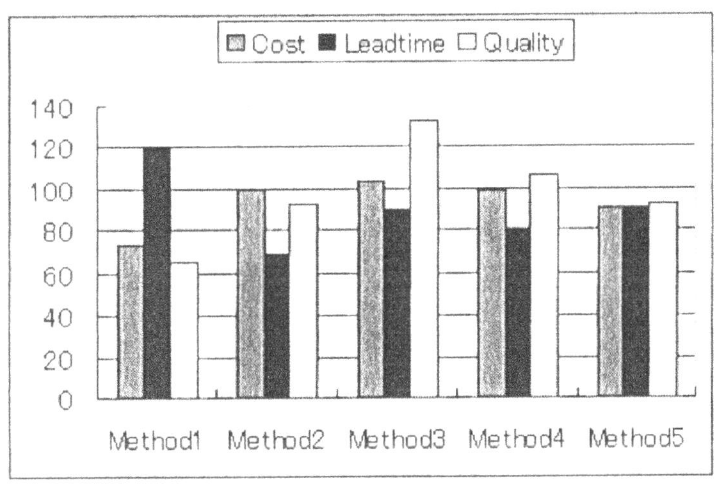

Figure 3 Unit structure

We summarise the characteristics of each method as follows:

Method 1: Cost minimisation

Since the negotiation amongst enterprises is cost-oriented in this method, cost parameter is the best of all the methods in Ave. Additionally Cost and Quality are better in St. Dev., because they are correlated to $E_{ij}^{k}, D_{ij}^{k}; P_{ij}^{k}$ shown in (1) and (3). It has been observed that all the utilities are small to minimise total cost in this method at Table 3.

Method 2: Lead time minimisation

Lead time-oriented method naturally conducts the minimal LeadTime in Ave. and St. Dev. Cost parameter is not good, because Leadtime and E_{ij}^{k} is in trade-off relation in (2), and that lead to higher cost.

Method 3: Quality maximisation

It is obvious that quality maximisation strategy caused the worst in Cost, and this result fits well to our general sense. In this method enterprises don't pay any attention to LeadTime shown in (2).

Method 4: Total utility maximisation

Generally the result is moderate in the balance amongst 3 parameters by trying to maximise total utility. In Figure 3 it has been observed that they are relatively better in its LeadTime and Quality, but worse in its Cost. That is because the general relationship amongst $E_{ij}^{k}, D_{ij}^{k}, P_{ij}^{k}$, in (1), (2) and (3), that means enterprise agents sacrifice LeadTime to increase Cost and Quality.

Method 5: Max-min strategy

Acquired result is completely well-balanced in Ave. It has also been confirmed that this strategy conducts minimal in St. Dev., and their negotiation is stable and robust enough to deal with agile trading situations. That is because each agent tried to minimise the risk based on the min-max theory.

Although our investigations have clearly not been exhaustive, it is already apparent that the agent behaviours have a great influence on autonomously formulated VE structure as a basic study. Proposed game theoretic formulation on agent decision mechanism with multi-agent paradigm is quite reasonable to realise negotiation process amongst enterprises.

4. CONCLUSIONS

In this paper, we focused on negotiation process in VE formulation as a basic research. Each enterprise in VE was defined as agent with multi-utilities and a framework of multi-agent programming with game theoretic is newly proposed as negotiation algorithm amongst the agents. Each unit is defined as agent in our VE model, and their decision-makings are formulated as a game theoretic methodology. Simulation results have proved that the proposed game theoretic formulation on agent decision mechanism with multi-agent paradigm is quite reasonable to analyse negotiation process amongst enterprises.

5. ACKONWLEDGEMENTS

This research was supported by International Research program IMS (Intelligent Manufacturing System) of MITI Japan, under contract No.0119 (HUTOP project).

6. REFERENCES

1. Camarinha-Matos, L. M. et al., The virtual enterprise concept, Infrastructures for virtual enterprises, Kluwer academic publishers, Boston, pp.3-14, 1999.
2. Durfee, E. et al., Coherent cooperation among communication problem solvers, IEEE Transaction on Computers, N 36, pp.1275-1291, 1987.
3. Fisher M. L., Making supply meet demand in uncertain world, Harvard Business Review, May/Jun, 1994.
4. Goldratt E. M., The GOAL, North River Press, 1983.
5. Kaihara, T. and S. Fujii, A proposal on negotiation methodology in VE, Collaborative Business Ecosystems and Virtual Enterprises, Kluwer Academic Publishers, Boston, pp125-132, 2002a.
6. Kaihara, T. and S. Fujii, IT based Virtual Enterprise Coalition Strategy for Agile Manufacturing Environment, Proc. of the 35th CIRP Int. Seminar on Manufacturing Systems, pp32-37, 2002b.
7. Von Neumann, J. et al., Theory of Games and Economic Behavior, Princeton University Press, 1947.
8. Smith, R., The contract net protocol, IEEE Transaction on Computers, C-29, pp.1104-1113, 1980.

PART 3

MULTI-AGENT AND HOLONIC MANUFACTURING SYSTEMS

24

IEC 61499 ARCHITECTURE, ENGINEERING METHODOLOGIES AND SOFTWARE TOOLS

James H. Christensen
Rockwell Automation Advanced Technology
JHChristensen@ra.rockwell.com

The IEC 61499 standard defines an architecture and software tool requirements for the encapsulation, embedding, deployment and integration of intellectual property (IP) in intelligent devices, machines and systems. A reference framework and engineering methodology is presented for the use of IEC 61499 in the design, development, simulation, testing and implementation of distributed control and automation systems employing intelligent mechatronic components.

1. INTRODUCTION

Advances in hardware and software technology have made possible the embedding of unprecedented levels of functionality in end devices (sensors and actuators) for industrial control and automation. In turn, this has generated significant technical and commercial opportunities for system architectures, engineering methodologies and software toolkits capable of supporting the cost-effective development and widespread deployment of intellectual property (IP) in such devices and their composition into scalable, flexible automated (SFA) systems. The principal requirements for such architectures, methodologies and toolkits include:

- *software component* orientation for IP encapsulation, reuse and portability;
- device *interoperability*;
- the ability to *distribute* and *integrate* applications;
- *functional completeness*;
- *scalability*;
- *extendability*; and
- flexible *reconfigurability*.

Over the past ten years, Technical Committee 65 (TC65) of the International Technical Commission (IEC) has been developing a series of architectural standards for the use of *function blocks* to meet these requirements (IEC, 2001, 2002). This paper presents an overview of this architecture and illustrates its use in conjunction with an appropriate engineering methodology and software tools to meet these requirements.

2. IEC 61499 ARCHITECTURE

The fundamental unit of software encapsulation and reuse in IEC 61499 is the *function block*, considered to be an *instance* of a function block *type*. As illustrated in Figure 1, an IEC 61499 function block type includes *event* inputs and outputs as well as the more traditional *data* inputs and outputs as seen, for example, in the IEC 61131-3 standard (IEC, 2002) for programmable controller languages. In this way IEC 61499 is able to account explicitly for the synchronization between data transfer and control algorithm execution in *distributed* as well as *centralized* systems.

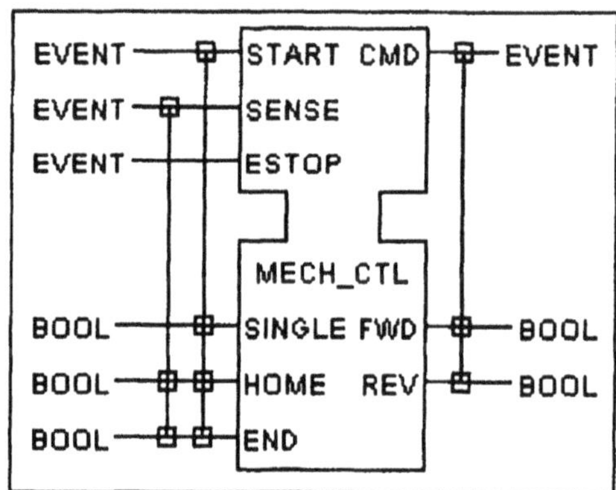

Figure 1 - Example of an IEC 61499 function block type

At the lowest level (the so-called *basic function block type*), intellectual property (IP) is encapsulated in the form of control *algorithms*. Each algorithm expresses a mapping from the current set of values of input, output and internal variables of the function block to a new set of values for its output and internal variables. These algorithms may be expressed in the programming languages of IEC 61131-3, or other procedural languages as appropriate.

Additional IP may be encapsulated in the *Execution Control Chart (ECC)* of a basic function block type. An ECC is an event-driven state machine determining the relationships among current state and input event occurrences, transitions between states, and the algorithm(s) to be executed and output event(s), if any, to be issued upon entering a new state.

IEC 61499-1 also provides *composite function block types* for the encapsulation of new IP developed through the functional composition of existing IP.

An important mechanism for interfacing to *services* provided by the underlying operating environment (called a *resource* in IEC 61499) is defined through the *service interface function block* (SIFB) construct of IEC 61499-1. This provides interfaces to such services as graphic user interface (GUI) components, timing and event handling, communications, and sensor/actuator interfaces. The externally visible behaviors of SIFBs are documented by their provider in the form of *service sequence diagrams* following the format defined by ISO 8509 (ISO, 1987), thus providing for complete protection of the encapsulated IP. The use of SIFBs in conjunction with basic or composite function blocks to provide the local portion of a distributed control application in a resource is illustrated in Figure 2.

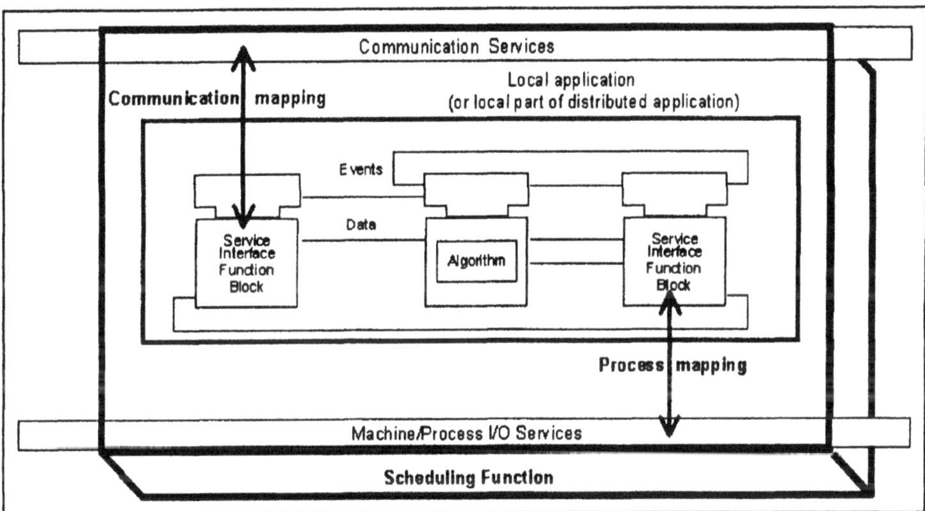

Figure 2 - IEC 61499 resource model (IEC, 2000)

The final element of the IEC 61499 architecture is the *device*, which serves as a container for multiple resources and provides them with *interfaces* to communication networks, sensors and actuators; the services provided by these interfaces are delivered by SIFBs in the resources to support the implementation of distributed applications. The communication networks in turn provide the means for integration of the devices into complete control and automation *systems*.

3. ENGINEERING METHODOLOGY AND TOOLS

IEC 61499-2 (IEC, 2001) defines general requirements for software tools for building elements defined in the IEC 61499-1 architecture (IEC, 2000). These requirements include but are not limited to: (i) reading and writing *library elements* (data types, function block types, resource types, device types, system configurations, etc.) in the standard XML (W3C, 1998) formats defined in IEC 61499-2; (ii) manipulating the *declarations* contained in the library elements; (iii) configuring *devices* and *resources* according the declarations contained in corresponding *system configurations*; and (iv) simulating and validating the operation of various library elements.

Specific software tool requirements will depend on the particular engineering methodologies employed. One such methodology (Christensen, 2000) proposed an extension of the well-known Model/View/Controller (MVC) user interface framework to encompass the development, simulation and deployment of IEC 61499-based systems. In this framework, each of the following elements would be represented as an *instance* of a function block *type*:

- **Model:** A function block that represents the time-dependent logical behavior of the system or device being controlled.
- **View:** A function block that represents the graphical display associated with one or more **Model** types.
- **Controller:** A function block that encapsulates the control functions to be performed on one or more instances of associated **Model** types, and presents

appropriate *event* and *data interfaces* for integration of its functions with those of other **Controller** blocks.

It was further suggested that as part of an associated engineering methodology, **Model** and **View** elements could be encapsulated together in composite **MV** function block types, and that a further encapsulation step could be used to produce **MVC** function block types. However, in practice this methodology has been found to have two major drawbacks:

1. The use of **MV** composite elements leads to *complex resource configurations* because graphic display configuration data is intermixed with model configuration data and interconnections. This complexity is further increased by the use of **MVC** elements.
2. The use of **MVC** composites makes it difficult to separate the **Controller** element from the **MV** element when configuring an actual system by replacing the MV element with appropriate actuator and sensor interfaces.

The layered architecture in Figure 3 overcomes these problems by placing functional elements of each type in a separate layer and explicitly adding a layer for human/machine interface (HMI). Elements within each layer communicate with each other via normal event and data connections. Communications between adjacent layers are implemented using communications service interface function blocks (CSIFBs) as defined in IEC 61499-1, enabling the contents of individual layers to be allocated to different devices as required. When adjacent layers are allocated to the same device, communications are implemented in an optimized way using specialized parameters of the CSIFBs.

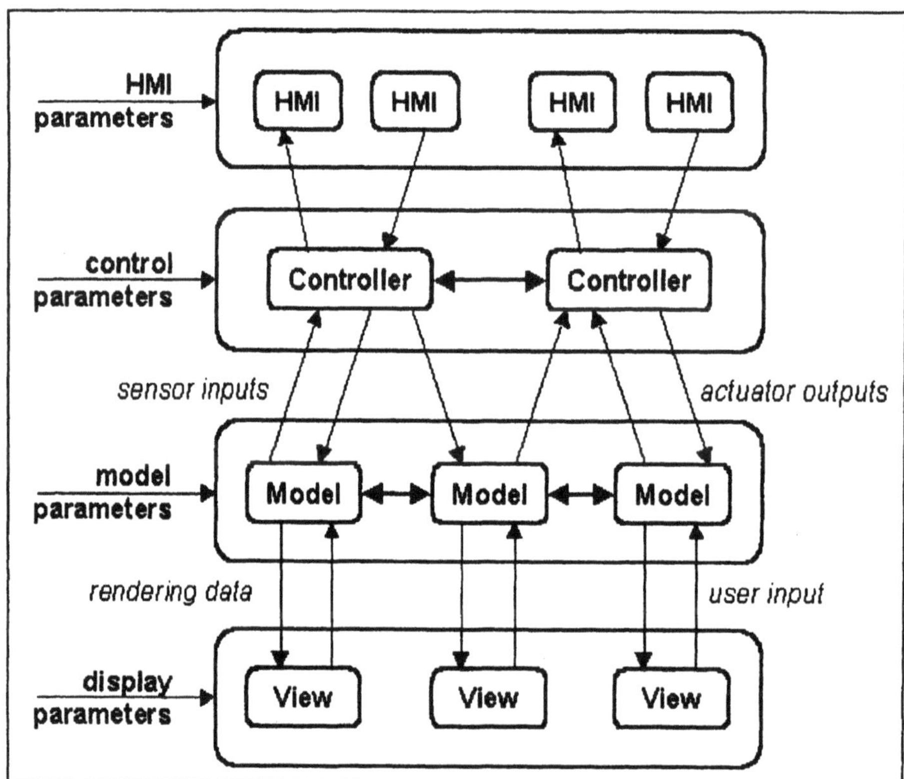

Figure 3 - Revised MVC framework

This framework enables the use of the following simplified version of the engineering methodology described in (Christensen, 2000), with the modified step numbers shown in **bold face**:

1. Start with a sketch of the machine or process to be controlled, along with a verbal description of the desired behavior.
2. From the sketch, develop and test a number of **Views** that present visually the essential information about the states of the controlled devices.
3. Utilizing the View testing mechanism in Figure 4(a), integrate the views into a static animation of the system to be controlled, and utilize the animation to develop descriptions of the desired operational sequences of the system under both normal and abnormal conditions.
4. For each view, develop and test one or more **Models** capable of simulating the dynamic behavior of the associated machine or process equipment in response to external stimuli and commanding the associated View to display the corresponding equipment states.

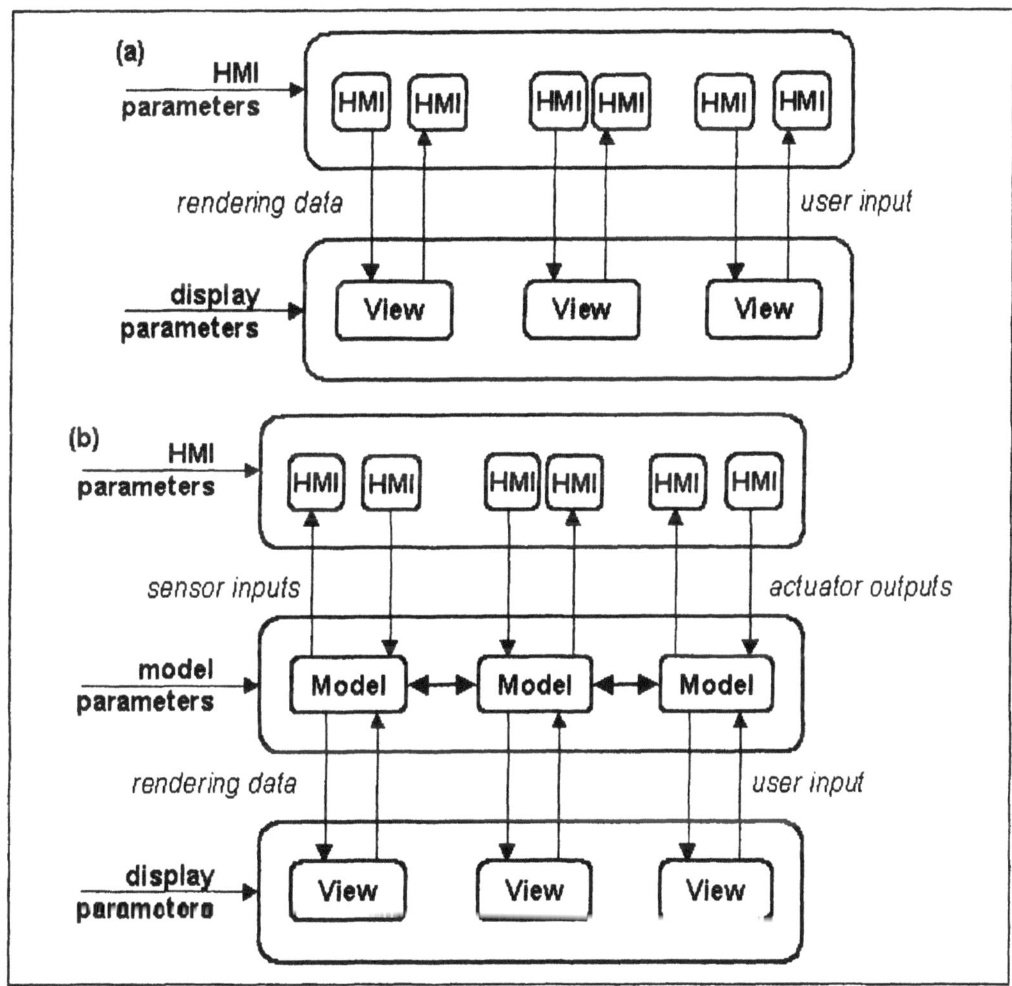

Figure 4 - Testing frameworks for: (a) Views, (b) Models

5. Use the Model testing mechanism shown in Figure 4(b) in conjunction with the previously tested Views to verify that the Models provide the correct behaviors in response to actuator inputs.
6. Develop **Controller** blocks as necessary to achieve required functions, e.g., sequencing of the simulated equipment, event and data interfaces for integration with other controller blocks. Test the Controller blocks, in conjunction with the previously developed Models and Vies, in the overall framework of Figure 4.
7. Implement the physical system as shown in Figure 5 by replacing the Model and View layers with the corresponding actual physical devices. Configure these devices to present to the Controller layer logical interfaces that are identical to the interfaces previously presented by the Model layer.

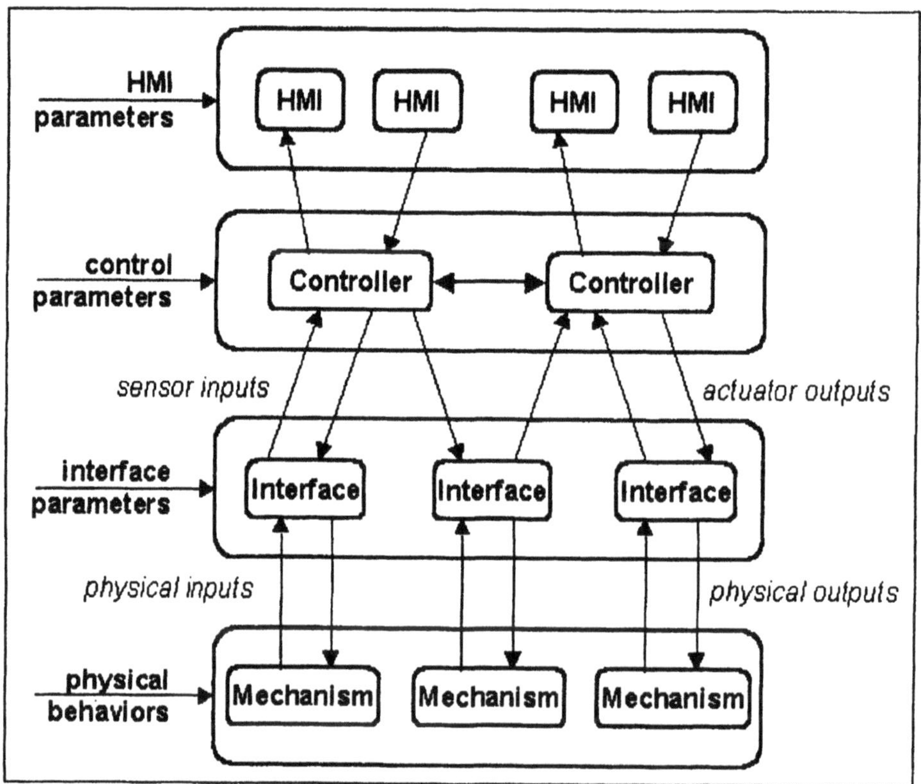

Figure 5 - Deployment framework

8. When possible, factor the Controller functions into **Low Level Control (LLC)** function blocks representing the control functions specific to physical devices and their interactions with other devices, and **High Level Control (HLC)** function blocks representing those functions which require interfaces with multiple devices, and which may utilize more complex technologies such as software agents. By allocating the LLC functionality to the physical devices, an architecture for intelligent "mechatronic" devices is created as illustrated in Figure 6, where the device boundaries are indicated by the dotted lines.
9. When possible, generalize the LLC function blocks and make them available, along with appropriate service interfaces, for reuse in libraries of intelligent mechatronic devices.

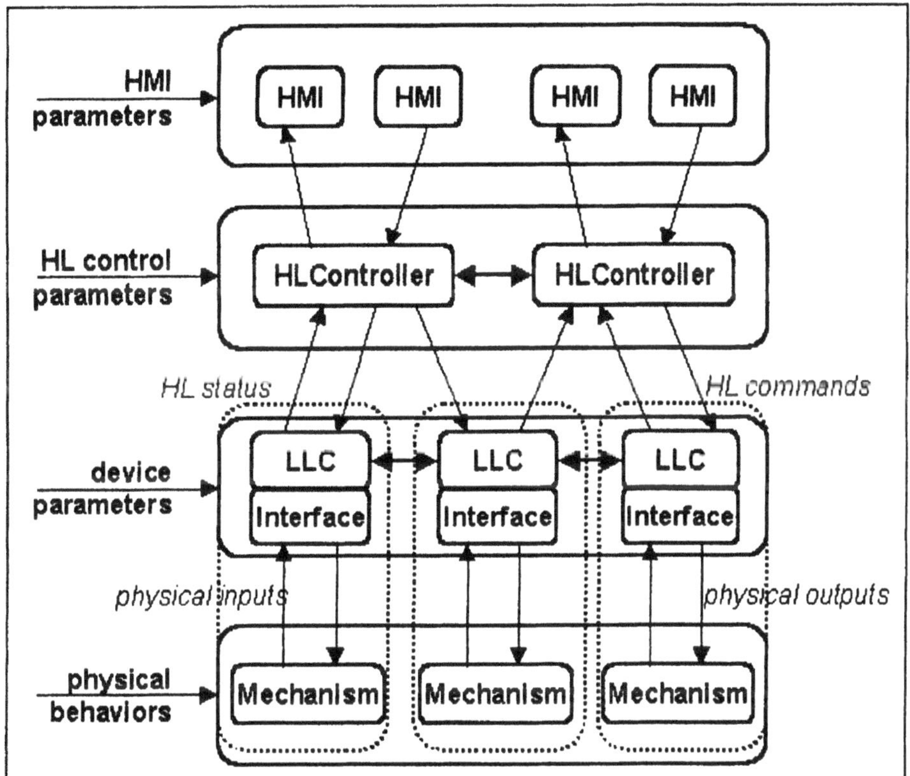

Figure 6 - Mechatronic device architecture

5. CONCLUSIONS

IEC 61499, with appropriate software tools and engineering methodologies, can be an effective way to meet the requirements for future scaleable, flexible automation. The original (Christensen, 2000) framework and engineering methodology have been successfully applied in a number of simulated and physical testbeds. A formal validation methodology and toolkit have also been applied to the original framework (Vyatkin, 2000). In addition, an electromechanical design workbench has been developed around this framework and methodology (Jain, 2002). The adaptation of this previous work to the improved framework and methodology presented in this paper, and the migration of the associated toolkits to an updated (Java 2) platform, are currently in progress.

6. ACKNOWLEDGMENTS

The author is indebted to Mr. Franz Auinger and Mr. Werner Rumpl of Profactor GmbH for pointing out the weaknesses of the original MVC framework and demonstrating the required refactoring of functionality. An immeasurable debt of gratitude is also owed to the late Dr. Odo Struger of Allen-Bradley and Rockwell Automation for his unflagging support and encouragement.

7. REFERENCES

1. Christensen, J. "Design patterns for systems engineering with IEC 61499." In Verteilte Automatisierung - Modelle und Methoden für Entwurf, Verifikation, Engineering und Instrumentierung, Ch. Döschner, ed. Magdeburg, Germany: Otto-von-Guericke-Universität, 2000.
2. IEC (International Electrotechnical Commission) 61499-1, Function blocks - Part 1, Architecture, Geneva, 2000.
3. IEC (International Electrotechnical Commission) 61499-2, Function blocks - Part 1, Software tool requirements, Geneva, 2001.
4. IEC (International Electrotechnical Commission) 61131-3, Programmable controllers - Part 3, Programming languages, Geneva, 2002.
5. ISO (International Organization for Standardization) TR 8509, Information processing systems - Open Systems Interconnection - Service conventions, Geneva, 1987.
6. W3C (W3 Consortium), eXtended Markup Language (XML) Specification, available at http://www.w3c.org/TR/1998/REC-xml-19980210, 1998.
7. Vyatkin, V., H.M. Hanisch, P. Starke, and S. Roch, "Formalisms for verification of discrete control applications on example of IEC 61499 function blocks." In Verteilte Automatisierung - Modelle und Methoden für Entwurf, Verifikation, Engineering und Instrumentierung, Ch. Döschner, ed. Magdeburg, Germany: Otto-von-Guericke-Universität, 2000.
8. Jain, S., C. Yuan and P. Ferreira, "EMBench: A Rapid Prototyping Environment for Numerical Control Systems," accepted for presentation, ASME IMECE, New Orleans, November 2002.

25

A LOW-COST EXPERIMENTAL SYSTEM AND ENGINEERING METHODOLOGY FOR IEC 61499 APPLICATIONS

Hirotsugu Tsunematsu[1], Hisashi Sasajima[1], Tatsuya Hojo[2]
[1] *Yamatake Corporation, {tunematu, sasajima }@atc.yamatake.co.jp*
[2] *Yamatake Corporation, hojo@atc.yamatake.co.jp*

IEC 61499, a new concept of control platform that consists of intelligent devices, has been proposed to resolve complications in system development and modification. However, there are few examples that have applied this architecture to a real system and the design methodology has not been established yet. This paper proposes a low-cost experimental system using LEGO® blocks for a feasibility study of design methodology based on IEC 61499 concepts. A method of system construction and technique to adopt features of physical machine factor, which was studied through using this experimental system, will also be presented.

1. INTRODUCTION

In general, conventional machine control systems consisting of centralized systems with PLC or distributed systems with some PLCs have been used. However, developing control software of these systems is very complicated, and system developers have sought a new control platform that can be configured and modified with ease.

To meet such requirements, a new concept of control platform with distributed intelligent devices has been proposed. It consists of intelligent devices such as axis controls or conveyance controls. Instead of a control program implemented in a centralized program, the control functions of each device are implemented in its own control unit as function blocks. Therefore, know-how of controlling devices can be embedded into each device. These devices will be easy to use, and the system developer doesn't have to open their knowledge. The system integrator can develop the system software in a cost-effective method of combining the distributed functions in the device. In addition, the software of these devices becomes highly reusable because it is isolated from the functions of other devices.

The International Electrotechnical Commission (IEC) is working to standardize this architecture as IEC 61499. However, only a few examples of applying this architecture to an actual system exist, and the design methodology has yet to be established. Also many of examples were shown with a simulation or discussed on conceptual design only.

In this paper, we propose a low-cost, experimental system using LEGO® blocks for the study of design methodology based on IEC 61499 architectures. This system consists of several sensors, motors and gears, and is controlled with two compact PCs. The devices are controlled with function blocks, which are compliant with IEC 61499. Because the controlled target is built with LEGO® blocks, the system can be developed and modified with ease. It also fits the IEC 61499 concept of building a whole system by putting parts, i.e., function blocks together like LEGO® blocks. We will also present a method of system construction and a technique to adopt features of physical machine factor, which was studied through using this experimental system.

2. BASIS OF IEC 61499

2.1 System Model

A system model of IEC 61499 concepts is shown in Figure 1. The controlled process consists of multiple devices. Each device is connected to a network and is able to communicate with each other. It also has its own functionality and control applications for this process, which are realized using functions on one device or combining functions distributed on multiple devices.

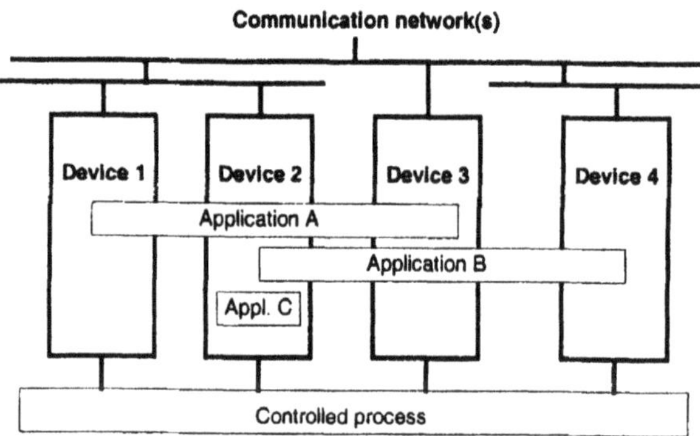

Figure 1 – System model

2.2 Application Model

Figure 2 illustrates an abstractive model of a distributed application. The application consists of one or more function block instances connected by event and data connections.

The function block instances may be distributed among devices. Execution sequence is decided by event flow, and data transfer among function blocks is represented by data flow.

In an executable model, event and data connections among devices can be represented by Service Interface function blocks.

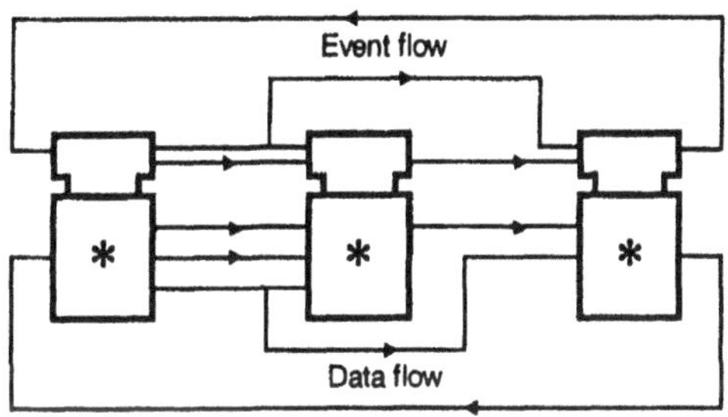

Figure 2 – Application model

2.3 Execution Control Chart

Execution of algorithm in Basic Function Block, which cannot be decomposed into other function blocks, is controlled by Execution Control Function which is represented by Execution Control Chart (ECC) as shown in Figure 3 (b).

In this example, *EC initial state*, which is active upon initialization of ECC, is START. In response to an INIT event input, *EC state* will be transferred to INIT state where *EC action* that initializes the function block INTEGRAL_REAL will be executed. First, the corresponding INIT algorithm is executed, and upon completion of execution, event output INITO will be generated. Condition 1 then sets the INIT state back to START state. Similarly in response to an EX event input, EC state is transferred to MAIN state followed by the execution of EC action, after which condition 1 sets the MAIN state to START state.

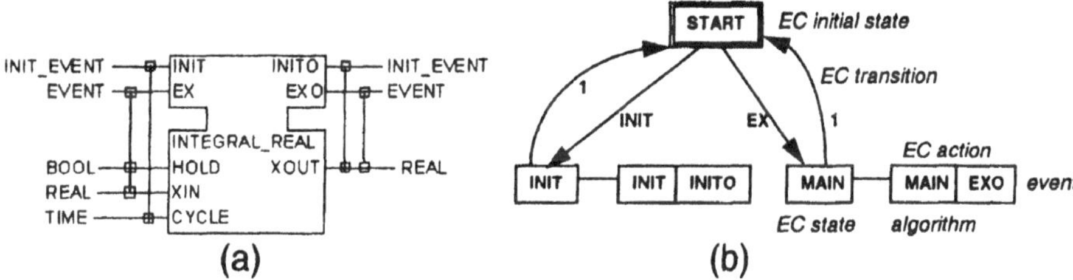

Figure 3 – Execution Control Chart

2.4 Composite Function Block

To avoid complexity of an application, the concept of *Composite Function Block* has been defined. In Composite Function Block, algorithms and their execution control are specified through event and data connections in one or more function block networks. It not only reduces the complexity of applications consisting of multiple function blocks but also encapsulates some specific know-how of control algorithms.

3. EXPERIMENTAL SYSTEM

3.1 Controlled Object

As illustrated in Figure 4, the controlled object was assembled of LEGO® blocks to assess IEC 61499 concept design methodology. The function of this machine is to feed and carry objects like an autonomous warehouse. It consists of three parts: one feeder and two conveyers. Each part is aimed to be an intelligent device and has sensors and a motor. These feeder and conveyer devices are controlled with low-cost AT-compatible computers running Windows 98/NT with PC 104-based digital input

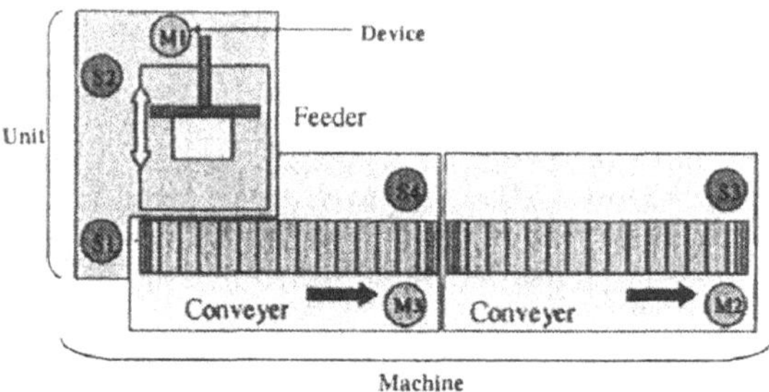

Figure 4 – Experimental equipment

and output control boards.

Supposing these devices are intelligent devices, each device should have an individual controller, however two conveyers are controlled by the same controller due to a restriction of the equipment.

3.2 System Overview

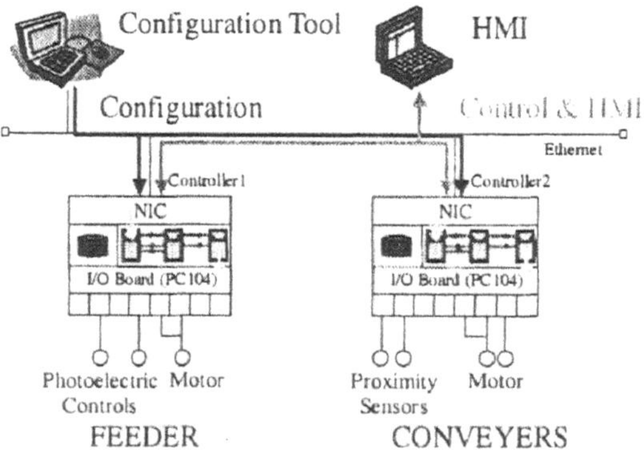

Figure 5 – System Overview

A system overview is shown in Figure 5. One PC is used for configuration of the devices and the other is used for operation.

In regards to configuration, each device has a function block library. According to the configuration message sent from the configuration tool, the function block instances and event/data connections will be created.

This configuration tool is not necessary for control and monitoring. Local applications on devices and HMI on remote PCs will communicate with each other through communication interface function blocks. Sensors and motors are controlled through process interface function blocks.

3.3 Operation

After a carried object has been set at designated place, the operator will press the "START" button on the HMI. This button will trigger a message sent to the "FEEDER" device, and the FEEDER will then push out the object onto the first CONVEYER. When the FEEDER accomplishes its work, a message will be passed to the first CONVEYER. In the same way, the first CONVEYER will take action to carry the object and send a message to the second CONVEYER. After the object arrives at the end of the second CONVEYER, a message will be forwarded to the first CONVEYOR and both conveyers will stop.

4. APPLICATION DEVELOPMENT METHODOLOGY

4.1 Overview

System development can be separated into several layers of physical interface, devices, units, and applications. In each layer, components supplied by the lower layer and some layer's specific know-how given by a developer will be encapsulated into a new composite function block.

This section describes the steps of feeder unit control design of the experimental system and the development of the overall application.

4.2 Physical Interface Layer

Introduction of service interface function blocks provides an application that is a useful interface in the physical world. In this experimental system, the network communication function block is furnished with the Function Block Development Kit (FBDK), an IEC 61499-compliant development environment provided by Rockwell Automation as a communication interface. This section discusses the process interface function block for digital input and output.

The controller has a digital input/output board with eight inputs and eight outputs. A driver of the interface board is installed on the OS, thus the function block is designed to encapsulate this driver. Due to restrictions of the driver, digital input and output interface have to be implemented into the same function block as Digital Input/Output interface.

Figure 6 describes the service sequences of this function block.

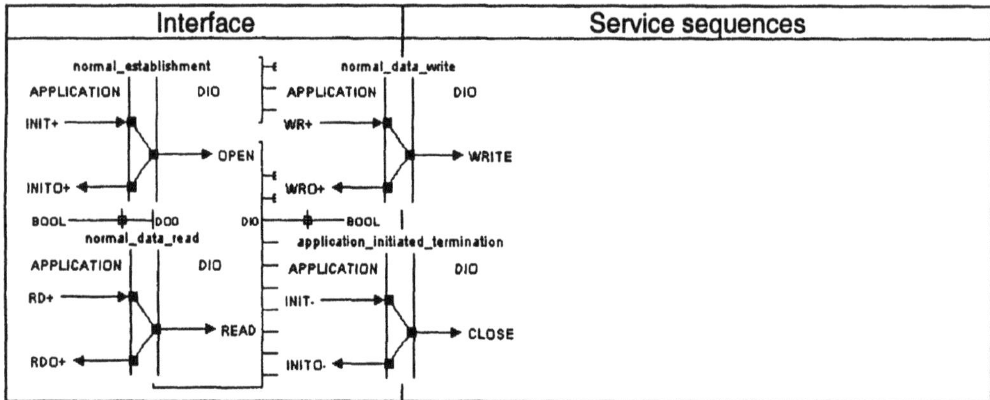

Figure 6– Digital Input/Output interface function block

4.3 Device Layer

4.3.1 Motor Control

A motor is a component device of the unit. Motor control function block implements know-how of the motor control designer.

A motor needs to move forward and backward, and stop at an exact location. As shown in Figure 7, this function block has M1_FW, M1_BW and M1_STOP event inputs. Each event initiates state transition to move or stop. In the M1_FW state, the M1_FW algorithm is executed in order to turn on the digital output port that specifies the motor direction. Then the REQ event is generated.

The "STOP" function includes a special sequence, which is a part of the know-how of motor control. When a motor stops, it should be reversed for a short time to brake. Duration of reverse depends on physical factors, such as mass. Therefore, this function block should be connected to the event delay function block that decides the reverse duration. The "STOP" event output is connected to the "START" event input of E_DELAY. After the duration of reverse, the E_DELAY generates "EO" event and will affect the state transition of the motor control function block to turn off the motor. Above two function blocks should be a composite function block.

4.3.2 Sensor Interface

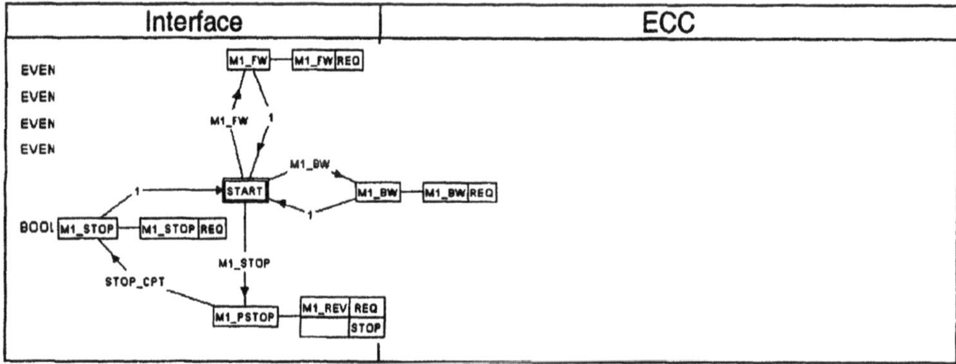

Figure 7 – Motor Control function block

For a machine control designer, state transition is the only necessary information with regards to sensors. Therefore, the sequence of reading the sensor cyclically, comparing the sensor's state and notifying the sensor's state transitions, is enclosed into the composite function block. In order to inspect sensor state change, the "MASK" function block is used. This function block compares the last and current states, and only when there are differences, it will output "IND" event.

4.3.3 Motor-with-Sensor Device

The above two devices can be composed into a function block of intelligent devices as shown in Figure 8. Know-how of using motor and sensor is encapsulated into a function block and it is a highly reusable software module.

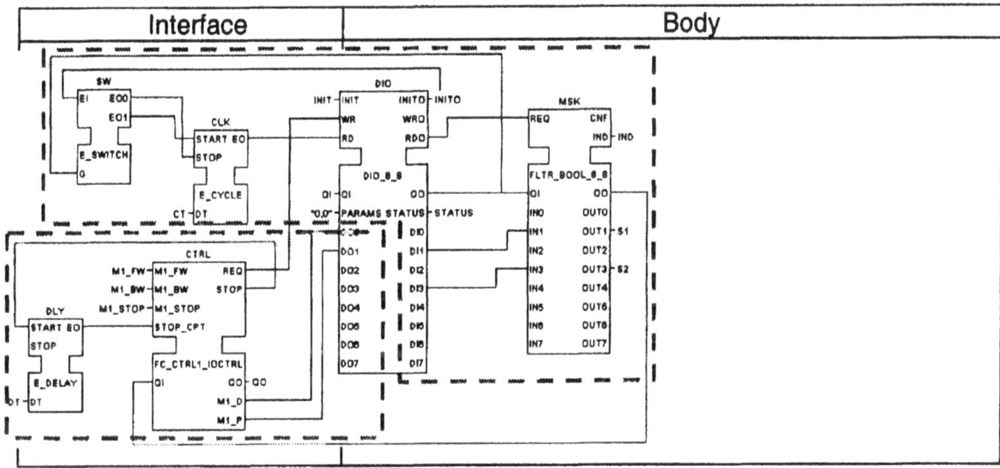

Figure 8 – Motor-with-Sensor function block

4.4 Unit Layer

There are four units in this experimental machine, i.e., FEEDER unit, HMI unit and two CONVEYER units.

Functions of the feeder unit can be implemented as the feeder control function block. This control function block is connected to a motor-with-sensor control function block. The combination of feeder control and motor-with-sensor control can be a feeder composite function block, FEEDER.

Considering this unit will be used under a distributed system, the local application in the feeder unit should provide the interface to get initiation of the feeder sequence and send a notification message confirming the sequence.

HMI unit and CONVEYER units can be built similarly.

4.5 Application Layer

Applications can be made combining HMI, FEEDER, and CONVEYER. Since every unit has a local application designed with function blocks and the local application has network interfaces, these devices can be combined easily through network.

5. CONCLUSION

An IEC 61499-compliant system design methodology using low-cost experiment system built with LOGO® blocks was discussed.

As shown in Figure 9, this methodology of developing machine control application will provide the hierarchy of system development of H/W, S/W suppliers, device vendors and system integrators based on IEC 61499 technologies. Control know-how of components can be hidden in function blocks, while it is available for upper layer users. As a result of know-how encapsulation repetition, the system integrator will be able to accomplish complicated system development with ease.

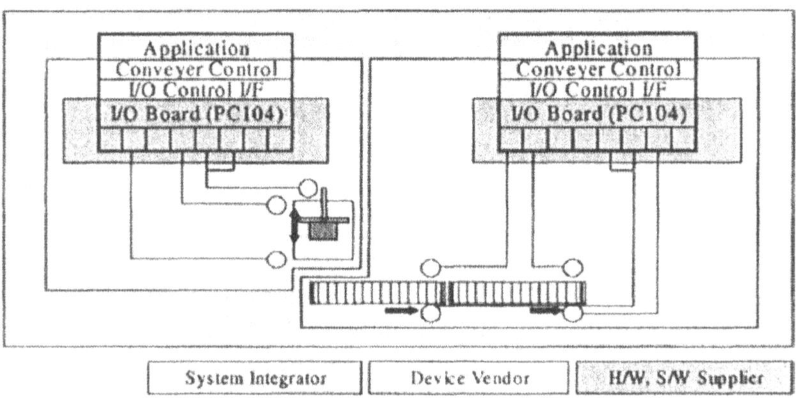

Figure 9 – Future System Development

For further research of IEC 61499 capabilities, we will study more complex and realistic examples including the case of system enhancement. Also, we will compare the scalability and development efficiency of IEC 61499 with conventional PLC programming or alternative implementation in C++, etc.

6. ACKNOWLEDGEMENTS

This work was accomplished using FBDK, which was provided by Rockwell Automation. The authors would like to thank Dr. J.H.Christensen for his fruitful suggestions.

7. REFERENCES

1. Christensen, James H. "Basic Concepts of IEC 61499"; Distributed Automation 2000.
2. IEC 65/248/PAS, Function blocks for industrial-process measurement and control systems - Part 1: Architecture, 19 April 2000.
3. Sasajima, Hisashi. "Fieldbus, The Digital Wave in Measurement, Control and Networks", ICAM ASIA 2001.
4. Tsunematsu, Hirotsugu. "IEC61499 Distributed Function Block Concept", ICAM ASIA 2001.

26

PLATFORMS FOR SCALABLE FLEXIBLE AUTOMATION CONSIDERING THE CONCEPTS OF IEC 61499

Werner E. Rumpl[1], Franz Auinger[1], Christoph Dutzler[2], Alois Zoitl[2]
[1] *Profactor GmbH, Wehrgrabengasse 1-5, A-4400 Steyr, Austria, werner.rumpl@profactor.at*
[2] *Institut für Automatiseriungs- und Regelungstechnik, Gusshausstr. 27-29, A-1040 Wien, Austria, cd@infa.tuwien.ac.at*

This work introduces approaches and embedded execution platforms for implementing the IEC 61499 (IEC, 2000) execution model. The IEC 61499 execution model is described as defined in the IEC 61499 standard. Issues that currently are not in the scope of the standard are discussed and by means of an illustrated IEC 61499 example application, it introduces different approaches that are beyond the standards' definition for embedding IEC 61499 on execution platforms with restricted memory, performance and operating system. Moreover the execution platforms as well as their implemented execution model are described and their advantages and disadvantages are illustrated.

1. INTRODUCTION

Currently industrial automation is divided into at least two main traditional domains: programmable logical controllers (PLC) and distributed control systems (DCS). Due to the trend of industrial automation equipping even small field devices with intelligent controllers in order to enable performing tasks autonomously, the concepts of PLCs and DCSs are merged and extended to distributed industrial process, measurement and control systems (IPMCSs). An IPMCS forms one base of Scalable Flexible Automation (SFA) (Christensen, 2002) and consists of a network of "smart" and heterogeneous field devices (different vendors, different applications) interacting with each other via standardized (field-) bus- connections. The IEC 61499 standard has been developed to enable and to ease engineering of IPMCSs by meeting the fundamental requirements for SFA such as reusability, configurability, portability of applications, scalability, flexibility, interoperability and reconfiguration, the last-mentioned especially for Holonic Manufacturing Systems (Christensen, 2002)(Holonic, 1998). As defined in IEC 61499 standard part 1 (IEC, 2000) the execution of IEC 61499 Function Blocks (FBs) is based on an event triggered methodology. However, currently the standard describes the execution of one IEC 61499 Function Block (FB). Considering a network of interacting FBs, also called an IEC 61499 application, there is the need to extend the IEC 61499 execution model by considering losses of overloaded events and its associated data that may cause unpredictable applications.

1.1 Motivation

Up to now there were only few trials to implement the execution model of the IEC 61499. Published approaches are based on PC based IEC 61499 runtimes using high performance processors (e.g.: Pentium or more) with sufficient memory and powerful operating systems (Holobloc, 2002). By considering embedded platforms with slower processors, less memory and without any powerful operating system or even no one, there is the need for alternative execution models in order to verify and validate the IEC 61499 execution model by means of realistic small and "smart" field devices that are realized with embedded systems.

2. THE IEC 61499 EXECUTION MODEL

2.1 Overview

The IEC 61499 standard describes architectures and models for distributed systems and is not primary considered being a programming methodology (Lewis, 2001). The IEC 61499 provides a set of models for the use of FBs in IPMCSs. These FBs encapsulate user-defined algorithms to perform different tasks (e.g.: measurement of temperature, control of a conveyor belt). The invocation of the algorithms processing data is triggered by events. Therefore one IEC 61499 FB consists of two main layers – one event layer and one data layer (see Figure 1). IEC 61499 describes different models of FBs, namely Basic Function Blocks, Composite Function Blocks, Service Interface Function Blocks, Adapters and a Subapplications Model. Here we focus on the relevant ones to provide a common understanding that is necessary for this work.

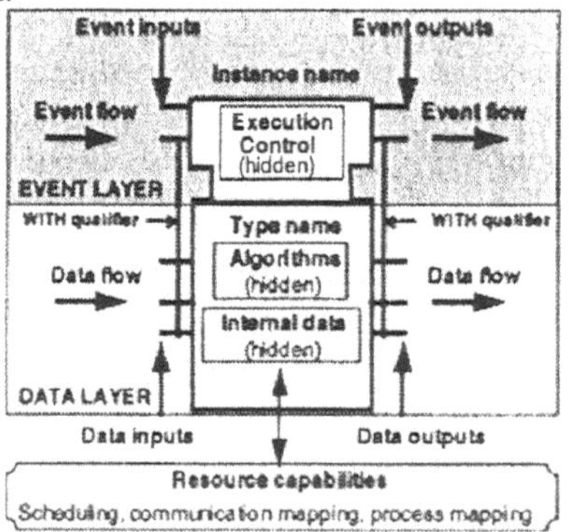

Figure 1 - Basic Function Block

As shown in Figure 1, each FB can be built up with zero or more event in- and outputs as well as with zero or more data in- and outputs. To get a network of interacting FBs, event/data outputs of one FB can be connected to event/data inputs of other FBs or even the same one - for detailed connection rules see (IEC, 2000). This network of FBs forms an IEC 61499 application that can be distributed among different Devices and Resources. One IEC 61499 system (equivalent with one IPMCS) consists of one ore more devices, resources and applications (see Figure 2) (IEC, 2000).

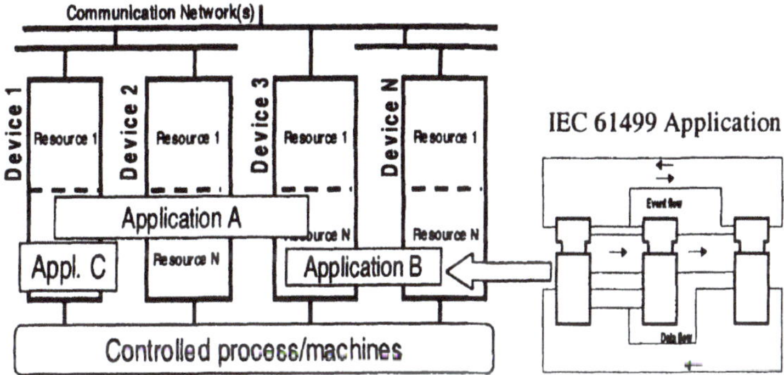

Figure 2 - Overview of an IEC 61499 system

2.2 The IEC 61499 Execution Model According to the Standard

As mentioned in chapter 2.1 IEC 61499 FBs are executed on the behalf of events. If an input event occurs, the algorithms may process input data, may update output data and may generate one or more event outputs. A so-called WITH qualifier is to determine, which data in- or output(s) to sample when its associated in- or output event(s) occurs - e.g.: REQ WITH SD, TEMP; means that the input variables SD and TEMP will be sampled if the event input REQ is invoked. The WITH qualifier is graphically represented by a line (see Figure 1). The IEC 61499 Standard Part 1 defines 8 times to illustrate the execution of **one Basic FB** with **a single event input**, **a single algorithm** and **a single event output** (see Figure 3).

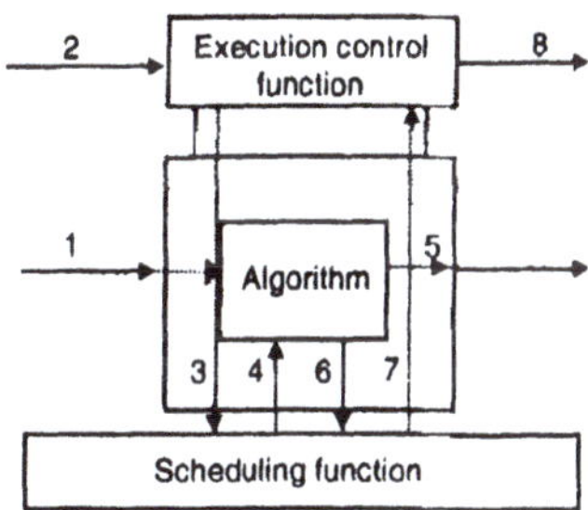

Figure 3 - Execution Model of an IEC 61499 Basic Function Block

Table 1 - Times according to IEC 61499

Time Nr.	Description of action
1	Relevant input variables, coming from other FBs, are stable at the input
2	The event occurs at an event input
3	The FB execution control function signals the resource scheduling function to schedule an algorithm for execution
4	The scheduling function starts the algorithm
5	The algorithm process input values, in some cases, also processes internally stored values and updates the output values that are written to the function block's outputs

6	The algorithm execution has finished and notification of the scheduling function to indicate that output data is stable at the output
7	The scheduling function invokes the execution control function
8	The execution control function signals an event at the event output

The IEC 61499 execution model implies that each FB has to have a scheduling function. This scheduling function refers to one FB and is to guarantee that each time occurs in the correct order, at the correct priority (Lewis, 2000) and to sample the right data with its associated event determined through the WITH qualifier. Considering one FB or a network of interacting FBs in one resource there has to be a mechanism to detect and handle event inputs that occur faster than the necessitated time between time slot 1 and 8. Additionally, the mechanism has to ensure that the resources' data of the network of FBs are consistent within the resource as well as to determine priorities and error handling for possible overloading of events in order to provide predictable IEC 61499 applications

Gaps of IEC 61499: Currently the IEC 61499 does not give detailed information what to do with overloaded input-events and its associated data and furthermore, it does not describe the characteristics and behavior of the scheduling function. It also does not include models for queuing input- or output events and its associated data. However, the standard points out these critical issues and mentions that "resources may need to schedule the execution of algorithms in a multitasking manner", but how to solve the existing problems is referred to be "implementation-dependent" (Part 1, 2000).

3. CONCEPTS FOR IEC 61499 EXECUTION MODEL BEYOND THE STANDARD

In this chapter we will introduce approaches for execution models that can be implemented on embedded execution platforms (slow processors, little memory and small or no operating system) in order to realize small and smart field devices. We also discuss the characteristics and behavior of the approaches to fill the gaps of the IEC 61499 standard (see 2.2).

All presented concepts shall be shown and compared via a little example application (Figure 4a) consisting of three Service Interface Function Blocks (SIFBs) and two Basic Function Blocks (BFBs). All of these FBs are located in one resource. The two SIFBs on the left generate events with their associated data (further referred as Input- SIFBs) that is processed by the two BFBs and finally published by the SIFB on the right (further referred as Output- SIFB). Each of these blocks is triggered by events. In case of the two Input- SIFBs this is any external event like a change of state of an external sensor. All other FBs are triggered by an event that is produced by another FB. So each FB has to be able to react on an event and autonomously start execution. If a multi- tasking system is used as suggested in the standard (see chapter 2) it seems to be obvious, at least in a first approach, to assign one task (- which may consist of one ore more threads) to each FB to allow parallel execution of all FBs containing one ore more internal algorithms. But this would definitely be too resource intensive to apply this concept on the embedded platforms we will introduce in section 4 below. So other solutions have to be found being able to run on these platforms. To overcome this problem two different approaches are discussed in the following subsections. In subsection 3.1 a single tasking and multi-threading concept with a definite reduction of the number of threads is presented, while the concepts in subsection 3.2 are based on conventional interrupt handling that can be found on small micro controllers.

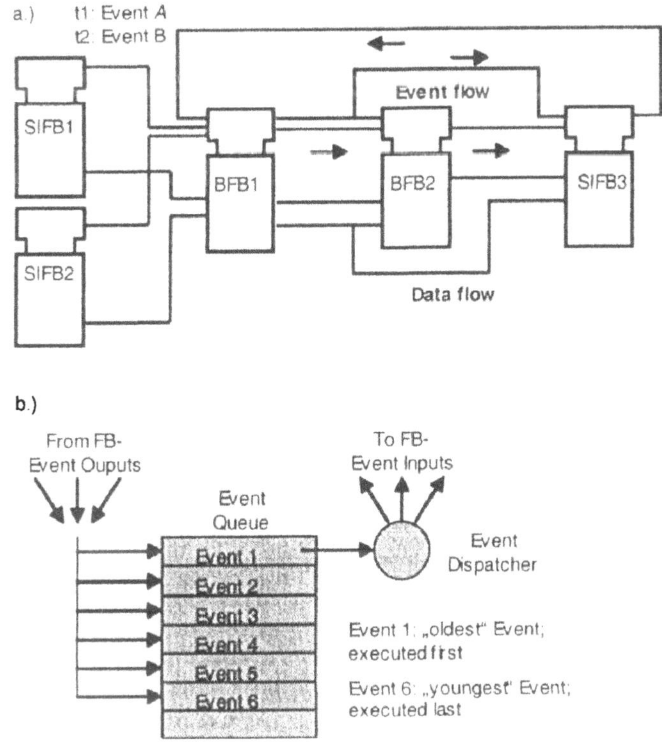

Figure 4 - Example a.) Application b.) Event Scheduler

3.1 Execution Model Single Tasking with Multi-Threading

The presented execution model of this chapter implies that the illustrated application (see Figure 4a.) runs in a single task containing several threads. Only one thread is to provide management services (Part 1, 2000) within one resource (e.g.: building up the application in the resources) and one thread is assigned to each Input- SIFB, to allow the IEC 61499 application to react to external events. After the application is built up the threads of the Input- SIFBs are initiated and can generate output events in two ways, either by an external interrupt or the thread itself polls for certain service it should provide (e.g.: 8 digital inputs of an I/O card). The following input- events of the BFBs are triggered by the generated output events of the Input-SIFBs based on event function calls in a nested manner.

With this concept absolute parallel execution of the BFBs and Output- SIFB is only possible if different Input- SIFBs would initiate their execution (and so trigger different threads) and these SIFBs would be a part of separate, independent FB-networks, latter because of the nested event function calls. If event outputs of different Input- SIFB are connected to the same FB (Figure 4a.) parallel execution is restricted caused by implemented threading mechanism based on the Java or C++ technology. To avoid data inconsistencies a synchronisation mechanism is implemented. This mechanism blocks an event coming from another thread to enter a FB while one thread is executing this block or succeeding blocks. The two restrictions to the parallel execution of FBs are:

- An execution triggered by an external event can only be done as long as the thread does not attempt to enter any FB that is blocked by another thread
- If a second input- event occurs at the same FBs while an initiated execution of a previous event has not finished this second event is ignored

The biggest drawback of this concept is that systems that support multi- threading are time and space consuming (see section 4.1 Java based systems). The benefit is that no central instance like a queue or scheduler is needed which reduces the complexity of implementing an IEC 61499 "like" execution model.

3.2 Execution Models with Event/Data Scheduler

In contrast to subsection 3.1 the following approaches are not based on multi-tasking or multi-threading operating system. Nonetheless, a method that allows an execution of FBs is achieved by scheduling events and data that are passed between FBs. Interrupt routines are used to trigger Input- SIFBs when a change of data is recognised at their inputs. All other FBs are executed according to different scheduler strategies described in the following subsections.

3.2.1 Scheduling of Events only

As illustrated in Figure 4b, all FB output events are set into a global event queue. The order of the events in the queue is equivalent to their order of occurrence. For example, event 1 shown in Figure 4b occurred first and so it was the first that was set into the queue. The dispatcher that knows the interconnection of the events takes event 1 first to trigger the corresponding FB. When the execution of this FB has terminated the dispatcher takes the next event from the queue and so on. A SIFBs' execution is triggered on external behalf at their service interfaces and not by any FB in the network. Due to that a SIFB cannot be triggered with t

he dispatcher. Instead interrupt routines are used for this purpose as mentioned above.

The concept has the drawback that events and corresponding data might be inconsistent. Consider the example shown in Figure 4a, The SIFB1 generates at t1 an event *A* at its event output to communicate the receiving of new input data. After a period of time it sends at t2 an event *B* at the same event output because input data changed again. Between the occurrence of event *A* and *B*, BFB1 was never executed because other function blocks were executed during that time. If after another period of time the dispatcher is able to take event *A* from the queue to trigger BFB1, the FBs' input data corresponds to event *B* and not to event *A*. Inconsistencies of data and events are the consequence, which may lead to undefined conditions in applications.

3.2.2 Scheduling of Events and *Data*

By storing not only events in a queue but also the corresponding data, it is guaranteed that when the dispatcher starts the execution of a definite FB by triggering it with an event the corresponding data is present at the data inputs of the block. To store also data in the global queue instead of just events (3.2.1) requires a lot of memory, time-consuming data copying and performance. If execution is too slow the dispatcher is not able to take as many events from the queue, as are put into the queue in the same period of time. This leads to unacceptable delays or even to an overload of the queue.

3.2.3 Definite Ignoring of Events

The standard defines that "multiple occurrences of an event at the same event input may be lost ... while waiting for ECC to finish ... The detection and processing of such loss is an implementation- dependent feature." (Part 1, 2000)

This is equivalent with the fact that an event may be ignored if the execution of the event's predecessor at the same event input of the FB is not finished when this new event occurs. This allows adopting the concept of event queues. Events are only put into the queue if no event of the same event output is already in the queue waiting to be executed. Otherwise the event is deleted. This leads to a shorter queue and so to the fact that waiting time of accepted events for getting executed is reduced.

Nonetheless it is important to provide mechanisms to detect event losses, as the number of lost events is a characteristic value for the user to estimate the systems workload. Another benefit of definite ignoring of events is that the problem of data inconsistencies like it occurred in 3.2.1 is significantly reduced. If all data inputs at a FB are assigned to their corresponding event by the WITH construct (see section 2), present data at the FBs data inputs may be used for execution; no matter if the ECC is executed immediately after the event occurred or if the execution is delayed because "older" events in the queue are executed first. Summarized advantages of this concept:

- Short event queue and so reduced waiting time for events to get executed
- Inconstancies of data and events can be avoided by proper use of the WITH construct
- No multi-tasking concept is required as SIFBs are handled with interrupts while all other FBs are executed sequentially

3.2.4 Hybrid Form

Due to the mentioned advantages the concept presented in 3.2.3 is most suitable for the aspired low performance execution platforms. Nonetheless one has to be aware that the ignoring of events like it is done in approach 3.2.3 is not acceptable for all applications. Consider a counter- FB whose task is to count its input events. In this case events may not be ignored even if the processing of the preceding event is not finished yet.

This can be solved by a hybrid form that is based on the concept of definite ignoring of events (3.3.3) with the extension of special event- and data- queuing for critical FBs.: Critical FBs whose input events may never be ignored have to be treated differently by the event queue. Every event that is calling such a special FB has to be put into the queue, no matter if a predecessor of this event is in the queue already or not. So it is guaranteed that all occurred events are handed on to the FB. As multiple occurrences of events are allowed for critical FBs additional data queuing for these FBs is required to avoid data inconstancies.

As a conclusion of this the hybrid form requires priorities of events with its associated data, which have to be set by the user. Therefore the user has to analyse his application before implementing it to be sure that the application is predictable.

4. CURRENT STATE OF WORK

Profactor and the Automation Control Institute are working intensively on the evaluation of the different execution models by means of various platforms. At the moment our work focuses on Class 1 devices (IEC, 2000). This chapter gives an overview of the platforms and describes their kernel (Java based or C/C++ based), interfaces and memory resources with respect to the execution model and problems.

4.1 Java-Based Execution Platforms

The Java technology for embedded systems attracts interest all over the world, due to its advantages (Sun, 2002).Therefore we introduce two small Java™ based execution platforms for the possible use of smart field devices.

4.1.1 TINI

TINI stands for Tiny Internet Interface and it is a small Java™ execution platform that is built up by one DS80C390 (a 8051 derivative) micro controller, one flash ROM, one static RAM, an Ethernet controller and a real-time clock. The micro controller itself is equipped with a CAN interface, 2 Serial ports, a 1-wire interface and several TTL IOs. The TINI runtime environment can be divided into two categories: native code execution directly by the micro controller and an API (Application Programming Interface) interpreted as byte codes by the TINI Java™ virtual machine (TINI, 2002) which size is less then 40 kilobytes. Applications can be executed in Java using the supported packages or if there exist stringent real-time requirements, native libraries can be loaded within an application.

The IEC 61499 runtime that allows the execution of IEC 61499 applications was implemented with the Java technology (runtime is currently available on http://www.holobloc.com). The TINI operating system provides facilities for multitasking and multithreading. Due to these features, each FB type is represented as a Java class with defined interfaces and the execution model is based on a multithreading methodology described in section 3.1 above. For verification purposes, we extended the TINI with starter kit boards providing a parallel interface with up to 24 discrete I/O points. Successful tests were done on a small assembly test bed..

Shortcomings: The bottleneck of the TINI platform is its memory that is limited to 512kByte Flash ROM and optional 512kByte or 1Mbyte SRAM and last but not least its slow performance. The Flash ROM is already used by the TINI OS, the TINI JVM, class libraries and command interpreter (TINI, 2002). The file system, the IEC 61499 runtime and the IEC 61499 FBs are stored in the non-volatile SRAM. The TINI board represents a device Class 1 (IEC, 2000). By downloading a programmed application from an IEC 61499 Editor, the application will be built up on the TINI's SRAM. This process is very resource intensive because of instancing the runtime's classes and the application's FB classes with all its interconnections to provide a runnable application. Additionally, the event-triggered methodology is based on Java synchronized function calls in a nested manner. This fact causes several problems with memory overflow and determinism if the system engineer doesn't consider these nested event function calls.

4.1.2 SaJe

SaJe stands for Systronix aJile Euroboard that is equipped with an aJ100 native Java™ processor (100MHz) from aJile systems, 1MB SRAM, 4MB FLASH and several communication interfaces including, among other things 2 Serial Ports, Ethernet, 1-Wire and expansion board socket. The J2ME CLDC (Sun, 2002) serves as runtime environment of the SaJe. The IEC 61499 runtime and the different FB types are implemented as on the TINI chip. For verification purposes we extended the board with a parallel interface with up to 24 IOs. By means of this interface we could also control a small assembly test bed.

Shortcomings: There are two main advantages compared to the TINI platform, namely the better execution performance and the size of the memory. Due to the 4MB of Flash ROM, there is the possibility to store the classes of both the runtime and the FB into the Flash in order to build up larger applications in the SRAM. Therefore the disadvantages regarding nested event function calls and the threading model are the same.

4.2 C++ Based Execution Platforms

The presented Java platforms are not capable of the defined requirements for small, distributed control platforms. Other approaches are necessary to reach real-time execution with low performance platforms. For instance, C/C++ implementations are less memory and time consuming than applications written in Java. Furthermore the number of embedded Java platforms accepted by automation industries is restricted. For these reasons an implementation in C++ was developed. To use existing know-how the implementation was based on the work done in Java.

Current state: Due to the wide distribution the C166 μ-controller from Infineon was chosen for a first implementation. Each FB is represented as a class in C++. These classes are compiled and linked into one executable file for the specific system (e.g. Intel hex file) that is stored in the flash. The application is built on instances of these classes in the RAM. The IEC 61499 execution model is implemented respectively to the methodology of Definite Ignoring of Events (3.2.3). SIFBs are triggered via hardware interrupts of the C166 μ-controller. For the communication between the devices communication SIFBs have been implemented using CAN .

Additionally the C++ execution platform has been compiled for the IPC@CHIP from Beck. On this system communication function blocks for Ethernet are available.

5. CONCLUSIONS AND FUTURE WORK

As described in chapter 3, a hybrid form of the introduced execution models may fulfill requirements like determinism, data consistence and event losses within one resource. Therefore events with their associated data may be classified according to the demands of the application (e.g.: a closed-loop control may need the latest event and the latest data, in contrast to that a counter may need all events with all associated data). System- engineers have to be aware of this classification while programming an IEC 61499 application.

Nonetheless, our test cases showed that with the presented concepts of the extended IEC 61499 execution models it is possible to run IEC 61499 applications on low-cost embedded systems in order to control several test beds, large and small sized ones.

In the near future our team will extend the variety of IEC 61499 embedded platforms and evaluate each of them by applying different execution models and test them with several test beds.

6. REFERENCES

1. Christensen J.H. "IEC 61499: An Open Architecture for Scalable Flexible Automation", http://www.holobloc.com/papers/sfarch2.zip
2. HMS European Module BPR-CT-97-9000 Deliverable D1.1-1/D1.1-1 Holonic System Architecture; University of Keele, 1998, Keele
3. Holobloc Homepage, http://www.holobloc.com
4. Lewis R.W. Modeling control systems using IEC 61499, ISBN: 0 85296 796 9
5. IEC (International Electrotechnical Commission): PAS 61499-1, "Function Blocks, Part 1 - Architecture". Geneva, 2000.
6. TINI software, http://www.ibutton.com/TINI/software/index.html
7. SaJe "Real Time Native Execution", http://www.systronix.com/saje/index.htm
8. "Embedded Systems go Real Time with Java™ Technology", http://java.sun.com/features/2001/04/embed.html

27

MANAGING FAULT MONITORING AND RECOVERY IN DISTRIBUTED REAL-TIME CONTROL SYSTEMS

Robert W. Brennan and Douglas H. Norrie
Department of Mechanical and Manufacturing Engineering
University of Calgary, 2500 University Dr. N.W. Calgary, T2N 1N4
brennan@enme.ucalgary.ca

In this paper we describe a holonic approach to managing distributed real-time control applications for manufacturing. The main feature of the architecture are layering (to support functional decomposition) and clustering (to support task propagation).

1. INTRODUCTION

The current trend toward higher levels of automation in the manufacturing and process industries has created a greater reliance on software. In particular, as devices such as controllers, sensors and actuators become "smarter", safety functions that were previously performed by mechanical or electrical interlocks have been assumed by computer software that may reside in a single device or distributed across multiple devices. Failures in these systems can have a significant impact on a company's bottom line (e.g., loss of equipment, production down-time), and more importantly, on the lives of many people.

As a result, as software begins to play an increasingly important role in safety-critical systems, it becomes increasingly important to understand the risks associated with these systems and how these risks can be managed. The objective of the research reported in this paper is to develop software techniques to achieve safe operation of these new distributed computer-based control systems.

We begin with background on distributed real-time control system, then outline the basic requirements for these systems in section 3. Next, we describe our layered architecture to support these basic requirements in section 4 then discuss our current and future work in this area in section 5.

2. BACKGROUND

Manufacturing control systems clearly fall in the category of safety-critical systems since these systems should not incur too much risk to persons or equipment. As well, the typical requirements of real-time systems such as timeliness, responsiveness, predictability, correctness and robustness are also of fundamental importance.

The primary distinction between non-real-time and real-time systems is that real-time systems tightly link correctness with timeliness. In other words, deadlines must be met under hard real-time (i.e., tasks must finish by a specified time) and soft real-time (i.e., tasks must meet deadlines on average) constraints (Douglass, 1999). Because of the more stringent requirements for latency, reliability and availability (Leveson, 1995), it follows that the step from the non-real-time or soft real-time domain is a large one. This is particularly true in light of the recent trend towards distributed process.

Although there has been a considerable amount of work in the area of fault-tolerant design of industrial control systems (Anderson, 1981; Siewiorek, 1982), fault-tolerant software, and particularly fault-tolerant *distributed* software is a relatively new area of research (Jalote, 1998). Recently, there have been a number of advances in distributed intelligent control that provide the tools to move away from the traditional centralized, scan-based programmable logic controller architecture towards a new architecture for real time distributed intelligent control. In particular, there have been a number of advances recently in programming languages (Lyons, 1998; Wang, 2001), models for distributed control (IEC, 2000) and software methodologies (Lyons, 1998; Odell, 2000). As well, there have been numerous advances in the development of intelligent field devices (e.g., sensors and actuators) that combine built-in processing capabilities with standard communication interfaces. These "Fieldbus" devices have been the focus of the IEC 1158 standard for a number of years, as well as the recent emergence of proprietary solutions such as Siemens Profibus and Allen-Bradley's DeviceNet.

The International Electro-technical Commission (IEC) 61499 standard is one example of this new trend (IEC, 2000). This standard addresses the need for modular software that can be used for distributed industrial process control. In particular, this standard builds on the function block portion of the IEC 61131-3 standard for PLC languages (Lewis, 1996) and extends the function block (FB) language to more adequately meet the requirements of distributed control in a format that is independent of implementation. A detailed description of the IEC 61499 standard is beyond the scope of this paper, however further details concerning this model and its relationship to multi-agent and holonic systems concepts can be found in (Brennan, 2001b).

3. REQUIREMENTS FOR DISTRIBUTED CONTROL

In this section we focus on the motivation for our work in distributed real-time control systems, which follows from three key requirements of these systems: (i) control application development, (ii) reconfiguration, and (iii) fault monitoring and recovery.

3.1 Basic Requirements

The first and most fundamental requirement is that our system should be capable of allowing the user to develop control applications using IEC 61499 function blocks.

Ideally, the development environment should comply with the standard's "class 2" (IEC, 2000): i.e., the user should be able to create completely new data types, function block types, and configurations of function blocks (Lewis, 2001). As well, to support ease of programming, the system should allow applications to be built from standard libraries of IEC 61499 function blocks as well as specialized, user-defined libraries. Once the control application is developed, the system should then be capable of arranging for compilation of the code into low-level application code and distributing this application code to appropriate resources for execution. For example, "resources" can be physical devices such as a robot, or may be individual microcontrollers on a physical device (e.g., for servo control). Once distributed, these function blocks must be executed, taking account of their timing and precedence relationships. This particular difficult when we consider distributed systems, since correctness must be maintained for applications that run over a number of CPUs, each with its own time base. Finally, if changes are required, the system should be capable of run-time reconfiguration. This may involve simply replacing portions of the running application at the granularity level of an individual function block or, the removal of a function block and the addition of a different function block or group of function blocks.

The configuration and reconfiguration of distributed function block applications is a key area of holonic systems research. This becomes particularly apparent when one considers that one of the fundamental holonic manufacturing systems ideals is the development of systems that can automatically adapt to change. A detailed explanation of our approach to configuration and reconfiguration of these systems, is beyond the scope of this paper, however one may consult (Brennan, 2001a) for further details.

Monitoring and fault recovery is a key requirement of any industrial control system, so it is not surprising that it is also critical for distributed real-time control system design. The purpose of monitoring is to ensure that the control system performs as intended. In other words, this involves ensuring that no unidentified, or latent, faults occur. Fault monitoring is basically the process of watching for failures and errors that may occur when the system is running or that are present (but possibly undetected) in the system itself. Before going any further, we should look at the terms "failures" and "errors" more closely. Failures relate to events that occur at specific times. For example, breakage or excessive wear of mechanical components or overloading of electrical components often manifests failures. Since software does not "break" or "wear" (though, arguably, data may "wear" by becoming obsolete), the notion of "component failures" has little relevance for control software. Errors, however, are a different matter: i.e., an error is an inherent characteristic of the system. As a result, this concept is more relevant to software systems since errors are often manifested in program "bugs".

Systematic errors can be, and almost always are, present in control software. As well, random failures can, and typically do, occur in the controlled system. Given these eventualities, the control system must be capable of recovering from the resulting faults. As a result, the types of responsibilities that our control system will have are: (i) diagnosis of program execution, (ii) monitoring for exceptions that are thrown by function block code during execution, and (iii) monitoring the system state for inconsistencies (e.g., deadline control).

To achieve a safe system, typically two general concepts are used (Leveson, 1995). The first approach involves separating the fault monitoring and recovery code (i.e., the "safety channels") from the control application code. This decomposition technique is typically referred to as the "firewall concept" (Leveson, 1995), since one may think of the safety channels as providing a firewall for the control code. The second approach involves applying redundancy in the control system. This is a very common means of fault recovery and can be achieved in two basic ways: homogeneous redundancy and diverse redundancy. Homogeneous redundancy, is the most basic form of redundancy, and involves "clones" or exact replicas of code to be used as backup code in the case of a failure. The main disadvantage with this technique is that it only protects against random failures. For example if a piece of hardware fails, a copy of the code that was running on the failed device can be moved to another device to allow the system to continue operating. However, if the failure was caused by a systematic error in the software (e.g., a command that causes the process to go into a deadlock state), this technique will not work: i.e., the same failure will occur on the new device. To overcome this problem and provide protection against random and systematic failures, diverse redundancy can be used. With this approach, the redundant code is implemented in a different way. For example, the redundant code for a PID controller could be implemented using fuzzy logic.

In the next sub-section, we propose an approach that builds on the "firewall concept" in order to address the issue of system safety (i.e., fault monitoring and recovery) as well as the basic requirements of control application development and reconfiguration for distributed real-time systems.

3.2 Methodology

The research presented in this paper is intended to address the basic requirements noted above by taking advantage of recent advances distributed control system models, software and hardware to realize a distributed process control system with intelligent control components to work in safety-critical environments.

In remainder of the paper, we describe a layered architecture to manage fault monitoring and recovery in distributed control systems based on the notion of "holonic agents" (Marik, 2001). Through their work with the IEC 61499 function block model, members of the Holonic Manufacturing Systems Consortium (HMS, 2002) came to the realization that the best approach is to encapsulate the function block solution into higher-level software when and where it is required to enable more sophisticated reasoning and a richer knowledge representation than function blocks alone. These resulting holonic agents can then integrate a holonic part (for hard real-time) and software agent part (responsible for higher level, soft real-time or non-real-time intelligent decision-making).

This paper extends this idea to a multi-layer architecture consisting of four temporally decomposed layers of agents and devices illustrated in Figure 1: execution control (EC), control execution (EC), execution (E), and hardware. As one moves down the layers, time scales become shorter and real-time constraints change from soft to hard real-time; as well, the degree of agency decreases (i.e., higher-level agents are more sophisticated but slower, while lower-level agents are fast and light-weight).

The EC and CE layers shown in Figure 1 support two fundamental system requirements: control application management, and fault detection and recovery. Since the real-time holonic control system is intended to meet hard real-time requirements, a temporal decomposition of the agents used for this purpose is necessary.

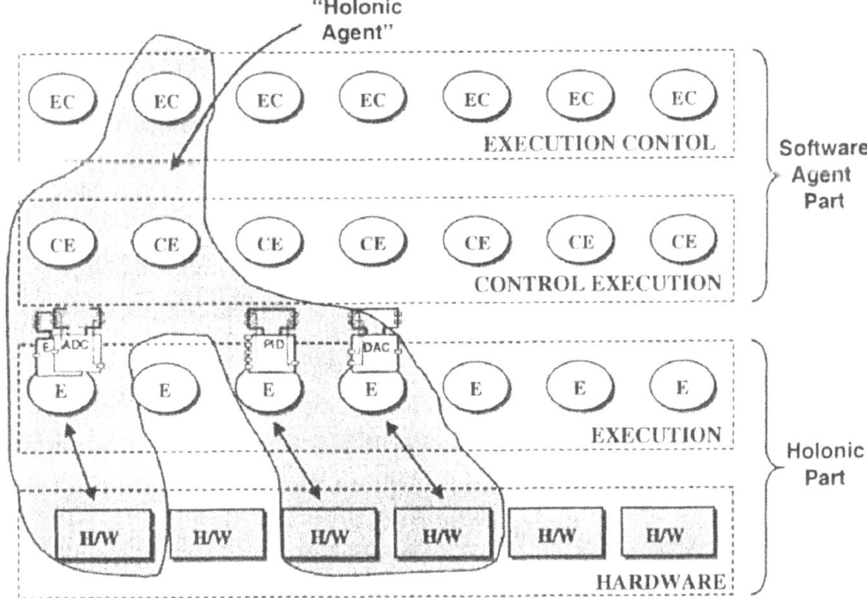

Figure 1 – Layered Architecture

The EC layer is composed of agents, or "holonic units" (i.e., the ovals shown in Figure 1), that are responsible for arranging control applications for execution as well as planning for reconfiguration, fault monitoring and fault detection. In general, CE holonic units are responsible for controlling what is being executed. In other words, the CE holonic units are concerned with distributing execution control code to the appropriate resources (shown as "H/W" in Figure 1), performing basic monitoring and alerts, and handling low-level fault recovery procedures. In cases where more sophisticated fault recovery decision-making is required, the CE layer will consult with holonic units in the EC layer (who may even have to consult higher-level agents). In the next section, we describe this decomposition in more detail.

4. AN ARCHITECTURE FOR DISTRIBUTED REAL-TIME CONTROL

One of the main features of our architecture for distributed real-time control is the concept of layering. The idea here is to identify various autonomous layers that appear to interact through API's (application program interfaces). On each layer, code is run asynchronously, resulting in clear functional separation across the layers. As will be discussed in section 4.1, clustering is another important feature of the architecture. In other words, everything happens through task propagation (and concurrently) through cluster formation.

Two general approaches can be used to execute applications using this general approach. First, all function blocks below the application level can be handled by a single level of controllers. Alternatively, function blocks can be distributed over the system for execution across a web of "holonic controllers" (i.e., the shaded area over the Execution and Hardware layers in Figure 1). In this case, higher-level function blocks (and/or software agents) run on "application level" controllers, middle-level function blocks run on "execution level" controllers, and low-level function blocks run on "control execution level" controllers and base level ("execution") controllers.

For the remainder of this section we can think of each layer as an independent set of controllers. Communication between the layers is facilitated by the layer interfaces.

4.1 Task Propagation

In Figure 1, the shaded boundary that extends from the EC layer down to the hardware layer is an example of a control application that is being run on a cluster of devices (for e.g., CNC's, AGV's, or Robots). The devices represent a virtual cluster (or virtual cell) of devices with a control application that is distributed across specific resources in each of the devices.

Figure 2 illustrates the concepts of "layering" and "clustering". First, a task is initiated by a command from a higher-level. For example, at the planning and scheduling level (not shown in Figure 2), a request may be made to move a part from point A to point B. At this stage, the first cluster of EC/CE agents is formed to handle the task execution. Next, a second cluster is formed, which represents the distribution of the control application. Finally, each bit of distributed code is executed on a specific hardware platform as shown by cluster 3.

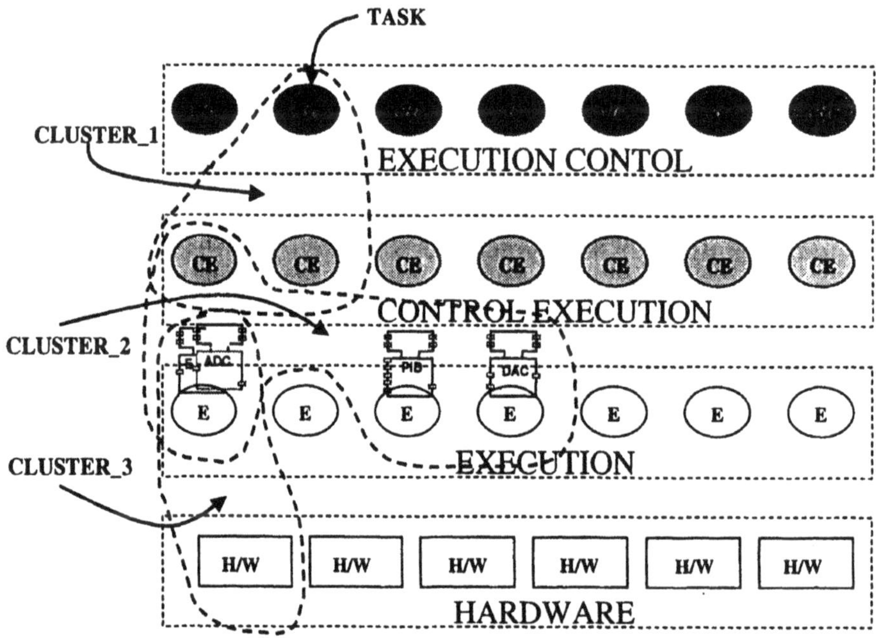

Figure 2 – Task Propagation

From a top-down perspective, layering and clustering allow us to manage the functional decomposition of high-level tasks and automatically determining the required distribution of function blocks. As will be discussed in the next sub-section, the resulting clusters can also be used for bottom-up fault-recovery management.

4.2 Fault Monitoring and Recovery

A primary advantage of this approach is that we can use the task sub-clusters illustrated in Figure 2 to track back as far as is required for fault monitoring and recovery. For example, Figure 3 illustrates what happens when a fault occurs at the hardware level. In this case, the fault is first caught at the execution level. For example, data corruption checks or reasonableness checks (i.e., comparisons using redundant software) may be used to catch the fault. The fault is then reported to the next higher level.

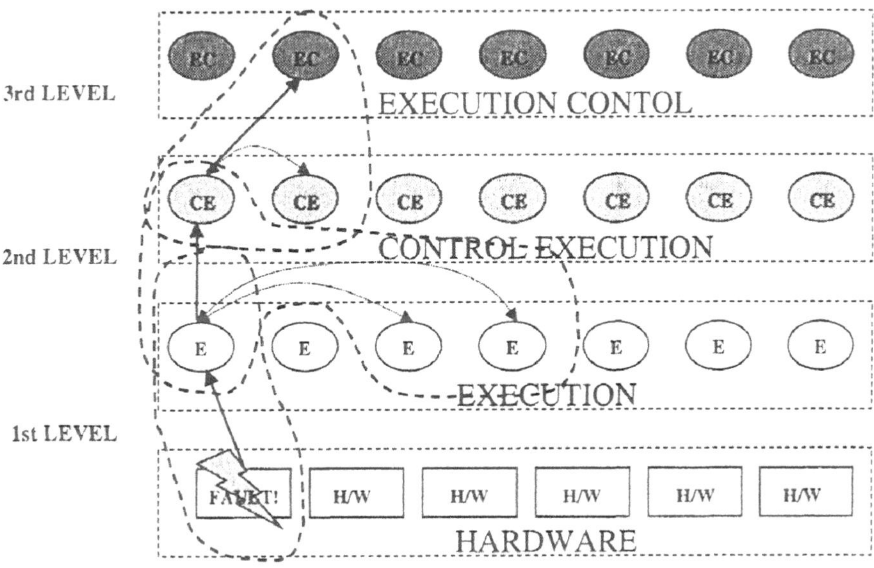

Figure 3 – Fault Monitoring and Recovery

Next, the CE level receives the fault information where the CE agents at this level first attempt more sophisticated means of recovery. For example, feedback error detection or feed-forward error detection may be used. In the first case, the fault is identified, but is not corrected. Instead, the sub-task (at the execution level) is redone or the hardware is placed in a fail-safe state. In the second case, the CE agents try to correct the error and continue processing. For example, "recovery" at this level may involve reconstruction of corrupt data. If the fault is unrecoverable however, the hardware would be placed in a fail-safe state and the CE agents would report to the execution control level.

Finally, at the EC level, more sophisticated techniques such as homogeneous or diverse redundancy may be used to recover from the fault. Of course, if this level is incapable of recovering (e.g., an operation cannot be done, so the batch will have to be rescheduled), higher levels may be consulted.

5. CONCLUSIONS

In this paper, we have provided a general overview of a layered architecture to manage the key requirements of distributed real-time control: i.e., (i) control application development, (ii) reconfiguration, and (iii) fault monitoring and recovery. At the most basic level, the architecture builds on the basic distinction between agents and holons: i.e., that a holon consist of a software part and a physical part. When considering the competing requirements of control application execution and system fault monitoring and recovery however, the architecture builds on the safety-critical systems' firewall concept. In other words, our layered architecture allows control channels (managed by a top-down task decomposition process) to be separated from safety channels (managed by a bottom-up fault monitoring and recovery process). Currently, we are working on a detailed approach to achieve dynamic and automatic reconfiguration of distributed real-time control systems (Zhang, 2001). Interestingly, we have found that the basic concepts from the general model reported in this paper are equally applicable to lower-level models. For example, in order to manage function block application reconfiguration, we have found that it is useful to also separate execution channels from "safety" channels. As a result, we represent function blocks using two flow paths: (i) an "execution control path" for control application management, and (ii) a "configuration control path" for configuration and reconfiguration control.

4. REFERENCES

1. Anderson, T, Lee, PA. Fault Tolerance Principles and Practice, Prentice Hall, 1981.
2. Brennan, RW, Fletcher, M, Norrie, DH. Reconfiguring real-time holonic manufacturing systems. Twelfth International Workshop on Database and Expert Systems Applications, IEEE Computer Society, pp. 611-615, 2001a.
3. Brennan, RW, Norrie, DH. Agents, holons and function blocks: distributed intelligent control in manufacturing. Journal of Applied Systems Studies Special Issue on Industrial Applications of Multi-Agent and Holonic Systems 2001b; 2(1): 1-19.
4. Douglass, B. Doing Hard Time: Developing Real-time Systems with UML, Objects, Frameworks, and Patterns, Addison-Wesley, 1999.
5. Holonic Manufacturing Systems Consortium, Website, http://hms.ifw.uni-hannover.de/, 2002.
6. IEC TC65/WG6, Voting Draft: Function Blocks for Industrial Process-Measurement and Control Systems, Part 1 Architecture, International Electrotechnical Commission, 2000.
7. Jalote, P. Fault Tolerance in Distributed Systems, Prentice Hall, 1998.
8. Leveson, N. Safeware, Addison-Wesley, 1995.
9. Lewis, R.Modelling Control Systems using IEC 61499: Applying Function Blocks to Distributed Systems, IEE, 2001.
10. Lewis, R. Programming Industrial Control Systems using IEC 1131-3, IEE, 1996.
11. Lyons, A. UML for real-time overview. Technical Report of ObjecTime Ltd, 1998.
12. Marik, V, Pechoucek, M. Holons and agents: recent developments and mutual impacts. Twelfth International Workshop on Database and Expert Systems Applications, IEEE Computer Society, 605-607, 2001.
13. Odell, J, Parunak, H, Bauer, B. Extending UML for agents. ERIM Center for Electronic Commerce, http://www.erim.org/~vparunak, 2000.
14. Siewiorek, DP, Wsarz, R. The Theory and Practice of Reliable System Design, Digital Press, 1982.
15. Wang, L, Brennan, RW, Balasubramanian, S, Norrie, DH. Realizing holonic control with function blocks. Integrated Computer-Aided Engineering 2001; 8(1): 81-93.
16. Zhang, X, Brennan, RW, Xu, Y, Norrie, DH. Runtime adaptability of a concurrent function block model for a real-time holonic controller. IEEE Systems, Man, and Cybernetics 2001. 164-168.

28

AN AGENT-BASED APPROACH TOWARDS THE DESIGN OF INDUSTRIAL HOLONIC CONTROL SYSTEMS

Boris Suessmann, Armando W. Colombo, Ralf Neubert
Schneider Electric, Automation Business, Development Central
Steinheimer Strasse 117, 63500 Seligenstadt, Germany
{boris.suessmann, armando.colombo, ralf.neubert}@modicon.com

After the description of the underlying principles on which the "multiagent-based production control" technology and the "holonic manufacturing control" concept within the intelligent manufacturing system paradigm are based, this work proposes an approach that supports the design of agent-based manufacturing control systems for different industrial holonic manufacturing scenarios. The results of the application to a pilot cell at industrial level are very promissory, showing that the approach seems to be very suited in accommodating heterogeneous hardware and software components in both their manufacturing control and information system, and in integrating existing/legacy systems.

1. INTRODUCTION

On one side, the recent production technologies reflect a world-wide trend towards both, batches of small and medium size, and product families of increased variety. Customers are more and more asking for personalised products. This tendency often comes in conflict with the demand on high productivity, i.e. on production-times/time-to-market minimisation and on simultaneous improvement of machine utilisation. For example, today's mass production systems like transfer lines in automotive-industry are suffering of poor capacity utilisation. Although the utilisation of individual machines can be as high as 98%, the overall utilisation of the factories is about 50 to 70%. This is due to the fact that there is typically only one linear line of production. So if somewhere at the shop floor a bottleneck exists, and every system has a bottleneck, the whole production line is influenced.

On the other side, current industrial control at the physical machine level is typically implemented using large, and often expensive, hardware platforms that support monolithic computer control applications. As a result, when the control system is installed, commissioning can take months to complete, and once the system is operational, changes are often complex and difficult. All these factors contribute significantly to the total cost of the industrial control project and of course, of the final product.

To redress this situation, new revolutionary manufacturing concepts and emerging manufacturing control technologies, which take advantage of the newest mechatronics, information and communication technologies and paradigms, are being researched and developed since the last decade of the 20th century (Tzafetas, 1997).

One promising structure, in this respect, is to have a conglomerate of distributed, autonomous, intelligent, fault-tolerant, and reusable manufacturing units, which operates as a set of co-operating entities. Each entity is capable to dynamically interact with each other to achieve both local and global manufacturing objectives, from the physical/machine control level on the shop floor to the higher levels of the factory management systems. This new generation of manufacturing systems is referenced as Intelligent Manufacturing Systems (IMS).

On one hand, several emerging concepts that advocate such structure have been reported in the literature (Tharumarajah et al., 1996). Holonic manufacturing (see (Hayashi, 1993) and the references therein) is an example of the new manufacturing paradigms. On the other hand, agent-based software systems are becoming a key control software technology for production control systems (Jennings, Wooldridge, 1998), (Parunak et al., 1998), (Shen, Norrie, 1999), (Colombo et al., 2001).

According to the practical experiences of the authors when working with agent-oriented production control technology in automotive-industry (Schoop et al., 2001), factors like the "time-to-market" can be decreased in a 10% order as a result of decreasing "start-up-time" and increasing "robustness" and "agility" of the system. Moreover, production systems that were developed for mass-production are capable, when they are agent-based managed and controlled, to accept prototype- and customer-oriented-production, without modifying their structure and without interrupting their normal production. An agent-controlled production system within a Holonic Manufacturing Systems framework provides rapid reactive and dynamic re-configurable manufacturing equipment to facilitate an agile, flexible and robust, management framework for the control over the system.

The so far available realisation experience and the scientific discoveries point out, that the further development requires a generic, systematic approach towards a common understanding of the technology versus the punctual developments of the past. The successful application of both, the "holonic manufacturing system" and the "agent-based manufacturing control system" technologies for making the Intelligent Manufacturing System at industrial level a reality necessitates new engineering methods, processes and tools. These must be on one hand as standardised as possible and on the other hand adapted to the conditions of the different production types and industrial scenarios.

In this paper the underlying principles on which the "physical agent" and "holonic" concepts are based are first described. After this description, the main specifications of an engineering methodology for the agentification of manufacturing systems, based on our last research results ((Colombo et al., 2001), (Schoop et al., 2001)), and in agreement with other studies ((Shen, Norrie, 1997), (Bohnenberger et al., 1998), (Parunak et al., 1998), (Bussmann, Schild, 2001), (Bussmann et al., 2001) and (Ritter et al., 2002)), are presented as a practical solution to the holonic manufacturing control paradigm.

This paper will show that this solution is compatible with other mechanisms and architectures for "Holonic Control" proposed recently, such as the "Holonic Control Device" presented in (Christensen, 2000) and/or "The Holonic Enterprise" proposed by M. Ulieru et al. in (http://www.fipa.org). The integration of our proposal and the above projects, although still in the early stages, is already in scope.

This paper is organised as follows: First, section 2 reviews the latest results in the field of agent-based industrial control design and presents issues relating to the synthesis of agent-based manufacturing control systems. Further this section shows a method of agentification. Section 3 details the main characteristics of the agentification method and a first analysis. Section 4 describes an extension to the existing method to remove the problems identified in section 0. Finally, section 5 rounds up the paper with conclusions and an overview of planned further developments related to the approach presented here.

2. AGENTIFICATION OF PRODUCTION SCENARIOS

This section discusses the integration of structural, functional and manufacturing management and control knowledge in agent-based industrial control system design. After an overview of reported results in the field, issues relating to the synthesis of agent-based manufacturing control systems (i.e., agentification of manufacturing scenarios) are presented.

As any other design activity, the design of agent-based manufacturing control systems consists of the creation and manipulation of objects, which are called here "production agents".

Agent system theories have been developed to innovating a number of control applications that are highly influenced by the exploding possibilities of new ICT-Systems. Today's most demanding operational areas for technical agents are:

- Telecommunications
- Data-mining
- Traffic control
- Distributed trade systems
- Management of huge heterogeneous information networks like the Internet

Unfortunately neither these agent systems nor the underlying theory can be used to design production agents, i.e., agent-based production systems. The main reasons are:

- Production agents are distributed physical agents while most of the current technology is dealing with software agents.
- Agent-systems in production are inhomogeneous multi-agent-systems while the so far realized applications are either homogenous or single agent systems.
- Production agents require a dynamic and controllable decision core to enable agile manufacturing system adaptation and (re)-configuration and support decision rule development.
- Production agents are self-reconfiguring; intelligent distributed automation elements that have to operate in a stochastic environment where hard real-time constraints must be met to achieve reliable system operation, while the software multi-agent-systems developed so far do not consider time as a problem at all.

These characteristics describe the transition from software agent-systems to Holonic Manufacturing Control Systems.

In any application domain, knowledge can be split between structural knowledge (about the objects and physical entities), functional knowledge (about how the objects behave and interact). This was the basic rationale underlying the structure-function paradigm proposed in (Cornelio et al., 1990). However, whenever the knowledge is used in a dynamic way for design purposes, a large gap, both practical and conceptual, exists between the structure-function specification and an implementation satisfying that specification as a constraint. Functionality represents complex behaviour whose achievement implies the realisation of suitable production control strategies. Many different control organisations compatible with the same high-level structural and functional specifications can be developed (Caselli et al., 1992).

These are the basic motivations leading to the proposal of an agent-based system-modelling paradigm oriented to the intelligent manufacturing domain, where proper consideration is given to management and control in the early modelling stages. The result is an engineering method, which supports a design synthesis of agent-based intelligent manufacturing scenarios, where physical, functional; and management and control specifications are integrated into an object called "production agent".

In Figure 1 an example of a production agent is shown, together with a picture of a flexible production cell, located at Schneider Electric Automation Business in Germany, which serves as pilot application of the approach outlined in this paper.

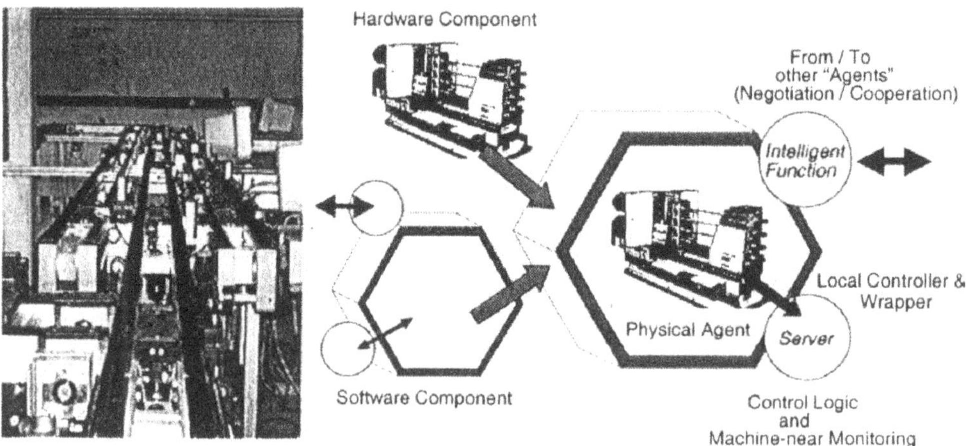

Figure 1 - Production agents and flexible production systems

In (Ritter et al., 2002), a method for identification of agents in a manufacturing system is described, which is mainly based on the following steps:

1. Identify all persistent manufacturing objects.
2. List all physical dependencies between the identified manufacturing objects.
3. List all logical dependencies between the identified manufacturing objects.
4. Aggregate all objects with physical dependencies into an object. (p-aggregation)
5. Aggregate all object with logical dependencies. (a-aggregation)

The resulting aggregates are the agents of the manufacturing system.

This method helps to find a suitable set of agents in the manufacturing system. As there are no dependencies between the agents, due to the method of aggregating object which depend on one another, there are also no deadlocks on the physical and logical level. We will call this method "IPA-method".

3. CASE STUDY

In the following is shown the application of the method proposed here, on a flexible manufacturing system. This case study is composed of both the pilot flexible production cell depicted in **Figure 1** (layout in **Figure 2**), and an existing agent-based production system for cylinder head manufacturing referenced in (Colombo et al., 2001). The system produces the end products (cylinder head) from the raw material with CNC machines. The CNC machines are all capable to execute different machining operations. A dispatcher assigns orders to raw workpieces mounted on pallets. The orders may define different machining resulting in different end products. Shift-tables shift pallets between conveyors to route them to their next destination. An unloader finally detaches the processed workpieces from the pallets and puts them into a storage.

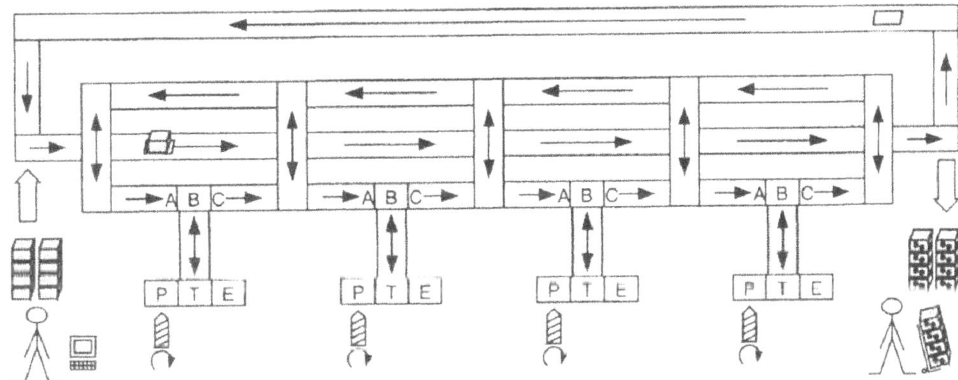

Figure 2 - Flexible manufacturing system

First, the manufacturing objects are identified (**Table 1**).

Table 1 - Manufacturing objects

Name	**Symbol**	**Manufacturing function**
Raw storage		Stores raw workpieces
Loader		Loads pallets with raw workpieces
Dispatcher		Generates orders for pallets
Conveyor belt		Transports pallets to shift-tables
Shift-table		Shifts pallets between conveyors
Loading conveyor	→A	Transports pallets to lifting place
Lifting place	B	Transports pallet to/from T-stem or passes pallets by
Unloading conveyor	B→	Transports pallets from lifting place
T-stem		Transports pallets to temporary place
Processing place	P	Holds pallets for processing
Temporary place	T	Moves pallets between T-stem, processing place, and exchange place
Exchange place	E	Holds pallets during exchange
CNC/Spindle		Processes workpiece (drilling, milling,...)
Unloader		Removes workpieces from pallets into exit storage
Exit storage		Stores processed workpieces

Next, the dependencies between the manufacturing objects are listed (**Table 2**). With these dependencies, the manufacturing objects are aggregated into agents. The main property of these agents is their independence from each other, by construction (see **Figure 3**).

Table 2 - Dependencies between manufacturing objects

Name	Physical dependency	Logical dependency
Raw storage	Loader	
Loader	Raw storage	Dispatcher
Dispatcher		
Conveyor belt		State of shift-table
Shift-table		
Loading conveyor		State of lifting place
Lifting place		
Unloading conveyor		State of lifting place
T-stem		State of lifting place, Temporary place
Temporary place		State of T-stem, processing place, exchange place
Exchange place		Temporary place
Processing place		Temporary place
CNC/Spindle		
Unloader		
Exit storage	Unloader	

Note: In this example the method aggregates all transporting objects into one huge transport agent. This is intended by the method. Give the transport agent a transport order for a given pallet and it cares for the transport.

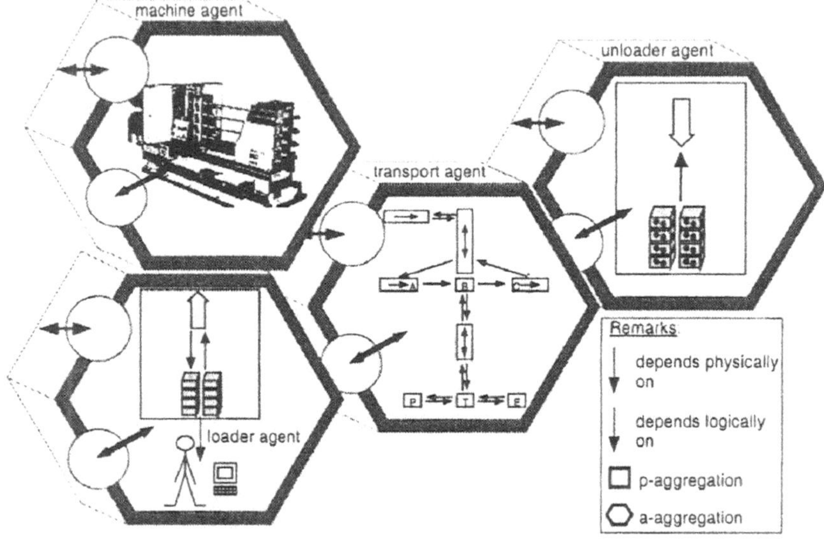

Figure 3 - Aggregation of manufacturing objects into agents

3.1 Analysis of the Method

The method identifies autonomous components. These components have to interact with each other to build the complete plant. The method does not handle the design of communication protocols for the identified agents. The result of the method is a flat agent community (**Figure 4** (a)).

As long as a physical or logical dependency is crossing physical boundaries, this flat agent community does not represent physical boundaries. This is an unwanted result, if you want to construct intelligent components for reuse. And it does not represent the reality, where you often have a hard unit of processing and loading and a soft unit of CNC- and PLC-programs. Another problem is the coarseness of the agent community. Flexible manufacturing systems depend on flexible transport systems. When there are dependencies between different modules of the transport system, the method will combine them all into one agent. With normal conveyor belt (or comparable) transport systems there are these dependencies resulting in one agent for the complete transport system. This makes the coding of the control logic difficult and error-prone. Also the extension of such a transport system is normally difficult. The agentified plant is not extendable by default.

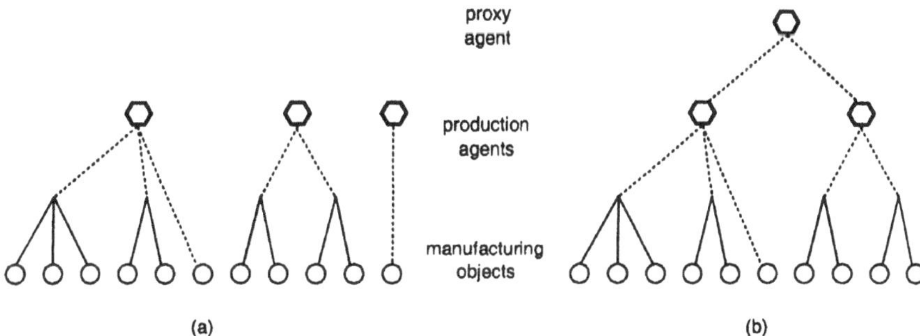

Figure 4- Flat versus hierarchical multi-agent system

In our case study this extension results in several transport agents. On top of these transport agents there is a facilitator. This facilitator is equivalent in functionality to the transport agent as identified in **Figure 3**.

4. SOLUTIONS TO THE IDENTIFIED PROBLEMS

To solve the problems identified in section 0, we suggest to extend the method with a degree of dependency based on identified physical boundaries. In the aggregation steps the degree of dependency defines which objects will be aggregated directly and which objects will be aggregated in the form of proxy agents. The degree of dependency leads to a hierarchy of agents. The top level multi agent system of the plant consists of the same agents as identified by the IPA-method, but some of these agents may only be proxies for lower level multi-agent system. These proxy agents are in this case study facilitators (Shen, Norrie, 1997).

5. CONCLUSION AND OUTLOOK

This work proposes an approach that supports the design of agent-based manufacturing control systems for different industrial holonic manufacturing scenarios. The first phase of such approach is related to the *"agentification"* of the production scenario when considering the definition of a "physical / production agent". The results of the application of the approach to a pilot cell at industrial level are very promissory, showing that the approach seems to be very suited in accommodating heterogeneous hardware and software components in both their manufacturing control and information system, and in integrating existing/legacy systems. Further work will be oriented to the study of different existing industrial scenarios and to test the possibility for their "agentification", i.e., the method for agentification will be further improved. We expect to find also mediating proxy agents with this method, and to extend the agentification path to other production resources like of workpieces and work-plans.

6. ACKNOWLEDGEMENTS

We would like to express our thanks to the colleagues of the Fraunhofer Institute for Manufacturing Engineering and Automation, Stuttgart, Germany, for their support during the realisation of this work.

7. REFERENCES

1. Bohnenberger T, Fischer K, Gerber C. "Agents in Manufacturing: Online Scheduling and Production Plant Configuration". In Proc. of 1st Int. Symposium on Agent Systems and Applications, 1998.
2. Bussmann S, Schild K. "An Agent-Based Approach to the Control of Flexible Production Systems". In Proc. of the 8th IEEE Conf. On Emerging Technologies and Factory Automation (ETFA'01), Sophia/Nice, France, 2001.
3. Bussmann S, Jennings NR, Wooldridge M. "On the identification of Agents in the Design of Production Control Systems". Agent-Oriented Software Engineering. Springer-Verlag, 2001.
4. Caselli S, Papaconstantinou C, Doty K, Navathe S. "A structure-function-control paradigm for knowledge-based modeling and design of manufacturing cells". Journal of Intelligent manufacturing, num. 3, pp. 11-30, 1992.
5. Christensen J. "Basic Principles of HMS Architecture". Proc. of the HMS'00 Int. Symposium, Kitakyushu, Japan, 2000.
6. Cornelio A, Navathe S. "Integration and cataloging of engineering design information". Proc. of the 1st Int. Conf. on Systems Integration, IEEE Press, 1990.
7. Colombo AW, Neubert R, Schoop R. "A Solution to Holonic Control Systems". Proc. of the 8th IEEE Conf. On Emerging Technologies and Factory Automation (ETFA'01), France, 2001.
8. Hayashi H. "The IMS International Collaborative Program". Proc. of the 24th ISIR, Japan Industrial Robot Association. 1993.
9. Jennings NR, Wooldridge MJ. "Applications of Intelligent Agents". Agent Technology: Foundations, Applications, and Markets, pp. 3-28. 1998.
10. Parunak VD, Baker A, Clark S. "The AARIA Agent Architecture: From Manufacturing Requirements to Agent-Based System Design". Working Notes of the Agent-Based Manufacturing Workshop, Minneapolis, MN. 1998.
11. Ritter A, Baum W, Höpf M, Westkämper E. "Agentification for Production Systems". To appear in Proc ETAPS'02, Grenoble, France, April 2002.
12. Schoop R, Neubert R, Colombo AW. "A Multiagent-based Distributed Control Platform for Industrial Flexible Production Systems". Proc. of the IEEE IECON'2001, Denver, USA, 2001.
13. Shen W, Norrie D. "Facilitators, Mediators and Autonomous Agents". Proc. of the 2nd Int. Workshop on CSCW in Design, Bangkok, Thailand, Nov. 1997, pp. 119-124.
14. Shen W, Norrie D. "Agent-Based Systems for Intelligent Manufacturing: A State-of-the-Art Survey". Int. Journal on Knowledge and Information Systems, 1(2), pp. 129-156. 1999.
15. Tharumarajah A, Wells AJ, Nemes L. "Comparison of the bionic, fractal and holonic manufacturing system concepts". Int. Journal Computer Integrated Manufacturing, vol. 9, num. 3, pp. 217-226.
16. Tzafestas S. "Modern Manufacturing Systems: An Information Technology Perspective". Advanced manufacturing Series – Computer-Assisted Management and Control of Manufacturing Systems. London. Springer Verlag. 1997.
17. http://www.fipa.org/docs/wps/f-wp-00009/f-wp-00009.html

29

A HOLONIC CONTROL APPROACH FOR DISTRIBUTED MANUFACTURING

Paulo Leitão[1], Francisco Restivo[2]

[1]*Polytechnic Institute of Bragança, Quinta Sta Apolónia, Apartado 134, 5301-857, pleitao@ipb.pt*

[2]*University of Porto, Rua Dr. Roberto Frias, 4200-465 Porto, fjr@fe.up.pt*

Manufacturing systems are complex and often chaotic environments, being collated with customer satisfaction, products shorter life cycle and new e-business trends, becoming the design of manufacturing control applications a complex and hard task. As the traditional control approaches present serious problems to handle simultaneously the distribution of functions, global production optimisation, reaction to disturbances and reconfiguration, it is necessary to introduce new approaches that support the new intelligent manufacturing control systems. The paper introduces an innovative holonic manufacturing control architecture to face some of these unsolved problems by supporting an increase of flexibility and an agile reaction to disturbances without compromising the global production optimisation, being regulated by a coordination mechanism that allow fast reaction and adaptation to disturbances.

1. INTRODUCTION

Nowadays, manufacturing systems are complex, concurrent, asynchronous and often chaotic environments. Customer satisfaction, products shorter life cycle and new e-business trends lead to mass customisation and to the need of agile adaptation to manufacturing volatility. The manufacturing systems must support production of several types of products, being capable to change quickly from one product to another, demanding the execution of set-up configuration in the machines. These characteristics require efficient planning and control systems to optimise the production process through the elaboration of optimised production plans. However, the occurrence of disturbances, both machine failures and manufacturing modifications, implies deviations from the original plans. The manufacturing control system should react quickly to the disturbances elaborating alternative plans in order to minimize the effects of the disturbance in the system and the propagation of the disturbance outside the local system neighbourhood.

To support the complexity of manufacturing environments, there is an important research effort to develop innovative manufacturing control systems that increase the production process efficiency and optimisation, and react quickly to the occurrence of disturbances, such as described in (Van Brussel *et al.*, 1998; Brennan *et al.*, 1997; Parunak *et al.*, 1998; Maturana and Norrie, 1996).

This paper intends to introduce an innovative holonic manufacturing control architecture that intends to support an increase of flexibility and agile reaction to disturbances without compromising the global production optimisation. The proposed architecture defines new concepts in manufacturing control systems, using a hybrid control structure and distributing the control and scheduling among several decision levels, being regulated by a coordination mechanism that allow fast reaction and adaptation to disturbances.

2. DISTURBANCE HANDLING PROBLEM

The occurrence of a disturbance can lead to a deviation from the initial and optimised plan and to productivity decrease due to the machine/system inactivity. In this case the system should respond dynamically and quickly to the disturbance, using appropriate mechanisms according to the type of disturbance.

The main types of disturbance are the manufacturing or work order cancel, the machine failure, the introduction of a new manufacturing order, and the layout re-configuration.

The manufacturing or work order cancellation comes from the need to abort the order due to the cancellation from the customer, a failure that provoked the destruction of the part, etc.. This disturbance causes a small impact in the system, because it is only necessary to release the operations already allocated and to re-schedule the other operations in order to optimise the local schedule. The modification of the work order attributes, such as the change of temporal window to produce, may lead to the need to re-schedule all the operations.

A machine failure can occur due a tool collision, a tool broken, mistake in the machine programme, etc, causing a temporary or longer out of service of the machine, becoming incapable to accomplish the allocated work orders. The objective is to recover quickly the machine and in parallel to find out alternative solutions that minimize the deviation from the initial plan.

The introduction of a new manufacturing order, usually with high priority, requires the interaction between the entities in the system in order to schedule all operations of the task. This type of disturbance is only a problem when it leads to temporal conflicts with already allocated work orders.

The layout re-configuration implies the re-organization of the manufacturing resources, like the addition of the new resource or the remotion of a resource. The addition of a resource causes small impact in the system, because it increases the alternative solutions for the execution of manufacturing order, solving in some cases some conflicts problems. On the other hand, the remotion of a resource, leads to a more complex problem, that can introduce conflicts in the system.

3. AGENT-BASED HOLONIC ARCHITECTURE FOR MANUFACTURING CONTROL

The capability of current control architectures to adapt with agility and quickly to internal disturbances and external environment changes is poor. Due to the rigidity of the control architectures, the changes on the behaviour of the control system have impact in different levels of the control architecture. As a consequence, the time spent with programming and debugging, in case of re-configuration, is high.

The manufacturing research community is faced with the need to develop new and innovative manufacturing control systems, which present more agility and flexibility, and higher robustness against disturbances. In ADACOR architecture (Leitão and Restivo, 2001) the authors propose a new holonic approach to manufacturing control, implemented on a set of autonomous, intelligent and co-operative holons, each one representing a manufacturing entity (Leitão and Restivo, 2002).

3.1 Internal Architecture of an ADACOR Holon

The architecture is based on a set of holons grouped in operational, supervisor, product and task holon classes. The operational holon represents the physical manufacturing devices, such as tool machines, robots and automated guided vehicles. The supervisor holon coordinates several operational and supervisor holons, introducing coordination features and global optimisation in the system. The product holon represents the product data, such as the product model and the process model, and is responsible for the process planning. The task holon controls the execution of a manufacturing order and contains the associated dynamic information.

The generic ADACOR holon comprises the physical resource, capable to perform manufacturing tasks (if applicable), and the Logical Control Device (LCD) implemented using agent technology (Leitão and Restivo, 2002). This logical part of the holon comprises a local knowledge base, decision component (DeC), communication component (ComC) and physical interface component (PIC), as represented in Figure 1.

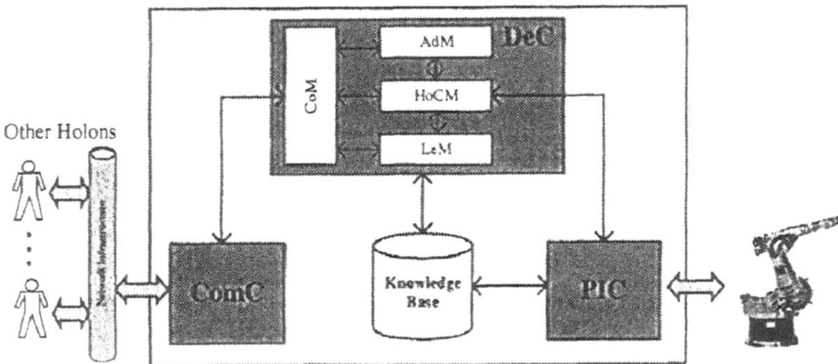

Figure 1 – Internal Architecture for an ADACOR Holon

The decision component, developed partially in a rule-based programming language, controls the activities of the holon and includes the holon control (HoCM), cooperation (CoM), adaptation (AdM) and learning (LeM) modules. The communication component deals with the interaction with other holons, making transparent the data exchange by using appropriate ontologies and the FIPA-ACL as communication language. The physical interface component comprises the mechanisms for the interaction with the physical devices that makes transparent the access to manufacturing resources. The local knowledge base stores all knowledge about the behaviour of the holon and the community where the holon belongs.

3.2 Distributed Control Concept

Aiming to achieve more flexible and agile features, the architecture proposes a distribution of the control by several decision-making levels, defining the local control, operational control and coordination control levels. The local controller level deals with the machine intrinsic control mechanisms and will not be described in this document.

3.2.1 Operational Control Level

Each operational holon in the architecture has abilities to perform local scheduling, dispatching, monitoring and reaction to disturbances functionalities.

The local scheduling module uses a scheduling engine and the local knowledge to implement the scheduling of the operations allocated to the holon. This module supports the optimised local schedule, the short term scheduling (when accepting the supervisor holon advices) and the agile reaction to disturbances. The local scheduling mechanism is a plug-in mechanism developed for the single machine scheduling problem, that uses a set of basic scheduling heuristics, such as EDD (Earliest Due Date) and SPT (Shortest Processing Time).

3.2.2 Coordination Control Level

The coordination control level introduces coordination in the control process, using the supervisor concept from bionic manufacturing systems. The coordinator entities are responsible for the global production optimisation, and are represented by supervisor holons. These supervisor holons, which can represent a manufacturing cell or a shop factory, have also a scheduling engine that deals with the multiple machines scheduling problem.

The optimised scheduling, elaborated at the coordination level, can be done in two different ways: task allocation process at supervision level or centralised scheduling. In the first approach, the supervisor holon launches several task allocation processes for the lower level, announcing the operations, and coordinates the negotiations in order to achieve the optimised schedule. In the second approach a centralised scheduling is executed by the supervisor holon using one algorithm for multiple machines problem.

The schedule elaborated by this holon eventually takes more time to achieve than the schedule obtained by each operational holon, but is optimised. The schedule elaborated is passed to the operational holons, in its coordination domain, as an advice.

3.2.3 Distributed Scheduling

There are scenarios where the control application can run without the presence of coordination levels, for example in heterarchical architecture or when there is a failure in the supervisor holon. The architecture defines a distributed and dynamic scheduling mechanism, Figure 2, which uses a multi-round Contract Net protocol

(Smith, 1980) with some extensions, such as supporting multiple iterations and bid partial quantities.

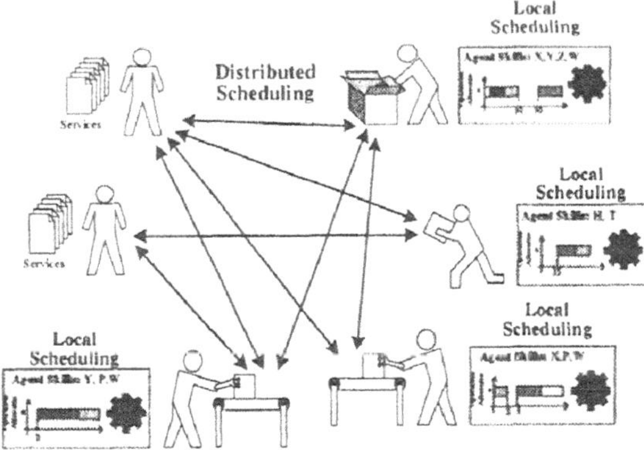

Figure 2 – Distributed and Local Scheduling

In this approach each operational holon has a local scheduling engine and is responsible for its own schedule, build from the local knowledge and goals. Operational holons verify the ability to execute the operation and find out their capacity to fulfil the operation due date before they submit their proposals. The global scheduling is achieved by the interaction between operational and task holons.

4. THE ADAPTIVE CONTROL APPROACH CONCEPT

The architecture allows different control approaches, such as hierarchical, federation and heterarchical, but in order to optimise the reaction to disturbances and the agility to unexpected events without compromising the global optimisation, it is necessary to evolve to a new control approach that combines those requirements.

The proposed control approach is based in holonic concepts, splitting the control into alternative states: steady state and transient state. In this holonic control approach the holons are organised in a federation structure and each holon has its own goals (the supervisor holons have the goal to achieve optimised schedule plans and operational holons the goal to optimise locally its behaviour) and evolves based in an autonomy degree, which is a dynamic factor that allows an operational holon to follow or not the advices sent by the supervisor holons.

4.1 Steady State

In the steady state, the supervisor holons that represent cells and/or the shop floor, have coordination functions through the elaboration of optimised schedule plans for the supervisor and/or operational holons in its coordination domain. The task holons interact with the supervisor holons, which will interact with other supervisor and operational holons, hierarchically in lower level, in order to allocate the manufacturing orders.

The supervisor holon elaborates optimised schedule for its coordinated resources, and dispatches it to the operational and supervisor holon that have enough autonomy to accept or reject the proposed schedule. If the operational holon rejects one or more proposed operations, the supervisor holon should re-schedule the production plan, trying to find alternatives, considering the previous rejection. If the operational holons accept the proposed operations, they are actualized in its local agenda.

4.2 Transient State

The need to react rapidly to a disturbance that requires the update to the original plans may not be satisfied by the steady state. In this case the system re-organise itself for a short period of time, with each operational holon adjusting its autonomy factor, applying a general mechanism that comprises three important steps.

Initially, the operational holon tries to recover locally the failure, increasing slightly the autonomy factor and re-scheduling its operations, in order to minimize the deviation to the original plan. In case of success, the operational holon reduces again the autonomy factor and the disturbance is recovered. If the operational holon cannot recover from the failure or it cannot fulfil the due date of an operation, the operational holon increases the autonomy factor, according with the type of disturbance, and disseminates the need for a re-organisation into a heterarchical organisational structure to other holons. In parallel the operational holon re-schedule the operations, interacting with the task holons if necessary to notify the disturbance.

After the recovery of disturbance the operational holon should synchronize its schedule with the optimised schedule, notifying the supervisor holon about the new schedule, and reducing again its autonomy factor. Since the autonomy factor is reduced the dissemination of disturbance is finished and the other holons doesn't sense anymore the occurrence of disturbance, reducing as well its autonomy factor, returning the system to the previous structure (hierarchical or federated form).

4.3 Autonomy Degree Mechanism

The autonomy degree of an operational agent evolves dynamically in order to adapt its behaviour to the external environment context. At moment, fuzzy logic and neural networks are being considered for the implementation of the autonomy factor mechanism.

In the stationary state, aiming the global production optimisation, the autonomy degree is low, allowing the operational agent to follow the schedule advices sent by the supervisor agents. The occurrence of a disturbance leads to an increase of the autonomy degree, decreasing the weight of the scheduling advices, in order to try to recover locally and quickly the disturbance.

The coordination between the holons, to perform the re-organisation to support disturbances, is performed using pheromone-like mechanisms. Thus, the need for re-organisation is disseminated to other supervisor holons, through the propagation and deposit of the pheromone to the neighbourhood supervisor holons, as represented in Figure 3. The holons associated to each supervisor holon perceive the need for re-organisation by sensing the pheromone, and increases its autonomy factor according with the type of disturbance, leading to an heterarchical organisation.

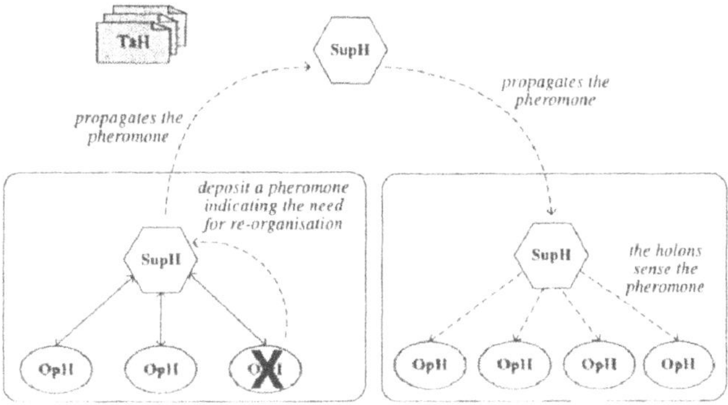

Figure 3 – Dissemination of a Disturbance

After the disturbance recovers, that should take short time, the autonomy degree decreases again in order to allow the operational holon to follow again the advices of the supervisor holons. Since the autonomy factor is reduced the dissemination of disturbance is finished and the other holons doesn't sense anymore the occurrence of disturbance, reducing as well its autonomy factor, returning the system to the previous structure.

The main advantage to use ant-based mechanisms to disseminate the need for re-organisation is to reduce the interaction level and communication overhead between the holons, improving the reaction to the re-organisation.

5. COMPARISON WITH OTHER APPROACHES

As referred before, other approaches for manufacturing control systems, such as PROSA architecture (Van Brussel, 1998), focus the agile reaction to disturbances. At this stage it is important to analyse some similarities and differences between the proposed architecture and the PROSA architecture.

PROSA is a reference architecture for manufacturing control and the ADACOR approach focus mainly in the distributed manufacturing shop floor control for job shop production type, with special attention to the agile reaction to disturbances, considering the set-up, maintenance and transportation operations.

In spite of both approaches have similar holon classes, the role of the holon responsible to introduce hierarchy is different in two approaches. The supervisor holon, used in ADACOR, coordinates several operational and/or supervisor holons, and implements the scheduling and control functions, representing manufacturing cell controllers or shop floor controllers. As the ADACOR approach supports federated control architectures, the supervisor holon coordinate the interactions between holons located in its coordination domain. In PROSA these functions are distributed by several staff holons, which doesn't have a specific role for cell controller. Additionally, in ADACOR approach the holons have learning capabilities in order to improve the performance of each holon during its life-cycle.

Both approaches use the holonic concepts to introduce more agility and flexibility in the reaction to disturbances maintaining the same levels of production optimisation. The solution adopted by both approaches is to introduce hierarchy in decentralised systems, and the dynamic re-configuration of the system. PROSA uses fixed rules and flexible strategies to change the control architecture supported by a meta-controller that define the basic re-configuration rules, while the ADACOR uses the autonomy degree mechanism associated to each operational holon to evolve between control architectures complemented by a pheromone-like mechanism to disseminate the need for the re-configuration.

6. CONCLUSIONS

The traditional manufacturing control systems have low capacity to adapt and react to the dynamic changes of its environment and to machine failures. The new generation of manufacturing control systems should comprise the high adaptation and reaction to the occurrence of disturbances and the optimisation of the global performance of the system, which require a global view of entire system.

This paper introduces an innovative holonic manufacturing control approach that intends to support an agile reaction to disturbances without compromising the production global optimisation and fulfilling the real time constraints.

The proposed approach to manufacturing control presents the following benefits: reconfiguration, flexibility, expansibility and fault tolerance. The reconfiguration capability is increased because the control approach allows a quick and agile reconfiguration to face the changes in production system strategy. The flexibility is increased due to the autonomy of the system entities and to the ability to support different organisational structures. In the ADACOR approach each component can be develop gradually and added to the system without stop or re-initialise the system, making easier the expansibility task. The reaction to disturbances is increased, because each holon is responsible for the execution of its tasks and for the recovery of the failures occurred in the resource that represents, minimizing the effects and propagation of the failure.

7. REFERENCES

1. Brennan R., Balasubramanian S. and Norrie D. A dynamic control architecture for metamorphic control of advanced manufacturing systems. In the Proceedings of the International Symposium on Intelligent Systems and Advanced Manufacturing, ed. by B. Gopaladrishnan, S. Murugesan, O. Struger, and G. Zeichen, 1997, pp. 213-223.
2. Leitão P. and Restivo F. Agent-based Holonic Production Control. To appear in Proceedings of 3rd International Workshop on Industrial Applications of Holonic and Multi-Agent Systems (HoloMAS), 2-6 September, Aix en Provence, France.
3. Leitão P. and Restivo F. An Agile and Cooperative Architecture for Distributed Manufacturing Systems. In Proceedings of IASTED Robotics and Manufacturing International Conference. Cancun, Mexico, 21-24 May, 2001, Cancun, Mexico, pp 188-193.
4. Maturana, F. and Norrie D. Multi-Agent Mediator Architecture for Distributed Manufacturing, Journal of Intelligent Manufacturing, Vol. 7, 1996, pp. 257-270.
5. Parunak, H. Van Dyke, Baker A. and Clark S. The AARIA agent architecture: from manufacturing requirements to agent-based system design, Workshop on Agent-based Manufacturing, ICAA'98, 1998, Minneapolis.
6. Smith R.G. The Contract Net Protocol: High-Level Communication and Control in a Distributed Solver. In IEEE Transactions on Computers, Vol. C-29, N°12, 1980, pp 1104-1113.
7. Van Brussel, H., Wyns J., Valckenaers P., Bongaerts L. and Peeters P. Reference Architecture for Holonic Manufacturing Systems: PROSA, Computers In Industry, vol. 37, 1998, pp. 255-274

30

DESIGN ISSUES IN HOLONIC INVENTORY MANAGEMENT AND MATERIAL HANDLING SYSTEMS

Martyn Fletcher
Agent Oriented Software Ltd, Mill Lane,Cambridge, CB2 1RX, United Kingdom,
martyn.fletcher@agent-software.co.uk

Vladimír Mařík
Department of Cybernetics, Czech Technical University in Prague, Czech Republic & Rockwell Automation Research Center, Americka 22, 120 00 Prague, Czech Republic,
marik@labe.felk.cvut.cz

Pavel Vrba
Rockwell Automation Research Center, Americka 22, 120 00 Prague, Czech Republic
pvrba@ra.rockwell.com

Holonic manufacturing systems (HMS) represent a novel paradigm for addressing the problems encountered by 21st Century engineering businesses. These next generations of decentralised AI-based shop-floor control systems are geared towards: (i) high-variety low-volume manufacturing, (ii) placing these customer-specific products into the market with short order-to-delivery times, and (iii) providing a fast return on investment. The paper presents a model of a Holonic Inventory Management System (HIMS) linked with an agent-based material handling within an agile manufacturing environment.

1. INTRODUCTION

Holonic manufacturing systems (HMS) represent a novel paradigm to address some critical problems faced by manufacturing businesses as they come to grips with the 21st Century market. Yet, the application of HMS principles places a severe strain on how inventories of raw materials, work-in-progress and finished goods are to be managed within the frame of a vision of a holonic factory. This is particularly so when there is demand for mass customization. This topic has not received much attention in the HMS community, but it needs addressing if businesses are to buy into the holonic vision and deploy holonic technologies in their factories.

Centralized solutions to controlling inventory, within the scope of such agile environments, do not work since they are slow to react, impose operational bottlenecks and are a critical point of failure. Holonics is a decentralized 'bottom up' approach and provides principles to ensure a higher echelon of responsiveness and handling of system complexity. The fundamental building blocks of a HMS are called *holons* to reflect the fact that these entities: (i) are both parts and wholes (Koestler, 1967), and (ii) behave simultaneously in an autonomous and cooperative fashion (Suda, 1989). Holonics is not just a new technology, but rather it is a system-wide philosophy for developing, configuring, running and managing the next generation of manufacturing business where flexibility is the paramount (Marik, *et al.*, 2002). Here we focus on the flexibility needed by the inventory management system inside a HMS and how holons can support these requirements. We propose that a holonic inventory management system (HIMS) can be characterized by several types of newly introduced holons:

- *Pick-and-Place robot holons* will distribute picking and placing tasks evenly amongst themselves, will select optimal routes to navigate along and will load different types of goods into the same collection bin attached to the robot (e.g. with the heaviest items at the bottom).
- Each item of stock being regarded as an independent *workpiece holon*. Thus it can play an active and intelligent role in getting itself manufactured on time, stored in the correct manner and so forth.
- *Shelf holons* will advertise how best their storage services can be used.

We also assume that there are the necessary *resource holons* to provide transformation, transportation and validation services (Van Brussel, *et al.*, 1999), as well as *order/product holons* to represent orders into the factory and provide knowledge on how these orders can be processed (Wang, 2001) (Xu, *et al.*, 1999). We get such holonic inventory management systems to work in the real world through investigating a number of design issues. The context for this pragmatic investigation is that a physical environment is provided by a variety of factories with different attributes. For example, the multi-cell holonic demonstrator (Chirn and McFarlane, 2000) being developed at the University of Cambridge's Institute for Manufacturing provides a machining and assembly environment. Meanwhile the lumber mill scenario of (Kotak, *et al.*, 2001) requires flexible storage for wood products during disassembly. Furthermore the automobile scenario of (Bussmann and Sieverding, 2001) has an agile engine assembly line where partially-complete engines must be stored while rush orders move through the line, or while assembly and inspection stations are busy/broken. Each of these, and other HMS test case environments need inventory management to varying extents. What is more, these physical environments are to be controlled using distributed artificial intelligence and so need a holonic solution to inventory management and material handling.

2. DESIGN CHALLENGES FOR A HOLONIC INVENTORY MANAGEMENT SYSTEM

A Holonic Inventory Management System (HIMS) is going to play a critical role in the next generation of holonic manufacturing systems because all of these systems demand flexibility to hold finished goods, work-in-progress (WIP), raw materials and any hybrid mixture in a unified fashion. Owing to space limitations in factories and the cost of installing the dedicated warehousing, an agile model for storing and retrieving goods is essential for smoothing out any peaks and troughs in demand.

This is especially so when dealing with assembly because some sub-ordinate workpieces must be held in the warehouse until all the constituent parts are available ready for aggregation. When the foundation for modelling, the decentralised control system needed to manage this warehouse is intelligent software agent-based holons then the solution is a HIMS. The key facets of a HIMS are illustrated in Figure 1.

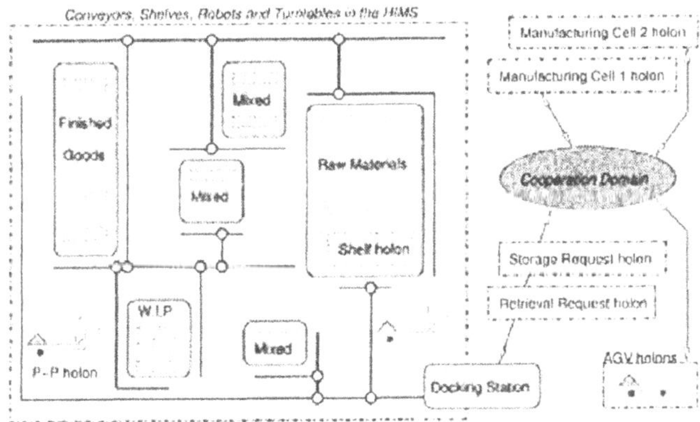

Figure 1 – Scope of a Holonic Inventory Management System

As can be seen in Figure 1, the HIMS interacts with the various manufacturing cell holons and groups of Automated Guided Vehicle (AGV) holons in order to collect, store, retrieve and deliver necessary inventory in a timely manner. These interactions take the form of structured negotiations and take place through a logical structure known in the HMS terminology as a *cooperation domain*. The gateway between the HIMS and the rest of the factory is one or more docking stations, at which AGVs may load and unload physical inventory.

The creation of a sequence of steps in which AGVs dispose of and collect goods is a classic scheduling problem. Therefore it is NP-hard when there are more than one AGV or when there are more than one docking station. This is another reason for adopting a holonic solution to the load/unload problem as holons have the facilities to deliberate, cooperate and act proactively in order to determine a feasible, if not optimal, strategy for sequencing and timing the arrival/departure of such AGVs. Within the confines of the HIMS, Pick-and-Place (P-P) robots move around the warehouse environment to: (i) transport recently-received inventory from the docking station and put it onto shelves; and (ii) take requested goods off the appropriate shelves and transfer them to the docking station for subsequent collection by an AGV. There are several routes that a Pick-and-Place robot can take from the docking station(s) to the appropriate shelf, and vice versa. Furthermore, the robot can collect and place several pieces of inventory on a single tour around the warehouse. For example it may visit shelf s12 to collect workpiece w4, then collect w8 from s32, deposit w90 onto s54, and then return to one of the docking stations. Hence we have a travelling salesman problem where the robot must visit a set of shelves and try to establish the least cost routes between subsequent shelves in order to minimise the overall journey time. Moreover, as conveyors break down, stock is moved by human personnel (also working in the warehouse environment) and the journey times between any two shelves may change over time.

Our solution is based on automatic identification (AutoID) technology (http://www.autoid.org) where an independent agent represents each workpiece and each shelf is a holon equipped with a tag reader. Each of the Pick-and-Place robots has four degrees of freedom: up/down, left/right, in/out of shelves, and between independent shelves within the WIP, mixed, finished goods or raw materials areas (see Figure 2). When gathering goods, these robots select one physical workpiece at a time and deposit it into their collection bins while ensuring that the biggest or heaviest items are loaded at the bottom of the bin and lighter/smaller items at the top. When depositing items into the shelves, the robot (in conjunction with other holons) selects the optimal slot into which the workpiece can be inserted, based on some heuristic algorithm with a view towards achieving global coherence.

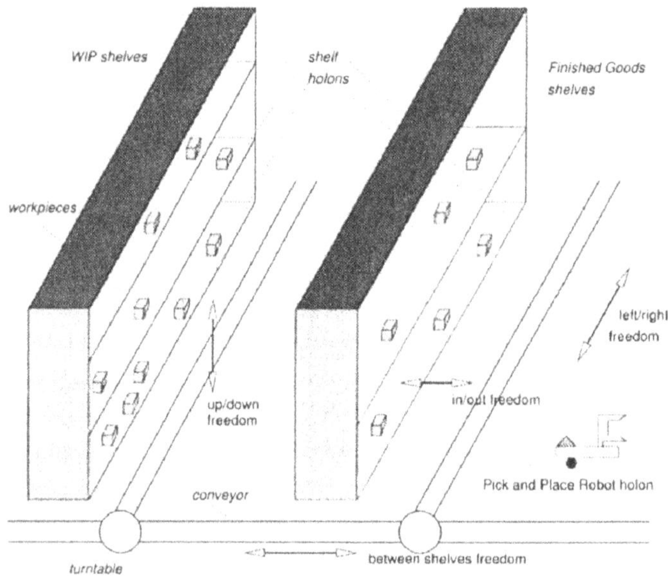

Figure 2 – Degrees of Freedom for the Pick-and-Place Robot Holons

A fundamental design issue in such a HIMS (with its associated decentralised control) is how to ensure global coherence when individual agent-based holons are acting to maximise their own, possibly mutually conflicting, goals. In the context of this mini-factory, coherence can be viewed as minimising any disadvantages of distribution, and would be measured in terms of performance. In other words, a coherent HIMS is one that behaves (from an external viewpoint) with a performance equal to that displayed by a centralised system capable of performing all the inventory management tasks needed. Hence the integration of *pathfinder holons* to act as expert systems on planning the travelling salesman circuit can contribute to such coherence (Jarvis, *et al.*, 2001). Moreover, they can be easily incorporated within the architecture proposed for the physical holonic demonstrators since the routes and item picking/placing sequences offered by these holons are recommendations that the Pick-and-Place robot holons can either accept or reject.

In this bottom-up or emerging behaviour approach, no central controller exists and the individual holons (with the aid of their agent-based decision-making software) act in an autonomous fashion in such a way that the behaviour of the entire HIMS emerges. This approach is similar to the way in which ant colonies operate with many (say 10,000) ants each searching for food in their environment.

There is no global commander (not even the queen ant) and every ant has very limited intelligence, in fact their can only obey a limited set of simple rules and communicate with each other using pheromones. Yet, from a global perspective, they appear to operate in both unison and smartly. The key problem with this purely bottom-up approach is that the behaviour that the ants, or the Pick-and-Place robot holons, workpiece holons, shelf holons and so forth in our HIMS, will produce cannot be predicted prior to execution, and neither can it be controlled in a top-down manner during execution, as there is only a limited hierarchical command structure. Therefore a compromise is demanded. Our solution is that:

- *A pathfinder holon* is put in charge of ensuring that the circuit that the robot will travel is as close to optimal as possible.
- The responsibility for ensuring all the workpiece insertions and removals required to store the factory's stock are handled by the corresponding *storage request holon* and *retrieval request holon*.
- Actual movement of physical items is governed in a distributed manner between the one or more Pick-and-Place holons, the workpiece holon, the multiple shelf holons and the product holon.

Therefore a *holarchy* is generated to best assign work amongst the holons of a particular class (e.g. allocating a storage job among the candidate shelves). This assignment is founded on various agent-based protocols like the classic 4-step contract net protocol, English or Dutch auctions, or market economy approaches.

3. HOLONIC INVENTORY MANAGEMENT SYSTEM

This section addresses one of the critical design issues for realising a holonic inventory management system regarding the storage and retrieval of workpieces. Decisions on where and when workpieces are to be stored/retrieved from the shelves is under the joint control of several distributed holons in the form of a *holarchy*. The holon types involved in the negotiations include: the retrieval/storage request holon, the Pick-and-Place robot holon, the workpiece holon, the team of resource holons (each representing an independent shelf), the pathfinder holon to help in selecting the optimal route the robot should take, and the product holon with its knowledge on how workpieces should be held in the warehouse. Cooperation domains are used to aid the holons in their negotiations. These concepts are illustrated in Figure 3. To insert an item into the HIMS (a storage request), the subsequent protocol is used:

1. The manufacturing cell holon that needs to store a workpiece w1 issues a request to the cooperation domain (see Figure 1). This request fully specifies what w1's characteristics are, how w1 is to be retained on the shelves, and what is its expected times of arrival/departure to/from the HIMS.
2. A new storage request holon is created to manage the transfer of the item and its subsequent storage. The storage request holon acts as an interface between the main holonic factory and the HIMS.
3. The storage request holon creates a new cooperation domain to orchestrate these management activities (see Figure 3) and so a new holarchy of HIMS holons will be generated.

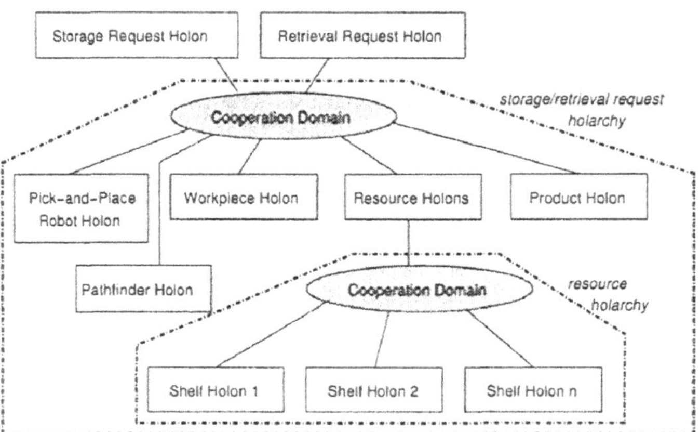

Figure 3 – Creating a Holarchy for a Storage or Retrieval Request.

4. A storage request is issued into the cooperation domain (where all of the available HIMS holons can receive information). This request contains the specification data provided by step 1.
5. A suitable product holon, of the same class as the workpiece being stored, joins the cooperation domain and provides knowledge about the types of shelves that can hold the workpiece.
6. The available shelf holons respond to the request indicating whether the workpiece can be stored (while satisfying the specified retention criteria given by the product holon) and what time it should be delivered to the docking station. They also inform the workpiece holon of how it is to be stored.
7. The storage request holon is told how much 'electronic money' that this storage will cost to hold the workpiece holon for the specified duration.
8. A resource holarchy is generated to find the appropriate shelf where the workpiece can be held. A market economy is used to support this pricing and to get the suitable shelf holons (sellers) to offer their storage capacity to the storage requester holon (acting as buyer) so that the workpiece will be assigned to the shelf holon offering retention at the lowest cost.
9. If the manufacturing cell holon and the storage request holon find this proposal satisfactory then a classic contract net protocol is established to get the workpiece to the docking station:
    a. A subsequent cooperation domain is created in order to arrange for an AGV to transport the said item to the docking station for arrival at the prescribed time.
    b. The storage requester holon invites bids from the AGV holons to perform the transport.
    c. AGV holons respond giving their bids in terms of collection time, availability and cost.
    d. The storage requester holon selects the best bid and awards a contract to the selected AGV.
10. The transport from the docking station to the correct shelf via a Pick-and-Place robot holon also must be arranged. Optimally, the workpiece should be

unloaded onto the docking station and loaded onto the robot with a minimal delay (i.e. the workpiece holon's objective) while balancing against the robot's objective (not being idle at the docking station waiting for the item to arrive).

11. The circuit around the shelves that the robot will adopt is created by the pathfinder holon based on the requests for storing and retrieving items, together with the times and sizes of these items. The robot will put larger heavier items at the bottom of its bin. The knowledge about how to perform such stacking is provided by the product holon. This problem is complex and is made even more complicated by the changes in workpiece delivery schedules and so forth.
12. When the workpiece arrives at the docking station, the attached AutoID tag is read and the physical item is either loaded into the waiting Pick-and-Place robot' collection bin, or is held at the docking station for a limited period until the robot arrives.
13. The robot then moves through its route so that it arrives at the assigned shelf with the workpiece easily available from its collection bin (i.e. at the top or close to it). The robot then takes the item out and places it onto the shelf.
14. As the physical workpiece is entering the shelf, the reader attached to the shelf reads the tag for the item's number. The shelf holon confirms that this item should be stored here and informs the workpiece holon, through the connected factory (wireless) network, that the corresponding physical item has been successfully deposited.
15. This concludes the storage activity and so the various holarchies, cooperation domains as well as the storage request holon are destroyed.

To remove an item from the HIMS (i.e. a retrieval request), a similar protocol is used. Yet in this case, a retrieval request holon is in charge of acquiring the desired workpiece from the shelves. Therefore a cooperation domain is established by either: (i) the workpiece holon (if it knows its deadline for being manufactured is quickly approaching); or (ii) by the manufacturing cell holon (if it will require the workpiece, say for assembly with another item, at some time in the near future).

4. AGENT-BASED MATERIAL HANDLING SYSTEM

This section provides a brief description of the ideas behind the multi-agent material handling system developed at the Rockwell Automation Research Center Prague. The attention is paid mainly to the transportation of workpieces among different manufacturing cells using AGVs. The first design of the agent-based FIPA (Foundation for Physical Intelligent Agents) compliant solution of the material handling problem, namely of the transportation of workpieces through the factory using conveyor belts can be found in (Vrba, Hrdonka, 2001). The basic material handling components such as a work-cell, conveyor belt, diverter/intersection and workpiece were identified and appropriate FIPA-compliant agents were developed. The behaviour of these agents was aimed at solving the discrete transportation task, i.e. the delivery of a particular workpiece from the source to the destination work-cell using conveyors. To accomplish such behaviour, the FIPA-compliant messages for inter-agent communication as well as an appropriate knowledge ontology providing agents with relevant semantics of messages were proposed.

The main stress was put on the dynamic reconfiguration capabilities, i.e. to be able to safely react to the failures of components. We call it *light-weight* reconfiguration – if a holon detects a failure of its physical device (e.g. conveyor stops for some reason), it sends a message to the other agents that a failure has happened. They update their routing knowledge and find other optimal routes throughout the factory avoiding the broken component. A kind of *heavy-weight* reconfiguration was considered as well to allow the physical restructuring of the system. It includes the removal of any component from and/or the integration of new components into the system at runtime without the need to stop the system. To demonstrate the functionality of this solution and to show the benefits of the agent technology in particular, the simulation tool was developed in the JAVA language using two open-source agent development toolkits, FIPA-OS and JADE.

Recently, the proposed multi-agent solution was extended to integrate another transport component – the AGV. As shown in Figure 4 we suggest that the AGVs follow a network of tracks (we call it *AGV path*) located on the factory's floor (a very usual approach used today). The AGV path comprises of the so-called *AGV sections* connecting *AGV nodes*, where a node can be either the *work-cell*, or the *junction* (a node where two or more AGV sections are joint) or a simple *curve*.

Unlike diverters or conveyor belts, the specification of the AGV agent and its behaviour seems to be much more complex task. The AGV must be able to find shortest routes through the AGV path, must be able to negotiate with the work-cells about the delivery and be capable of avoiding collisions with other AGVs. To accomplish all of these requirements we decided to equip the AGV with the complex knowledge about its environment.

First, the AGV is provided with the precise knowledge (ontology) regarding the AGV path it follows. When the AGV agent is created it is given the XML description of the path specifying where the AGV nodes are located (x, y coordinates), what is their type (work-cell, junction, curve) and how these nodes are interconnected via the AGV sections. The AGV translates this description into an appropriate object model and consequently performs a searching algorithm to find all the possible routes to work-cells from each junction node. A *home section* is specified for each AGV – when the AGV has completed the delivery task and/or it has currently nothing to do, it returns to its home section and waits there idle. When integrated with a HIMS, the home section might be an appropriate docking station.

Second, while the AGV moves it has to be aware of other AGVs to predict and avoid possible collisions. On one hand, a collision in the area around a junction node can occur as two or more AGVs try to enter it simultaneously (each of it from different section). On the other hand there can be a collision called *head-to-head deadlock* when the AGV wants to enter some section in a particular junction, but there already is another AGV moving in this section heading to the same junction

To solve the former type of collision, we had to introduce a special agent for each junction node responsible for the scheduling of the AGVs' movement in the area around the junction. When some AGV is about to enter such an area it sends a message to the *junction agent* asking whether the area is free or not. If the area is free, the node agent gives the AGV a permission to enter the node whilst locking the area for this AGV for appropriate time period (after this period the lock is automatically released). No other AGVs are allowed to enter the junction within this period – they have to wait until the area is made free.

Solving head-to-head deadlocks is an even more complicated issue. When the AGV approaches a junction node it chooses one of the sections connected to this junction which should be used next to get to the AGV's intended destination. But a collision can happen in this section if there already is another AGV moving in the opposite direction. To predict such a situation the AGV should know in advance, if the section is free or not. To accomplish it, two different approaches can be used. Each AGV holds the information about where all the other AGVs currently are (and in which directions they move). This information is updated via messages sent by each AGV to all others when it leaves a section for another one. The disadvantage of this approach we are using now could be a huge amount of messages with the increasing number of AGVs. To reduce the communication traffic we plan to extend the abilities of the junction agents by applying the 3bA acquaintance models for organising and maintaining social knowledge (Marik, *et al.*, 2001).

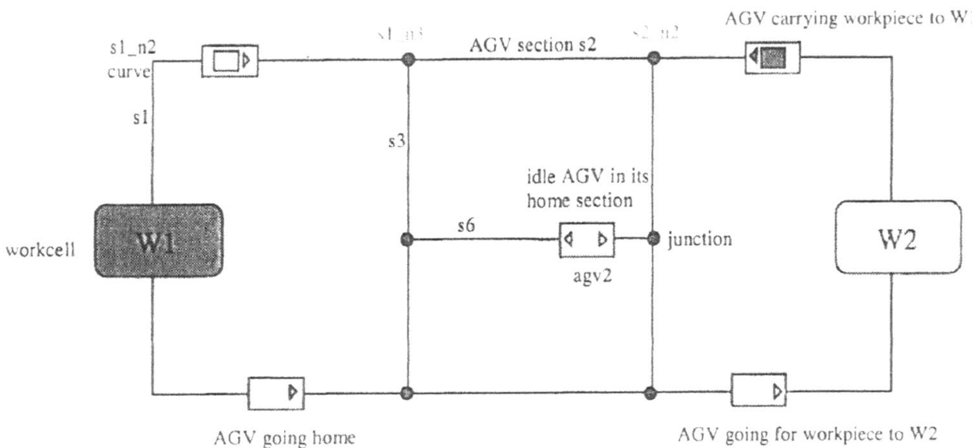

Figure 4 – Material handling using AGVs.

If there is a colliding AGV (lets say A2) in the section where A1 wants to continue, A1 sends a <deadlock?> message to A2. If A2 plans to continue towards the section, occupied by A1, it replies <deadlock!> saying that there is a head-to-head deadlock, otherwise replies with <noDeadlock>. In both these cases, A2 adds an estimate of the time period in which it will take to reach the junction node. A1 then decides, whether it is better to choose another section with respect to the time period it will have to wait until the colliding AGV reaches the junction. If it decides to wait and there is really a deadlock, the AGV moves to another (third) section (if available) where it stops and waits until A2 enters the freed section.

According to ideas presented in §3 for the workpiece delivery purposes the contract-net-protocol negotiation is used (see step 9 of the protocol mentioned in the section 3). Let us note, that the behaviour of pick-and place robots can be easily described using the same patterns as in the case of AGVs presented in this section. Each group of shelves depicted in Figure 2 can be treated as a single source or destination work-cell. The only extension needed is to define a communication scenario determining which shelf (i.e. additional *up-down* movement) and what position on this shelf (*left-right* movement) that must be reached in order to store/retrieve the workpiece correctly.

5. CONCLUSIONS

The paper presents a new (holonic) approach to inventory management as an extension of the holonic visions into the area, which is usually out of the main stream of attention of the holonic research. Here each item of inventory, every shelf and every Pick-and-Place robot is treated as a holon. The other decentralised holons (i.e. the pathfinder holons, storage request and retrieval request holons) considered here are rather software (information) agents as they are not directly connected with any physical transportation/storage hardware. They are expected to "live" just temporarily, for the period needed to accomplish the given storage/retrieval mission.

Overall the proposed approach works well with a high degree of agility (especially with respect to stock movement planning) and is more reactive to environmental changes than existing approaches. Future work will focus on the implementation of this HIMS model with each holon modelled as an autonomous agent, and holon actions/interactions represented using well-established *belief-desire-intention* and *coalition-formation* ideas. Moreover we intend to deploy our generic model into a physical environments and conduct experiments to prove our hypothesis that holonic inventory management is needed to support the flexibility required by 21st Century manufacturing businesses.

6. REFERENCES

1. Bussmann S, Sieverding J. Holonic Control of an Engine Assembly Plant: An Industrial Evaluation. In Proceedings of the IEEE International Conference on Systems, Man and Cybernetics, 2001.
2. Chirn JL, McFarlane DC. Building Holonic Systems in Today's Factories: A Migration Strategy. . Journal of Applied System Studies, special issue on Holonic and Multi-Agent Systems, **2**(1), 2000.
3. Jarvis D, Jarvis J, Lucas A, Ronnquist R, McFarlane DC. Implementing a Multi-Agent Systems Approach to Collaborative Autonomous Manufacturing Operations. In Proceedings of IEEE International Conference on Systems, Man and Cybernetics, 2001.
4. Koestler A. The Ghost in the Machine. Arkana, 1967.
5. Kotak DB, Fleetwood M, Tamoto H, Gruver WA. Operational Scheduling for Rough Mills Using a Virtual Manufacturing Environment. In Proceedings of IEEE Int. Conf. on SMC, 2001.
6. Marik V., Fletcher M., Pechoucek M.: Holons & Agents: Recent Developments and Mutual Impacts. In: Multi-Agent Systems and Applications II. LNAI No. 2322, Springer Verlag, Heidelberg, 2002
7. Marik V, Stepankova O, Pechoucek M. Social Knowledge in Multi-Agent Systems. *Multi-Agent Systems and Applications.* LNAI No. 2086, Springer Verlag, 2001
8. Suda H. Future Factory System. In Japan. Journ. of Advanced Automation Technology, vol. 1, 1989.
9. Van Brussel H, Bongaerts L, Wyns J, Valckenaers P, Van Ginderachter T. A Conceptual Framework for Holonic Manufacturing: Identification of Manufacturing Holons. Journal of Manufacturing Systems, **18**(1), 1999.
10. Vrba P, Hrdonka V. Material Handling Problem: FIPA Compliant Agent Implementation. In Proceedings of the Twelfth International Workshop on Distributed and Expert Systems Applications DEXA, 635-639, 2001.
11. Wang L. Integrated Design-to-Control Approach for Holonic Manufacturing Systems. Journal of Robotics and Computer Integrated Manufacturing, vol. 17, 2001.
12. Xu Y, Brennan RW, Zhang X, Norrie DH. A Genetic Algorithm-based Approach to Holon Virtual Clustering. Technical report of the Mechanical and Manufacturing Engineering Department, University of Calgary, Canada, 1999.

31

AGENT-BASED, DISTRIBUTED DIAGNOSIS FOR SHIPBOARD SYSTEMS

Gregory Provan, Yi-Liang Chen
Rockwell Scientific Company,1049 Camino dos Rios, Thousand Oaks, CA 91320, USA
{gprovan,ylchen}@rwsc.com

The ability to reconfigure a ship's engineering plant in response to changing mission or equipment conditions can dramatically increase a ship's capability and survivability. We describe the agent-based, distributed diagnostic aspects of a distributed control architecture that integrates multiple ship systems and provides resource- and diagnostic-driven reconfiguration at multiple system levels, such as mission-level, process-level and component-level. We embed system- and sub-system models in distributed, agent-based components to provide distributed diagnostics. We demonstrate this architecture using a shipboard chilled water system application.

1. INTRODUCTION

Improving the fight-through capability of future combat ships necessitates an integrated ship control system that can monitor all shipboard engineering assets and adaptively reconfigure these assets during battle conditions. For example, if a chilled water supply unit is damaged during combat, a ship control system may temporarily overload another chiller to provide the required cooling capacity or shed non-combat heat loads to reduce cooling requirements. If the chilled water system still cannot satisfy combat cooling demand, the ship control system may allow certain combat systems to moderately overheat or selectively reduce the performance of combat systems (e.g., reduce gun firing rate) to avoid complete system shutdown. To achieve such intelligent ship responses, all the various shipboard subsystems (e.g., chilled water system, fire-main, propulsion, generator, combat system, etc.) must be tied together under an integrated control hardware and software architecture. To maximize fault/damage tolerance, the integrated ship control system must also be a physically distributed architecture with intelligent autonomous behavior embedded in low-level system components.

We use an agent-based approach to guarantee global system properties, such as mission achievement, while distributing inference for fault-tolerance and sub-system autonomy. To this end, we have developed a hierarchical, distributed software architecture based on agent technology. Agents are self-contained software entities capable of communicating and making individual decisions (6). They work autonomously, handle goals, maintain beliefs, and cooperate through negotiation to create solutions.

An agent's decision logic is usually implemented using rule-based reasoning similar to an expert system. Rule-based reasoning has two main drawbacks: (1) difficulty of ensuring the completeness of the rule set for handling all situations, and (2) difficulty of maintaining the rule set when the controlled system expands or changes. To overcome these drawbacks, we use a model-based framework for the agents' decision logic. A model not only captures an expert's knowledge, but is a rigorous description of how a system works based on first principles. Given a model, model-based diagnostics algorithms can guarantee soundness and completeness of all diagnoses generated (1).

We embed within each agent system and sub-system models to provide diagnostics and assist in system reconfiguration when problems are detected. In the following sections, we describe the autonomous cooperative agent and model-based reasoning methodology, and the integration of these two methodologies within a distributed, reconfigurable control architecture. We use a chilled water system as a demonstration test-bed of this agent-based architecture.

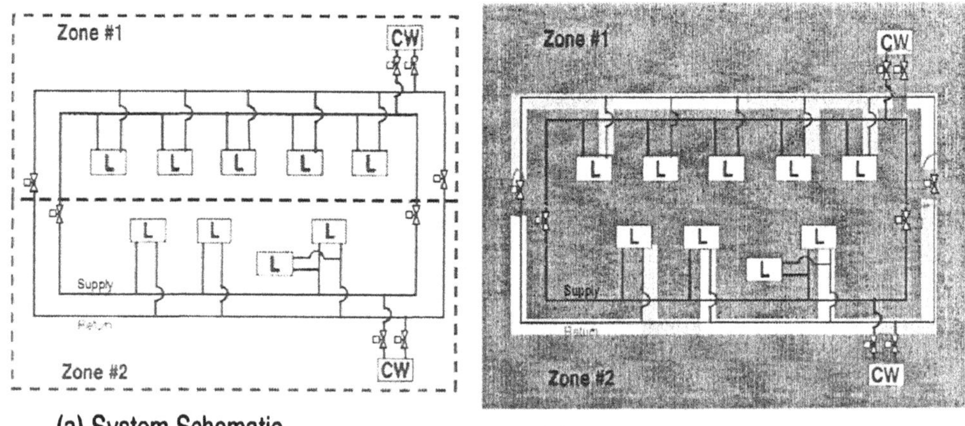

Figure 1: *Figure (a) shows a simplified diagram of chilled water system test bed. L = Load, CW = Chilled Water Production Unit. Individual valves for each load are not shown. Figure (b) shows how we partition regions of the system into functional units. The partitioning of segments of the return piping system are shown .*

2. CHILLED-WATER SYSTEM APPLICATION DOMAIN

In this article we apply our agent-based diagnostics architecture to a chilled water system testbed. This system provides multiple types of services across two physical zones, and contains redundant pumps and valves to allow for control reconfiguration in case of equipment failure. Figure 1(a) shows a highly simplified diagram of the chilled water system. The heat loads (marked by "L") are divided into three types: non-vital, vital, and combat system heat exchanger. The non-vital loads have a single path for supply water and a single path for return water; the vital loads have a single supply path and dual (redundant) return paths, the combat system heat exchangers (critical loads) have either a single or dual supply paths and dual return paths. The loads are also located in two different physical zones. The key objectives of control reconfiguration are to segregate the zones, shut down low-priority services in combat conditions, and to manage the loads upon detection of a chiller machine failure.

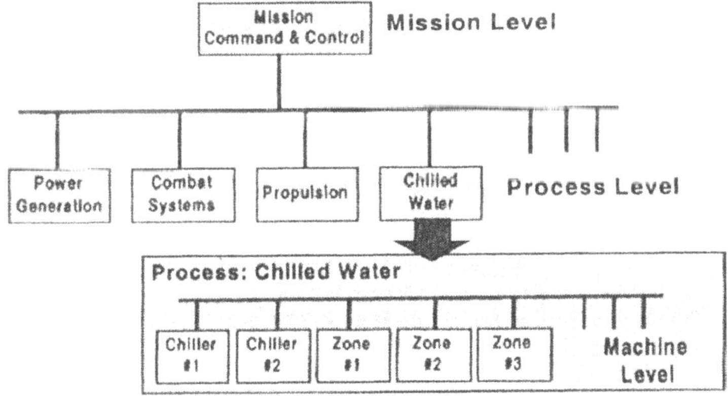

Figure 2: Control system hierarchy is composed of three levels.

2. DISTRIBUTED AGENT FRAMEWORK

We break our architecture into three levels, based on the functional requirements and control techniques which must be employed at each level. These levels are:

1. Mission Level – This is the highest level in the control architecture; the mission-level controller sets priorities and performance objectives for all ship engineering systems based on the overall mission goals. For example, in a damage control situation, resources would be shifted from less critical services, such as drinking water production, to fire-fighting systems. Similarly, control and use of the ship's resources for the various system functions can be optimized for dockside, normal steaming, battle stations, and damage control conditions. Inference at this level typically consists of tradeoff analysis of system requirements and optimization of mission-level parameters, such as overall fuel usage.
2. Process Level – Each process-level controller provides a general ship service (e.g., chilled water service, propulsion service, etc.), and will reconfigure its system operation based on the performance objectives set by the higher level (i.e., mission-level) controller. For example, the chilled water service may temporarily overload a water chiller unit when it senses another unit is down, in order to maintain the cooling rate objective set by the mission-level controller. This will result in optimized machine and energy use, and automatic reconfiguration of resources to maintain service availability in the event of faults or damage. Inference at this level typically consists of optimization of process-level parameters, together with discrete-event control.

3. Machine Level – Controllers at this level monitor and control individual machine units (e.g., a chiller) to maintain machine availability and achieve the machine setpoints requested by the process-level controller. For example, if excessive motor vibration at a pump is detected, the machine-level controller may alter the motor speed to avoid exciting a critical frequency and thus avoid damage. Inference at this level typically consists of optimization of process-level parameters, together with discrete-event and/or continuous control.

In the agent-based control system, each agent (called an Autonomous Cooperative Unit, or ACU) represents a physical process or equipment and coordinates its operation with other agents. Control actions are the result of coordinated decisions among all ACUs.

Figure 3 shows the control software architecture, composed of a collection of mission-level ACU, process-level ACUs, and machine-level ACUs. Each ACU at each level receives performance goals from a higher level ACU, and uses its internal model (whether it be a mission-level, process-level, or machine-level model) to diagnose problems and achieve the desired performance goal.

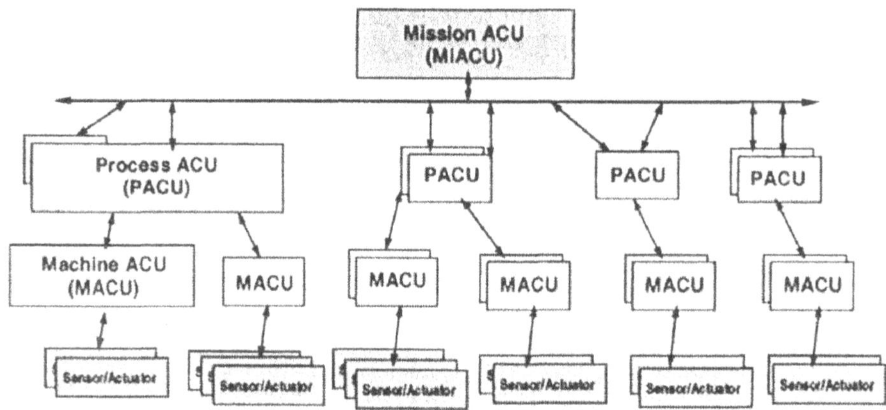

Figure 3: Hierarchical software architecture showing three ACU levels, corresponding to Mission, Process and Machine. The machine level ACU interacts with sensors and actuators.

When a requested performance goal cannot be achieved, ACUs initiate distributed problem solving actions to find alternative solutions that best meet the system's goals. The technique is comprised of 2 steps. The first step consists of discovering the physical relationships among Machine ACUs. The second step involves developing feasible plans that satisfy both local and shared constraints.

Machine ACUs contain models that provide self-awareness and self-assessment capabilities. The interaction of Machine ACUs is founded on the creation and dissolution of *virtual control clusters.* Within these clusters, Machine ACUs negotiate to obtain the near-optimal solutions, while considering both local and system conditions. The sequence of communication is as follows: Machine ACUs provide Process ACU with a number of solutions to be prioritized according to goals and constraints. Process ACUs use local (process) goals to select the best settings. In the same way, when a process-level goal cannot be achieved, Process ACUs also negotiate and provide the Mission ACU with a number of possible solutions.

Cooperative software agents permit the creation of highly flexible control systems based on both autonomy and cooperation. The ACU framework is well suited for solving resource allocation problems on distributed hardware. The resultant software is easily scalable to large systems. When a new machine is added to a system, the overall software is updated simply by adding a corresponding agent to represent the new machine. Autonomous capability is directly designed into an agent so that it can continue to operate in the event of failures in the other agents.

To ensure generality of our approach, we have developed a Job Description Language, called JDL (5), for inter-agent communication. This language enables agents to communicate for all activities using a single, unified framework.

3. DISTRIBUTED MODEL-BASED DIAGNOSTICS

This section summarizes our distributed framework for model-based diagnostics that can generate a distributed system model, and then integrate the diagnostics computed by each distributed component into a globally sound and complete system-level diagnosis (4). We first show how we create a distributed model, and then how we use agents to integrate the distributed diagnoses into a system-level diagnosis.

3.1 Distributed Model-Based Diagnosis

A model-based diagnosis approach works as follows. The algorithm uses the system model to simulate sensor values, and compare these with the actual sensor readings. If there is a discrepancy, the diagnostic engine is invoked to determine the most likely cause of this discrepancy.

We have extended the same causal-network diagnostics approach such that it can be used for both diagnostics and for assisting control reconfiguration (3). For diagnostics, the actual sensor values are propagated through the causal-network model to determine the faulty component and the operational mode(s) that would produce the abnormal sensor values. Conversely, for system reconfiguration, the desired machine or process output values are propagated through the causal network to determine the equipment settings necessary to achieve the desired output (subject to the constraint that certain components are unavailable or are in failure mode). When multiple diagnostic solutions or reconfiguration solutions are found in the model, the best solution can be determined by evaluating probabilities or costs associated with the various component modes or settings.

Our distributed diagnosis technique transforms a centralized model into a distributed model, and then synthesizes the minimal diagnoses computed by the distributed components into a global minimal diagnosis using formally sound principles. We use the topology, both functional and physical, of the system to partition the model into distributed components. For example, for the shipboard chilled-water system shown in **Figure 1**, we can create components for the major subsystems (e.g., chillers and loads) and piping segments (according to the physical connectivity of pipes).

For each distributed component, we also record the entities that are inputs and outputs. For our chilled water application, for each distributed component we have water (with properties like temperature, pressure and flow) as the inputs and outputs. In addition, each component may have control entities, which include requirements placed *on* the component, e.g., a chiller being required to provide x units of chilled water, or requirements placed *by* a component, e.g., a load requesting y units of chilled water. For this chilled-water application, we decompose the system into a set of functional units, as shown in **Figure 1**(b). A functional unit is defined to be a load, valve, chiller, and pipe segment; we then assign an agent to each unit.

Unlike previous approaches, which compute diagnoses using the system observations and a centralized system description (1; 2), we use a distributed approach. We build a causal network model for the high-level component interactions. A causal-network model consists of interconnected component models in which each component has various operational modes; for example, a valve component may have the following operational modes: normal, stuck open, and stuck closed. An input/output behavior is defined for each mode of the component. For example, if a valve is in normal mode, then the output pressure is equal to the input supply pressure when the valve is open.

We assume that each component can compute a local minimal diagnosis based only on sensors internal to that component and knowledge only of the component system description; note that we place no restriction on the technique used to compute that local diagnosis, e.g., neural network, Bayesian network, etc. Given a set of least-cost or most-likely local diagnoses, we can compute a globally sound, complete and minimal diagnosis for the complete system (4). The algorithm uses a graph-based message-passing algorithm that passes diagnoses as messages and synthesizes local diagnoses into a globally minimal diagnosis. We employ agents to handle the message-passing and diagnostic synthesis. By compiling diagnoses for collections of components (as determined by the system topology), we can significantly improve the performance of distributed embedded systems.

3.2 Agent-Based Diagnostic Synthesis

This section outlines how the agents facilitate the diagnostic synthesis process. Figure 4 shows the internal functions within an ACU. The ACU entity consists of three main components: a data table, middleware, and a set of application components. The data table contains input/output data for sensing/controlling the devices attached to the control hardware as well as data for the embedded applications. The middleware supports the agent services, enabling inter-agent communication across networked hardware. The application components are:

1. *equipment simulator* (Equip. Sim), which simulates the behavior of the associated machine or process;
2. *diagnostics engine* (Diag), which computes the fault status of the associated machine or process;
3. *coordinator* (Coord), which computes optimal control reconfiguration plans whenever a fault condition arises or system goals change;
4. *execution control* module (Exe. Ctrl), which controls the attached devices and can execute the reconfiguration control plans.

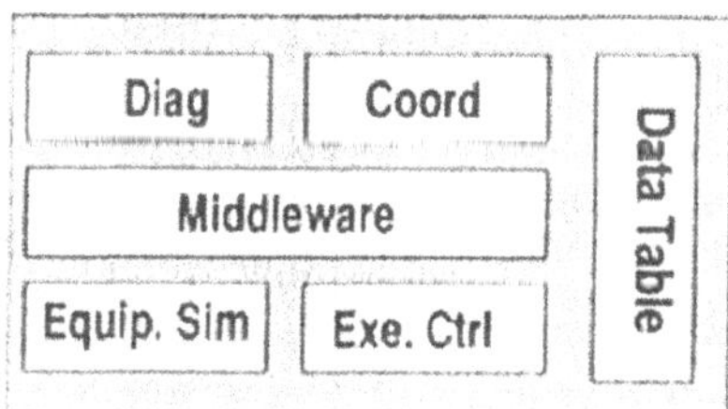

Figure 4: Internal functions within an ACU

The equipment simulator and diagnostic engine are both implemented using a causal-network model. The equipment simulator takes equipment settings (or commands) as input, and simulates the machine or process behavior with all components assumed healthy. The equipment simulator thus computes the values of the expected sensor readings by propagating the equipment setting values through the model. These simulated values are stored in the data table, and compared with the actual sensor values retrieved by the agents (and also put into the data table). If there is a discrepancy between the simulated and actual sensor values, the agent invokes the diagnostic engine to update the local machine's health state. Given any local fault, the agents communicate appropriate health status data, and then invoke the diagnosis synthesis algorithm to generate a global system health status. Finally, if a fault prevents the mission from being achieved, the agents invoke the control reconfiguration algorithm to reconfigure the system controls, and then the Execution Control module (via agent messaging) modifies the equipment control settings.

4. DISTRIBUTED DIAGNOSIS OF A CHILLED-WATER SYSTEM

ACU Type	Number	Description
Non-Vital Load	2	Provides low priority cooling that is shut off during combat mode.
Vital Load	9	Provides high priority cooling that needs to be maintained under any operation mode.
Combat Sys. Heat Exchanger	4	Provides high priority cooling during combat mode.
Chilled Water Producer	2	Provides cooling capacity.
Water Transport Pipe	1	Provides water transport path under open and segregated zone conditions.
Chilled Water Service	1	Oversees the chilled water process.
Zone	2	Oversees the areas within a zone.

Table 1: Agent types for chilled-water testbed

We have developed parameterized component models for pump, motor, pipe, valve, chiller, and heat load. We also identified 7 types of ACU associated with the chilled water test-bed; these ACU types are listed in Table 1 along with the number of ACUs required for controlling the simplified chilled water system.

For this testbed, we can use this agent-based framework to demonstrate the diagnostics and control reconfiguration capabilities for several scenarios, such as:

1. *Mode changes*: moving from one system mode to another, such as from cruise to battle mode, requires readjustment of chilled water supply due to differences in chilled-water demands, and to differences in system segregation between the different modes.
2. *Faults*: we can simulate the incidence of a fault in the system, such as the failure of a chiller unit, or a pipe fault (blockage or leakage). In such fault scenarios, the fault is first identified by a distributed agent, which then must consult with other agents to compute a global diagnosis.
3. *Control Reconfiguration*: Given a global diagnosis, the agents then must reconfigure the control settings in order to see if the goals (both local goals and chilled-water system goals) can still me met. The coordinator module of each distributed entity then executes the control reconfiguration.

5. SUMMARY

We have described an architecture for using agents to compute diagnoses and reconfigure control for a distributed system. Our approach uses a novel agent language, called a Job Description Language, for the agent interactions, and a novel model-based diagnostics technique for distributing diagnostics models and computing system-level diagnoses. We have applied this approach to a chilled-water test-bed, and have shown how our approach can handle a variety of mode changes and faults within the test-bed.

6. REFERENCES

1. A. Darwiche Model-based diagnosis using structured system descriptions. *J. of AI Research*, 8:165- 222, June 1998.

2. J. de Kleer and B. Williams. Diagnosis with Behavioral Modes. In *Proceedings of the International Joint Conference on Artificial Intelligence*, pages 1324—1330, August 1989. Morgan-Kaufmann Publishers.

3. Provan, G. and Y.-L. Chen, "Model-Based Diagnosis and Control Reconfiguration for Discrete Event Systems: An Integrated Approach," Proc. 38th IEEE Conf. on Decision and Control, pp. 1762-1768, December 1999.

4. G. Provan. A Model-based Framework for Distributed Embedded Diagnostics. In *Proc. Conf. on Principles of Knowledge Representation*, Toulouse, France April 2002.

5. Tichý P., Šlechta P., Maturana F., and Balasubramanian S.: *Industrial MAS for Planning and Control*. In: Multi-Agent Systems and Applications II, LNAI 2322, Springer Verlag, Heidelberg, 2002, pp. 280-295.

6. Wooldridge, M. and N.R., Jennings, "Intelligent Agents: Theory and Practice," *Knowledge Engineering Review*, 10(2), 115-152, 1995.

32

SERVICE-ORIENTED CONCEPT OF A HOLONIC ENTERPRISE - ENABLING ADAPTIVE NETWORKS ALONG THE VALUE CHAIN

Georg Weichhart, Alexander Hämmerle, Kurt Fessl
PROFACTOR Produktionsforschungs GmbH, Wehrgrabengasse 1-5, A-4400 Steyr
{Georg.Weichhart | Alexander.Haemmerle | Kurt.Fessl}@Profactor.at

In this paper we are discussing a holonic architecture for a management and control software, supporting users within enterprises and networks of enterprises in their co-ordination tasks. Holons are extended with functionality identified by intelligent software agent and multi agent systems research. This improves communication capabilities, flexibility, and the overall system robustness. Furthermore we discuss the need for a service oriented approach, which enables us to let the same agent kernel, which is handling mainly co-ordination and communication, be applied to hierarchy levels ranging from the virtual-enterprise-level to the shop-floor level.

1. INTRODUCTION

"Recently the manufacturing industry is facing a continuous change from a supplier's market to a customer's market" (Bussmann 1999). Customers are asking for complex and personalized products. The first demand adds to the complexity, that the production machinery needs to handle. This wouldn't be too much of a problem, if the second wouldn't imply that the batch size is decreased to one in the worst case. Therefore the time to set-up a new product version has to be reduced towards zero, at almost no cost. "These effects can be summarized as increasing complexity and continuous change at no cost" (Bussmann 1999).

1.1 Alternate Approaches

Traditional control and management approaches are optimistic. A plan is created, where each unit follows the optimal way through the system. There is one implied precondition: Everything is working correct.

Even if only a small degree of complexity is reached, but there is only one way through the system, it can been proven that it is almost impossible to guarantee a working system:

If two or more independent systems have to be used one after the other, the probability that the whole system functions can be calculated by multiplying the sub-systems probability to function (P(A and B) = P(A) · P(B)). For the following calculations we assume to need a 99% probability of the whole system working:

Table 1 – Needed availability of subsystems

Number of subsystems	Necessary probability of subsystem to work has to be at least
2	0,9949874371
20	0,9994976094
200	0,9999497496

The conclusion is that the probability of a malfunction of the whole system gets higher the more subsystems are involved. To fight this problem redundancy has to be introduced. Since there is more than one possible way through the system, the probability of success is higher. Redundancy allows flexibility, but increases complexity. Scheduling and Planing is getting harder because of a increased number of possible solutions and interdependencies.

To fight this complexity, different groups have conducted research on decentralized systems (see for example Weiss 1999, Walsh 1998, Tönshoff et. al. 2000 and research on Multi Agent Systems in general). In these approaches independent systems have knowledge about their local subsystem. To reach a solution that satisfies all participating sub-systems' local optimization function, intense communication has to be conducted. With decentralized approaches in general it can not always be guaranteed that a common satisfactory point can be reached. Additionally the amount of communication is high compared to centralized approaches.

Centralized systems introduce other problems. A scale-up of such a system often leads to an overload of the central unit, where most of the decisions are made. Flexibility and robustness are additional problems with centralized approaches.

We therefore use a holonic approach to balance the advantages of those two approaches (see also for different domains Ulieru et. al. 2001, Fischer 1999, Bongaerts et. al. 2000).

1.2 Holonic and Software Agents

Our view of a Holon is that it is a Software Agent, embedded in a recursively designed Multi-Agent-System. All the attributes identified by (Wooldridge and Jennings 1995) and (Nwana 1996), for example, will be implemented by our holons (see also Gerber and Russ 2001), by a varying extend, dependent on the system level, which the individual holon is part of.

Since holonic architectures are typically designed to work on the shop floor, on lower holarchy levels the holons will degenerate to simple agents, having less autonomy, but focus on reactiveness. The problems tackled by holons interfacing hardware are simple enough to allow a more centralized but time efficient control.

The higher the level the holon is located within the holarchy, the more intelligence is necessary to make decisions. For example the time frame considered is increased, or the number of system variables that have to be considered for a decision is higher. The tasks to be done, and the problems tackled on theses levels are complex, but on the other side do not have real time constraints as hard as on hardware close levels. It shall be possible to integrate a holon in a multi agent system where it won't be distinguishable from any other intelligent agent.

2. THE ARCHITECTURE

2.1 The Constructs (Objects) Used

Our Software-Architecture is based on two constructs:
- the Resource-Holon and
- the Service-Object.

Resources are necessary to apply services to a (intermediate-) product according to some plan. This application of services generates additional value. Two types of resources are identified. On the one hand machines, persons and the like, that are actively applying services to products. On the other hand electrical power, cooling water, construction material and sub- products like tires consumed by the product and after being applied might not be disunited from the product without damaging it.

A service describes the process of a resource to apply some material or energy consuming operation that in the long term adds value, which in turn is sold to the world outside by finally selling the product (i.e. the enterprise gains profit).

2.2 The Holons

2.2.1 General

Basic resource holons encapsulate a piece of hardware or an external system. These holons join to form a super ordinate system (e.g. machines form a shop floor).

We refer to this system as super holon. When considering this super ordinate holon we label the building blocks sub holons. Each level, but the lowest and the highest, is formed by holons that are sub-holons when considering higher level holons, but are super-holons for lower level holons.

We do not assume anything about the internal architecture of a basic holon. A basic holon in our words is a holon, that does not consist of sub-holons.

Several super-holons formed by basic holons will join again to reach a common goal. The recursive architecture leads to a holarchy, where holons are formed over several levels.

The formation may happen dynamically and temporary. Each holon might provide its services to more than one super-holon (see for example Wyns 1999, Christensen 1994). The offered services might be clusters of services offered by sub-holons, atomic services, and, of course, a combination of those possibilities.

Service clusters are used to reduce complexity. We do not define the methods how the sub services are clustered, or even force a holon to cluster the services of it's sub-holons. In a worst case scenario the Holon might offer all possible permutations of sub-services as separate clusters.

The resource-holons in this architecture are autonomous. They decide on their own which services when to offer. However an efficient way to influence decisions of sub-holons, especially on the lower levels is needed. These influences could be based on parameters like priority and cost, which are provided by holons that have better knowledge of the overall system (i.e. the global objective function).

The following picture gives an overview of our architecture:

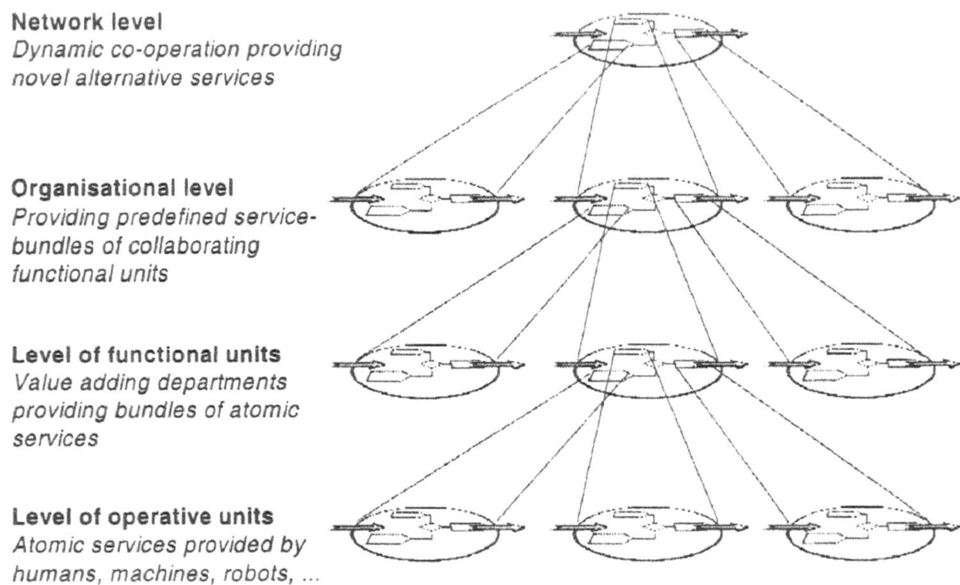

Figure 1. Holarchy levels

Holons on the network level are formed dynamically and temporary. The resource holons on the organisational level are rather longer lasting systems. On the levels below, time-consuming decisions are reduced, and it is gradually focused on run-time efficiency. Despite this picture might suggest a strict hierarchy, this is not the case. Each holon may be part of multiple holons.

2.2.2 Identification of Basic Holons

Recently research has been carried out to create a methodology that supports system designer in identifying Software Agents (see Wooldridge and Ciancarini 2000 for an overview). As recognised by (Bussmann et. al. 2000) "none of these methodologies is applicable to the design of agent-based production control systems; they either provide analysis models that are inappropriate for production control or else they lack comprehensive design rationales".

In our architecture, the physical objects (e.g. machines, work-pieces) are represented by holons. This is possible, since, our architecture allows a gradually degeneration from intelligent agents to eventually even passive objects. The services provided depend on the possibilities and permissions the hardware has. Theses basic holons will join and form higher level holons with a dedicated mission (e.g. shop floor). Our service oriented architecture is flexible enough to blur the borders between real-time requirements and (time-consuming) intelligence, and allow a gradually introduction of intelligent agents. It also allows to implement load-balancing algorithms as described later.

2.2.3 Basic Types of Holons

Guided by the basic PROSA architecture (Wyns 1996), we identified the following types of holons in a production enterprise: 1) Order-holon, 2) Product-holon, 3)

Resource-holon (e.g. Enterprise-holon, Shop-Floor-Holon, Machine-holon, Raw-Material-Holon, Energy-Holon), 4) Work-piece-holon.

The following use case shall demonstrate the knowledge and possibilities possessed by each:

A customer request triggers the generation of an Order-Holon. This holon contacts the "Yellow Pages" Service of the virtual. It looks up standard products directly and additionally all the services (processes) necessary to build the desired product. A compatible product-holon is found. This holon provides information services about the represented product. The product-holon might offer an ontology describing in detail which services are applied. If this process is considered to be of competitive advantage for thc providing enterprise, this holon will interactively decide what information to provide.

The enterprisc-holons known by the product holon are contacted. Eventually an auction is held to sell the order (the interaction protocol has to be agreed by the participating holons and is not predetermined by our architecture). However, the order-holon finally contacts one enterprise holon able to produce the desired product. Depending on the interaction protocol, the price, time of delivery, and quality might be already negotiated, or this is done now with user support.

The winning enterprise-holon contacts the holon able to provide internal co-ordination services necessary to organize the production process. The order-holon is not allowed to get into the enterprise. This would weaken the encapsulation, and introduce security risks. Instead an internal representation, a work-piece-holon, is started. Additionally to the knowledge it inherits from the order-holon, it has detailed information about the production process. This holon mainly provides information services about its current state, and the resources it has used. It might consist of intermediate products, or parts (tires of a car for example), and is therefore also organized as holon. These work-piece-holons contact the machines necessary to apply the desired services, according to the process-description. The sub-holons of the work-piece-holon communicate with different resource-holons to co-ordinate the production process.

The machine-holons subcontract other resource-holons if necessary. We do not address scheduling and other problems raised on the shop-floor here. In our architecture these are services needed by the shop-floor holon.

2.3 The Services

2.3.1 Services, Ontologies and the Product-Holon

The provision of services is the possibility of enterprises to generate value. We consider a product for example as the aggregation of several services (cluster of services).

Service objects are not holons or agents because the lack of autonomy and intelligence. For efficiency reasons they should be as lightweight as possible.

Resource-holons decide which services (or service clusters) to provide to its peers. The distinction between a service and a service cluster is only possible by checking against the according ontology. It shall not be determinable by just querying the service-object. Because each holon encapsulates its sub-holon it is possible that each holon might have its own ontology. For efficiency reasons one single centralised ontology, which is referred to by each holon, is preferable at least within an enterprise or even better within the enterprise network.

Product-holons represent the products as described by the ontology to the holons outside the originating enterprise. This holon has a detailed description of the services needed, and the order in which they will be applied (i.e. the production-process). This encapsulation of the ontology by the product-holon makes it possible to determine at runtime the extend to which the production process is visible to a specific order-holon.

In addition to the above mentioned value generating services other (sub-) services are necessary. These services are information, communication and co-ordination services, necessary for internal use of the system. These services do not generate an addition value by them self.

The demanded robustness of the systems needs co-ordination mechanisms to allow plugging in of new resources (hardware) at any time. Additionally a breakdown of the hardware needs to be communicated to other holons by either logging off the whole machine or not providing the affected services anymore. Since a breakdown eventually implies that the holon has no change to logoff, control strategies are necessary.

2.3.2 Value generating Services

Depending on the task to be fulfilled, or product offered, the resource-holons provide different services. A drilling machine may provide the service "Drill hole with a diameter of X mm". A cooling-water-holon might offer the service "Provide cooling-water in quality A".

The work-piece holon has knowledge about the production process. To apply the services according to the process description, the resources and the application of their services have to be coordinated.

2.3.3 Co-ordination Services

Each resource holon needs co-ordination services to co-ordinate its internal sub-holons, and to present the internal services to the super system (gateway functionality).

These services are often jointly provided by a mediator agent or holonhead (e.g. Haemmerle 2002, Shen et al 2000) in other architectures. We don't use a Mediator, any holon able to do so may offer co-ordination services. This means that internal co-ordination and gateway functionality could be provided by different holons. The service-oriented approach allows to implement load-balancing and fallback algorithms. At runtime a resource will identify dynamically whose service to use.

The decision might be based on attributes like workload of individual holons. For a fallback support, to have the system stable even if the co-ordinator goes offline, duplication of co-ordination information is necessary. The primary co-ordinator duplicates its "database". If it fails, the backup co-ordinator will be promoted to be the primary co-ordinator. The same holds true for other types of services.

Necessary co-ordination services are yellow-pages and white-pages services. These are needed to contact the right holons if a special type of service is needed.

Another required set of services allows plug and play capabilities. A standard login-process needs to be designed to automate the process of entering (joining) a holon and publish the new available services in the white- and yellow-pages. If new services are introduced by the entering resource they might also be communicated (i.e. offered) to the outside.

The encapsulation of the sub-holons in one holon (the super holon) guarantees that the addition or subtraction of some holon has no direct impact on the peers of that (super-)holon. Holons might experience a difference only if a type of service is not available any more or a new one is available.

2.3.4 Information Services and Advanced Decision Support

When stepping up the holarchy more and more holons are clustered indirectly (i.e. more and mores system variables are introduced). Therefore the amount of data available and probably needed for a decision is increased. The clustering of offered services will help to decrease the level of detail. Data Mining algorithms may be implemented utilising the information services provided by sub-holons.

The service concept allows the ease introduction of heuristic optimisation functions. Depending on parameters like priority or available system resources, different more or less resource consuming algorithms might be chosen.

3. CONCLUSION

We have proposed an architecture that allows to control and automate processes within the whole enterprise and even dynamic networks of enterprises. The service-centered approach allows flexibility and robustness. Contrary to other architectures, co-ordination and information services are not provided by a single mediator. This allows the easy implementation of load balancing and fallback algorithms, which adds to robustness.

The fine granularity that is provided by the services centered approach is to be used to gradually decrease the intelligence, and increase time-efficiency on lower enterprise levels. A broad spectrum of different implementations is made possible.

4. ACKNOWLEDGMENTS

The authors are grateful for financial contributions of the VPTÖ, the Austrian association for promoting manufacturing sciences

5. REFERENCES

1. Sivaram Balasubramanian, Robert W. Brennan, Douglas H. Norrie, "An architecture for metamorphic control of holonic manufacturing systems", Computers in Industry 46, 2001.
2. Luc Bongaerts, László Monostori, Duncan McFarlane, Botond Kádár, "Hierarchy in distributed shop foor control", Computers in Industry 43, Elsevier, 2000.
3. Stefan Bussmann, Duncan C. McFarlane, "Rationales for Holonic Manufacturing Control", Proceedings of 2nd International Workshop on IMS, Leuven, Belgium, 1999.

4. Stefan Bussmann "An Agent-Oriented Architecture for Holonic Manufacturing Control", First Open Workshop IMS Europe, Lausanne Switzerland, 1998.
5. James H. Christensen, "Holonic Manufacturing Systems: Initial Architecture and Standards Directions", First European Conference on HMS, Hannover, Germany, 1994.
6. Klaus Fischer, "Agent-Based Design of Holonic Manufacturing Systems", Journal of Robotics and Autonomous Systems 27, Elsevier Science, 1999.
7. Andreas Gerber, Christian Russ, "A Holonic multi-agent Infrastructure for Electronic Procurement", Proceedings of the 14th International FLAIRS Conference, 2001.
8. Alexander Haemmerle, Kurt Fessl, Georg Weichhart "The MaBE Project: An Agent-Based Environment for Business Networks", submitted to HOLOMAS, 2002.
9. Hyacinth S. Nwana, "Software Agents: An Overview", Knowledge Engineering Review, Vol. 11, No 3, Cambridge University Press, 1996.
10. Weiming Shen, Francisco Maturana, and Douglas H. Norrie "MetaMorph II: an agent-based architecture for distributed intelligent design and manufacturing", Journal of Intelligent Manufacturing, Kluwer Academic Publishers, 2000
11. Weiming Shen, Douglas H. Norrie, Jean-Paul A. Barthès, "Multi-Agent Systems for Concurrent Intellignet Design and Manufacturing", Taylor and Francis, London, New York, 2001.
12. H.-K. Tönshoff, I. Seilonen, G. Teunis, P.Leitao, "A Mediator-Based Approach For Decentralised Production Planning, Scheduling, And Monitoring", Proceedings of CIRP International Seminar on Intelligent Computation in Manufacturing Engineering (ICME), Italy, 2000.
13. Mihaela Ulieru, Scott S. Walker, and Robert W. Brennan, "The Holonic Enterprise as a Collaborative Information Ecosystem", Proceedings of the Workshop on Holons: Autonomous and Cooperating Agents for Industry, Autonomous Agents 2001, Montreal, May 29, 2001
14. Paul Valckenaers, Henrik Van Brussel, Jo Wyns, Luc Bongaerts, Patrick Peeters, "Desining Holonic manufacturing systems", Robotics and Computer-Integrated Manufactruing 14, 1998.
15. William E. Walsh, Michael P. Wellmann, "A Market Protocol for Decentralized Task Allocation", Extended version of a paper in Proceedings of the 3rd ICMAS, Paris, France, July 1998.
16. Gerhard Weiss (editor), "Multiagent systems: a modern approach to distributed artificial intelligence", Massachusetts Institute of Technology, 1999
17. Michael Wooldridge and Nicholas R. Jennings, "Intelligent Agents: Theory and Practice", Knowledge Engineering Review Volume 10 No 2, Cambridge University Press, 1995.
18. Michael Wooldridge and Paolo Ciancarini, "Agent-Oriented Software Engineering: The State of the Art", Agent-Oriented Software Engineering, Paolo Ciancarini, Michael J. Wooldridge (editors), Lecture Notes in Computer Science Vol. 1957, Springer 2000
19. Joe Wyns, "Reference Architecture for Holonic Manufacturing Systems", Phd. Thesis, Katholieke Universiteit Leuven Faculteit Toegepaste Wetenschappen, Arenbergkasteel, B-3001 Heverlee (Belgium), 1999

33

HOLONIC MANUFACTURING WITH INTELLIGENT OBJECTS

Eddy Bajic, Frédéric Chaxel
Research Center for Automatic Control, University of Nancy
CRAN - CNRS UMR 7039
BP 239, 54506 Vandœuvre-les-Nancy, FRANCE
eddy.bajic@cran.uhp-nancy.fr
frederic.chaxel@cran.uhp-nancy.fr

This paper presents and analyzes different approaches in the implementation of the Intelligent Manufacturing System concept, with a main focus on the holon paradigm proposed by the HMS project. After a survey of manufacturing systems evolution, it deals with the holon-product concept and its instantiation to the physical part product as a key issue to novel manufacturing system. Propositions are discussed to enrich products with new capabilities in order to decide and deal actively with their environment, such as intelligent objects. Several methodologies are described to implement this approach and an original one is proposed to promote holonic control of production systems driven by intelligent products. New perspectives of process reactivity and robustness, product tracking, and product life cycle information management are depicted, as also problems still not solved.

1. INTRODUCTION

Since the last decade, tremendous changes have occurred in the field of manufacturing systems research activities considering production control and organization. To manage product diversity and rapid changes in production demands, research effort of the nineties have been focused on manufacturing systems architectures satisfying productivity, flexibility, openness characteristics for integration aspect and cost reduction, widely based on automation increase (Dilts, 1991).

Originally represented in the eighties by the CIM concept (Computer Integrated Manufacturing), new approaches emerged to remedy to the limits hit by such hierarchically and centrally controlled organization suffering from rigidity in response to fast production changes and adaptations. Then, priority have been put on decentralization and distribution of decision-making activities and information flow with an expected downsizing of manufacturing systems. Fully distributed structures were proposed (Duffie, 1986) involving concurrent mechanism for job decision and coordination support, based on network communication procedures, contract nets. Although heterarchical architectures were promoted to provide manufacturing systems with decentralization, modularity, robustness and cooperative functionnalities.

Beyond those approaches characterized by system-based functionality, and machine-centered decision making, strong demand appears for new formalizations of manufacturing systems to break off from conventional system organization to satisfy autonomy and individualism along with cooperation capabilities amongst all components of a manufacturing system. Emphasis was put on coordination, self-organization, hyper-flexibility, adaptation and product-orientation.

2. NEXT GENERATION MANUFACTURING SYSTEMS

Several new paradigms for manufacturing system description were formulated drawing inspiration from the real world mainly over the two aspects of social organization of human societies and natural rules and environment.

Biological metaphor have been proposed by Okino (Okino, 1994) to fit autonomous distributed manufacturing system description, so called *Bionic Manufacturing System* (BMS) in CAM-I/Japan. BMS concept lays on a system theory involving self-organization rules over distributed components with quasi-life functions copying genetic behavior, allowing freely adaptive and flexible connections in response to changes of system conditions. Ueda (Ueda, 1994) specified a model of BMS as a pseudo ecosystem built around works and manufacturing cells thus mimicking biological organisms carrying DNA (Deshoxyribo Nucleic Acid) gene type and BN (Brain and Neuron) type behavior and information. In a Bionic world environment, works and tasks are considered as organisms that grow up to become or generate products, manufacturing cells are other types of organisms that process works. DNA type information is supporting inherited information and transformation as "growing up" objectives of products, while BN type information governs works activities. In this, a manufacturing system control behavior should be described by evolution strategies with mathematical model based expressions.

A social organization metaphor has been derived from the socio-philosophical proposition of a Hungarian journalist and philosopher Arthur Koestler, specified early in 1971 in the book "The ghost in the machine", as the holonic concept (Koestler, 1989). Based on the observation of self-regulation capabilities of social organization, a social holonic behavior involves very few characteristics supported by elementary entities named *Holon,* acting and cooperating to assume living of complex and ruled organization named *Holarchy*. Koestler adds that holonic argument can be applied to biological, social or cognitive hierarchy which manifests rule-governed behavior and structural consistency.

The holonic metaphor have been applied to manufacturing system organization by the International joint program IMS (Intelligent Manufacturing System) with the thematic research consortium HMS (Holonic Manufacturing System) as a promising response to provide production systems with robustness and adaptability to condition changes and disturbances, modularity and flexibility capacities. Underlying principles of holonic application to manufacturing systems have been defined as follows by the HMS consortium (Van Brussel, 1995) : *Holon :* An autonomous and co-operative building block of a manufacturing system for transforming, transporting, storing information and physical object. *Holarchy :* An assembly of holons which act in cooperation having a specific set of objectives and common goal. *Autonomy :* Ability of an holon to control its own execution plan associated with its own strategy. *Co-operation* : Capabilities of systems entities to communicate, negotiate and execute actions plans in order to reach a global objective.

The previous paradigms are actually drawing up the next generation manufacturing systems to come. Scientist research community have to cope with formalization and resolution of the aiming capabilities of the real world to validate and prove efficiency of metaphorical paradigms and concepts within the production world. Agent technology derived from artificial intelligence research fields have emerged to support distributed intelligent control within manufacturing system architecture (Jennings 1995, Shen 2000). So the Holon, previously an imitation metaphor of social and human organization has become consequently a pragmatic element of agent technology implementation represented by an intelligent software agent (Fletcher, 2001).

A major goal is to fit the abstract world mainly focused on information management, treatment and decision-making capacities, to the real world represented by physical product-parts, machines and resources. By joining bits to atoms, BMS and HMS paradigms could take shape. In that way the need for distribution of information system onto individual product and objects requires tools and methods to manage and provide automatic or human-based interaction to product related information for manufacturing and logistic systems.

This conducts to a conceptual dilemma to answer : does the product itself need to be intelligent, or instead do intelligent services have to be offered to the product ? The following paragraphs analyze different solutions and focus on a validation approach of the holon concept supported by part product and resources cooperating in a manufacturing environment as intelligent objects.

3. PRODUCT ORIENTED MANAGEMENT

A common characteristic is revealed in both approaches BMS and HMS, with the duality of elementary organisms performing in complex systems. A holon consists of an information processing entity allied to a physical processing entity, as also biological organisms are unified entity of information and substance. This characteristic contributes to the emergence of an autonomous behavior appearance in complex systems, on the basis of internal structure of holon as described in Figure 1. The holon-product as an intelligent object concept can be seen as an entity created by real or forecasted market demand, ruling a servicing environment in a competitive and cooperative manner. At the first stage, the intelligent object should embed the necessary knowledge to assure the realization of the associated product, with the capacity of disseminating individual customer and product specifications directly within the process.

An essential characteristic of the described holon-product formalization is the merging of bits and atoms on one host, the product, in order to maintain consistency and coherency in between abstract world (manufacturing plan order and scheduling) and real world (material flow, physical production process or distribution environment) (Brock 2001).

Product information and knowledge is basically defined at the design level in words of product specification and process operations as quality criteria, manufacturing plan, maintenance procedure, ... This knowledge need to be constructed step by step and structured through a life cycle product information model, to be shared by all the actors tools operating on the product. At the manufacturing stage, this knowledge is conceptually duplicated to fit to each individual product, so that product definition data set is cloned, and then follow its own life.

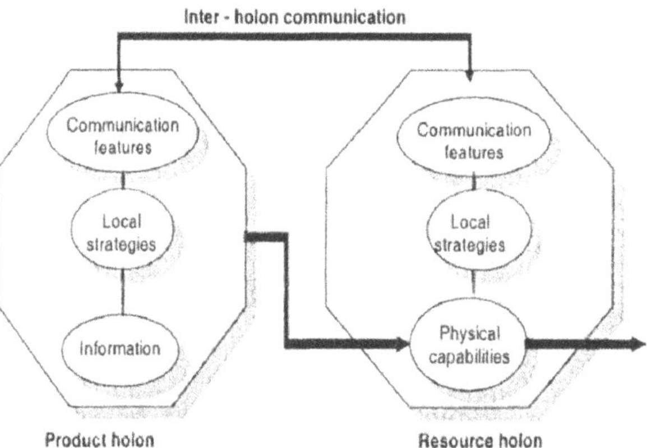

Figure 1 - Resource and Product Holons structure

In the intelligent object approach, a product as a holonic entity object carry its own information on a programmable electronic tag (R/W mode) communicating with each user involved in its development process (Bajic 1999, MacFarlane 2000). Advantage of this approach is in machine capacities to focus on operations control (transport, measures, ...) and not on coherency maintenance of product related information, this point is conceptually assumed by each individual product. A dialog can be imagined in between machine and product as follows : *"Part 17843, where are you ?"* says the machine , *"I am currently at Machine 4 for a 10 minutes operation and I expect to be soon served by you"* replies the product. This leads to the emergence of claims contracts between customers and suppliers in a concurrent client/server formalism.

Thus intelligent Tracking in manufacturing and supply chain environment is affordable, offering two new concepts for product mobility management known as postponement and merge-in-transit (Brewer 1999). Postponement is the capability to assign destination or final realization of a general purpose object (i.e. a semi-finished product) at the latest time in the process when production availability or client demand occurs. Merge-in-transit involves combining various objects (product-parts to be assembled), thus merging information system and objects capabilities at a common place to be delivered as a whole to the customer site.

The major issues of the proposed intelligent object approach lie on one hand in the management of information and object mobility, and on a second hand on decision-making capabilities associated to each holon-product. Automatic identification technologies using electronic data carriers and radio frequency techniques have now gain in maturity and have been industrially proofed, so they are currently the target technologies to implement attended functionality to the product. But still limitations in these technologies, mainly du to the current market size, bounds the physical implementation of the holon-product concept, by mean of lack of storage capacity (up to Mbyte needed by automotive application Bajic 1999), and lack of user-program and method encapsulation within tag. Nevertheless the today technological barrier, enhancement and refinement of the intelligent object concept still have to be continued with the objective of a full embedding on the product.

As results of research conducted at CRAN since several years, an intelligent product design and formalization methodology, still under development is proposed in the following chapter as a logistic support to manufacturing system control. The following chapters shows part of this methodology concerning holon-product data management. Holon-Product specification will assume both vertical integration up to the design level and the horizontal integration over the process organization by supplying methodology and support tool allowing each part carrying electronic tag, to act as a communication vector of process information system, in charge of the overall application management, and information coherency, consistency and accessibility.

4. PRODUCT DRIVEN PROCESSING

In the way to reach the formalization of the holon-product concept as an intelligent object, individual an dmobile information management is one of the key challenges. For this purpose, international research activities currently running are investigating two approaches.

The Auto-ID center (Brock 2001) based at MIT Lab and Cambridge University UK, propose an information system infrastructure centered on the product-part which is tagged with a 96 bits RFID smart tag. Products are virtually connected to internet, where life cycle product information is stored and indexed by mean of a code number named ePC (electronic product code) tagged on the product, and representing a pointer to distributed data bases over internet network (Figure 2). The ePC approach works together with a Product Markup Language (PML), describing the object with XML (eXtended Markup Language) syntax and Object Naming Services (ONS) implemented on Internet machines, thus assuming the routing of product information request to appropriate distributed web sites as Domain Name Servers actually do in Internet philosophy. The Auto-ID project is mainly focused on retail supply chain applications with low cost passive tag.

Research on intelligent product concept conducted at CRAN tends to implement information management capacity directly on the product, assuming Mobile Database Nodes infrastructure for intelligent objects management. Figure 3 depicts the concept adapted from a client/server local model, where the object is the manager of its own information and gives them to the process after it received a service request (*"What is the next operation to be proceed on yourself"* for example).

Requests issued from the process are sent to an object interface application supporting product access methods in an object-oriented requesting semantic such as *Object_Selector.Message (Parameters), SystemMessage(Parameters)*: color.getvalue() ; color.putvalue(Red);

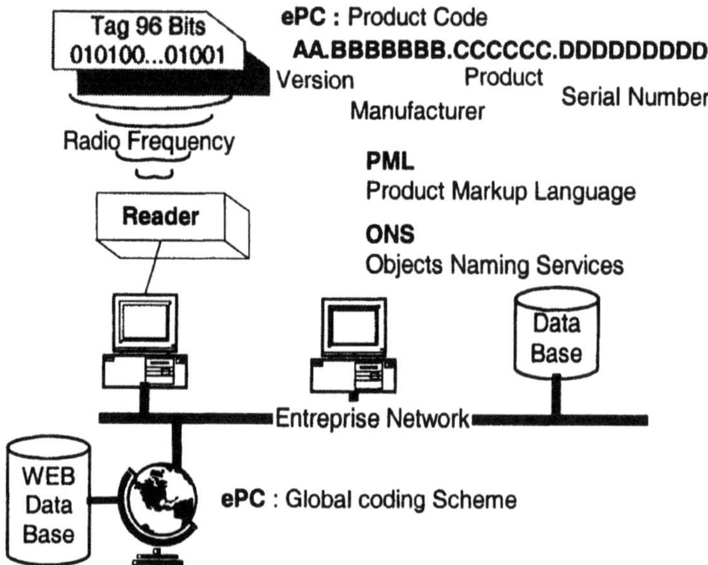

Figure 2 - ePC product-tagged information infrastructure

A the STEP-based methodology (Standard for Exchange of Product data Model) allows translation of product models, described in the EXPRESS language into :

- a library of product-information access functions, allowing easy application-oriented requesting of product according to the EXPRESS data model;
- an external repository database structure definition, to assume a full description of product information model when storage capacity on the product is limited. This is an optional service of the methodology.

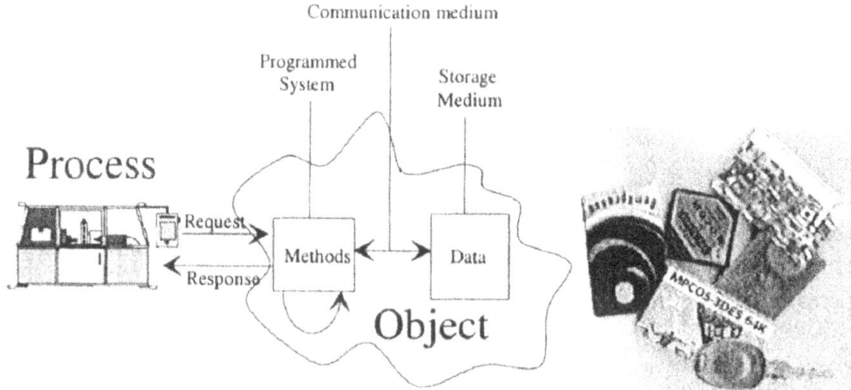

Figure 3 - Intelligent object in manufacturing system & RFID tags embedded

The product definition within the STEP neutral file is used on one hand to create the tag memory image, for the first state of a product associated to the current phase of its life cycle in the manufacturing environment, and on a second hand if needed, to populate the previously created database schema. Although holon-product definition is the result of a first phase supplying both a holon-product data model and holon data in the form of an EXPRESS data model and STEP files. Product information is split into two categories, one is managed on the product and the other is distributed over a networked database as shown on Figure 4.

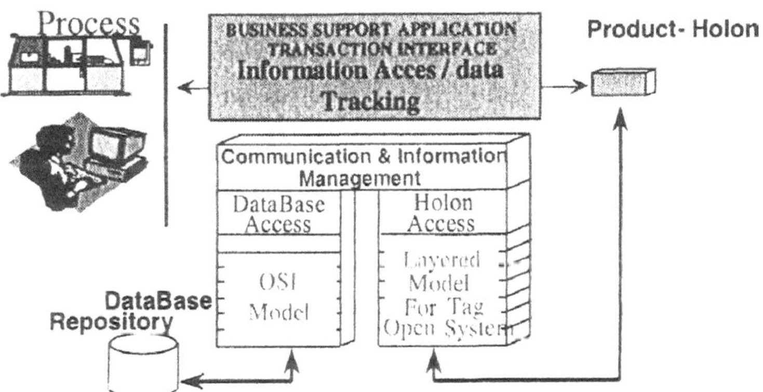

Figure 4 - Dual access to intelligent product data models

This information dichotomy of the proposed methodology firstly assumes a high degree of autonomy to assume product-based process management, with time-response efficiency for real time process activity on the object independently of any information computing complex infrastructure, and secondly it allows accessibility to large volume of data to cover product life cycle management, according to product data models stored on the product. Figure 5 shows the implementation process assuring intelligent object management and information system distribution over both the product and distributed database.

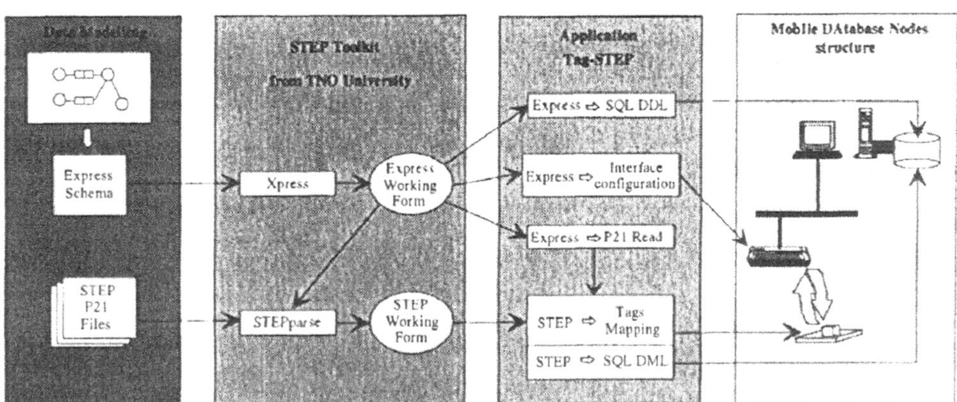

Figure 5 - Product Information system implementation processing

Current storage capacity of modern tags offers up to 128 Kbytes, which can be considered as huge but often not enough as regard to the needs in automotive industries for example, and at expensive price per part. The dichotomic methodology presented before have been successfully validated in automotive application with Renault car manufacturer research project resulting in no-key car vehicle Laguna II (Bajic 2002).

5. CONCLUSION

The intelligent object concept is promising significant benefits in automation applications to cover the full product life cycle management from production up to after sale services and recycling. Manufacturing system control activities and supply chain management are the meaningful targets. From the concept to its instantiation, several approaches are currently investigated providing different ways for distribution of competencies in between the product and its environment. Manufacturing automation and devices are certainly not yet matured enough to integrate such innovative control and give intelligence to the product. Cost matter is currently orienting research activities towards less intelligence on product, but robustness, reactivity, and object autonomy suffer from this. But there is still limitations in the Auto-ID technologies, mainly due to a small market size, bounds the practical implementation of the intelligent object concept performing holon product metaphor, that needs incorporation of computing power into tags. Applications have been investigated by the authors with smart java card, with virtual java machine inside the object, promising high efficiency. Conceptual development still have to be enhanced, with a need for formal modelling of intelligent product, independently of technological platform. Even multi-agents technology do not give yet formal solution, without deep embedding in software platform.

6. REFERENCES

1. Bajic E, Chaxel F, Auto-ID Mobile Information System for Vehicle Life Cycle Data Management, IEEE SMC, October 6-9 2002, Hamamet, Tunisia
2. Brewer A, Sloan N, Intelligent tracking in manufacturing. Journal of intelligent manufacturing, 1999, 10: pp 2 45-250.
3. Brock D, The electronic product code. Auto-Id center, MIT, Cambridge, 2001.
4. Bajic E, Chaxel F, Richard J. Automotive vehicle data management based on holon-product paradigm IEEE SMC, pp 122-132, October 12-15 1999, Tokyo, Japan.
5. Dilts D.M., Boyd N.P., (1991). Whorms H.H. The evolution of control Architecture for Automated Manufacturing systems. *In Manufacturing Systems*, Vol 10, N° 1, pp 79-93.
6. Duffie N. A. , Piper R. S. . Non-hierarchical Control of Manufacturing Systems. *In Manufacturing Systems*, 1986, Vol 5, N° 2, pp 137-139.
7. Fletcher M, Deen M. Fault tolerant holonic manufacturing systems. Concurrency and computation : practice and experience, 2001, 13:43-70.
8. Jennings N. Coordination techniques for distributed artificial intelligence. Foundations of distributed intelligencec ch. 7, O'Hare GH, Jennings N (Eds); Wiley, 1995
9. Koestler A. The ghost in the machine, *Arkana books*, 1989, London.
10. Lonc B., Bajic E. "Design and exploitation of communicating escort memories for automotive applications". Int. conf. on Advanced Microsystems for automotive applications, VDI-VDE-IT, pp. 142-150, 19 96, Berlin, Germany.
11. MacFarlane D, Bussmann S. State of the art of holonic systems in production planning and control. Production planning and control, 2000, V11, N6,: 522-536
12. Okino, N. Bionic manufacturing system. *In Manufacturing Systems*, 1994, Vol. 23, pp. 175-187
13. Shen W, Maturana F, Norrie D. Metamorph II : an agent based architecture for distributed design and manufacturing. Journal of Intelligent manufacturing 2000: 11, 237-251.
14. Ueda K . Biological-oriented paragidgm for artifactual systems. *Japan symposium on flexible automation*, Kobbe, 1994, pp 1263-1266
15. Van Brussel H., Wyns J., Valckenaers P., Bongaerts L., Peeters. Reference architecture for holonic manufacturing systems : PROSA Computers in industry, 37, N°3, pp225-276, 1998

34

DISTRIBUTED SELF-SIMULATION OF HOLONIC MANUFACTURING SYSTEMS

Naoki Imasaki[1], Ambalavanar Tharumarajah[2], Shinsuke Tamura[3]
[1] *Toshiba Corporation, Japan, naoki.imasaki@toshiba.co.jp*
[2] *CSIRO Manufacturing Science & Technology, Australia, rajah.tharumarajah@csiro.au*
[3] *Fukui University, Japan, tamura@fuis.fuis.fukui-u.ac.jp*

This paper details the development of a distributed simulation capability for holonic manufacturing systems based on the concept of self-simulation. Every holon in the system would function similar to an autonomous simulator that maintains its own clock and event execution. This paper discusses synchronization and other technical issues in designing such a simulator and puts forward the basic requirements and design options for its implementation. These are results of HMS project in IMS (Intelligent Manufacturing Systems) program.

1. INTRODUCTION

Simulation is an effective tool for examining how a system works. For Holonic Manufacturing Systems (HMSs; Christensen, 1994), simulation becomes critical because HMSs are often too large-scale and distributed to handle their behavior analytically. Further, holons in HMSs exhibit non-deterministic behaviors and deal with discrete events like human operations, thus the simulation should be of discrete-event naturally.

Simulation of HMSs fulfills four core capabilities that are critical for designing and operating HMSs. First, it is used to test the functional and logic correctness of a proposed system during design. Second, it is used in analyzing faults during operation. Third, it is used for implementing intelligence in the holons. This enables a holon to assess future performance and decide on a course of actions. Lastly it is used to test task execution performances, e.g. response time and throughput.

To provide the above capabilities, a simulator of HMSs should ideally be modifiable and extendable as and when changes in design or operation of the system takes place. Also, it should permit easy switching between normal (i.e. actual operation) and simulation modes of operation of a holon. A distributed self-simulator is proposed to satisfy these features. The idea behind a distributed self-simulator is firstly to provide holons with their own simulation capabilities (their operation mode can be changed by their mode switch, i.e., "normal" and "simulation"), and secondly to create a simulation capability as a set of independently acting self-simulators having their own processes and that can be remotely connected over a network. A single self-simulator (hereafter called a logical process or LP (Fujimoto, 2000)) would process events in strict time sequence, generate new events and communicate with other LPs. In a holonic system, an LP can be representative of a holon or a sub-set of holons. Compared to the traditional centralized approach of using a single sequential simulator for the entire system, this approach has the following advantages: system simplicity, modularity, extensibility, maintainability, and high computation performance.

This paper is structured as follows. Section two describes the architecture and the high level functional requirements of the proposed distributed simulator. Section three elaborates the requirements for the development of the distributed simulator. Next features a prototype is briefly described followed by conclusion

2. GENERAL REQUIREMENTS

2.1 Architecture

The architecture of the distributed self-simulator is shown in Figure 1.

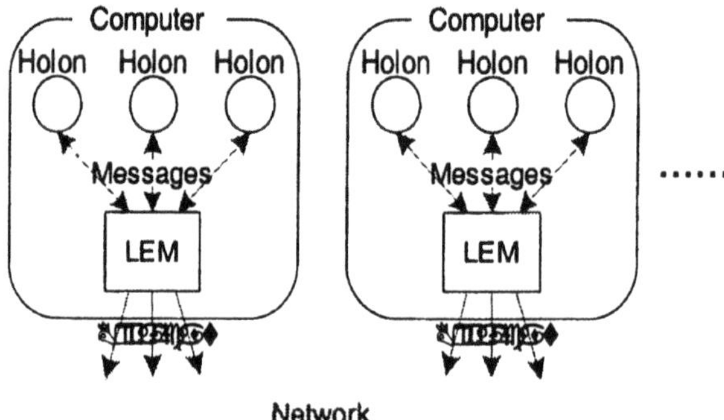

Figure 1 - Communication Architecture

In this architecture, a set of holons is defined to operate under a single Local Event Manager (LEM). Likewise, another set of holons can be defined to operate under a different LEM. This architecture and the development are based on JDPS (Seki, 1991), a Java based HMS execution platform. A member holon wishing to send a message would forward it to an LEM to which the holon belongs. The LEM would broadcast the message to other LEMs and also check whether the receiver holon is one of the members. If it were the latter, the message would be internally forwarded to that holon. On receiving a message from another LEM, an LEM would check whether the receiver holon is a member and if so would forward it to the holon. If this is not the case, the message will be ignored.

This architecture is used to define and construct the holons of the distributed simulator. Two distinct configurations are possible:

LEM as an LP (LEM-LP): An LEM acts as a single simulator. It manages the ordering and execution of incoming events and maintains its own local clock. The holons would receive the events, process them and any new events generated would be forwarded to the LEM. Inconsistencies among events are detected by the LEM and appropriate actions are taken to correct such inconsistencies.

Holon as an LP (Holon-LP): A holon acts as a single simulator and, hence, manages the ordering, execution and generation of events. Each holon maintains its own clock and any inconsistencies among events are detected and rectified by the holon. LEM acts purely as a message router.

The simulator that this paper proposes is the mixture of LEM-LP and Holon-LP configurations, i.e., local clocks are managed by LEMs and event inconsistency is detected and corrected by holons.

2.2 Functional Requirements

An overriding requirement on the performance of a distributed simulator is that it must produce the same result as that of a single sequential simulator for the same data. This requires the LPs (i.e. distributed simulators) to correctly synchronize their local clocks with each other as well as to maintain perfect consistency of states. However, a distributed simulator is markedly different in its architecture and its performance depends on the adequacy of the underlying communication network and memory. The following sub-sections first describe the assumptions followed by the requirements on synchronization.

2.2.1 Assumptions

The following assumptions are made with respect to the underlying communication network and the computational environment of LPs (modified and extended from p. 98, Fujimoto, 2000):

Assumption 1: There are no state variables shared between LPs: This is to say that LPs manage their state dependencies primarily through communication.

Assumption 2: Communication among the LPs is reliable: That is, every message that is sent eventually arrives at the receiver.

Assumption 3: An LP sends messages in its local-timestamp order.

Assumption 4: A communication network guarantees that messages are delivered in the same order as they were sent.

Assumption 5: LPs may be destroyed or new LPs created during the execution of simulation.

Assumption 6: Memory at each LP for storing states is limited: Memory overflow when storing states can cause fatal errors and should be avoided.

2.2.2 Requirement of Synchronization

In the distributed simulation environment an LP manages the ordering and execution of local events and maintains the local simulation clock. There are two kinds of events in the simulator, one is a *pure*-simulation event that signifies the start or finish of an activity, and the other is an event corresponding to a message delivered. The types of activities can be associated with the LPs (or holons representing physical devices) and include processing activities with time delays and other message sending/receiving actions. An event would have a timestamp (local clock time) for its occurrence and a recipient for its execution.

An LP chronologically orders the events according to time of occurrence (i.e., the timestamp), and posts the first event for execution. The time in the local clock is incremented to the timestamp of the event that is being executed. This way, the time within an LP is maintained (i.e. local synchronization)

However, along with the local synchronization, a mechanism should exist to assure synchronization of events among the LPs. The problem of non-synchronization occurs due to the independent adjustments of local clock times by the LPs. To elaborate this problem, consider a message sent to LP_A at time t_3 from another LP as shown in Figure 2. LP_A finds that the event #3 (hereafter referred to as a *straggler* event) is in the past (current time at LP_A is $t_A > t_3$). This means that there is a difference of $t_A - t_3$ between the clock time of the LP that sent the message and the local clock time. An immediate consequence of the straggler event is that the state of LP_A in this time period is invalid or has to be re-validated. The consistency among the simulated states of LP_A can be assured only up to time t_3.

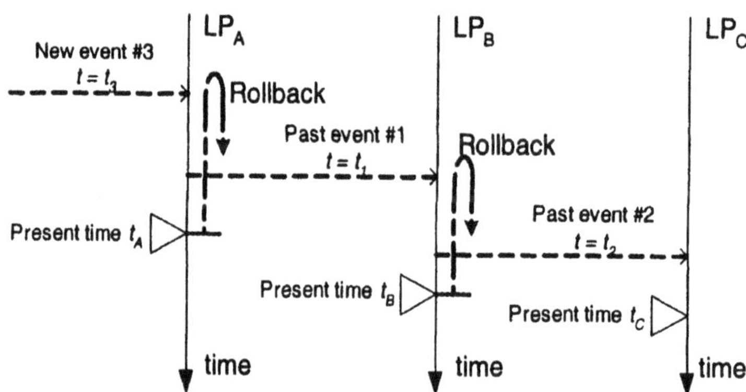

Figure 2 - Event synchronization and rollbacks

To remove the inconsistency, LP_A should ideally rollback its state to that which prevailed at time t_3 and re-execute the events (including the one received) that occurred in the intervening period $t_A - t_3$. The rollback would cancel all the events that the holon posted with a timestamp later than t_3, execute the straggler event and then re-execute the simulation from t_3. The rollback in a one holon, however, can lead to retraction of events that were previously scheduled for other holons and a consequent propagation of straggler events. For instance, the retraction of event #1 posted from LP_A to LP_B at time $t_1 > t_3$ would cause LP_B to rollback. This, in turn, would cause a retraction of the event posted by LP_B to LP_C at time t_2 and so on. The local detection and correction of inconsistencies using rollback, thus, provides a mechanism for ensuring the states of the LPs are globally consistent with each other.

In order to satisfy the requirements of synchronization and to perform adequately under the above assumptions, a simulator needs the following essential functions:

1) Detection of inconsistencies
2) Rollback of events to maintain a consistent state within and across LPs
3) State saving that conserves the memory
4) Recursive rollback avoidance (RRA)

These functions are elaborated in the next section.

3. REQUIREMENTS SPECIFICATION

This section elaborates the functions required to construct the distributed simulator and suitable strategies for their implementation.

3.1 Detection of Inconsistencies

As observed before, a distributed simulator should be capable of producing the same final result as a sequential simulator. This could be guaranteed by ensuring that each holon satisfies the local causality constraint, i.e., when each holon is able to process the events in timestamp order and thereby ensures the correct mapping of the state space of a holon. However, in a distributed implementation of LPs, there can be occurrence of straggler events, thus violating the local causality constraints.

When an LP receives a straggler message it has to first detect the inconsistency and correct it by undoing the inconsistent events, i.e., through a rollback. The possible ways to detect inconsistencies are as follows.

Time inversion inconsistency detection (TIID): If the timestamp t_S of a received event satisfies $t_S < t_C$ where t_C is the local simulation time of the LP, it is unconditionally judged as an inconsistency occurrence.

Semi-semantic inconsistency detection (SSID): If the timestamp t_S of a received event satisfies $t_S < t_C$ where t_C is the local simulation time of the LP *and* the action invoked by the event changes the state of the LP, it is regarded as an inconsistency occurrence. However, if there are no events that fetch the state during $t_S < t \le t_C$, then there is no inconsistency.

Obviously SSID can reduce redundant rollbacks though it may require additional computation.

Because rollback can be computationally intensive, inconsistency is detected at the level of a holon, instead at the level of an LEM as in conventional distributed simulators. Holon-wise inconsistency checking connected with LEM-wise event ordering reduces the frequency of inconsistency. Namely time inversion in an LEM does not always imply time inversion in individual holons. On the other hand, an LEM insures that events posted by holons within itself are consistent.

3.2 Rollback

Retraction of events due to a rollback can employ one of two methods, viz. *aggressive* and *lazy* cancellation (Fujimoto, 2000). Aggressive cancellation is when an event E that is being retracted by an LP sends a cancel message to retract all events that the LP posted after E. In lazy cancellation, no such message is sent until the rolled back event is recreated and the validity of the previously scheduled event is examined. Thus, lazy cancellation offers the advantage of avoiding retracting events that are recreated when rolled back events are reprocessed, though more computation is required. The semi-semantic inconsistency checking can be directly implemented for lazy cancellation.

It should be noted that if the assumption on correct network delivery is violated (i.e., the network cannot guarantee the delivery of messages in the same order as they are sent), then an additional cancellation of all processed events with a timestamp equal to that of the straggler event becomes necessary.

A holon can initiate rollback a) locally, b) LEM-wide or c) system-wide. Types b) and c) help to re-synchronize clock times of a sub-set of holons. However, a similar effect can be obtained with local rollback through propagation of event cancellation with less computation.

Holon-wise (local) rollback: When a holon rollbacks to time t_s, it sends rollback requests only holons that received events from it.

LEM-wide rollback: When a holon belonging to an LEM rollbacks to time t_s, it sends rollback requests to all holons belonging to the LEM to rollback to time t_s.

System-wide rollback: When a holon rollbacks to time t_s, it sends rollback requests to all holons in the system to rollback to time t_s.

A rollback operation is when a holon, detecting inconsistency, re-initializes its state at the current clock time $t_c = t_c'$ to a previous state (at time t_s) and then proceeds to re-construct its state-space up to the current clock time. The followings show the comparison between the aggressive cancellation and the lazy cancellation.

Aggressive cancellation (with local rollback):

Step 1. A straggler event $E_j(t_s)$ received by holon H_j causes rollback to t_s

Step 2. H_j sends cancellation events $E_k^c(t)$ to holons H_k of previously scheduled events $E_k(t)$ where $t_s < t \le t_c'$

Step 3. H_j executes straggler event $E_j(t_s)$ and resets the local clock time $t_c = t_s$

Step 4. H_j executes an RRA (discussed in Section 3.4) procedure

Step 5. H_j re-executes a previously received event or executes a newly received events (includes a resent event) $E_j(t_0)$ where $t_0 \le t_c'$ in ascending order of time and resets the local clock time to $t_c = t_0$

Step 6. H_j schedules new events $E_k(t_0)$, if appropriate, to holon H_k

Step 7. Goto Step 5

Lazy cancellation (with local rollback):

Step 1. A straggler event $E_j(t_s)$ received by holon H_j causes rollback to t_s

Step 2. H_j executes straggler event $E_j(t_s)$ and resets the local clock time $t_c = t_s$

Step 3. H_j re-executes a previously received event or executes a newly received events $E_j(t_0)$ where $t_0 \le t_c'$ in ascending order of time and resets the local clock time to $t_c = t_0$

Step 4. H_j re-validates a previously scheduled event $E_k(t)$ where $t_s < t \le t_c'$ and if $E_k(t)$ is not valid, H_j sends a cancellation event $E_k^c(t)$ to holon H_k

Step 5. H_j schedules new events $E_k(t_0)$, if appropriate, to holon H_k

Step 6. H_j executes an RRA procedure

Step 7. Goto Step 3

3.3 State Saving

When a straggler event occurs and events are cancelled, an LP should ensure that a consistent state-space mapping prevails. This is achieved by rolling back the state variables in time. Thus, rollback operation requires storing the states at each state change or event execution (called *checkpoint saving*) in order that the desired state at some point in time in the past can be restored.

Checkpoint saving at each event consumes more and more memory as new events are created, but it seldom releases memory. This situation is not acceptable due to the finite availability of memory (assumption 6) at an LP. Therefore, a mechanism should be constructed to limit the storing of state variables over the simulated period. While infrequent saving of state can reduce memory needs, it too cannot be used to reclaim memory.

This problem can be overcome by determining the events that cannot be rolled back and hence the time before which no checkpoint saving is necessary. Computing the lower bound on the timestamp among all unprocessed and partially processed messages in the system referred to as Global Virtual Time (GVT) could identify these events. Thus, a requirement for an efficient checkpoint saving is the computation of GVT using an appropriate algorithm, though it should be pointed out that this may or may not be implemented in preference to simpler local methods.

3.4 Recursive Rollback Avoidance

In (re) scheduling an event after a local rollback, a holon can face the following situation. If a cancelled event is found to be valid, the holon will schedule a new event. However, due to the previous cancellation, the holon can expect to receive a response event. It is possible that the timestamp of the response event happens to be smaller than the local clock time. Such a case would require another rollback during a rollback procedure. This is computationally quite ineffective.

The following are some of mechanisms that can be explored to avoid or minimize recursive rollbacks.

Local Fixed Wait: A simple mechanism to avoid a recursive rollback is for the holon to wait (in real-time), after it re-executes scheduled events.

Controlled event execution: A holon controls the speed of re-execution after rollback, thus, permitting other holons to respond.

Conservative execution: Holons involved in the rollback adopt conservative event handling strategy to eliminate time inversion during rollback operations. In this case, events that are received before the rollback can be used as *look-ahead.*

To select the best method that guarantees the synchronization of rollback is one of the most important topics. Local fixed wait method is simplest, though investigations are required to determine its performance.

3.5 Design options

The following summarizes the design options that are selected to minimize communication and computational loads and to achieve adequate performance:

Configuration:	LEM-LP
Detection of inconsistencies:	Holon-wise SSID
Rollback:	Lazy cancellation
State saving:	Event-wise saving with GVT estimation
Recursive rollback avoidance:	Local fixed wait

However, further investigations will be carried out to ascertain the sufficiency of performance, and if necessary other appropriate options may be investigated.

4. PROTOTYPING

A prototype of the distributed self-simulator, called *simJDPS* is developed based on the architecture we discussed above. Each holon is endowed with simulation capabilities to maintain their respective local clocks and event lists. Communication is indirect and is mediated by a Site Manager, acting as an LEM. In essence, the holons function similar to their actual counterparts, except for the passage of time that is simulated rather than real.

simJDPS is implemented on JDPS by extending existing classes and by adding new classes. For example, `simHolon` class extends the Holon class of JDPS to implement the self-simulation capability in holons, and `SiteManager` class is modified to act as LEM. The first prototype model incorporates Holon-LP configuration, TIID, aggressive cancellation with local rollback and event-wise check point saving. This model was tested for its functionality and run for a 2-site multi-holon situation.

This model will be extended to include mechanisms for lazy cancellation, computation of GVT and RRA.

5. CONCLUSION

Distributed self-simulation of holons in a HMS has many advantages, both during design and operation. However, there are many technical challenges in developing such a simulator including ensuring perfect synchronization, minimizing rollback situations, preventing memory overflows and above all maintaining a performance that at least matches that of a single centralized simulator. The model and the specifications detailed in this paper attempts to address these challenges by proposing a novel distributed self-simulation approach.

6. REFERENCES

1. Christensen, J. Holonic Manufacturing Systems – Initial Architecture and Standards Directions, 1st Euro. Conf. on HMS, Hanover, Germany, 1994.
2. Fujimoto, RM. Parallel and Distributed Simulation Systems, John Wiley & Sons, Inc., 2000.
3. Seki, T, Hasegawa, T, Okataku, Y, Tamura, S. An Operating System for Intellectual Distributed Processing System – An Object Oriented Approach based on Broadcast Communication -. J. of Information Processing, Vol. 14, No. 4, pp.405-413, 1991. EMBED

35

COMPONENT DESIGN AND FORMAL VALIDATION OF SFA SYSTEMS: A CASE STUDY

Valeriy Vyatkin, Hans-Michael Hanisch
Martin Luther University of Halle-Wittenberg
Valeriy.Vyatkin@iw.uni-halle.de
Hans-Michael.Hanisch@iw.uni-halle.de

In this paper we present a case study of component based automation system design using IEC61499 accompanied by subsequent application of the formal modeling methods and the corresponding verification tools.
Our approach to validation is based on the results of formerly conducted research and development works on formal modeling of distributed control systems. The validation tool VEDA (Verification Environment for Distributed Applications) is intended on integration with IEC61499 engineering tools by means of using standardized source-code syntax and XML-based document types.

1. INTRODUCTION

The new developing international standard IEC61499 [1,2] provides an architectural framework for development and deployment of scalable flexible automation systems powered by distributed intelligence.

In this paper we attempt to illustrate the component based automation system design using IEC61499. The *component* is understood as a container that encapsulates heterogeneous properties of real industrial objects, such as dynamic models, the intelligence needed to control the underlying equipment in order to solve the predestined tasks, and the interfaces to process and to other objects constituting industrial systems. In this sense, the concept of component is somewhat complementary to the mechatronic approach e.g. [3], which serves as a framework to combine mechanical and electronic circuitry elements and properties of the equipment.

The goal of the component-based design is to facilitate development, deployment and, particularly re-engineering of automation systems. The key goal is to optimize testing of the modified configurations by application of automated validation methods. Testing of the resultant system, if it is done according to state-of-the-art simulation methods, could nullify such gains of the component-oriented design as fast re-configuration.

However, along with new challenges, IEC61499 has created new opportunities of formal methods application in order to improve reliability of flexible automation systems. Thus, the formal verification tools can be easier applied for automated check of the validity of a pre-given set of safety properties for the modified system architectures, finding erroneous situations arising from the integration of different objects. In this paper we present a case study of component based automation system design using IEC61499 accompanied by subsequent application of the formal modeling methods and the corresponding verification tools.

2. COMPONENTS

We will illustrate the component structure on the drilling station represented in the following Figure 1 with the functionality as follows:

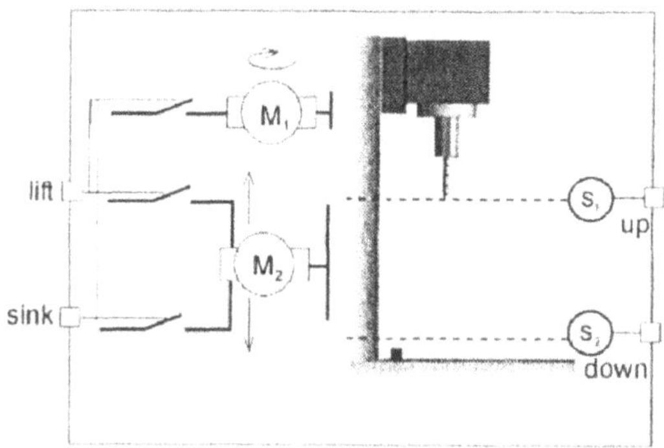

Figure 1. A drilling Station.

The spin motor M_1 rotates the bore of the drill. The step motor M_2 moves the head of the drill in vertical direction. The motor is controlled by two Boolean level signals: lift and sink. These signals are connected in parallel to the spin motor: thus the drill rotates always when the step motor moves the head. Position of the head is detected by two logic sensors: up and down

The corresponding *component* is presented in Figure 2. It serves to encapsulate heterogeneous control-related properties and functions of the object. The interface of the component is unified with the interface of IEC61499 function blocks. There are pre-defined classes of inputs/outputs, e.g. Input Commands, uniting the pulse signals, representing the commands from operator, or from the other components; or State Information, representing the parameters of the object or of the environment.

The cornerstone of the component is one or several sub-applications, defining as the structure, as well functionality of the object. The sub-application is an architectural unit defined in IEC61499 for distributable compositions of function blocks. Several sub-applications may be necessary for different configurations such as a pure run-time configuration, or a configuration with real object substituted by its simulation model, or combination of those allowing comparison of the outputs of the real process with the simulated ones.

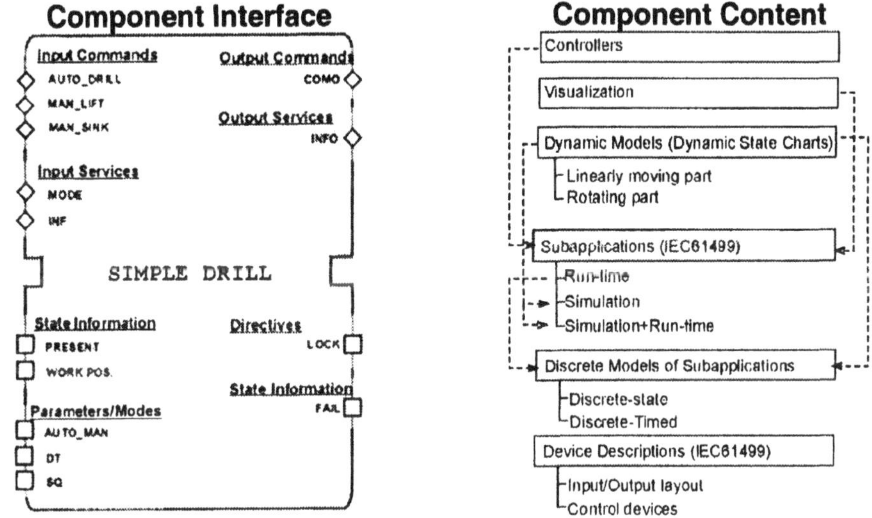

Figure 2. Interface and Constituent Elements of the Component "SIMPLE DRILL".

All these configurations may share common control and visualization functions. The corresponding simulation function blocks may be generated from the formal models of the object's behavior. The models and repositories cannot be encapsulated directly in the framework of IEC61499, so the component serves as a container for all these loosely connected elements. The common XML-based presentation will facilitate integration of elements with the component.

The formal models of the whole sub-applications contained in the component are intended for the use in the automated validation of applications, generated as a result of several components interconnection. These models can be generated from the sub-application descriptions. For the blocks, representing the models of objects within the sub-applications the corresponding "verification-oriented" models can be generated more efficiently with the help of the formal models of objects.

The contained sub-applications are built according to the MVC (Model/View/Control) methodology suggested in [4]. The Figure 3 shows the hierarchical structure sub-application combining the simulation and interaction with the real object. The upper level of the hierarchy is represented by the DM_MVC sub-application. The interface of the component is mapped onto the interface of the contained sub-applications.

Model/View/Controller

The sub-application is constituted from the blocks OBJECT and CONTROLLER interconnected in closed loop to each other, and also connected to the inputs and outputs of the component.

The block OBJECT of type DM_MV (Drill with Motor Model and View) represents the functionality of the equipment, while the block CONTROLLER stands for the control logic. The execution modes include the MANUAL and the AUTOMATIC mode, determined by the AUTO_MAN qualifier. If the qualifier is TRUE (automatic mode) then the OBJECT block receives the control commands (LIFT,

SINK, TURN) from the CONTROLLER. Otherwise these signals are taken from the inputs of the block itself, which can be connected to manual control buttons.

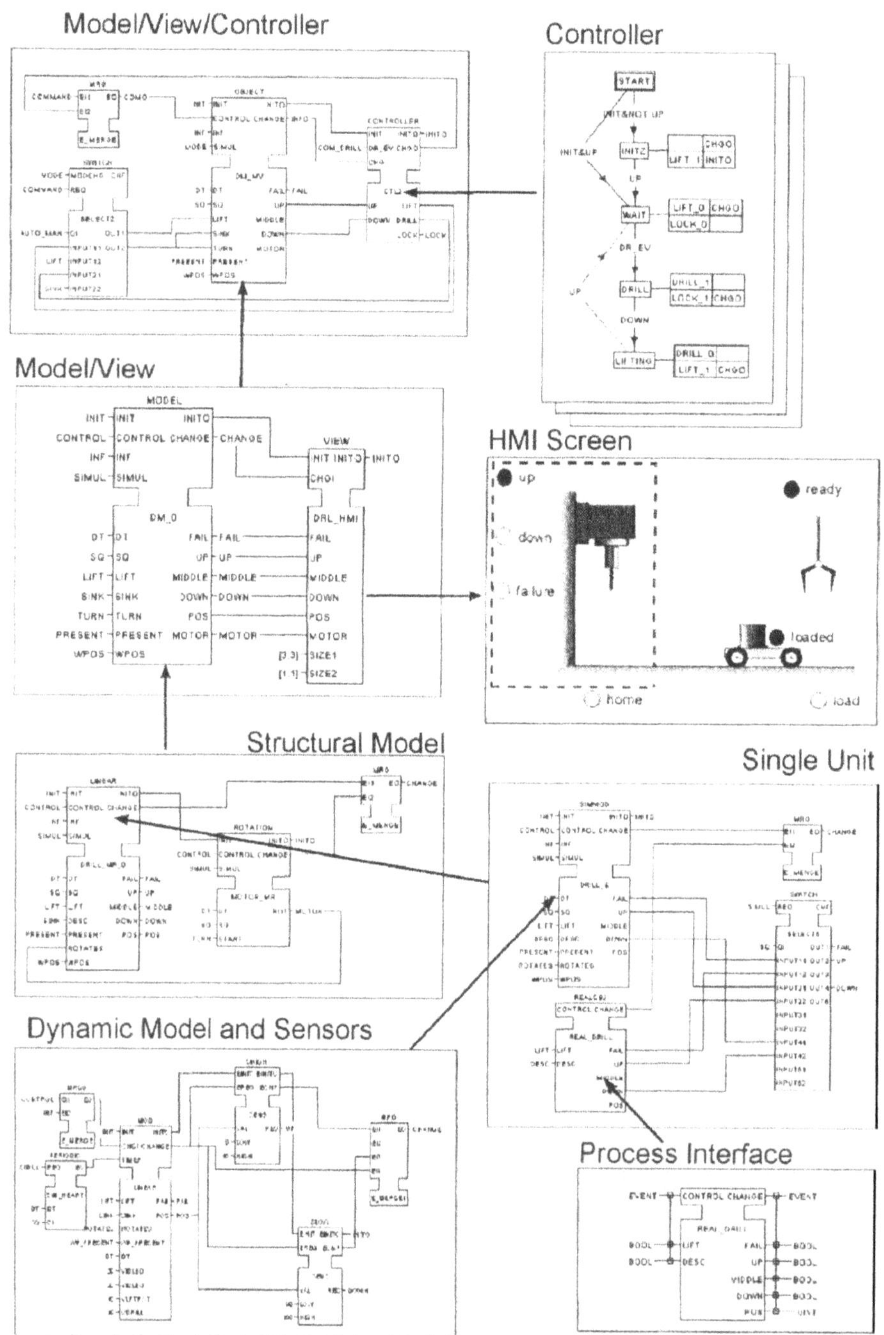

Figure 3. Hierarchical Structure of the MVC Sub-Application.

Model/View

The block VIEW is responsible for displaying of the image of drill on the operator station screen. At every event CHGI the outlined part of the HMI display as shown in the Figure 3, is refreshed given the values obtained from the OBJECT block. Location of the drill's head is displayed according to the coordinate POS.

The block OBJECT of type DM (stands for Drill with Motor) represents the drill itself. Its interface almost copies the interface of DM_MV: all commands and data coming from the controller are directly transferred to DM.

Controller

The sequential control of the drill is defined in the form of sequential function chart. A repository of controllers may be necessary to implement several behavior scenarios of the object.

Structural Model

This level represents the structure of the object. Thus, the DM block represents the model of drill composed from two components: a model of the head as a vertically moving object, and a model of spindle's rotation.

The model reflects the fact of relative independence of the components: axis position of the head has no influence on its rotation, however the rotation status of the motor influences the results of drilling. For this reason the ROT (rotation) output of the ROTATION (Motor) block is connected to the ROTATES input of the model of the head. The blocks LINEAR (of type DRILL_MR_0) and ROTATION encapsulate the functionality of real component units of the object: they receive control inputs and generate the output parameters such as axis position of the head and turning speed of the spin of the motor. They also produce the values of Boolean and analog sensors, e.g. the position sensors UP and DOWN.

Model of a single unit

Next level of the component hierarchy is represented by single functional units of the equipment, such as vertically moving head and rotation motor of the drill. These components can be either further defined by means of dynamic models and models of the corresponding sensors, or can be substituted by direct interfaces to real devices.

The model and the interface to the real process are combined within one function block DRILL_MR (Model + Real object). The event input SIMUL with qualifier SQ controls the way of the outputs assignment: if SQ=TRUE then the SWITCH relays outputs of the simulation model (SIMMOD). Otherwise, if SQ=FALSE, the outputs are taken from the block REALOBJ serving as an interface to the actual DRILL.

Dynamic model

The block MOD (of type LINEAR) encapsulates discrete implementation of the dynamic model of the vertically moving head driven by the motor M_2. State of the model is re-evaluated at every event TIMER. These events are generated by the block PERIODIC with frequency defined by the time discretization parameter DT as long as the simulation qualifier SQ is TRUE. The model produces the numeric parameter POS (in the interval from 0 to 100) indicating vertical position of the head. Blocks SHIGH, SLOW of type SENS represent the discrete sensors, that indicate correspondingly up and the low positions of the head. The LOW and HIGH parameters of the SENS block represent the interval in which must fall the numeric input value VAL in order to the logic output RES to be produced.

3. BUILDING SYSTEMS

3.1 Integration

We illustrate the component-based system design on the following prototype of an automated manufacturing cell, consisting of 3 units as shown in the Figure 4.

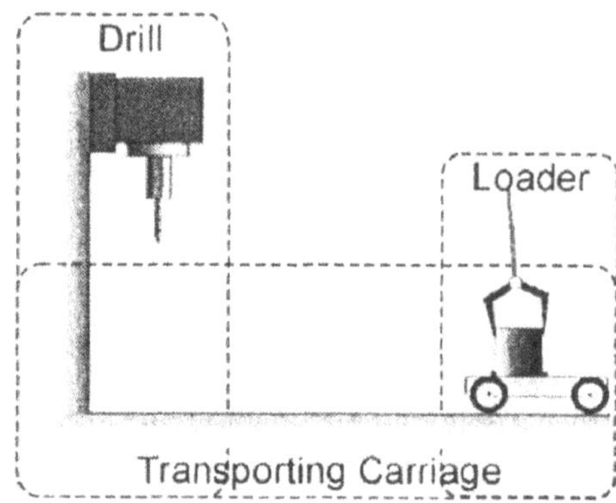

Figure 4. A Prototype of a Modular Manufacturing Cell.

These are the boring machine (*drill*), *carriage*, which delivers workpieces to the home position of the drill, and the *loader* that loads/unloads the carriage in the *loading* position that is opposite to the home position.

The appearance of the workpiece on the carriage is detected by an embedded sensor, so no particular communication between carriage and loader is necessary. Arrival of a new workpiece may serve as a signal to the carriage to approach the drill and request the processing service from it.

This object can be built using constituents from different vendors, having diverse dynamic characteristics, sizes, layouts of sensors/actuators, and other differences. In our case-study we have considered 3 models of drills, and 2 models of loaders and carriages. All the differences between the equipment units are encapsulated within the component descriptions.

Visual tools can facilitate the design process, reducing it to interconnection of components as shown in the following Figure 5. The resultant application is built automatically from the corresponding sub-applications contained in the given components.

The application is appended by the HMI panel, that can be designed with the help of a visual editor and placed into repository is as a component.

In our example, the panel has one button to control switching the simulation mode, and two LEDs indicating failures in drill and in the carriage.

The panel is selected from the repository and added to the Design Screen, that implies the appearance of the corresponding component in the Application window.

This description is enough to generate the application. In this stage the application is independent from the architecture of hardware, where it will be executed.

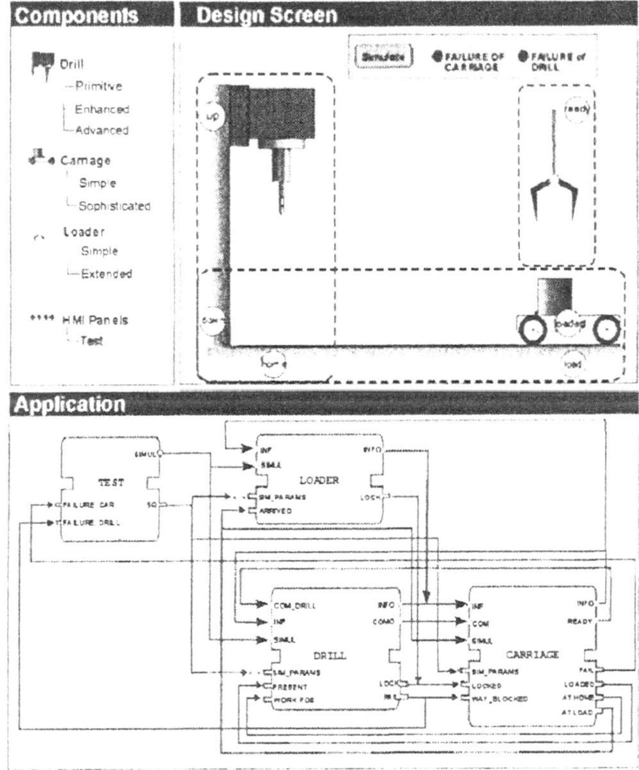

Figure 5. Application Design in a Visual Tool by Plug-And-Play of Components.

3.2 Distribution

Next step of system's implementation is the planning of the architecture. Some possible architectures can be considered with respect to our example. In the architecture, presented in Figure 6 the control is distributed over the constituent parts of the system, while the simulation is conducted on the PC-based station.

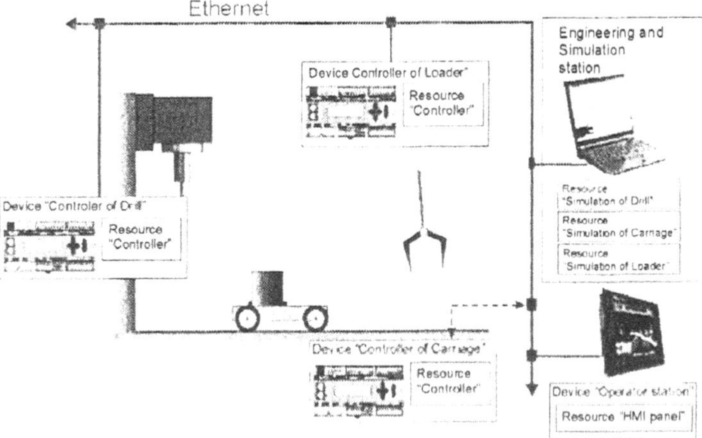

Figure 6. Distributed Control System Architecture.

System configuration in IEC61499 consists of the description of the set of container devices and their resources, and of the mapping of the application's parts onto the containers.

4. MODELING AND VALIDATION

Testing of scalable, flexible automation (SFA) systems having distributed architecture of control is complicated by the following reasons:

- Asynchronous event-driven logic of execution, statically unpredictable combinations of concurrent processes in plant and dynamic scheduling of algorithms in controllers;
- Communication phenomena: use of different protocols, influence of delays, etc.
- Reconfiguration phenomena: the same application could be executed on different architectures;

Dynamic models of controlled equipment are indispensable for simulation, verification, and for interpretation of the verification results by simulation. It is important to unify the modeling process by using a standard self-explanatory problem-oriented visual modeling language.

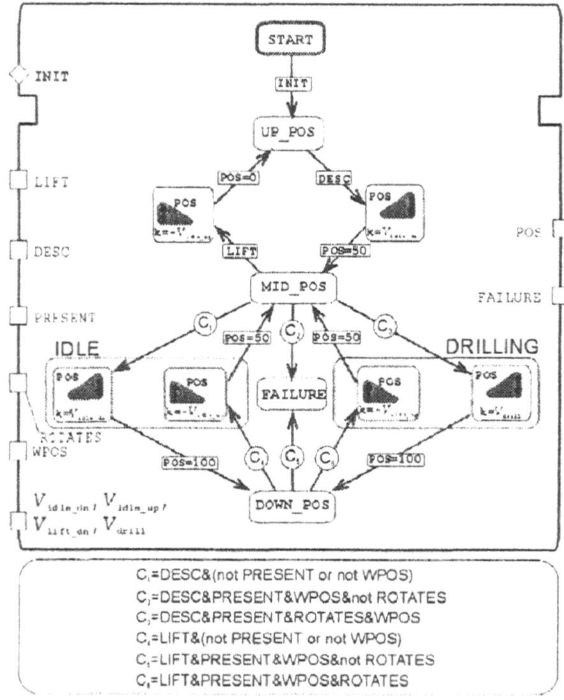

Figure 7. Modular Dynamic State Chart Model of the Linearly Moving Part of the Drill.

We apply for this purpose a customized form of State Charts (the same as used in UML). The customizations concern the set of state shapes, corresponding to particular dynamic properties of parameters, and modular interface, compatible with interface of IEC 61499 function blocks.

The modular interface is unified also with the interface of hybrid and discrete state modeling formalisms, such as: Condition/ Event Automata [5] and Net Condition/Event Systems [6], that simplifies the transformation of state-chart models to these formalisms. The dynamic state chart is built from states (rectangular shapes) and state transitions (arcs) marked with Boolean conditions.

In the chart in the Figure 7 there are two types of states: fixed position states UP_POS, MID_POS, DOWN_POS and dynamic states with linear change of parameter POS as $POS=POS_{old}+kdt$, where the coefficient k is the speed of moving, dt – time increment.

The model describes the following behavior. The head moves free in the upper part of the axis, no matter present the workpiece or not. When the middle position is reached and the control signal DESC remains ON, the head continues its moving downwards. Should the workpiece be in the home position, and the bore spins, then normal drilling goes on. If the drill does not rotate, then it just hits the blank workpiece and a failure occurs. If no workpiece is present, then the drill moves down idle, with the speed higher than that of drilling. The same applies to the moving upwards. Thus the presented model defines *uncontrolled behavior* of the drill (its vertically moving part).

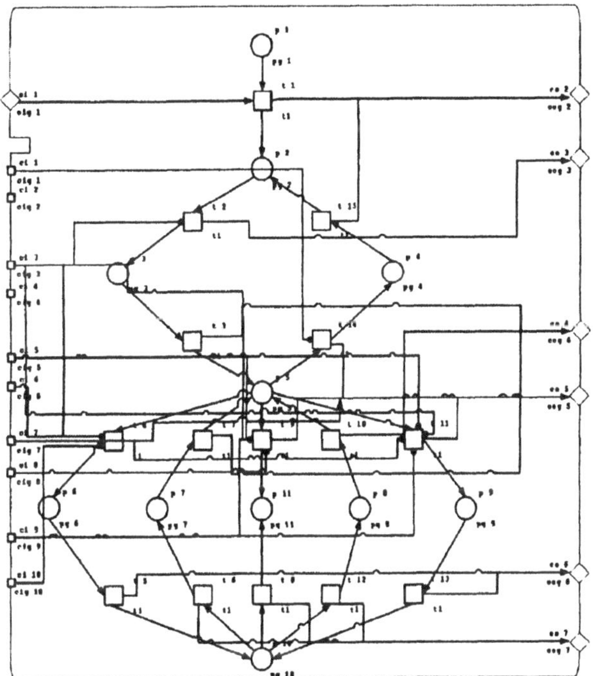

Figure 8. Net Condition/Event Model of the Linearly Moving Part of the Drill.

Note, that the presented model generates the numerical value POS and can be re-used as a core of models for several types of drills with different number of logic position sensors.

The State Chart model can be used to generate discrete state model in Net Condition/Event Systems as presented in Figure 8. The latter is required for conducting the formal validation procedure using the tool VEDA, as it is described in [7].

The module modeling the drill is incorporated into the modularly built NCES model of the application, substituting the block DRILL_M in Figure 3.

The tool VEDA inputs the applications, generates the NCES models for the remaining blocks (not explicitly presented in NCES) and verifies the compliance of the models behavior with the set of pre-given specifications of permitted/forbidden behavior.

6. REFERENCES

1. *Function Blocks for Industrial Process Measurement and Control Systems.* Publicly Available Specification, International Electrotechnical Commission, Tech. Comm. 65, Working group 6, Geneva, 1998.
2. R. Lewis: Modeling Control Systems using IEC 61499, IEE, London, 2001
3. M. Bonfe, C. Fantuzzi: *Mechatronic Objects encapsulation in IEC 1131-3 Norm,* Intl. Conf. on Control Applications, Anchorage, 2002
4. J.H. Christensen: *Design patterns for system engineering with IEC 61459.* Proc. Of Conference "Verteile Automatisierung" (Distributed Automation), pages 63--71, Magdeburg, Germany, 2000
5. S.Kowalewski, P.Herrmann, S.Engell, R.Huuk, H.Krumm, Y.Lakhnech, B.Lukoschus, and H.Treseler: *Approaches to the formal verification of hybrid systems.* Automatisierungstechnik, 2:66--73, 2001.
6. Rausch, M., H.-M. Hanisch. *Net condition/event systems with multiple condition outputs.* In: Symposium on Emerging Technologies and Factory Automation, 1995. Vol.1., INRIA/IEEE. Paris, France. pp.592--600.
7. Vyatkin V., Hanisch H.-M.: *Verification of Distributed Control Systems in Intelligent Manufacturing,* Journal of Intelligent Manufacturing, special issue on Internet Based modeling in Intelligent Manufacturing, *to appear as No.1, 2003*

36 A PRACTICAL REPRESENTATION OF HOLONIC MANUFACTURING SYSTEMS

Shahin Rahimifard
Wolfson School of Mechanical and Manufacturing Engineering
Loughborough University, United Kingdom
S.Rahimifard@lboro.ac.uk

Holonic manufacturing systems is now a well established research area with a significant body of work being undertaken which has resulted in generation of a large number of holonic manufacturing system configurations, architectures and reference models, together with various holonic approaches to the shop floor control, production scheduling, and machine control. There is now a common belief amongst the research community that the application of such holonic concepts would result in meeting the responsiveness and agility of manufacturing activities, necessitated by the modern pressures of the global market. However, the most important challenge remains the persuasion of decision makers within manufacturing companies and in particular small to medium enterprises to adopt these research results in their daily operation. The work reported in this paper is directed at addressing this challenge through realisation of a practical representation of holonic concepts to support a typical machining facility in a form of a laboratory-based demonstrator. In this practical presentation a conscious effort has been made to utilise commercially available and commonly used manufacturing software packages.

1. INTRODUCTION

The term holon was used initially by Koestler (1967) to describe an identifiable part of a system that possesses an individual identity and comprises of sub-ordinate parts. Another concept which Koestler introduced was that of a "holarchy", which is a stable, self-contained system consisting of holons as building blocks (Leeuwen and Norrie 1997). These concepts were adapted and applied to manufacturing systems by Suda (1990) and the Intelligent Manufacturing Systems (IMS) TC5 program to form the contemporary paradigm known as Holonic Manufacturing Systems (Matthews 1995, Van Brussel et al. 1996). In this contemporary paradigm, holons aim at both the co-operation with peer holons to achieve global manufacturing goals and also act autonomously as self-reliant units.

A number of interpretations of holonic concepts for manufacturing may be encountered in literature, and in recent years there has been a significant build up of holonic research initiatives. The most relevant of these to research reported in this paper are the use of holonic concepts in production planning (Sugimura and Moriwaki 1996, Gou et al. 1998, Sousa and Ramos 1999), shop floor control

(Tonshoff and Winkler 1996, Balasubramanian et al. 2000), and developing intelligent controllers for manufacturing workstations (Wyns et al. 1996, Tanaya et al. 1997, Shin and Cho 2001). Furthermore, a number of researchers including the author have explored the application of holonic concepts in human centred systems within Small to Medium Enterprises (SMEs) as outlined in this paper. The research has investigated an innovative approach to management and control of manufacturing SMEs based on a conglomerate of distributed and autonomous holons which operate as a set of cooperating entities based on holonic concepts. In this paper the development of a comprehensive laboratory-based demonstrator is outlined based on implementation of three areas of research, namely a holonic information network, a holonic production planning and control structure and holonic manufacturing workstations. It is intended to utilise this holonic manufacturing demonstrator for *(a)* industrial illustration and visualisation of complex issues related to an autonomous co-operative working practices within a distributed system and how such practices improve the flexibility and performance of manufacturing activities, and *(b)* the training of managers and production operators to be able to adopt this new working culture.

2. HOLONIC REPRESENTATION OF AN SME

SMEs represent the largest proportion of the manufacturing sector, generating more than half of the total production output, in every industrial country. The production system of SMEs are typified by human centred manufacturing systems where the flexibility introduced through utilisation of often multi-skilled operators plays a major role in the agile performance and responsiveness of the company. The major assertions made in this paper are: that the familiar information system hierarchy and range of IT tools employed in larger companies are inappropriate for SMEs. In pursuit of realisation of more efficient IT tools for SMEs a new innovative approach is adopted based on groups of distributed and autonomous holons, operating in a collaborative manner. A holonic business model is developed to represent activities of a typical manufacturing SME, as depicted in figure 1. This model represents an enterprise as an enhanced organisation holarchy which can be viewed to consists of three main holons namely: the executive holon that represents the ultimate decision-making process within the company; the business holon that covers administration activities such as order processing, finance, costing, process planning and scheduling etc.; and the manufacturing holon involving the implementation and monitoring of the production plans produced by the business holon.

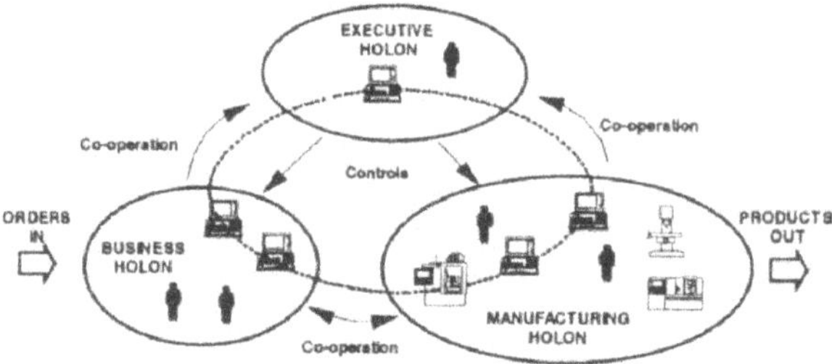

Figure 1 - The Conceptual Holonic Representation of an IT Supported SME

Due to the vital role of individual operators within SMEs, the research is committed to realising the information and planning systems that support the human activity rather than enveloping them. The research was structured around three major work streams as outline below.

2.1. The Generation of a Holonic Information System.

The goal for the specification and design of the holonic information system was to reduce all information subsystems into a one homogeneous integrated system. As the basis for the development of such a homogenous information network, a SME enterprise model is constructed. To capture the holonic perspective within this SME enterprise reference model, a novel three phase approach of control, co-operation and autonomy has been utilised. Readers are referred to Toh *et al.* 1998 for more detailed information on this novel three phase approach which not only enables the information requirements to be modelled but also allows the human centred behaviour of the SME organisation to be represented. The realisation of a holonic information system (HIS) based on this SME enterprise model comprises of a number of node holons, which are defined as a composite of human, manufacturing equipment or software systems and their IT interfaces is depicted in figure 2. The HIS network is supported by a manufacturing and an order database which store and maintain data required to facilitate the functionality of such homogenous information system.

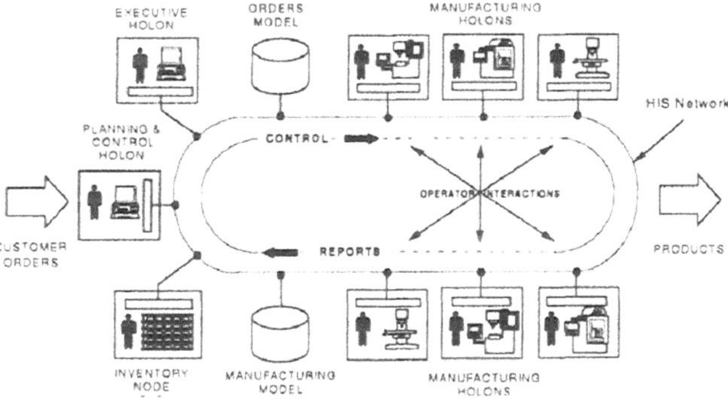

Figure 2 - Holonic Information System

2.2 A Holonic Structure for Planning and Control of SMEs

A heterarchical structure in which a collection of loosely coupled autonomous planning systems are co-operating to achieve an overall manufacturing goal is adopted to develope a planning and control solution tailored to the needs of SMEs, referred to as 'Distributed Autonomous Real Time' (DART) planning and control system (Rahimifard *et al.* 1999). DART utilise a simpler view of SME organisations which classifies these planning and control tasks into two categories of factory level and workstation level. Factory level tasks include the executive and business support activities, carried out by holons such as an executive holon, inventory holon and scheduling holon. The workstation level tasks represent the manufacturing activities, undertaken by manufacturing holons. The factory level tasks convert the customer orders into a set of production orders and the workstation level tasks execute these production orders to generate the required products. In DART a real-time planning approach is utilised based on generation of a 'production order list' (POL). Access to the POL is made available to both the planners and operators across the HIS network. The planner within the scheduling holon has the capability of forcing a production order onto a specific manufacturing holon, or allow them to be selected and processed by one of the manufacturing holons. At workstation level, a large number of criteria, such as priorities, due dates, slack times and commonality with present machine and tool set ups are taken into account to select and process a production order. The completion of the production order is then flagged, and appropriate information with regard to processing of the order is recorded.

2.3. The Holonic Manufacturing Workstation

A holonic manufacturing workstation in this research is considered as the coupling of the human operator with a manufacturing workstation, which has been enhanced through implementation of a specially designed IT support system to aid the operator for the effective operation of the workstation in an autonomous and co-operative manner. This is achieved through the design of a modular software structure consisting of mainly commercial manufacturing software tools which are integrated with other modules across the HIS. As stated, these software modules are grouped at each manufacturing holon to support :-

a) **Autonomous Functions** : These are specific to each and every workstation and are required for local control of the workstation. For example within the machining facilities of a typical SME, such functions could include the modifications of existing part programs, generation of inspection code, management of tools and fixture set-ups, work sequencing, and material planning. Such local functionality enables operators to utilise their skills more effectively in responding to changes in demands and increasing the overall performance of the workstation.
b) **Co-operative Functions** : These are related to the common business and manufacturing goals across the HIS network which are supported by individual operators such as updating shared information relating to customer orders, process planning, manufacturing operations, production planning and inventory control. In addition, co-operative functions enable the operator to view and communicate with other holonic nodes attached to the HIS , as depicted in figure 3.

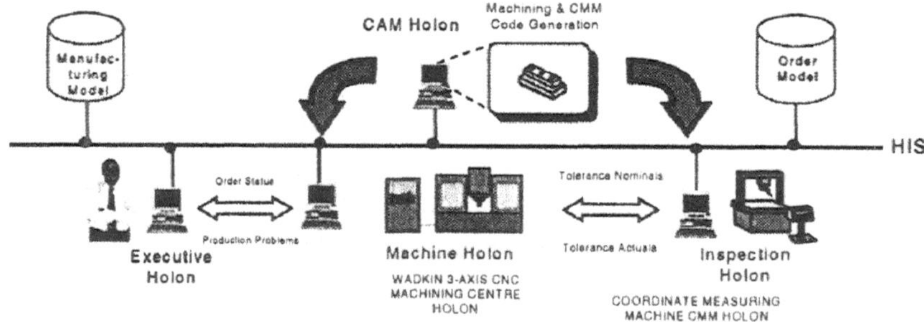

Figure 3 - Autonomous co-operative operations of holonic workstations within HIS

3. LABORATORY-BASED DEMONSTRATOR

One of the main objectives of the research has been the development of visualisation and training tools to facilitate the wide adoption of unfamiliar and complex holonic concepts within contemporary industrial applications. Therefore, a comprehensive laboratory based demonstrator based on the configuration of a typical machining cell within a small metalworking enterprise has been developed, as shown in Figure 4. This production facility consists of a number of computer numerical control milling and turning machines, CNC vertical and horizontal machining centres, a range of conventional machine tools, a co-ordinate measuring machine, and a tool pre-setting workstation. The manufacturing facilities are linked together via a computer network (Microsoft NT network) and each area of manufacturing activity (a manufacturing holon) is equipped with a computer (running Windows NT 4.0). Each of these manufacturing holons is manned by one or more operators. It should be noted that such manufacturing holons could consist of a single workstation (e.g. a PC based CNC machining centre) or a collection of workstations grouped together around a computer node which is linked to the information network (e.g. conventional machine tools or tool prestters). In addition, a number of other computers within the design office, planning office, part and tool store and managers office are linked to this information network which represent the CAD/CAM holon, scheduling holon, inventory holon and executive holon (see figure 4). A special purpose user interface has been designed and implemented which is hosted by every computer linked to the network. This user interface not only provides access to all the software modules supported by the information network, namely the order database, the manufacturing database, the inventory module and the DART scheduler, but also enables the operators of various holons to execute a range of special purpose software packages which are required to support their daily functionality. In addition, this user interface supports a range of bi-directional messaging activities between the various holons within the system, so that not only the instructions can be downloaded by the executive holon or planning holon to the manufacturing holons, but also various types of queries (negotiations) can be made between each holon in the system. In this demonstrator, the typical functions supported by the machining centre holon are:-

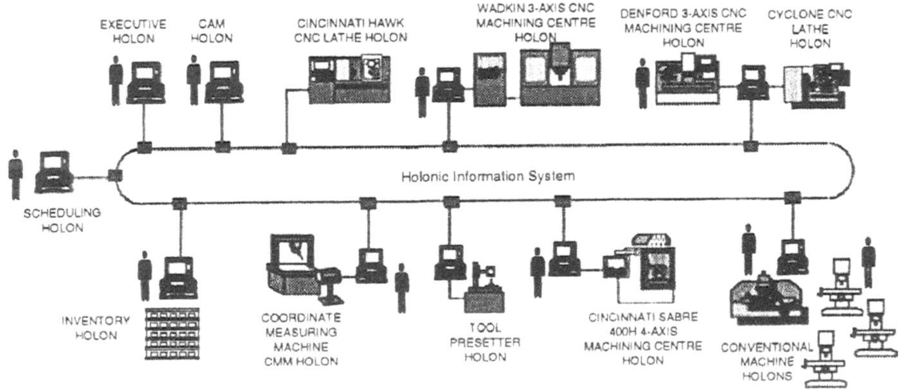

Figure 4 - Schematic of a Laboratory Based Demonstrator

- **NC Program Re-generation :** enables operator to modify part programmes due to changes regarding the size of the raw material billet, tooling configurations, or even small alterations to the design of the component to be machined. There are several commercial systems for the purpose of regeneration of part-programs. One such system is the Mazak CAMWARE (MAZAK 2000) which provides functions such as minor design modifications, tool path simulation and machine code regeneration. Another important feature of this approach is the tool selection being based on the existing tool configuration with the machine tool magazine thus reducing the need for tool exchange and moving the tool to a different pocket number due to restrictions in a part program.
- **NC Program Validation & NC Machine Simulation** : the importance of validation and simulation at the machining processes is very high, as any errors may potentially be very costly due to tool breakage and machine down times, wasted material and delays in delivery times. Therefore a commercial package called VERICUT (CGTech 1998) is used to verify modifications and give the operator confidence before the re-generated part programs are executed.
- **Tool Management** : is used to allow the operator to locate tools and fixtures, from their machine without having to physically go and search through various buffers and storage. Again, a commercial software package, namely ISIS-ATMS (ISIS 2000) is used. This system is capable of informing the operator of the location of a tool item and if it is available for use, assigned to another machine, or actually in use. It can also provide the information concerning whether a particular tool is in a suitable state for the job, i.e. the level of wear it has incurred and whether it has enough life left. To this end, any tool can be swapped locally by the operator, within the workstation or between workstations, to maximise the potential of any set of tools.
- **Material Planning :** allows the operator to have visibility of the material flow and inventory control, and to change some aspects of the material allocated to a specific job e.g. billet size due to a temporary material shortages. A commercial MRP II package, namely Alliance / MFG (1999) has been incorporated within various holons in the HIS to support such functionality.
- **Work Sequencing** : the DART software has been developed using a commercial finite capacity planning system, called PREACTOR (Preactor International 2000). It consists of a number of PREACTOR modules that have been significantly reconfigured to generate a scheduling holon together with a number of local work sequencing modules hosted by each of the other holons within the HIS. This facility enables the workstation holon to receive work orders and instructions from the executive or scheduling holons, whilst at the same time permitting changes to be made locally to the work sequence. The operator may want to change the work sequence for a variety of reasons - from minimising the tool and fixture changes, to slotting in a high priority job.
- **Local Performance Monitoring** : is used to assess any deviations in performance of the machine tool, which may provide an early indication of a problem or fault with the machine. Typical monitoring issues are the accuracy of the machine tool and the set-up and cycle times which are recorded to allow analysis of the amount of time spent actually cutting material, and also the converse of this to view where the majority of non-machining time is spent.

4. CONCLUDING DISCUSSIONS

In the contemporary global market, SMEs must consider the use of modern IT tools and networking to maximise productivity and responsiveness to customer orders. The requirements for such responsiveness to customer requirements have intensified in recent years, as manufacturing SMEs have experienced an urgency for greater flexibility to deal with highly individualistic customer desires for participation in the design and production procedures within the 'engineering-to-order' sector, and the unpredictable pattern of demands in the 'make-to-order' sector. In the late 1980's, and early 1990's, it was commonly assumed that the implementation of CIM concepts would provide such flexibility. This notion is now being challenged by the increasing belief that the implementation of CIM results in manufacturing systems which are in general too rigid and that the attributes of such highly integrated systems with totally predictable patterns of operation will not meet the needs of a modern SMEs.

In pursuit of this greater reactivity, there is a growing opinion that current CIM based organisations should be replaced by more innovative structures based on a conglomerate of distributed and autonomous units which operate as a set of cooperating entities, such as those defined by holonic concepts. This paper has illustrated the development of an IT facility which has been designed and implemented based on holonic concepts for the small manufacturing enterprise. However, the effective utilisation of such novel IT tools and working practices necessitates a significant transition from traditional methods. One of the major tasks facing the researchers of holonic concepts is convincing the industrial decision makers and strategists in particular those within SMEs that their operators can improve performance with such IT facilities and provide the desired flexibility and responsiveness to the customer demands. Identification of the most effective method for description and demonstration and of complex holonic concepts to busy production managers, engineers and operators with varying manufacturing and business knowledge and skills provides tough and interesting challenges. The laboratory-based demonstrator described in this paper is believed to provide a powerful visualisation facility to meet these challenges. Furthermore, this can be used as an efficient training tool for the operator of typical SMEs to familiarise themselves with the modern autonomous co-operative working environment, before adoption of such concepts within their daily operations. The author acknowledges the difficulties in introducing such significant changes in working cultures, but argues that the utilisation of such holonic structures and systems provide a number of commonly desired operational characteristics within SMEs, i.e.

- Reducing delays in processing of customer orders within the pre-production activities.
- Supporting distributed decision making to strengthen the role of the skilled and experienced production operators.
- Supporting frequent interactions between planners and operators via an information network.
- Incorporating a dynamic real time approach to enable extreme agility in responding to customer pressures.

5. ACKNOWLEDGEMENTS

This work has been carried out as part of a collaborative research programme at Loughborough University and funded by the Engineering and Physical Science Research Council (EPSRC), entitled 'IT Tools to Improve Manufacturing Performance of Metalworking SMEs' (GR/L/27077). The author would also like to acknowledge the contributions Dr N Shires of PREACTOR International, Mr G Herrington of ISIS Informatics Ltd and the colleagues of the Advanced Manufacturing Technology Centre at Loughborough University.

6. REFERENCES

1. Alliance Manufacturing Software International, 1999, Warrens Business Park, Leicester – UK, http://www.alliancenfg.com.
2. Balasubramanian S, Zhang X, Norrie DH, 2000, Intelligent control for holonic manufacturing systems, Proceedings of Institution Mechanical Engineers Part-B: Journal of Engineering Manufacture, 214 (B10), 953-961.
3. CGTech Ltd, 1999, The Coach House Shipwright's Yard, Brighton – UK, http://www.cgtech.com.
4. Gou L, Luh PB, Kyoya Y, 1998, Holonic manufacturing scheduling: architecture, co-operation mechanism and implementation, Computers in Industry, 37 (3), 213-231.
5. ISIS Informatics Ltd, 1999, Woodside Park, Godalming – UK, http://www.isistool.co.uk.
6. Koestler A, 1967, The Ghost in the Machine, (Arkana Books, London).
7. Leeuwen EH and Norrie D, 1997, Holons and Holarchies, Manufacturing Engineering, 76 (2), 86-88.
8. Matthews J, 1995, Organisational foundations of intelligent manufacturing systems- the holonic viewpoint, Computer Integrated Manufacturing Systems, 8 (4), 237-243.
9. Preactor International, 2000, Cornbrash Park, Chippenham – UK, http://www.preactor.com.
10. Rahimifard S, Newman ST and Bell R, 1999, Distributed Autonomous Real Time Planning and Control of SMEs, Institute of Mechanical Engineer – Part B : Journal of Engineering Manufacture, 213 (B5), 475 – 489.
11. Shin J, Cho H, 2001, Planning and sequencing heuristics for featured-based control of holonic machining equipment, International Journal of Flexible Manufacturing Systems, 13 (1), 49-70.
12. Sousa P, Ramos C, 1999, A distributed architecture and negotiation protocal for scheduling in manufacturing systems, Computers in Industry, 38 (2), 103-113.
13. Suda H, 1990, Future Factory Systems Formulated in Japan, Japanese Journal of Advanced Automated Technology, 23 (3), 51-61.
14. Sugimura N, Moriwaki T, 1996, Modelling of holonic manufacturing system and its application to real-time scheduling, Proceedings of CIRP Seminars - Manufacturing Systems, 25 (4), 345-352.
15. Tanaya PI, Detand J, Kruth J.-P., 1997, Holonic machine controller: a study and implementation of holonic behaviour to current NC controller, Computers in Industry, 33 (2-3), 323-333.
16. Toh KTK, Newman ST, Bell R, 1998, An Information Architecture for Small MetalWorking Companies, Proceedings of Institution Mechanical Engineers-Part-B: Journal of Engineering Manufacture, 212, 87-103.
17. Toh KTK, Newman ST, Bell R, 1998, An Information Architecture for Small MetalWorking Companies, Proceedings of Institution Mechanical Engineers-Part-B: Journal of Engineering Manufacture, 212, 87-103.
18. Tonshoff HK, Winkler M, 1996, Shop control for holonic manufacturing systems, Proceedings of CIRP Seminars - Manufacturing Systems, 25 (3), 227-281.
19. Van Brussel H, Valckenaers P, Wyns J, Bongaerts L, Detand J, 1996, Holonic Manufacturing Systems and LiM, in Brown et. al. (Eds.) : IT and Manufacturing Partnerships, 185-196.
20. Wyns J, Van Brussel H, Valckenaers P, Bongaerts L, 1996, Workstation Architecture in holonic manufacturing systems, Proceedings of 28th CIRP International Seminar on Manufacturing Systems, Johannesburg, South Africa.

37 HOLONIC MANAGEMENT SYSTEM FOR HIERARCHICAL ROBOT GROUPS

Yasumichi Aiyama
University of Tsukuba, aiyama@esys.tsukuba.ac.jp

This paper introduces a management system for robot groups with "holonic architecture" which is one of distributed and hierarchical system architectures. In order to manage collaboration of many robots, we put sub-management system on each work sub-space. A management system on a sub-space divides a task given by upper space into some sub-tasks and gives lower sub-spaces those sub-tasks. With this architecture we obtain distributed and hierarchical management system for the whole work space. We made a demonstration system and showed an example of task division and execution.

1. INTRODUCTION

There are several studies of multi-agent system. In the field of robotics, one of the most efficient targets of multi-agent system is production plant. In the production plant, there are several assembly robots, AGVs, machining tools, storages etc. They are considered as agents that have various characteristics.

Current production plant systems adopt central control method. It is because that the most efficient method is the lowest cost method and it can neglect the cost to make system motion plan. It depends that once we make a production line, it is not changed long time and also it products very large number of product.

But today, consumers' needs have become diversified. The life cycle of products has been shorten in the area of manufacturing. So, in these days, several researchers have started various studies with multi-agent system concept for highly flexibility against change of production plan. For example, Iwata et al. introduced RMS (Random Manufacturing System) (Iwata, 1994) and Ramos introduced similar structured distributed production system (Ramos, 1996). In Denso Corp., Hanai et al. realized practical autonomous mobile robot system APS (Adaptive Production System) (Hanai, 2001).

As an international joint research program, there is IMS (Intelligent Manufacturing System) program. IMS has several projects. One of them is HMS (Holonic Manufacturing System) project that was started at 1996 and it aims to research flexible and agile production system. Concept of holon is proposed by Koestler, a philosopher in 1967 (Koestler, 1967). Holon is an agent that has autonomy and cooperability. It is a component of hierarchical system; that means that all system components is a part of a stratum and acts as the whole for lower stratum component and as a part for upper component. For example, a human body consists of various organs, an organ consists of several cells, a cell consists of various small elements, and so on. Koestler names these elements as "holon"' and this hierarchy as "holarchy."

In HMS project, we introduce the concept of holon and holarchy into production system to give flexibility and agility against demand. Production plant can be regarded as one of holonic system. Factory holon that manages the whole of the factory consists of some division holons that manage manufacturing, material management, design et al. They cooperate to achieve the function of the factory. And each division holon also consists some sub-divisions with cooperation for achievement of the function of the division.

There are several systems of HMS. Valckenaers compared holonic architecture, holarchy, to hierarchy and heterarchy and the three are assessed according to six criteria (Valckenaers, 1997). Ramos studied dynamic scheduling on the holonic system (Ramos, 1996). Arai et al. constructed holonic robot system that has similar architecture with Ramos's system (Arai, 1997)(Arai, 1999).

These researches are mainly concerned with a single production cell. In this paper, we pay attention to hierarchy of the production plant elements; factory, shop, cell and robot. We will introduce management architecture that has recursive structure for each hierarchical layer.

2. HOLONIC MANAGEMENT SYSTEM FOR HIERARCHICAL ROBOT GROUPS

2.1 Management of Robot Groups by Hierarchization

In case we intend to manage a number of cooperation tasks by two or more robots, two major methods can be considered. One is that a single management system manages intensively. The other is that each robot manages in autonomous distributed control. However, by these methods, there are some problems such as fault tolerance and increase of the amount of communication. So in these methods, to manage of great many robots is difficult.

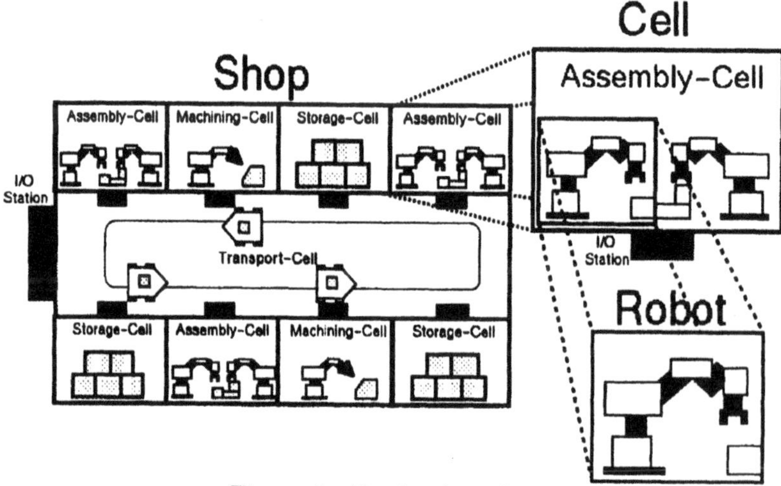

Figure 1 – Production plant

One example of management system that adjusts to great many robots is a production plant. Figure 1 shows a conceptual figure of working area called "Shop" in a production plant. Shop consists of one or more cells, and each cell consists of one or more robots. Inside of a cell, robots execute cooperation tasks such as machining, assembling, and storing. Inside a shop, cells cooperate mutually and execute more complicated tasks. A production plant handles complicated tasks by dividing a task hierarchically in this structure. Therefore it mitigates the complexity of a task in each working area. This mechanism is expected to be effective in managing cooperation tasks that are executed by great many robots. This architecture is suited for the holonic concept. So we adopt holonic system to manage this hierarchical system.

2.2 Unit and Sub-unit

When we intend to manage great many robots with distributed and hierarchical architecture, it can manage more efficiently if it has the same mechanism on each layer. Therefore, we defined a basic unit that manages tasks in a layer and subunits that compose the basic unit.

Unit is a set of subunits and manages tasks by making subunits cooperate mutually

Subunit is an element that composes the upper unit. A subunit is a unit itself and has subunits in its inside.

2.3 Tasks Executed in a Unit

Tasks executed in a unit are cooperation tasks of subunits. In this research, we defined two kinds of tasks. They are abstracted tasks of production plants. They are classified into the following two tasks.

Proper task is proper action that a unit gives to target objects

Transport task is delivering a target object to adjoining unit

A task can be divided into subtasks called operations, which are distributed to subunits.

3. UNIT MANAGEMENT HOLON

3.1 Architecture of a Unit Management Holon

We embraced the concept of the holonic system on unit management system in order to manage hierarchical architecture. Elements shown in the Figure 2 with ellipse are holons. They manage a unit by mutual cooperation.

A unit management system divides a task into one or more operations and distributes them to subunits. Then they execute and manage the tasks. If the task is a proper task, the system distributes operations by contract net protocol with blackboard model. By this model, a unit management system does not have to have status of subunits. If the task is a transport task, the system contracts with subunits directly without the blackboard model.

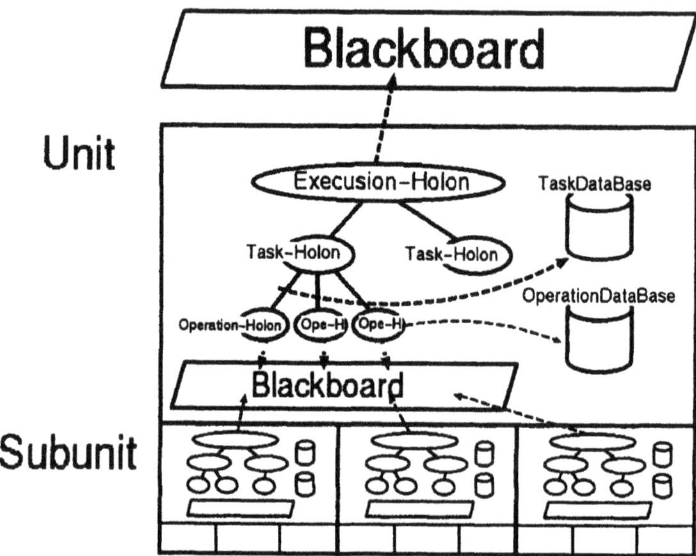

Figure 2 – Unit Management Holarchy

And the system makes a route for transportation based on contiguity relation of subunits. The relation is described in a database. So all the subunits laying on the route join into a group for transportation.

A unit management system has following 4 layers inside. They have hierarchy for management.

Unit Execution Layer (Execution Holon)

In this layer, there is a single execution holon. The execution holon negotiates with operation holons that exist in its upper layer. And it manages all the tasks that are executed in the unit.

Task Layer (Task Holon)

In this layer there are some task holons. Each task holon manages a single task. A task holon divides a task into operations and manages them.

Operation Layer (Operation Holon)

In this layer there are some operation holons. Each operation holon manages a single operation. An operation holon negotiates with execution holons of its subunits. Then it selects one or more suitable execution holons and distributes the holons the operation.

Subunit Execution Layer (Execution Holon)

In this layer there are execution holons of subunits. Each subunit has a single execution holon. And each execution holon negotiates with the operation holons of the unit.

In a unit management system, there are some other elements. They are blackboard, task database and operation database. A blackboard is place on which operation holons put public offerings to subunits. And a task database is a database in which data of proper tasks are stored. Operation database is a database in which the data of contiguity relation of subunits are stored.

A unit management system is a part of the whole management system. And the whole system has hierarchical connection of unit management systems.

3.2 Algorithm of Task Management

In a unit management system, holons manage the unit by communicating mutually. The communication of holons travel from upper layer to lower layer hierarchically.

Following explains a process of task management in a unit.

1. An operation holon in an upper layer puts a public offering on the blackboard in the upper layer.
2. The execution holon checks the blackboard. When it finds the public offering, it uses the task database and searchs data of the task.
3. If the execution holon succeeds to find, it generates a task holon for estimation of execution time.
4. The task holon starts the estimation. It divides the task into operations. Then it generates operation holons as many as the operations.
5. Each operation holon begins to search suitable subunits by putting public offerings on the blackboard to reserve them.
6. The task holon is observing the operation holons. If all the operation holons succeed to reserve, then it waits request from the execution holon. It is the completion of the estimation.
7. The execution holon is observing the task holon. If the task holon succeeds to estimate, it bids the public offering with the estimation and negotiates with the operation holon in the upper layer. Then it is reserved by the upper operation holon and begins to wait for the request from it.
8. If the execution holon receives request for executing the task from the operation holon in the upper layer, it sends request for executing the task to the task holon.
9. If the task holon receives request from the execution holon, it sends request for executing the operations to each operation holon according to the work procedure.
10. Each operation holon sends the request for executing to subunit execution holons.

Task holons and operation holons show the progress of the tasks and the operations as their states. For example, a task holon takes state of "estimate" when it is in estimation. And an operation holon also takes the state of "estimate" when it puts public offering and waits for bids. And if it succeeds to reserve suitable subunits, it takes state of "ready".

Holons have some other states such as "execute", "complete", and so on. "Execute" states that a holon is executing a task or an operation. "Complete" states that a holon has already completed a task or an operation.

4. SIMULATION

4.1 System Construction Using Java

To construct a simulation system, we used Java language that is an object oriented-language. By using an object-oriented language, we can efficiently develop elements of system as independent modules. If we intend to update a module, we don't have to mention all the system and just to update the single module. Being compared with other languages such as C, Java provides advanced functions for networking. And we can use easily functions such as two way communication by using a platform provided by Java.

4.2 Composition of the Simulation System

The composition of the simulation system is shown in Figure 3. A shop consists of an assembly cell, a transport cell, and 2 I/Os (I/O is a transport buffer). The assembly cell consists of 3 manipulators (Rob1, Rob2, Rob3), 2 storages (St1, St2) and 2 I/Os (I/O1, I/O2). The transport cell consists of an AGV. Each manipulator has a proper task that the manipulators inserts Part B into Part A. The shop and the assembly cell have a proper task of assembling P. In the shop, task assembling P divides into a single proper operation of assembling P that is a proper task of the assembly cell. In the assembly cell the task assembling P is divided into 4 operations, transporting A, transporting B, inserting B into A and transporting P.

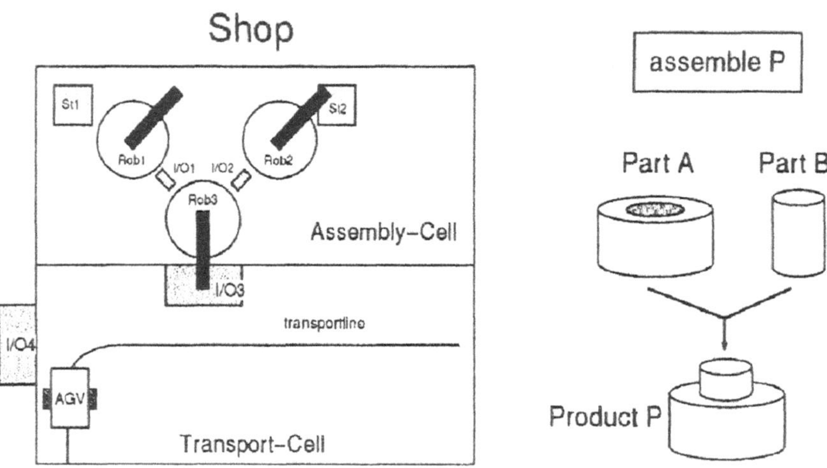

Figure 3 – Composition of Simulation System

4.3 Simulation and Result

In the simulation system, a user is the top level of the hierarchy. The user orders the shop to execute tasks by putting public offerings on a blackboard for the shop. We carried out the simulation on following condition. Time limit of public offerings to a shop is 10[sec], time limit of public offerings to cells is 5[sec], time limit of public offerings to robots is 1[sec], time required by robots for inserting is 10[sec] and time required by AGV for transporting is 20[sec]. Parts required for assembling P exist in the assembly cell beforehand.

The user puts the public offering for assembling P at 0[sec]. Then, 1 second later for completing assembling P, the user puts the public offering for transport P. We carried out this simulation for several times.

Figure 4 shows two results of the simulation. The states of task holons and operation holons in each unit and the actions executed by each unit along time are shown in the figure. The two cases are chosen from various results of simulation.

Comparing result (1) with result (2), it becomes clear that although we carry out the same simulation several times, different results have come out. The reason is that 3 manipulators have the same performance and we do not optimize in negotiation of operation holons and execution holons. So in the assembly cell, the robot group that executed the task had different compositions each time.

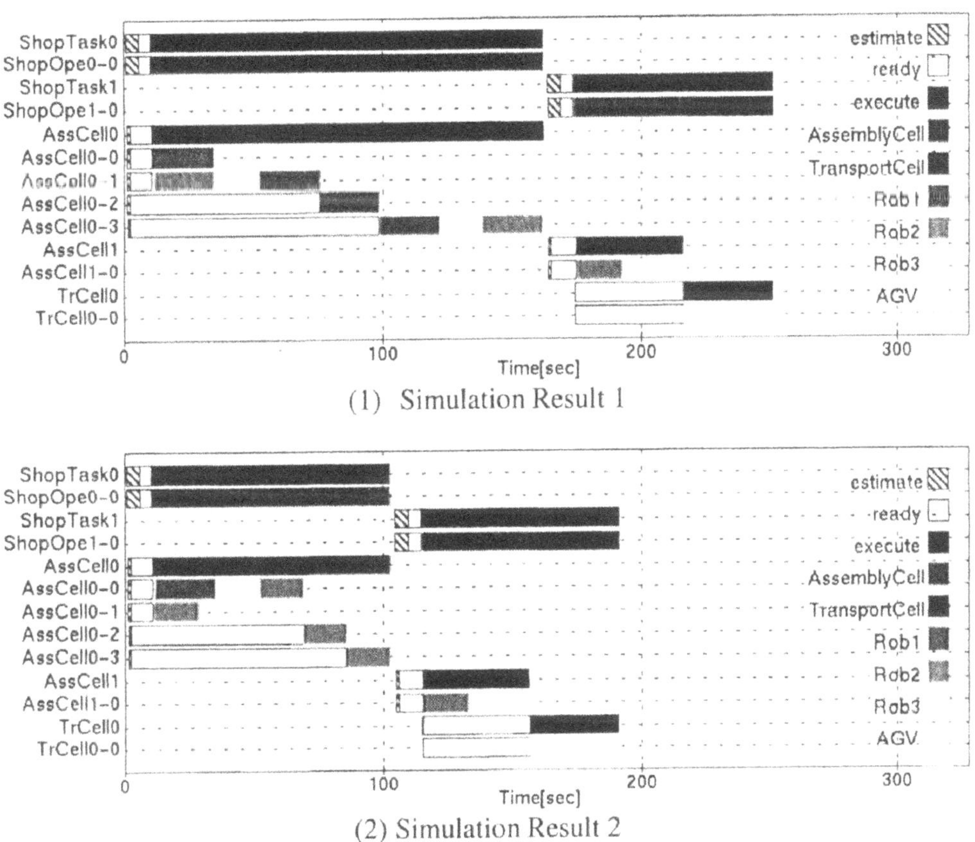

(1) Simulation Result 1

(2) Simulation Result 2

Figure 4 – Two Results of Simulation

4.4 Demonstration System

We have made a demonstration system for visualization of simulation result by using LEGO Mindstorms. LEGO Mindstorms are toy blocks and we can create various mechanisms with them. As they provide motors and sensors, we control them by using the programmable control device called RCX. We have created robots such as manipulators, conveyer and so on. By using LEGO Mindstorms, it needs much less cost for construction of a demonstration system comparing with using actual industrial robots.

5. CONCLUSION

In this research, we noticed the distributed and hierarchical architecture of production plants and suggested a technique for cooperation tasks by great many robots. Then we constructed a simulation system and visualized it on a demonstration system.

When we carried out simulation, the usage of subunits brought differences of working term. So what remains to be done are following.

- Introduction of a scheduler that manages middle or long term plans.
- Introduction of negotiation based on difference of performance of robots.

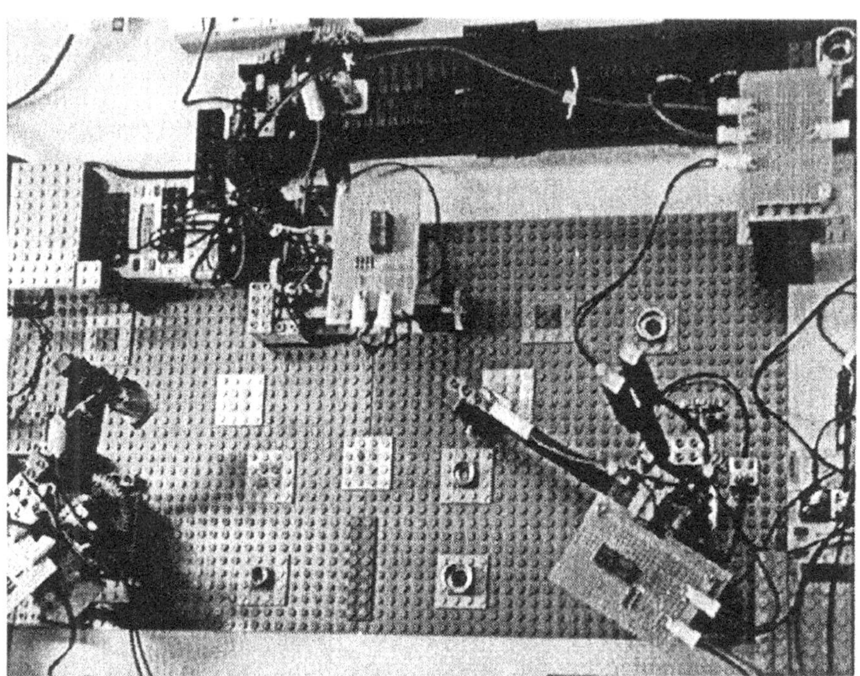

Figure 5 – Overview of the Demonstration System

6. ACKNOWLEDGEMENT

This research is supported by IMS (Intelligent Manufacturing System) / HMS (Holonic Manufacturing System) project.

7. REFERENCES

1. Arai, T et al. "Holonic Storage: An Assembly and Storage Cell by Manipulation using Environment". Proc. 29th CIRP Int. Seminar on Manufacturing systems, 1997: 221-226.
2. Arai, T et al. "Holonic Assembly System with Plug & Produce". Proc. Second Int. Workshop on Intelligent Manufacturing Systems, 1999: 119-126.
3. Hanai, M et al. "Development of Adaptive Production System to Market Uncertainty – Autonomous Mobile Robot System --". Proc. Int. Symp. On Assembly and Task planning, 2001: 61-66.
4. Iwata, K et al. "Random Manufacturing System: A New Concept of Manufacturing System for Production to Order". Annals of the CIRP, Vol.43, No.1, 1994: 379-383.
5. Koestler, A. "A Ghost in the Machine". Arkana, 1967.
6. Ramos, C et al. "A Holonic Approach for Task Scheduling in Manufacturing Systems". Proc. Int. Conf. on Robotics and Automation, 1996: 2511-2516.
7. Valckenaers, P et al. "Holonic Manufacturing Systems". Integrated Computer Aided Engineering, No.4, 1997: 191-201.

38

PROCESS PLANNING AND SCHEDULING WITH MULTIAGENT SYSTEMS

Berend Denkena
Hans Kurt Tönshoff
Michael Zwick
Peer-Oliver Woelk
Institute of Production Engineering and Machine Tools, University of Hannover, Germany
{denkena|toenshoff|zwick|woelk}@ifw.uni-hannover.de

This paper deals with the approach of application of intelligent software agents to improve information logistics in the area of process planning and production control. Thus, enterprises will be able to fulfil the requirement of flexible, reliable and fault-tolerant manufacturing. Fulfilment of these requirements is a prerequisite for successful participation in modern business alliances like supply chains, temporal logistic networks and virtual enterprises. Thus, agent-based improvements of information logistics enable enterprises to face the challenges of competition successfully. Current research activities focus on the development of agent-based systems for integrated process planning and production control. They led to the "IntaPS" approach, which is presented in this paper.

1. INTRODUCTION

Since the last decade is characterized by far-reaching changes in global economy and liberalization, modern management trends such as just-in-time manufacturing, or reduction of vertical range of manufacture are of increasing importance to realize shortened time-to-market and a more flexible consideration of customer' demands. However, modern industrial products are often characterized by a high complexity of design, functionality and necessary manufacturing and assembly processes. Computer systems for the support of process planning, production control, and scheduling tasks have to handle critical paths, bottlenecks and risk of failures within real-time. On the one hand, this situation provides the opportunity for small and medium-sized enterprises (SME) to improve their competitiveness within global economy. They participate in supply chains and form virtual enterprises to fulfil specific customer demands. On the other hand, the ability to perform efficient handling and processing of all necessary information is of increasing importance.

Thus, so-called "information logistics" is one of the crucial factors for business success of enterprises. This paper presents the approach to improve in-house information logistics in the field of process planning and scheduling by the application of intelligent software agents.

2. SITUATION IN THE APPLICATION DOMAIN

2.1 Existing Challenges in the Application Domain

Companies participating in supply chains and virtual enterprises have to meet several requirements such as providing a specified product at a defined time to the customer reliably. Since customers will switch to other contractors for their orders in future if their requirements are not met (e.g. by repeated delivery delay), unfulfilled requirements will weaken the market position with a lasting influence. From a holistic point of view ("top-down point of view"), the supply chain as a whole is as efficient as the weakest "link", respective an inefficient enterprise. Thus, each enterprise aims to reach a high economic viability and to become a strong and reliable link of the supply chain. Therefore, it is important to take all necessary organisational measures to keep estimated manufacturing costs and due dates as well as to meet contracted quality of the product. One of these organisational measures deals with the improvement of internal information logistics, because availability of information is a crucial factor for modern enterprises in a dynamic environment.

This challenging situation is enforced not only by dynamic behaviour of the supply chain itself but also by other trends in modern product design and manufacturing. It effects internal structures of the enterprise ("bottom-up point of view"). For example, customers demand highly customised products even in serial production ("mass customisation") which leads to a large number of variants. Thus, modern manufacturing systems must be able to handle several products and variants with small lot sizes simultaneously. Furthermore, modern products are characterized by a high complexity of design. They take advantage of an integrated design of mechanical, electrical and information processing components ("mechatronics"). In conjunction with innovative product design, manufacturing processes need to be improved as well. These optimisation procedures depend on information about constraints and suitable parameters of all involved manufacturing processes (Tönshoff & Siebert, 2001). Thus, improvements of internal information logistics are not only a demand resulting from the holistic point of view of the supply chain as a whole. From a bottom-up point of view, these improvements are necessary for every modern manufacturing system, too. Consequently, modern manufacturing is in need of new and innovative concepts for improved information logistics.

2.2 Current Situation in the Area of Process Planning and Production Control

With respect to the manufacturing domain, attention has to be drawn to process planning and production control. The traditional approach of separating planning activities like process planning from executing activities like production control and scheduling is characterized by strong borderlines. These borderlines result in a gap between involved systems which implies a loss of time and information. This situation becomes obvious for example in the strict spatial as well as temporal separation of process planning and production control. In most cases, static linear process plans are used for information exchange. Thus, the current situation in industrial application is characterised by several disadvantages like:

- Information about capacity and current load of resources as well as further economic aspects remain disregarded while generating conventional static process plans.
- In case of unexpected events like machine breakdown, missing devices or tools etc. at the shop floor, process plan modifications are carried out on shop floor level. This will lead to feasible, but not to optimal results. On the other hand, modifications carried out by a centralised process planning group are very time-consuming.
- Complexity of manufacturing processes and the knowledge necessary for process planning increase. Due to well-trained workers, this knowledge is available at shop floor level mostly. It often takes a long time until this knowledge is available at a centralised process planning group.
- Due to the lack of knowledge exchange, quality and reliability of planning results will be reduced on a long-term basis.
- Advantages of the application of innovative manufacturing technologies, which are often more suitable regarding ecological aspects, remain unused.

Since it is indispensable to improve information logistics in process planning and production control, several research activities tried to find suitable solutions. A very promising approach is the use of multiagent systems. Ongoing research activities at the Institute of Production Engineering and Machine Tools, Hannover, focus on this field and are carried out in cooperation with the Center for Computing Technologies, Bremen. These activities led to the "IntaPS" approach.

2.3 Existing Approaches to Overcome Known Limitations

2.3.1 Integration of Process Planning and Production Control

The aim of integration of process planning and production control functionality is well known for several years. Since the end of the 1980ies, several research projects worked on this problem, but most of these projects based on centralised system architectures and used approaches like bulky, non-linear process plans, e.g. the EC joint-research projects FLEXPLAN and COMPLAN (Tönshoff *et al.*, 1989, Kruth & Detand, 1992). Current research activities use flexible process plans for scheduling of flexible manufacturing systems or apply AI techniques to improve the procedure of process planning (Teti & Kumara, 1997). A very interesting approach ("EtoPlan") is presented by Kals, Zijm and Giebels (Giebels *et al.*, 1998, Giebels, 2000).

2.3.2 Application of Software Agents in the Manufacturing Domain

Very interesting and promising developments deal with intelligent software agents to improve information logistics in the manufacturing domain. First applications of multiagent based concepts are implemented yet. Most of these applications aim at scheduling problems and resource allocation like the "MAPS" system (Wellner & Dilger, 1998). "MAPS" is a multiagent production planning system, which was part of a joint-research project called "INKAD". The system comprises functionality for middle-term and short-term scheduling with regard to the current shop floor situation as well as an interface to communicate with a commercial PPC system ("Production Planning and Control"). Further approaches focus on applications with a less detailed but wider scope like plant design, inter-enterprise relationship and supply-chain management.

Another important application is the design of "Holonic Manufacturing Systems" (HMS). The idea of HMS is promoted by an international IMS research project ("Intelligent Manufacturing Systems") for instance. A "Holon" is an autonomous and co-operative building block of a manufacturing system. It consists of an information processing part, and can also contain a physical processing part or even a human being. Thus, the concept of holons has a wider scope than a pure intelligent software agent. Furthermore, a holon can be part of another holon. Thus, the presence of hierarchies (called "holarchies") is a basic concept of HMS. Furthermore, a holon may belong to more than one holarchy at the same time which is an important difference to the traditional concept of hierarchies. A very comprehensive overview of holonic scheduling technologies is given by L. Bongaerts (Bongaerts, 1998). Current HMS research activities at IFW focus on holonic scheduling algorithms (Zwick & Brandes, 2001).

3. AGENTBASED ARCHITECTURE FOR INTEGRATED PROCESS PLANNING AND PRODUCTION CONTROL

3.1 Basic Architectural Concepts of the "IntaPS" Approach

Since most applications of software agents in the manufacturing domain focus on planning and scheduling tasks from a logistic point of view, the main topic of the current research project "IntaPS" is set to agent-based integration of process planning and production control. Thus, technological information about various products and product variants are handled in addition to economic information in a very flexible and distributed way.

Since the application of co-operative multiagent systems (MAS) and intelligent agents seems to be very promising, MAS also open up risks for the safety and security of enterprises and the robustness of the (distributed) production. The security issues associated with agents in real-world industrial applications fall into three major groups: integrity attacks, privacy attacks, and denial of service attacks. Therefore, it is necessary to establish adequate security mechanisms (e.g. certification mechanisms for dynamic trusted relationships in supply chains) or to restrict MAS to trusted cooperation partners only (e.g. "rational agents" and "closed markets"). Recent research deals with the first issue, but for implementation of MAS in today's production processes, it seems to be necessary to apply the latter security approach and to restrict MAS to trustful participants.

The "IntaPS" approach is based on the application of co-operative agents and in-house electronic marketplaces. The basic architecture of "IntaPS" consists of two substantial components, which link information systems of earlier stages of product development and the resources on the shop floor (see Figure 1). This link is realised by decentralised planning on shop floor level and by rough level process planning.

3.2 Decentralised Planning Unit on Shop-Floor Level

A multiagent system implements decentralised planning on shop-floor level. The co-operative agents act very closely to the shop floor and have access to production data at any time. Within this architecture three different types of agents are used, resource, order, and service agents.

Each relevant resource of the production system and its environment is represented by an *resource agent*. In contrast to a "Holon", the real world entity is not part of the artificial concept of the agent. Agents exist for e.g. machines, assembly workplaces, transportation devices as well as virtual resources like business information systems, CAM systems for NC code generation or legacy information systems. Resource agents provide local knowledge bases of associated resources. The entirety of all resource agents represents the shop floor model of the whole production system.

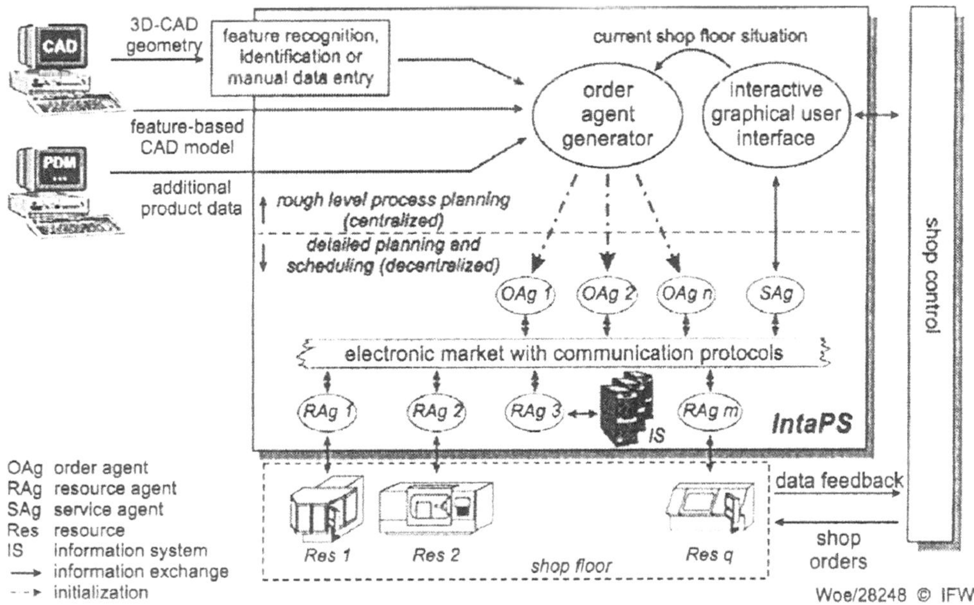

Figure 1 – Basic architecture of the "IntaPS" approach

Order agents represent orders for manufacturing and pursue the goal of market-based optimisation (i.e. optimise utility functions representing their individual goals). Different order agent types vary in divergent weights of goals within their utility functions: An order agent representing a rush order will rate the goal "finished on scheduled due date" higher than the goal "using cost-efficient manufacturing processes", for example. An order agent representing a stock order should prefer the opposite weight of goals. Thus, the individual utility function is used to evaluate possible action alternatives of the order agent. Since lead times in single or small-batch manufacturing of high-sophisticated products may be very long compared to mass production, boundary conditions of the production environment can change significantly. Thus, orders are represented by agents, not as passive objects resources have to work on. Due to their autonomy and pro-activity, purposeful acting order agents recognise these changes and are able to react appropriately and reorganise their plans and goals if necessary.

Service agents are used for human interaction, transparency and maintenance purposes. Thus, human users like process planners are enabled to track actions performed by agents and to interact with the system. Users can inquire for information concerning the status of current orders or the system's performance. Processes hidden inside the agent system are made visible and comprehensible. Furthermore, the user is able to adapt the system to new boundary conditions e.g. by generating new resource agents in case of putting new machines into operation at the shop floor. Some service agents perform system monitoring tasks and will request user interaction under particular conditions, e.g. if the knowledge of some agents is insufficient or if the agent communication comes to a "deadlock situation" which has to be solved by external intervention.

The detailed process planning and scheduling takes place co-operatively within an electronic marketplace, which is realised as a "closed market" due to the security issues above. Order agents and resource agents are interacting according to a "three-phase-model":

- Communication on required manufacturing skills, due dates, capabilities, and capacities results in identifying of suitable sequences of manufacturing. The optimal sequence of manufacturing operations is accepted as a detailed plan ("negotiation phase")
- Order agents examine continuously whether detailed plans are executable under the current conditions to ensure the feasibility of plans ("verification phase").
- If necessary, order agents tender parts of the detailed plan for new auctions. The improved alternative detailed plan substitutes the previous plan. Afterwards the verification phase is resumed and lasts until the order is finished ("re-negotiation phase").

Since "IntaPS" focuses on internal coordination of an enterprise, it does not contain particular agents to represent customers or products as known by the HMS architecture. Only information about the product and customer demands, which are relevant for the manufacturing process, are passed to the order agent during initialisation. All other information about products and customers would increase the amount of necessary communication for the MAS and may lead to a reduced performance of the system. Nevertheless, product agents and customer agents are useful to represent supply chains or customer relationships. In these cases, a workshop, a plant or a whole company may be represented by e.g. a resource holon, which has to deliver a specific product to a specific customer in time. The internal structure of the resource is immaterial in this case, but a system based on the "IntaPS" architecture may be used for this purpose.

The electronic marketplace as well as the agents of the JAVA-based "IntaPS" prototype implementation are realised using a FIPA-compliant agent platform called "FIPA-OS" (Buckle, 2000). In addition to standardised components of the agent platform, further enhancements (e.g. adaptive communication protocols and knowledge representation) are part of the "IntaPS" project (Timm *et al.*, 2001).

3.3 Centralised Rough-Level Process Planning

The second essential component of the "IntaPS" approach is the centralised rough level process planning which processes the incoming data and generates a rough process plan in the context of a rough planning. These data are geometrical or technological information about the workpiece (e.g. from CAD systems) as well as further organizational information related to products and orders (e.g. from PDM or ERP systems). Order agents are instantiated with respect to these information and to current production data like machine skills and load. After their instantiation, order agents possess a rough level process plan which defines their scope and contains geometrical, technological and organisational information. The rough level process plan only contains information which the agent is not able to recognize from its environment. Examples for this kind of information are manufacturing features, which have to be processed during manufacturing, constraints between separate manufacturing operations (e.g. compelling manufacturing sequences) and constraints with other orders. Thus, order agents get all necessary information for decentralized detailed process planning and scheduling and obtain a maximum scope for the allocation of suitable resources and time slots for manufacturing.

3.4 Modelling of the Application Domain

One important aspect of "IntaPS" is the structured modelling of the application domain. Thus, a modified modelling method based on "MAS-CommonKADS" (Iglesia *et al.*, 1998) has been used for this purpose. This method consists of three phases: Conceptualisation, Analysis, and Design. During the first phase called *Conceptualisation*, the analysed domain is examined from a user-centric point of view. Typical use-cases are identified as well as some basic communication requirements. The objective of this phase is to get a basic idea of relevant interaction between participating entities. The results of this phase a documented using UML charts (Use-case diagrams, Message-Sequence-Charts) and will be refined in the second phase.

The second phase is called *Analysis* and results in five mostly formalised detailed models which serve as a basis for prototype implementation. These five models are:

- *Organisational model.* Description of the organisational structures in which the MAS has to be used (in this case: process planning department and shop floor of an enterprise) such as hierarchical structures, relationship between agents and their environment and agent society structure, identification of agents and roles.
- *Task model.* Determination of goals of the individual agents and their tasks.
- *Agent model.* Detailed model (e.g. represented as a UML class diagram) and (semiformal) textural description of the agents.
- *Coordination model.* Model of the agent interaction and coordination including specification of suitable communication protocols (e.g. based on state diagrams and detailed sequence message charts).
- *Expertise model.* Modelling knowledge of the domain, agents and environment.

These models are represented in UML mostly. Some descriptions of individual agent properties contained in the agent model are based on a semiformal textual patterns.

The last phase is called "Design" and deals with detailed design of the agents as well as the agent platform respective the electronic marketplace. Thus, the third phase leads to implementation activities for realisation of the MAS and in our case to the "IntaPS" prototype.

In context of the expertise model the „Ontology Inference Layer“ (OIL) is used for specification of an ontology which is common to all agents participating in the electronic marketplace. Thus, formalisation of necessary knowledge for rough-level process planning as well as for decentralised detailed planning is an important task of the “IntaPS” project. Therefore, common information models of the manufacturing domain are analysed (see Figure 2). Relevant information as well as other information concerning the domain are represented by three major information models: product model, resource model and process model. For example, appreciable information models are: a formal description of manufacturing features from ISO 14649 “STEP-NC” (e.g. as a basis of negotiations between order agents and resource agents and as a basis for time calculation for resource agents), product structure definitions based on ISO 10303-4x “STEP” and a classification of manufacturing processes according DIN 8580.

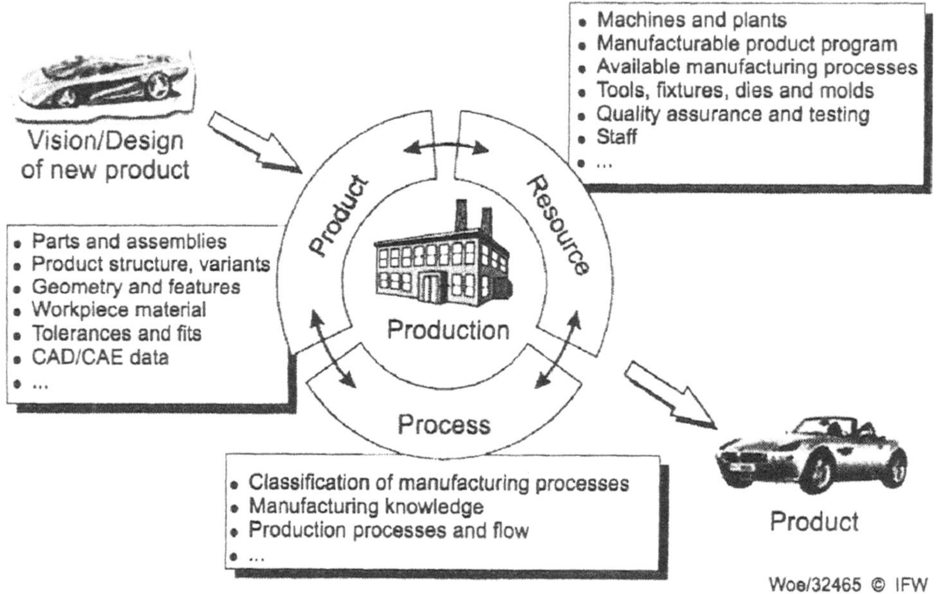

Figure 2 – Relevant information models in the production engineering domain

4.3 Evaluation Concept

The evaluation concept for the “IntaPS” prototype implementation is based on reference data sets which are part of a realistic scenario. They contain technical information about the products and orders (e.g. data of manufacturing features) as well as economic and logistic information like due dates and order quantities. Reference data sets will be processed in two different ways: With conventional tools as well as using the “IntaPS” prototype. Using conventional tools (see Figure 3, left side), sets of static process plans will be created using a standard process plan editor and scheduled by a conventional scheduler. The scheduled manufacturing orders are "manufactured" in a simulated ("virtual") shop floor environment. The "virtual" shop floor will be realized using “Tecnomatix eM-Plant” (former “SIMPLE++”). Simulation results are logged by “eM-Plant” and will be used for statistical analyses.

In addition, the same reference data sets will be processed using the "IntaPS" prototype. Therefore, the "IntaPS" systems communicates with the "virtual" shop floor using a TCP/IP connection and the TCP/IP socket interface of "eM-Plant". Thus, the MAS serves like a "remote control" for the "eM-Plant" simulation. As in the first case, "eM-Plant" logs all relevant events and simulation results. Finally, statistical data like average and maximum load of resources, lead times or delay of delivery will be compared and evaluated.

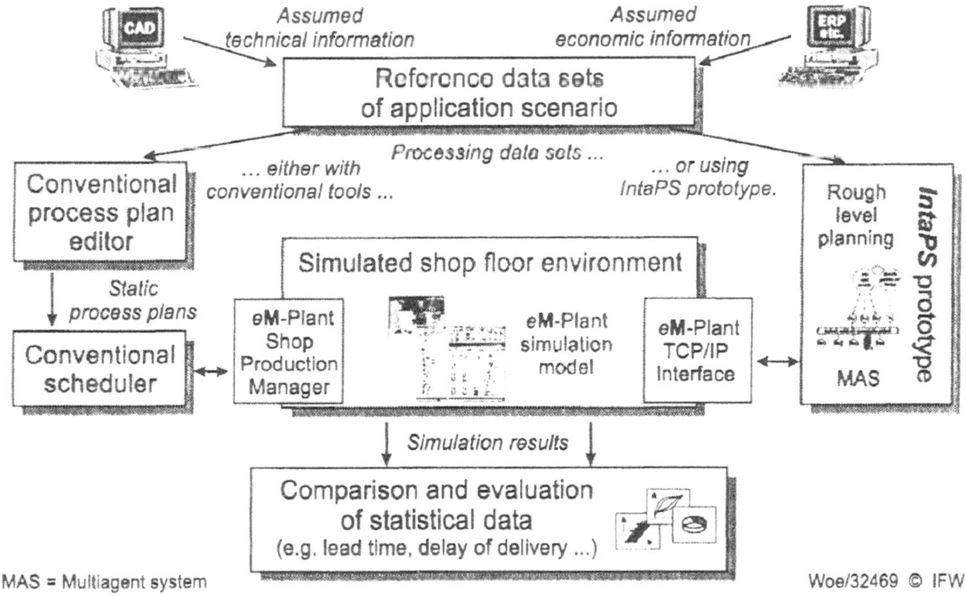

Figure 3 – Evaluation concept for the "InaPS" prototype

The reference scenarios used for evaluation purpose are not only used for the "IntaPS" project. They are specified using a document structure which is very similar to the FIPA template for application specifications. Since the "IntaPS" project is part of a German priority research program and all projects of this program agreed to use a FIPA-compliant specification to describe their scenarios, a library of several scenarios is under development and will be available at end 2003. On a long term basis, the application scenarios of the priority research program will lead to FIPA-compliant application specifications. Some aspects of the "IntaPS" approach are specified according to patterns which are used for agent-oriented software engineering, too.

5. SUMMARY AND OUTLOOK

This paper proposes a system architecture based on the application of co-operative agents for optimising information logistics in the field of process planning and production control. Due to the approach of a wide integration, capacity information and due dates will be taken into consideration for early stages of process planning. On the other hand, process planning knowledge will be used for short term scheduling decisions at the shop floor. Therefore, problems will be eliminated which result from time-delayed return of manufacturing knowledge and capacity data or other lacks of information flows e.g. from the use of static process plans.

Our current research activities deal with a structured application domain model which is a representative sample of a real-world production system. The evaluation is based on a prototypical implementation. Further developments are planned for a second project phase starting in summer 2002. Some of the addressed topics of "IntaPS-2" are enhancements for co-operative manufacturing (e.g. subcontracting of single manufacturing process steps). Since the current shop floor model is capable to represent job shop production only, "IntaPS-2" will consider integration of principles like manufacturing islands which may lead to hierarchical structures in the multiagent system.

6. ACKNOWLEDGEMENT

The presented work results partly from "IntaPS" joint research project, which is funded by the Deutsche Forschungsgemeinschaft (DFG) within the projects He 989/5 and To 56/149 as part of the Priority Research Program 1083 "Intelligent Agents and Realistic Commercial Application Scenarios". "IntaPS" is carried out in cooperation with the Center of Computing Technologies (TZI), University of Bremen. Further information is available at http://www.intaps.org

7. REFERENCES

Bongaerts L. "Integration of Scheduling and Control in Holonic Manufacturing Systems". Ph.D. thesis, Katholieke Universiteit Leuven, Belgium, 1998.

Buckle P. "FIPA and FIPA-OS Overview". Holonic Manufacturing Systems and FIPA Workshop, London, September, 2000.

Giebels M. "EtoPlan – a Concept for Concurrent Manufacturing Planning and Control", Ph.D. thesis. University of Twente, Netherlands, 2000.

Giebels M, Kals HJJ, Zijm WHM. "Dynamic manufacturing planning and control" In Production Engineering – Annals of the German Academic Society for Production Engineering, Vol. V/2, pp. 107-110, 1998.

Iglesia GA, Garijo M, Gonzalez JC, Velasco JR. "Analysis and Design of Multiagent Systems using MAS-CommonKADS". In Singh *et al.* (eds.) "Intelligent Agents IV –Agent Theories, Architectures and Languages". Berlin: Springer, 1998.

Kruth JP,. Detand J. "CAPP system for nonlinear process plans". In Annals of the CIRP, vol. 41/1, pp. 489-492, 1992.

Teti R, Kumara SRT. "Intelligent Computing Methods for Manufacturing Systems". In Annals of the CIRP, Keynote paper, vol. 46/2, pp. 629-652, 1997.

Timm IJ, Tönshoff HK, Herzog O, Woelk PO. "Synthesis and Adaptation of Multiagent Communication Protocols in the Production Engineering Domain". In Proceedings of the 3rd International Workshop on Emergent Synthesis (IWES01),Bled, Slovenia, pp. 73-82, March 12th – 13th 2001.

Tönshoff HK, Beckendorff U, Andres N. "FLEXPLAN – A Concept for Intelligent Process Planning and Scheduling". In Proceedings of the CIRP Int. Workshop, Hannover, 1989.

Tönshoff HK, Siebert K. "Positioning of Technological Interfaces". In Proceedings of the International Conference on Competitive Manufacturing (COMA' 01), Stellenbosch, South Africa, pp. 105-110, January 31th – February 2nd 2001.

Wellner J, Dilger W. "MAPS - A Multi-Agent Production Planning System". Intelligent Agents in Information and Process Management, Workshop at the 22nd German Annual Conference on Artificial Intelligence (KI98), Bremen, pp. 71 –78, 1998.

Zwick M, Brandes A. "Scheduling Methods for Holonic Control Systems". In Katalinic B. (Ed.): "Intelligent Manufacturing & Automation – Focus on Precision Engineering", Proceedings of 12th DAAAM International Symposium, Jena, pp. 531-532, October 24th – 27th 2001.

39

FROM INTRA-ENTERPRISE TOWARDS EXTRA-ENTERPRISE PRODUCTION PLANNING

Aleš Říha, Michal Pěchouček, Jiří Vokřínek, Vladimír Mařík
Gerstner Laboratory, Department of Cybernetics
Czech Technical University in Prague
Technická 2, Prague 6, 166 27 Czech Republic
{riha, vokrinek, pechouc, marik}@labe.felk.cvut.cz

In the domain of production planning multi-agent systems there is a strong demand for extending the solution beyond the borders of a single enterprise in order to meet future business requirements: (i) to manage the extra-enterprise production planning effectively, (ii) to create and reconfigure flexible dynamic configuration of virtual enterprises (e.g. among collaborating business partners). The concept of extra-enterprise agents helps to facilitate secure remote access and manage the production planning processes from outside the factory, inspect the current and the future load of particular production units, modify already running customer-projects, or include/invoke a new customer-project into the system remotely.

1. INTRODUCTION

The application domain of the research described here is oriented to support a project-oriented type of production. Unlike mass-production, in the case of the project-oriented production there is always a limited series of complex products of one type manufactured (e.g. space shuttles, power turbines, TV broadcasters or patterns and forms). Accordingly, an important part of resources has to be devoted to design-related activities such as quotation and configuration, design, and production planning. Production-oriented planning consists of three separate (while interrelated) phases:

- **quotation and configuration**, where the quotation engineer negotiates with a customer on a detailed specification of the product [1],
- **project specification**, where the complete product configuration is transformed into specifications of a project and required resource and
- **resource allocation**, where the required resources are allocated in time to appropriate resource providers.

Even though different areas of artificial intelligence, such as constraint programming, theorem proving, or evolutionary computing [2] very often support the first phase, we have relied on the human expertise in both the quotation and configuration as well as the project specification phases. The research described in this paper concerns primarily the last phase, where appropriate resource providers, such as machines, technicians, departments etc., allocate the required amount of resources. It becomes rather difficult to allocate project-related resources provided by partially booked resource providers and to allow re-planning due to resource malfunction or due to scheduling of higher priority projects. In this paper we will comment how the ExPlanTech [3] multi-agent technology addresses both the intra-enterprise and extra-enterprise aspects of the resource allocation problem.

2. INTRA-ENTERPRISE PRODUCTION PLANNING

ExPlanTech [3] is a physically **distributed multi-agent system** that exploits latest research achievements in the fields of distributed artificial intelligence, agent based computing and production planning. It builds upon the theoretical concept of social intelligence representation, acquaintance models, meta-agents and community monitoring, agentification and others. These concepts were originally studied, implemented and tested in the ProPlanT multi-agent system [4]. A full, stable and approved implementation of the ExPlanTech system has been partially supported within the ExPlanTech project (IST-1999-20171). The resulted multi-agent system has been implemented in JAVA and complies with the latest standards in agent based computing – **FIPA** (Federation of Intelligent Physical Agents – http://www.fipa.org/) [6]. The **JADE** (Java Agents Development Environment - sharon.cselt.it/projects/jade/) platform has been adopted [7]. The system has been tested in the Liaz Pattern Shop factory that produce moulds, forms and dies.

ExPlanTech was originally designed for the purposes of **intra-enterprise production planning** in the project oriented manufacturing environment – especially for managing resources and estimating delivery times and costs of a possible project. ExPlanTech integrates existing software systems that administer the production processes within the enterprise (such as enterprise resource planning systems (ERP), material management, human resource systems, CAD/CAM systems) by the **agentification** process. The agentified software system is encapsulated within the agent **wrapper** that administers agent-to-agent communication and collects the agents' social knowledge [5]. Such a software system becomes an agent – a fully-fledged member of the multi-agent system. The factory management does not need to replace the entire operational information systems by a new technology. Instead, they can make a best use of a combination of (i) the software infrastructure they already have and (ii) the novel, agent-based production planning technology.

The organizational structure of the ProPlanT (and also ExPlanTech) multi-agent system mirrors the organizational structure of the given enterprise. The agents have been divided into two fundamental super-classes: intra-enterprise (IEA) agents and extra-enterprise (EEA) agents. We distinguish among the following basic classes of IEA agents: **Production Planning Agent** (PPA), which is in charge of the product configuration and project specification, **Production Management Agent** (PMA), which accounts for decomposition of the project/task into several (sub)tasks and for contracting the best possible collaborator and **Production Agent** (PA), which belongs to the lowest level production units that simulate or encapsulate shop floor production processes.

Meta agent (MA) – a special monitoring agent visualises information, material and work flows across the agents' community. Shall be noted that the operation of the community of agents is completely independent of the meta-agent. Besides monitoring, the meta-agent can carry out independent reasoning and analyse the community overall behaviour. Such reasoning may result in suggestions aimed at efficiency improvements.

Apart from agentification and meta-agents, there is another important theoretical concept that is a vital part of the ProPlanT/ExPlanTech technology. The agents' wrappers are equipped with an *acquaintance model* that is a social knowledge container. A social knowledge of an agent (its computational model of behaviour of the rest of the multi-agent system) allows accurate while fast production planning, efficient re-planning in the case of a malfunction, or on-line community reconfiguration when some of the encapsulated software/hardware components fail to operate [5].

While integrated within the company internal ERP system, ExPlanTech elaborates an optimal production plan for a particular project. The plan, which is visualized in the graphical form, is provided to a human decision maker who can either confirm the plan or invoke an automated re-planning. The production plan can be re-planned either by changing priorities of the particular project, increasing or decreasing capacities of the respective production unites or redefining project specification. After testing in the factory floor, it has been identified that this technology provided more optimal production plans than the human planning expert. This is why the management can be provided with more accurate estimations of the required resources and due dates, by which the overall competitiveness of the factory increases and resources are used in the most optimal way.

3. EXTENDED ENTERPRISE

The optimal production plan should balance the available resources, maximizing the number of orders to be processed and minimizing their due times. As the workshops capacity is not unlimited, the decision has to be made whether the specific task/subtask will be implemented internally or subcontracted externally (e.g. within the frame of a virtual enterprise). Such a decision might be crucial in order not to threaten successful completion of other orders and not to misbalance the whole production flow. The efficient supply chain management can be handled by extending the original agent-based solution out of the boundaries of a single enterprise [8]. Moreover, orders are categorized by an internal priority value ensuring that orders with a higher priority are manufactured before those with lower ones. The ExPlanTech system monitors loads of workshops and other resource providers and consequently it 'measures' how suitable is the requested order.

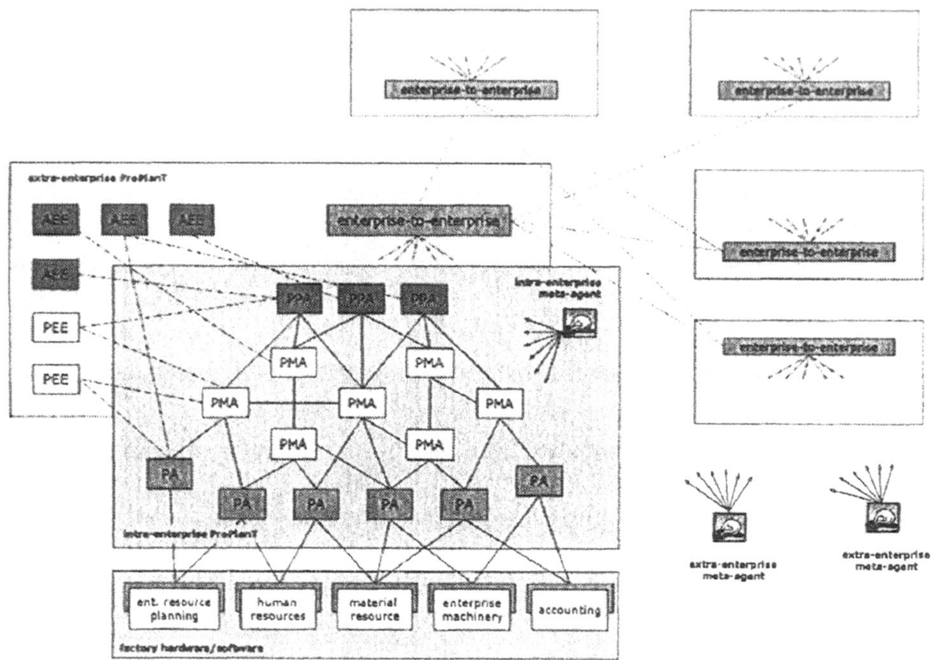

Figure 1: ProPlanT/ExPlanTech Architecture for Intra/Extra-Enterprise Production Planning

The extra-enterprise concept of the ExPlanTech technology provides several other classes to the agent community (see Figure 1):

- **Passive Extra-Enterprise Agent** (PEE) which may passively access the production planning data from outside of the company. These data can be accessed either by (i) customers, who (if the access rules permit) may inspect the status of their order manufacturing or (ii) managers who may want to monitor the load of production unites and available resources,
- **Active Extra-Enterprise Agent** (AEE) which may trigger from outside of the enterprise the entire course of production planning. AEE agent negotiates with the PPA agent in order to specify the production requirements, the deadline and the budgetary constraints. It can also subcontract individual PMA or PA agents for only parts of the products.
- **Enterprise-to-Enterprise Agent** (E2E) connects two enterprises that want to participate in a supply chain. E2E agent models the cooperating enterprise as an instance of a PA agent. The E2E agent acts on behalf of the cooperating enterprise and allows the PMA or PPA agents to subcontract it for a specific part of the supply. The E2E agentifies the whole enterprise.

Either a user or the AEE agent usually communicates with the PPA agent. The PPA agent constructs a component list and delegates further responsibilities to the PMA agents who contract either the best possible PA agents or via the E2E agent the best possible supplier or a collaborating entity. Costs and due times, that represent the distributed production plan, are then back-propagated to either the AEE agent or the user.

The extra-enterprise agents can be appreciated either by production managers when traveling (monitoring of the production, competitive planning etc.) or by customers (observing production progress of their orders). The extra-enterprise (EE) technology provides accessibility of the production planning data to the management of the enterprise while they are out of the enterprise using modern information/communication standards. This technology is primarily designed for accessing the production data (occupancy of workshops, list of orders, material etc.) via the Internet by an ordinary web browser. Apart from the portable or the desktop PC, the extra-enterprise agents can be installed on the mobile PDA devices that are based on the Windows CE platform. The extra-enterprise agents' wrappers can be adapted for communication using the Wireless Application Protocol (WAP) for running in the cell-phone devices. Only authenticated agents/human users can access and manage the intra-enterprise production planning data.

The E2E agent extends the ExPlanTech technology for managing outsourcing and capacity sharing across various enterprises. In the simple case, a supplier/collaborator can be represented as a virtual workshop by a simple E2E agent that advertises (and administers) only the services and capacities it is able to provide. Such an E2E agent represents either one physical workshop or can be viewed as a wrapper of the entire collaborating enterprise. The shared (public) knowledge about currently available resources should be prepared in a standard form with respect to the agreed and shared knowledge ontology. The agent could, for example, read the data from the partner's enterprise database or could be provided with this data by the ERP system. If there are not enough resources locally available, the planning system is able to contract such an agent and avoid failing to meet the deadline.

The second option is to use the E2E concept for interconnecting several enterprises that use the ExPlanTech technology on the intra-enterprise level. In such a case, the E2E agent does not simply represent services, the collaborator offers to the community, but serves as proxy to its own multi-agent community. Each intra-enterprise ExPlanTech system maintains one E2E agent that periodically checks with its intra-enterprise agents for their available resources and advertises these to the other E2E agents. Once the production planning agents within one enterprise are threatened by a possibility of failing to meet the deadline, they immediately contact their E2E agent which initiates negotiations with the other E2E agents representing the outsourcing resources and finds the most suitable subcontractor.

4. EXTRA-ENTERPRISE PLANNING SCENARIOS

Firstly, we will comment the technology migration phase when the agent-based system is integrated within the factory information infrastructure. Initially, the set of orders is defined in the factory information system. Orders specifications are propagated to the PPA agent, that starts planning by broadcasting the requests to the set of PMAs according to the specifications of the orders. Each order is represented in the planning system by a partially ordered set of tasks, required resources and priority of the order. The PMAs start negotiating aimed at finding the best configuration of the PAs for each task. The PA schedules the tasks on their resources. The final plan is propagated through the community back to the information system. As the result of this initial stage, the system contains all the orders to be carried out in the factory and is ready for receiving (planning) new orders.

4.1 Passive Access

The current status of the production planning system can be inspected via an ordinary internet browser, mobile PDA, or WAP cell phone using the passive extra-enterprise agents (see Figure 2). These agents are created and connected to the multi-agent system in real time. According the access rights, the customers can inspect "their own" orders or the company managers can access all the orders being processed by the agents. This information is downloaded directly from the agents via standard inter-agent communication. It is possible to inspect plans for the selected tasks or the entire load allocation of some PA (workshop, machine). For example the plan for the task "Z_211-0005 Seat model" can be seen only by the customer from the company "AUTO GD" or by the factory manager.

4.2 Active Access

Active extra-enterprise agents can be created and connected to the system in the same way as the passive extra-enterprise agents. The AEEs provide convenient functionality to factory managers. The manager, when traveling, can define a new order on the server side and ask the system to plan it. According to the resulting plan, the system either books the capacities – **permanent planning** (by sending the `achieve` speech-act messages) or, more often, only checks possibility of acceptance of a new order (by sending the `query` speech-act messages) – **competitive planning**. The competitive planning can be used for comparing alternative plans for several tasks. In the case of the 'Seat model' task, the manager (or a trusted customer from the "AUTO GD" company) can try to plan production within the manufacturing enterprise or with subcontracting parts of the project externally (e.g. using cooperating CAD studio). The manager will find out differences between two obtained plans and decides not to use external resources for the "Z_211-0005 Seat model" and will plan this order permanently on internal resources only (See Figure 2).

4.2 E2E Connecting

The enterprise-to-enterprise agent is used for linking suppliers into a virtual enterprise. The cooperating enterprise can offer the available resources via the E2E agent. Other enterprises can use these resources transparently like their own resources. An E2E agent plays the role of trustful active EEA on the side of one enterprise and the role of the PA on the side of the other enterprise. The planning system can only operate with available resources of the other enterprise that are accessible via the E2E. For example, the cooperating enterprise (CAD studio) integrates their resources within the factory via E2E representing CAD studio in the virtual enterprise and can be used instead of the standard factory department ("CAD konstrukce") when it is more efficient.

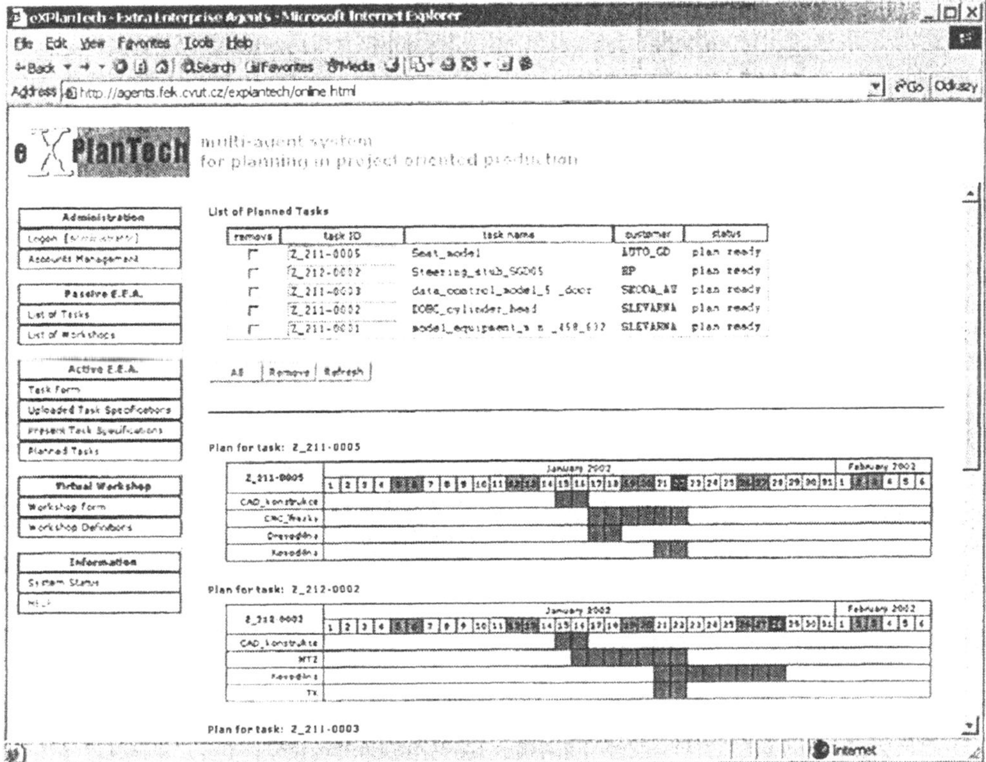

Figure 2: Screenshot of the internet browser window. On the left there is an access panel to the functionality of the PEE, AEE and E2E agents, while in the main frame, there is a result of the selected action - a list of planned tasks from AEE agent.

5. CONCLUSIONS

In this paper we have illustrated strengths of the multi-agent approach to intra-enterprise project-driven production planning and potentials of extending the general technology to the extra-enterprise level. The ExPlanTech multi-agent community has been originally designed so that each agent represents/models a particular manufacturing unit within the respective factory (e.g. department, workshop, CNC machine, warehouse). Agents' interaction simulates possible variations of the course of manufacturing. Such a model facilitates interaction-based production planning and flexible, intelligent replanning/reconfiguration once a production unit fails to operate, gets overloaded or simply a high priority order is in conflict with an already planned order. The agents may represent not only the in-house production actors but also other members of the supply chain which contribute to manufacturing of a required product. This is why the concept of agentification that has been designed for integrating legacy systems and encapsulating hardware machinery can be used for integrating suppliers as well.

This research work has been supported by the European Commission contract No. IST-1999-20171 (ExPlanTech) and by the Ministry of Education, Youth and Sports of the Czech Republic within the frame of the project No. MSM212300013.

6. REFERENCES

[1] Wielinga, B. J. and Schreiber A.:Configuration-design Problem Solving. *IEEE Expert*, 12(2), 1997, pp. 49-56

[2] Kubalík, J., and Lažanský, J.: Genetic Algorithms and their Tuning. In: *Proceedings of CASYS '98 (Dubois D., ed.)*, Liege, Belgium, 1998, pp. 217-229

[3] Říha, A., Pěchouček, M., Vokřínek, J. and Mařík, V.: ExPlanTech: Exploitation of Agent-based Technology in Production Planning. In: *V. Mařík, et. Al, (Eds.), Multi-Agent Systems and Application II*, LNAI 2322, Springer Verlag, 2002, pp. 308-322

[4] Mařík, V., Pěchouček, M., Štěpánková, O., and Lažanský, J.: ProPlanT: Multi-Agent System for Production Planning. *Applied Artificial Intelligence*, vol. 14, No.7(2000), pp.727-762

[5] Pěchouček, M., Mařík, V., and Štěpánková, O.: Towards Reducing Communication Traffic in Multi-Agent Systems. In: *Journal of Applied System Studies*, Cambridge International Science Publishing, Cambridge, UK, No.1, 2001

[6] FIPA: Agent Management. In: *http://www.fipa.org*, Geneva, Switzerland, 1998

[7] Bellifemine, F., Poggi, A., and Rimassa, G.,: Developing Multi-agent Systems with JADE. In: *Seventh International Workshop on Agent Theories, Architectures, and Languages (ATAL-2000)*, Boston, MA, 2000

[8] Camarinha-Matos, L.M., Afsarmanesh, H., and Lima, C.: Hierarchical Coordination in Virtual Enterprises. *Journal of Intelligent and Robotic Systems*, vol. 26 (1999), Issue 3/4, pp. 267-287

PART 4

INTEGRATION OF PRODUCT AND SERVICE LIFE CYCLES

40

DESIGN OF PRODUCT ORIENTED MANUFACTURING SYSTEMS

Sílvio Carmo Silva*, Anabela Alves**
Universidade do Minho, (*)scarmo @dps.uminho.pt (**) anabela@dps.uminho.pt

A Product Oriented Manufacturing System is designed for the manufacture of a product or a family of similar products. POM may be seen as a development of traditional Cellular Manufacturing and tends to involve more than one cell. A POMS may either be physically organized in a single place or be made of distributed manufacturing or servicing units, thus comprising a virtual system. To be efficient, the POMS design should identify design phases and point to the data, methods and tools that should be used to obtain good design solutions. In this paper, one such methodology is proposed, together with an analysis of the conceptual configuration of the cells that are the building blocks of POM systems.

1. INTRODUCTION

Cellular Manufacturing Systems (CMS) (Gallagher, 1973), (Burbidge, 1996), (Suresh, 1998) although designed for a variety of parts, grouped into families, rarely take into consideration the need for parts production coordination and synchronization for meeting customer orders of end items. Thus, the need for rapid response to customer requirements, which is recognized as an important strategic objective, is not adequately taken into account. This limitation, however, has been addressed in recent years through a variety of systems interlinking a number of cells. A paradigmatic example of this is what Black calls a linked-cell manufacturing system (Black, 1991). This may be seen as a Product Oriented Manufacturing System (POMS), as may many manufacturing systems currently referred to as JIT, lean, flexible and virtual manufacturing systems (Silva, 2001(a)). POM can also be associated with concepts such as focused factories (Skinner, 1974) and OPIM systems (Putnik, 1995).

To be efficient, POMS should be designed in a way that easily identifies design phases, data, methods and the tools that should be used. This is important for helping the user to obtain good design solutions, taking into consideration all the relevant restrictions.

Here, one such methodology is put forward, together with the definition of a set of conceptual cell configurations seen as building blocks of POM systems.

2. PRODUCT ORIENTED MANUFACTURING SYSTEMS

A POMS is defined as *a set of interlinked manufacturing resources and cells that simultaneously and in a coordinated manner address the manufacture of a product or a range of similar products, including the necessary assembly work.* A product may be simple, like a part, or complex, having a product manufacturing structure of several levels. This may be represented in a multilevel bill-of-materials. When the product is simple, a POMS may simply take the form of a cell. Otherwise, it comprises a coordinated set of interlinked resources and cells. The coordination of work between manufacturing cells, towards production of end items, is one of the most distinguishing aspect of POMS. A set of cells that does not work under such a coordination setting does not form a POMS.

POM may be seen as a development of traditional Cellular Manufacturing in the sense that a set of interrelated manufacturing cells may be necessary to completely manufacture a product, or a set of similar products, including assembly.

The Design of POMS needs to take logistic operations into account. This is particularly critical when manufacturing resources are distributed in space.

Directing systems to the manufacture of specific products can provide competitive advantages that include short production times and improved product quality. This may be enhanced through the application of recent technical and technological advances in the internal and external logistics of production. In this sense, several strategies to the control of materials, based on the pull and push paradigms, or combinations of these, can be used.

To be successful, POM must be able to fully and dynamically use resources and services available to a company over time, locally or globally, whether they be the company's own or those available in the market. Under changing product demands, frequent, i.e. dynamic, reconfiguration of POMSs will probably be necessary. This is particularly so because POMSs are dedicated to a specific mix of products which, changing over time, calls for new arrangements of resources and services to ensure high levels of operational and economical performance.

A POMS may be built by putting together, in a localized site, manufacturing resources or cells that may be physically dispersed or, alternatively, by organizing them into virtual POMS. Today these can benefit from intranet and internet based technologies, a prerequisite of the widely discussed Virtual Enterprise concept (Camarinha-Matos, 1999). This approach to the virtual configuration of manufacturing systems was initially put forward in 1982, by McLean, Bloom and Hopp (McLean, 1987) (Drolet, 1996) and also by Simpson, Hocken and Albus, according to Ratchev (2001).

POMS are very different from Functional Oriented Manufacturing Systems (FOMS). These are organized in functional departments and are normally oriented towards providing servicing functions for a whole set of different parts and end items with varying processing requirements.

Due to the product oriented nature of POMS, in relation to FOMS, not only can higher productivity, lower WIP, lower throughput time and better production control be expected, but also higher volumes of production.

3. DESIGN METHODOLOGY FOR POMS

Here we propose a methodology for POMS design, identified as the GCD methodology. It is composed of three design phases or functions, namely the Generic, the Conceptual and the Detailed, Figure 1. The methodology is presented in this paper with the support of the IDEF0 modeling technique (FIPS, 1993).

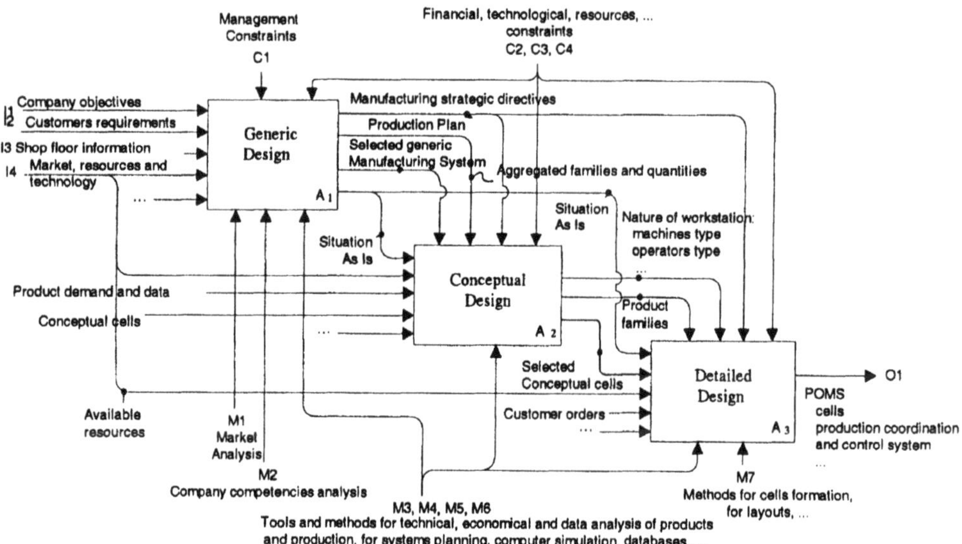

Figure 1 – Overview of the GCD design methodology for POMS

In the GCD methodology, we seek to use all relevant data, restrictions, tools and methods, and to provide for the expandable and up-dated databases and knowledge bases that are relevant to the POMS design. This is in line with design approach of Suh (1995).

Several decisions at strategic, tactical and operational level are used both successively and iteratively in the design process aimed at reaching suitable POMS organizational and operational configurations.

3.1 Generic Design

One important decision to be taken at this design phase is to choose the generic manufacturing system configuration. We can identify two extreme and fundamentally different types of generic configurations: the POM configuration and the FOM configuration (Silva, 2002). A third one must be considered, namely the hybrid configuration, which integrates the FOM organization, usually at parts and possibly at some subassemblies manufacturing, and the POM organization. Although we think that efforts must be made to reach pure POMS whenever possible, the hybrid configuration should be considered in the design and decision process. If the FOM configuration is to be used, the GCD methodology's design purpose terminates here. On the other hand, if POM or hybrid arrangements are to be investigated, then the next steps of the methodology should follow.

When we consider using frequent systems reconfiguration for adapting to changing market demands and product manufacturing requirements then, the POM organization is, most probably, very suitable. This is what happens, for example, in

virtual manufacturing systems. By definition, these are ephemeral systems oriented and designed for addressing a single business opportunity. They are usually identified as a product or a service and, therefore, product oriented.

Another important piece of information generated at the Generic design stage is a production plan. This is essential for developing the subsequent design activities.

Strategic directives must also be given in relation with the sources of manufacturing resources, keeping in mind that a network of cooperating manufacturing units, cells or partners may be involved.

The choices at this design phase are determined by many factors related with company's manufacturing strategy. Particularly relevant are the production requirements resulting from the product forecasted demand, market available resources and services and company present manufacturing position and situation. Product variety and volumes of production should also be identified and a first level analysis of similarities, leading to aggregated product families, should be made.

Thus, we can identify three interrelated design activities at the Generic design phase: *Strategic Production Planning (A11), Analysis of Company and Market Manufacturing Situation (A12)* and *Generic Manufacturing System Selection (A13).*

In order to carry out this design phase a variety of tools and methods for technical, economical and data analysis of products and production are required. Examples of these include, clustering methods, ABC analysis, multi-attributes decision analysis (Canada, 1989) and computer simulation.

A more detailed description of this design phase can be seen in Silva (2001(b)).

3.2 Conceptual Design

The main and fundamental purpose of this design is selecting conceptual cell configurations that, once implemented in practice, will lead to real POMS configurations. Additionally, a first approximation to product and part families' formation, based on both forecasted and settled customer orders and process plans, must be made. It is also important to specify the nature of workstations and operators. Based on such purposes two main activities must be carried out, namely, *Conceptual Cell Configurations Selection (*A21) and *Workstation Selection (*A22), see Figure 2. Clearly matters such as workstation functions/flexibility and operators skills must be defined at this stage.

The conceptual cells that can be used are the *basic* ones, shown in Figure 3, and their shared cell counterparts, called *non-basic* (Silva, 2002). These are cells that need to do work on products or parts initially allocated to other cells, or need work to be done in other cells, or both. The adoption of non-basic cells leads to intercellular workflows. The virtual version of conceptual cells should also be considered at this design phase.

Workstations can have a variety of configurations dependent on resource combination and flexibility. Thus the type and quantity of manufacturing resources, such as machines, auxiliary resources, operators and tools, change the nature of workstations. This leads to different versions of each identified conceptual cell, posing different problems for both the design and operation of the POM systems. The following versions of each conceptual cell can be identified (Silva, 2002): *flexible conceptual cell, multiprocessor task conceptual cell* and *multifunction processor conceptual cell* for workstations with parallel processors, with multiple

resources or processors and with multifunction processors respectively. This classification is derived and adapted from the theory of scheduling (Brucker, 1995), (Blazewicz, 1996), (Pinedo, 1995). In practice we might expect to see other versions of conceptual cells, which might combine different types of workstation configurations.

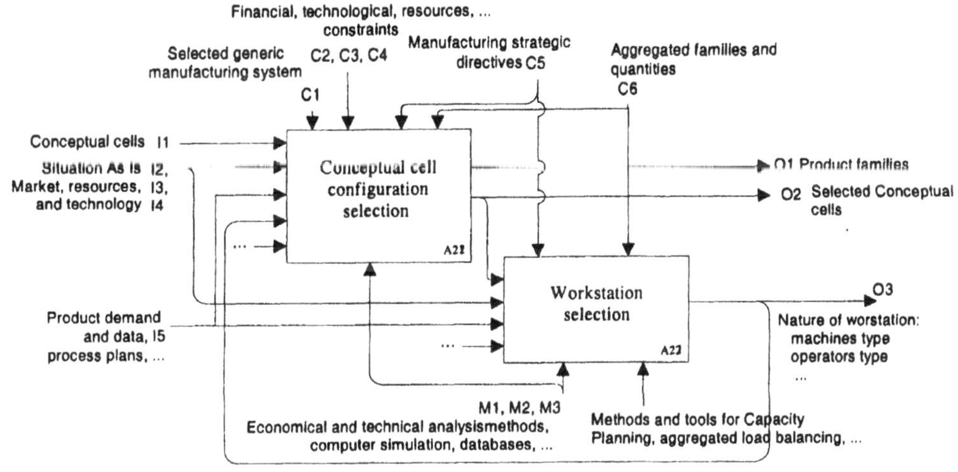

Figure 2 –Conceptual design activities

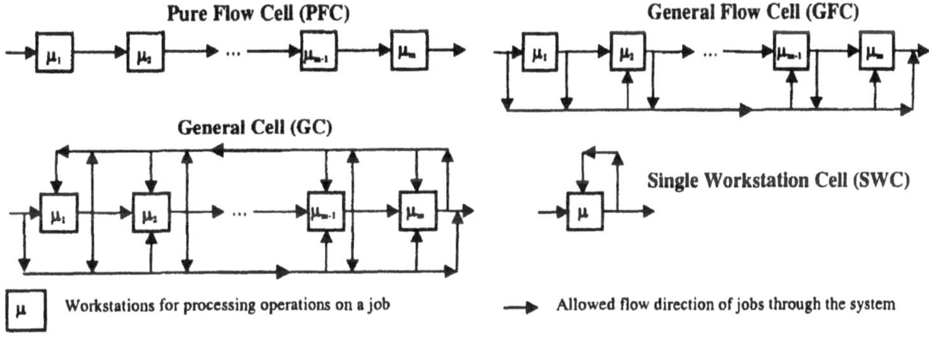

Figure 3 – Schematic representation of the four basic conceptual cell configurations

A typical analysis to be done at this design stage includes workflow analysis associated with the products and processes, which is essential for choosing system configuration based on conceptual cells. This choice requires evaluation of alternatives, which can initially be made through computer simulation.

A range of input data, restrictions and mechanisms for obtaining and evaluating solutions must be used at conceptual design stage as shown in Figure 2.

Important restrictions, information and guidelines are provided by the previous design phase. These include a production plan based on manufacturing aggregated families and guidelines for production capacity mix which take into consideration the company's actual manufacturing position and its strategy for accessing and involving market resources and partners. Decisions in relation to shifts, overtime, outsourcing and make or buy decisions must be put forward too.

Tools that may be used in this design phase, in addition to database systems and computer simulation, include methods for economical analysis, multi-attributes technical analysis (Canada, 1989), capacity planning and aggregated load balancing.

The results from this design are already a good approximation to the POM system for the product or the family of products selected. However, the real, detailed system configuration is obtained at the next design phase, i. e. at Detailed design.

3.3 Detailed Design

The design of POM systems is a dynamic activity at all levels. However, it is at this detailed design level that frequency of design is high. This design should be made every time a new product order is released for production. This order may join together a few customer orders of the same product or of similar products.

At the Detailed design, instantiation of conceptual cells is made, that take into consideration forecasted and customer orders for products. Thus, families of parts, subassemblies and end items, based on actual orders and due dates, are allocated to each conceptual cell and coordinated control of work among cells for POM is devised. Therefore, detailed specification of the production system is achieved, including the design of its physical or virtual configuration.

We identify the following activities at Detailed design phase: *Formation of Families of Parts, Subassemblies and End Items (A31), Instantiation of the Conceptual Cells (A32), Instantiation of Workstations (A33), Intracellular Organization and Control (A34) and POM System Organization and Intercellular workflow Coordination and Control (A35).*

Activity A31 has to do with manufacturing requirements for the near future. It must deal with an in depth analysis of processing requirements based on actual production orders and existing sources of manufacturing capacity or services, either inside or outside the company. This activity is simplified due to the first level clustering analysis of production previously done at conceptual design stage.

Activity A32 performs the detailed design leading to the manufacturing cells to be implemented in practice. Thus, the allocation of parts to cells and cell configuration is established. This is based on the conceptual cells selected at the previous design phase and on results from the previous design activity. Manufacturing service providers and materials suppliers should also be considered, in design process, at this stage. This is particularly necessary for large and multi site POM systems.

The number of workstations and their manufacturing resources, together with a detailed arrangement of each, is established by activity A33. This involves a detailed knowledge of the main and auxiliary, pieces of equipment available, not only for processing but also for handling, transport and storage. Operators should also be selected, based on skills and on cell operating modes. Activity A33 makes, therefore, the necessary adjustments to the workstations selected at the conceptual level, having in consideration existing manufacturing resources and results of detailed load balancing and of previous Detailed design activities.

Although the conceptual configuration chosen restricts cell arrangements that can be made, there is still a need to clearly define the detailed, intracellular organization and control, achieved by activity A34. This involves the precise location of workstations, machines and auxiliary devices, including workstation decouplers (Black, 1995). A clear definition of how materials flow and how operators work within a cell is also required, it being possible to evaluate several layout configurations (Arvindh, 1994), such as the well known U shaped one, which should fit into the conceptual configuration chosen. Moreover, operating cell modes exploring strategies such as teamwork and time-sharing resources (Suri, 1998), rabbit chase, TSS and working balance (Black, 1995), should be considered for implementation.

Finally the POM system can be attained. This culminates with the activity A35 dealing with the total system integration and organization. An important part of this is the selection of the POM intercellular coordination and production control system. This should focus on the need to coordinate and synchronize production of the several items required by each specific product order. This coordination and control system should explore the push and pull paradigms and novel combinations of them such as the POLCA (Suri, 1998), the DBR (Goldratt, 1986), the CONWIP (Spearman, 1990) and SYNCRO-MRP (Hall, 1981) systems, to mention only a few.

It is very clear that, once again, no single design activity can be performed in isolation. All these five-detailed activities are closely interrelated and must be developed in an iterative manner. Moreover, in order to carry them out, a range of methods and tools should be used for technical and economical evaluation of alternative solutions. This means solving problems such as those of detailed clustering of work, equipment selection, intra and intercellular workflow and workload analysis, system flexibility and operations scheduling.

Most probably, detailed computer simulation can be of great use at this design stage. This would certainly help fine tune the resources required including machines, operators and tooling, the evaluation of operating strategies and establishing work schedules.

4. CONCLUSION

To keep up with the increasing and ever-changing market demands of today and tomorrow, companies must be able to efficiently manufacture and quickly deliver good quality products to customers. To achieve this, manufacturing companies cannot rely on traditional organization and the operation of systems based on functional departments. Moreover, cellular manufacturing based on uncoordinated or loosely coordinated manufacturing cells is also inappropriate. Present requirements indicate that a more holistic approach to manufacturing is necessary. This can be achieved through Product Oriented Manufacturing Systems (POMS) dynamically built from cells or manufacturing resources, locally or globally available. These must be interlinked and closely coordinated for the total and rapid production of complete products, not parts only. These products may preferably bear manufacturing similarities. Although a localized, physical set-up for such purpose should be sought, POMS are likely to be more dependent on virtual reconfiguration when resources are dispersed or are uneconomical to rearrange.

Designing POM systems is a complex task that requires a methodology that both takes into account the different steps in the design process and points to updated restrictions, data, tools and methods that should be used in the design. The summarized methodology presented in this paper is a contribution to this, emphasizing the interrelated and iterative nature of POMS design functions. We call it the GDC methodology because of its three main design phases addressing respectively the Generic, the Conceptual and the Detailed design. We suggest that Conceptual design should concentrate as much as possible on conceptual cells, which may be seen as classes of the different cell configurations, based on complexity of workflow that we may encounter in practice.

5. REFERENCES

1. Arvindh B, Irani SA. Cell formation: the need for an integrated solution of the problems. Int. Journal of Production Research, 1994; 32; 5: 1197-218.
2. Black JT, Chen JC. The role of decouplers in JIT pull apparel cells. International Journal of Operations & Production Management, 1995; 7, 1: 17-35.
3. Black JT. The Design of the Factory with Future. McGraw-Hill, Inc., 1991
4. Blazewicz J, Ecker KH, Pesch E, Schmidt G, Weglarz J. Scheduling Computer and Manufacturing Processes. Springer Verlag, Heidelberg, 1996.
5. Brucker, P. Scheduling Algorithms. Springer, 1995.
6. Burbidge JL. Production Flow Analysis for Planning Group Technology. Clarendon Press, 1996.
7. Camarinha-Matos LM, Afsarmanesh H. "The Virtual Enterprise Concept". In Working Conference on Infraestructures for Virtual Enterprises (PRO-VE'99), L. M. Camarinha-Matos and H. Afsarmanesh, ed., Kluwer Academic Publishers, 1999.
8. Canada JR, Sullivan WG. Economic and multiattribute evaluation of Advanced Manufacturing Systems. Prentice-Hall1, 1989.
9. Drolet JR, Montreuil B, Moodie CL. Empirical Investigation of Virtual Cellular Manufacturing System. Symposium of Industrial Engineering - SIE'96, 1996.
10. FIPS PUBS - Federal Information Processing Standards Publications. Draft FIPS Publication 183 Announcing the standard for Integration Definition for Function Modeling (IDEF0). http://www.sdct.itl.nist.gov/~ftp/idef/idef0.rtf, 1993.
11. Gallagher CC, Knight WA. Group Technology. Butterworths, 1973.
12. Goldratt EM, Fox RE. The Race, North River Press, Inc, 1986.
13. Hall, RW. "Syncro MRP: Combining Kanban and MRP – The Yamaha PYMAC System" In Driving the Productivity Machine: Production Planning and Control in Japan, APICS, 1981: 43-56.
14. McLean CR, Brown, PF. "The Automated Manufacturing Research Facility at the National Bureau of Standards". In New Technologies for Production Management systems, H. Yoshikawa e J. L. Burbidge, ed., Elsevier Science Publishers B. V. North – Holland, 1987.
15. Pinedo, M. Scheduling – Theory, Algorithms and Systems. New Jersey: Prentice-Hall Inc, 1995.
16. Putnik GD, Silva SC. "One Product Integrated Manufacturing". In Balanced Automation Systems, L. M. Camarinha-Matos, H. Afsarmanesh, eds. Chapman & Hall, 1995.
17. Ratchev, SM. Concurrent process and facility prototyping for formation of virtual manufacturing cells. Integrated Manufacturing Systems, 2001; 12: 4, 306-315.
18. Silva SC., Alves, AC. SPOP - Sistemas de Produção Orientados ao Produto. Células Autónomas de Produção - TeamWork'2001 Conferencia, Lisboa, 2001 (a).
19. Silva SC, Alves AC. Uma Metodologia para o Projecto de Sistemas de Produção Orientados ao Produto. VII Int. Conf. on Industrial Engineering and Operations Management, Brasil, 2001 (b).
20. Silva SC., Alves, AC. A Framework for Understanding Cellular Manufacturing, accepted to CAR&FOF Conference, Porto, Portugal, 2002.
21. Skinner, W. The focused factory. Harvard Business Review, 1974.
22. Spearman ML., Woodruff DL, Hopp, WJ. CONWIP: A Pull Alternative to Kanban, International Journal of Production Research, Vol. 28, N. 5, 879-894, 1990.
23. Suresh NC, Kay JM. Group Technology and Cellular Manufacturing – State of the Art Synthesis of Research and Practice. Kluwer Academic Publishers, 1998.
24. Suri, R. Quick Response Manufacturing – A Companywide Approach to Reducing Lead Times. Oregon: Productivity Press, 1998.
25. Suh NP. Design and Operation of Large systems. Journal of Manufacturing Systems, 1995; 14; 3: 203-13.

41

INTEGRATED DEVELOPMENT OF PRODUCTS AND SERVICES

Karin Auernhammer, Matthias Stabe
Fraunhofer Institute for Industrial Engineering
Karin.Auernhammer@iao.fhg.de
Matthias.Stabe@iao.fhg.de

This article focuses on innovation patterns in product-service systems and presents a conceptual framework for the integrated development of products and services. Traditionally, research in innovation patterns has dealt primarily with manufacturing systems. Since the early eighties, service innovation and its impact on economic growth increasingly went into focus of scientific interest. Although more comprehensive, commonly accepted, concepts still remain to be elaborated, innovative solutions in manufacturing and services - especially in product-service systems – can be argued to show an increasing tendency towards pattern convergence. This hypothesis results in the research question how the integrated development of products and services impacts the innovation systems of companies.

1. INTRODUCTION

Recent investigations into growth patterns in companies did not merely point on efficiency increase – achieved intensively or extensively - in production processes but emphasized changing roles of innovation and fast technology progress as key drivers, too (OECD, 2000). On a macro-economic level, this was as well revealed by the research results of Romer (Romer, 1995): after investigating various differing national growth rates he developed a "new growth theory", stating that differences in growth patterns cannot be explained by natural resources and capital goods alone anymore, but rather by ideas and knowledge resulting in innovation.

Innovation does not only relate to new products or technically advanced or superior systems, but increasingly covers intangible aspects in the corporate product and service portfolios, too. In contexts of international competition, successful companies gain decisive advantage not only by cost-leadership, quality or traditional technology, but in particular by differentiation through innovative products offering value-added services. The relationship between services and manufacturing seems to have changed in the last years (Miles, 2000). Many companies perceive themselves not only as product-oriented, but more and more as solution-oriented, which implies services as intrinsic parts of solutions (OECD, 2000). Consequently, simultaneous development of products and services for perceivable combination of tangible and intangible assets gains increasing importance. In this, services form not only add-ons to products, but strike as valuable part in the value proposition of a company.

An approach for integrated development of products and services is meant on the one hand to overcome the traditional difficulties in investigating the growth patterns of manufacturing and service industry. On the other hand, the purpose of the approach is to provide a sound methodological framework and toolset for companies managing their product-service system.

2. PECULARITIES AND CHARACTERISTICS OF INNOVATION PROCESSES IN PRODUCTS AND SERVICES

2.1 Innovation in Manufacturing

Traditionally, innovation research has been focused on manufacturing industries. Accordingly, the Oslo Manual of OECD (OECD, 1992) defined innovation in the following way:

"Technological innovations comprise new products and processes and significant technological changes of products and processes. An innovation has been implemented if it has been introduced on the market (product innovation) or used within a production process (process innovation). Innovations therefore involve a series of scientific, technological, organization, financial and commercial activities."

Furthermore, OECD differentiates between major and incremental product innovation.

Innovation in manufacturing industry is mainly driven by new technologies or new materials applied in production processes or products. Due to predominantly technological orientation, the innovation function is organizationally realized by R&D departments that implement new technologies or materials in products and /or processes. The overall objective for product innovation is a superior competitive position in the relevant market. Accordingly, new products or production processes aim strategically either on cost-reduction or functional improvements. The relevant knowledge incorporated into a new product or a new production process can be protected by patents.

2.2 Innovation in Services

Innovations in services show specific characteristics, that primarily relate to specific characteristics of services. They can according to Hipp (Hipp et al., 2000; Sirilli and Evangelista, 1998) be described as

- Close interaction between production and consumption
- High information content and the intangible nature of service output
- The key role of human resources in the pro-vision of services
- Critical role of organizational factors in firms performance

In contrast to the rather homogeneous essential nature of services, the service sector itself shows a great heterogeneity with respect to output composition, branches, processes or company size. Furthermore, a number of sectors are still regulated while others are relatively open with low barriers of entry and keen competition (OECD, 2000).

Many authors (such as Preissl, 2000; Soete and Miozzo, 1989) argue that traditional innovation indicators are not applicable to investigate the characteristics and implications of service innovations. Moreover, they emphasize upon differences between manufacturing and service innovations in organizational design, process, impetus and general management models. The provision of services as well as the cost structure show significant differences to those in manufacturing (Preissl, 2000). While knowledge-based services do not require large investment in early phases of development, other types of services such as scale-intensive physical networks (Soete and Miozzo, 1989) require investments to a large extent. This limits the value of using investment figures for innovation measurement. Furthermore, services put a high emphasis on intellectual capital which is difficult to measure. The quality of service innovation output as a measure for productivity growth, as well as a proper differentiation between product and process innovation for services are major elements of difference, too. Furthermore, R&D in service sectors is only rarely comparable to manufacturing as it mostly spreads over all actors and is not located in a specific group of actors or a department. Therefore, the R&D expenditure is difficult to measure and the protection of knowledge by patents does not seem appropriate for services as well.

3. DETERMINANTS AND TYPOLOGY OF INNOVATIONS IN PRODUCT-SERVICE-SYSTEMS

3.1 Relations between Products and Services

Besides the differences in characteristics of manufacturing and service innovation, however, convergence of innovation patterns of products and services is recognizable with several respects. For example, some key factors such as appropriation of knowledge, learning organization or changing qualification needs do not differ significantly. However the knowledge intensity and the strong emphasis on human factors and skills still differentiate most service innovation from manufacturing innovations.

The interactive nature of information and communication technologies (ICT) changes the way in which economic agents exchange - virtual and real - value information (Antonelli, 2000). Preissl (Preissl, 2000) points on the importance of ICT use on modularization and standardization potentials in services. New technologies change services in ways increasingly similar to those in manufacturing in the past (Licht et al., 1999); e.g. services types that traditionally were provided by human agents are automated through technology applications such as self-service terminals etc. Products and services seemingly depend on each other in particular with respect to the increasing implementation of ICT.

Although these signs of convergence do not erase the major differences between manufacturing and service innovation patterns the arguments above show that both concepts have as well similar features. Due to their heterogeneity, though, the specific relations between products and services cause challenges and obstacles for establishing an integrative framework that require more detailed investigation.

3.2 Business Models

Within the context of combining innovations in products and services, several development opportunities for related business models can be identified:
- First is that an enterprise with products innovates via adding services to the former on their own
- Second is that a service provider refers to a "platform" product to develop and market a specific service that adds value to this product
- Third is that both the product manufacturer and the service provider bundle forces in concurrently optimizing and innovating their respective tangible or intangible offer to the other.
- Fourth would be alliances of inter-dependent services

Within these different (general) types of product-service relations, the innovation impetus derives from the focus of main business activity.

To identify patterns of innovation in service industries, (Den Hertog, 2000) suggested observation of specific inter-relations between a) supplier of – technical as well as non-technical - innovation input, b) individual service firm and c) type of clients of innovative service (intermediate – manufacturer or service provider - or final user). Subsequently five patterns were presented:
- (Product-) supplier-dominated innovation
- Innovation in service (calling onto product innovation)
- Client-led innovation (calling both product as well as service innovation)
- Innovation through service (e.g. knowledge-intensive)
- Paradigmatic innovation (completely new product & service system model)

According to these types, specific innovation processes and related organizational models can be established. As is obvious, furthermore, holistic understanding of product-service solutions is required for appropriate business design.

4. CONCEPTUAL FRAMEWORK FOR INTEGRATED DEVELOPMENT OF PRODUCTS AND SERVICES

4.1 Concept Fundamentals

The research project "Pro(duct) Se(rvi)c(e) Co-(design)" (also: ProSecCo, PSCD) combines research partners and other solution providers as well as industrial partners from several European countries. For the conceptual framework for above project, it was understood that holistic solutions to customer demands require conception spaces that extend beyond mere product or service innovation models. Consequently, the initial framework was conceived as set of qualitative and quantitative entrepreneurial goals and content interests, based on interrelations of products and services as perceived by both customers and providers. As the emphasis here laid on socio-economic issues rather than on (e.g. technological) instrumental means, the initial concept was then detailed in more practical terms of market, product & service, technology etc. This resulted in a model for design of product-service systems as shown in Figure 1 below. Integrated conception of product-service system architectures is understood to be an integrative cluster of at least partially iterative processes, involving multiple technical and non-technical issues and requiring continuous scanning of business environments in multi-dimensional way (following innovation patterns as mentioned in chapter 3 already).

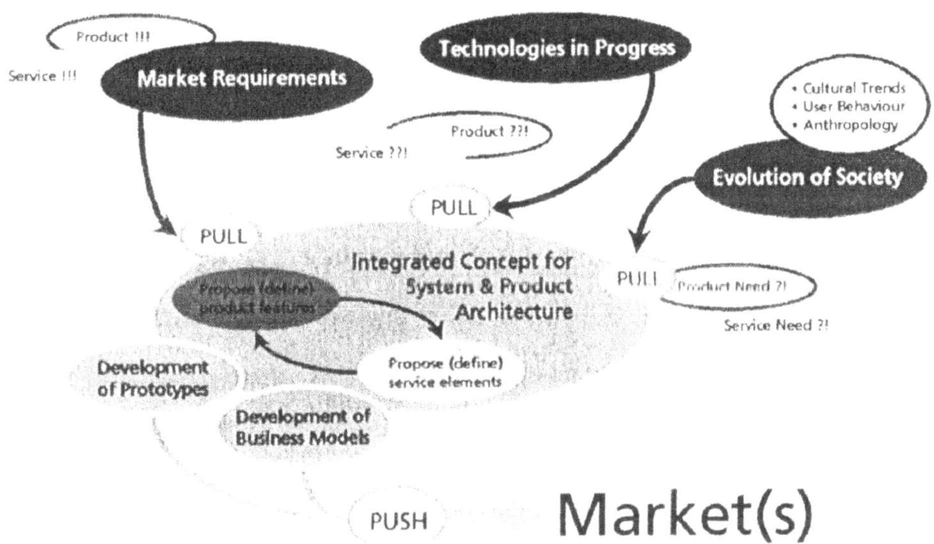

Figure 1 – Product-service system innovation scheme

The ProSecCo industrial partners relate to three industrial clusters – "Culture and Entertainment", "Medical Technology and Applications", and "Health Care and Food Safety" - where co-development of product and services is of increasing importance and where, due to the cross-border markets and competition for products and services, transnational collaboration has become critical for success. Industrial partners from small and medium companies (SME) participate, with different levels achieved in implementing ICT, experience in inter-company collaboration and working in production development, innovation management etc.

In the current article, the third of the clusters above shall be described. Here SMEs typically form chains of companies providing electronic control equipment for quality surveillance, transportation and tracking, related maintenance, handling and packaging etc. of perishables. Thus, product-service hybrid innovation has to realize interrelating functionalities by means of structures in space and / or time (see Figure 2). Food safety and health care are perceived as issues differing mainly with regard to aspects of security standards and scales. Firstly, this may imply that rather simple products have to be combined with peculiar, if complex, services to fasten the logistics as well as the management of mass (eg. food) or very low lot (eg. synthetic or organic implants) production. Secondly, to offer a value proposition may include assistant functionality to be realized by rather specific technical PSCD innovation. Additionally, Figure 2 reveals that product-service innovation implies and cross-branch, cross-sectoral collaboration efforts. For this reason, it is proposed to group networks according to related solution themes rather than along traditional branch or sector models. Therefore, the chosen approach refers to networks of product manufacturers and service providers belonging to different typologies of innovation impetus as presented in chapter 3.

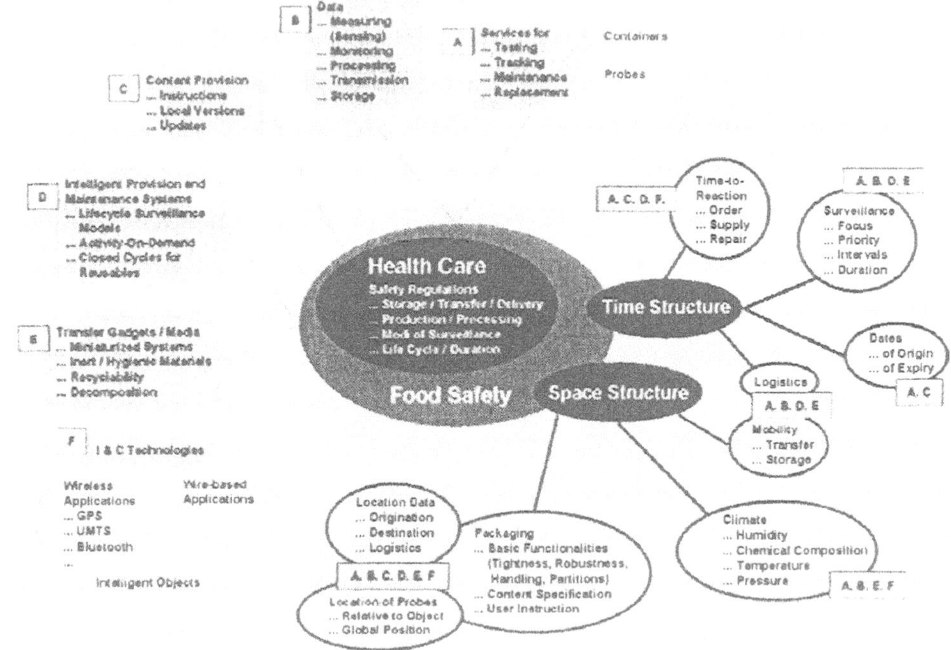

Figure 2 - Potential product-service network in the area of "Health Care and Food Safety"

Finally, solution spaces as depicted in Figure 2 shall encourage entrepreneurial creativity in SMEs to further evolve current business profiles or to forge strategic alliances in areas of (future) interest.

4.2 Dimensions of Convergence

In the following, first thoughts of a conceptual framework of an integrated approach for innovation in product-service systems are presented. It is based on hypotheses still to be tested and refined within the ongoing research in this field.

The approach is based on the convergent factors of technology and knowledge related to products and services. The strategic context forms an overall framework for the integration. The concept refers to Hertogs four-dimensional model of service innovation (Hertog, 2000), but focuses upon linking dimensions in product-service systems that are fundamental to an integrated approach.

Dimension 1: The value proposition concept
The composition of product and services within a system constitutes the value proposition that the company or the network is offering: to provide a solution to a specific customer problem implies combining tangible and intangible elements. In fact, integrated development of product and service systems is likely to cause shifts in corporate image and strategy regarding the means to create value for customers because holistic problem solutions must cover tangible and intangible components in a manner appropriate to corporate economical interests as well as responding the

customer (or market) needs in best-possible way. Business design is required to cover both relevant contents as well as establishment of networks of partners with complementary competences (e.g. related to branch / sector models) required for holistic problem solutions. Accordingly, business strategies and - in particular - the development methods have to focus product and service issues integratively, too.

Dimension 2: Product and service system interface and technological options
Whereas an increased demand for customer-tailored products leads to incorporation of services in products (e.g. remote maintenance), other solutions feature specific service models that may require particular hardware for being enabled / delivered to final customers (e.g. location-based information services). In both cases, technology significantly shapes the area of intersection between a system's particular products and services. While large companies may be capable of developing those sub-systems integrally, SMEs intending to establish equivalent cross-branch, inter-organizational competence and strategic networks need to set-up the functional and content-related interfaces between their particular ranges of contribution in ways that both result in sufficient critical mass for setting new standards as well as open chances for further "plug-ins" solving specific problems of other final users innovatively but within a particular product - service system's paradigm. Whereas dimension 1 relates to the system interface for relations to the (external) customer, the current dimension affects more the internal routines and specifications that finally enable an integrated product-service system at all. This, of course, strongly affects organizational design as well. The flexibility of a company to meet various specifications and openness to technological progress or shifts constitutes a competence area critical for success. Technology forming a link between product and service, is not only required to focus requirements of final user but also those of service partners. This widens e.g. the set of criteria for assessing alternatives.

Dimension 3: Role of knowledge
Bodies developing value propositions via specific composition of products and services into systems inevitably have to establish and manage the competences (capabilities in terms of resources, processes and values (Christensen, 2000)) required in the related business models. In doing so, critical knowledge regarding technologies, delivery and applications is developed through interaction both internal of the value-creating network and – even more important - through its direct encounters with final customers (as the very way of delivering services). Due to the tacit nature of knowledge involved in developing and delivering services, management methodology as well as ICT-based tools addressing the issues above strongly rely on the "human factor" to become supportive at all. Especially knowledge-intensive services form a critical link between products and services. within a product-service system

5. CONCLUSION

Based on considerations of research in the innovation patterns in manufacturing and service industries, the current work proposes a conceptual framework for integrated design of products and services in terms of proposing more holistic solutions. The presented approach in particular relates to the convergent factors of technology and knowledge and conceptually incorporates the dimensions of value proposition, system interface design and role of knowledge. To successfully develop product-service systems, companies are required to adopt a holistic solution perspective and to consider implications for managerial practice regarding strategic issues of business development (emergent versus intended approaches), organizational design to achieve necessary capabilities in terms of networking adaptiveness and efficient innovation processes. These issues need to be further investigated by combining expertise from various fields of expertise such as service engineering, design and innovation management, R&D management and advanced marketing.

6. ACKNOWLEDGEMENTS

This work has been sponsored by the European Commission through the Growth Project No. G1RD-CT-2002-00716: ProSecCo, "Product & Service Co-Design". The authors wish to acknowledge the Commission for its support as well as all the ProSecCo project partners for their contribution during the development of ideas and concepts presented in this paper. However, the text presented here is in the sole responsibility of the authors and the usual disclaimers apply.

7. REFERENCES

1. Antonelli C. Recombination of the production of technological knowledge: some international evidence. In Melcalfe JS, Miles I. Innovation Systems in the Service Economy. Measurement and Case Study Analysis. Boston /Dordrecht /London: Kluwer Academic Publ., 2000.
2. Christensen, Clayton M. The Innovators Dilemma, New York: HarperCollins Publ. Inc., 2000.
3 Hertog den P. Knowledge-Intensive Business Services as Co-Producers of Innovation. In International Journal of Innovation Management, Vol.4 No.4 (Dec 2000) , pp. 491-528
4. Hipp et al.. The incidence and effects of innovation in services: Evidence from Germany. In Journal of Innovation Management. Vol. 4, No. 4 (December 2000): pp. 417-453.
5. Licht et al.. Innovation in the service sector – selected facts and some policy conclusions. Mannheim: Center for European Economic research, 1999.
6. .Miles, I. Service Innovation: Coming Age in the Know-ledge-based Economy. In Journal of Innovation Management. Vol. 4, No. 4 (December 2000): pp. 371-389.
7. Melcalfe JS, Miles I. Innovation Systems in the Service Economy. Measurement and Case Study Analysis. Boston /Dordrecht /London: Kluwer Academic Publ., 2000.
8. OECD. Proposed Guidelines for collecting and interpreting technological innovation data - Oslo Manual 1992.
9. OECD. The Service Economy, Business and Industry Policy Forum, 2000. http://www.oecd.org/dsti/sti/industry/indcomp/act/services/forum.htm
10. Preissl B. Service innovation: what makes it different? Empirical evidence from Germany. In Metcalfe JS, Miles I. Innovation Systems in the Service Economy. Measurement and Case Study Analysis. Boston /Dordrecht /London: Kluwer Academic Publ., 2000.
11. Romer, P.M. (1995) Economic Growth The Fortune Encyclopedia of Economics, David R. Henderson (ed.)
12. Sirilli G, Evangelista R. Technological innovation in services and manufacturing: Results from an Italian survey. In Research policy Vol. 27 (1998), No. 9, pp. 881-899.
13. Soete L, Miozzo M. Trade and development in services: a technological perspective. In MERIT Report 89-031, Maastricht: MERIT, 1989.
14. Ramaswamy R. Design and Management of Services processes. Keeping Customers for Life. Reading MA: Addison-Wesley Publ. Comp., 1996.

42

AGILE E-BUSINESS PROCESS ASSEMBLY AND DEVELOPMENT

Thomas Schmidt, Karl Fürst, Gerald Wippel
Automation Control Institute – TU Vienna
ts@infa.tuwien.ac.at, kf@infa.tuwien.ac.at, gw@infa.tuwien.ac.at

A collaborative enterprise uses Internet technology to achieve dramatic improvements along the whole life cycle by integrating the business processes of collaborating partners. Therefore it is necessary to describe the public aspects of business processes in a standard way using international standardized languages like WSFL, XLANG, BPML, or ebXML. In this paper the architecture for automatically program code generation to realize the business process tier of the FLoCI-EE system architecture is discussed. This tier uses feature rich business Web Services to realize business processes as a composition of Web Services and provide the business processes as Web Services.

1. INTRODUCTION

The ultimate goal of companies is the delivery of high quality products and services to the global market within the shortest possible time (time-to-market) and lowest costs (time-to-money) in order to be competitive. Because more and more enterprises focus on their core-competencies, they have to collaborate to support the whole life cycle of complex products or services. Such collaborations are temporary or permanent networks of independent enterprises that cooperate with the aim to design, manufacture, and sell a product or service independent of enterprise borderlines. Each member contributes specific core know-how to the collaboration network. This concept enables very fast and flexible reactions to changed market conditions or new opportunities.

Enterprise Application Integration (EAI) follows the aim to integrate isolated application implementations among each other or with central and enterprise-wide systems like ERP. Such realized integration solutions are often selective and restricted application integration approaches which means that data-oriented one-way integration solutions without synchronization of the underlying business processes stand in the foreground (Linthicum, 2000). To support the integration of enterprise-wide and enterprise-spanning business processes, we need the next step in the EAI-evolution: the process-centric EAI called business integration.

2. BUSINESS INTEGRATION

With the growth of e-commerce there is an emerging need to integrate and automate business processes that span enterprise boundaries (the so-called B2C and B2B processes). A business process can be defined as a collection of business transactions between partners and/or internal activities within one business. A typical business process may consist of up to 100 IT transactions. Coordinating the entire process correctly and efficiently places severe demands on the organization's IT infrastructure.

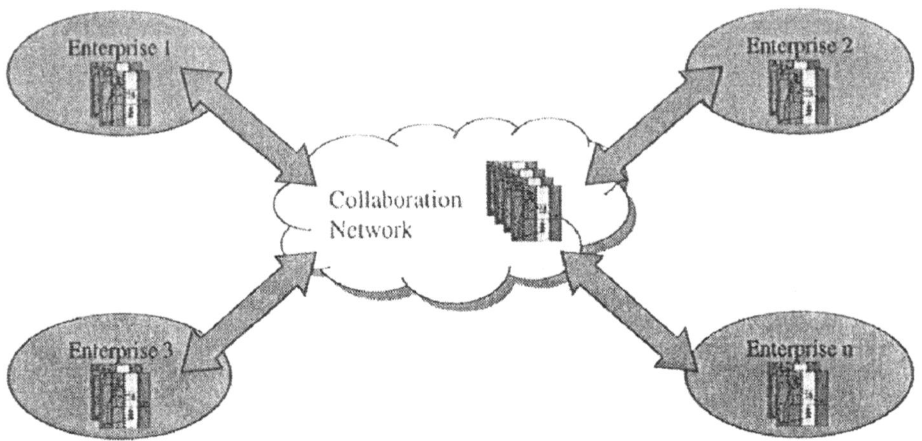

Figure 1 – Business Processes in the Collaboration Network

Figure 1 shows the collaboration network scenario with internal enterprise specific and common business processes. All processes are networked to achieve the common goal of delivering high quality products and services to the customers. Each enterprise inside the network has their own core-competencies like engineering, production, or marketing and sales. Members of the collaboration network are also the suppliers with the core-competence to deliver specific raw materials and semi-finished goods. A tight integration of the customers is needed especially in the case of creation complex products and services.

The currently running international research and development project FLoCI-EE (Flexible Low-Cost Internet Extended Enterprise) aims at the development of an easy to use, component based software system to support the whole lifecycle of products in extended enterprises (Fürst, 2001). Extended enterprises are special forms of collaboration networks where one dominant enterprise "extends" its boundaries to all or some of its suppliers. During this project, more precisely at architecture design, the need for a separate business process tier was detected (see Figure 2). This tier uses feature rich business Web Services (e.g. Document Management, Project Management, etc.), which are provided by the lower tier, to realize business processes as a composition of Web Services. These business processes are provided as Web Services to the upper tier.

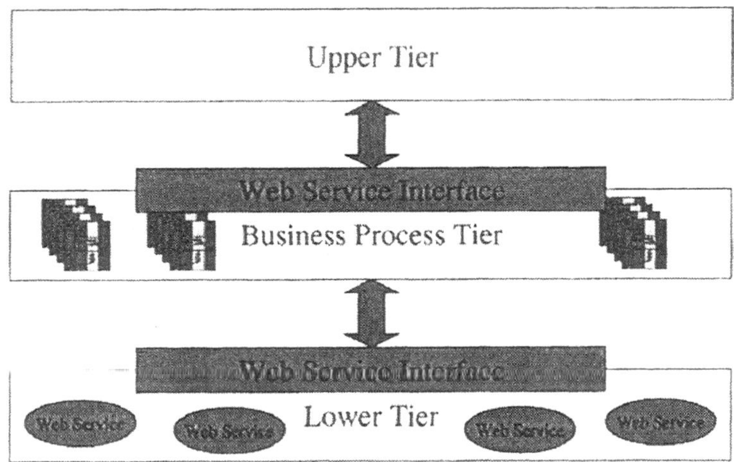

Figure 2 – Business Process Tier

The following chapter gives a short introduction into the up-to-date topic Web Services. In chapter 4 the current available Web Service based business process modeling standards WSFL, XLANG, and BPML are discussed. Additionally mentioned is the promising standard ebXML. In chapter 5 the vision of automatically program code generation using the description of the business processes is described.

3. WEB SERVICES

A Web Service represents a unit of business, application, or system functionality that can be accessed over the Web. Web Services are applicable to any type of Web environment, whether Internet, Intranet, or Extranet, whether with a focus on business-to-consumer, business-to-business, department-to-department, or peer-to-peer communication. A Web Service consumer could be a human user accessing the service through a desktop or wireless browser; it could also be an application program or another Web Service (Sun, 2002).

A Web Service exhibits the following basic characteristics:

- Web Services communicate using XML messages over standard Web protocols. SOAP (Simple Object Access Protocol) provides an extensible XML messaging protocol and also supports an RPC (Remote Procedure Call) programming model (SOAP, 2000). An extended variant of SOAP, called SOAP Messages with Attachments, is using MIME to be able to transport also non XML-payload.
- A Web Service exposes an XML interface description. WSDL (Web Service Description Language) is a common XML framework for describing a Web Service (WSDL, 2001).
- A Web Service is registered and can be located through a Web Service registry. The UDDI (Universal Description, Discovery, and Integration) initiative is an industry consortium that is developing specifications for

a universal, Web-based business directory called the UDDI Business Registry (UDDI, 2002).

Figure 3 shows the cooperation between a service provider, who has published the Web Service at a service registry, and a service requestor, who has found the Web Service at this service registry.

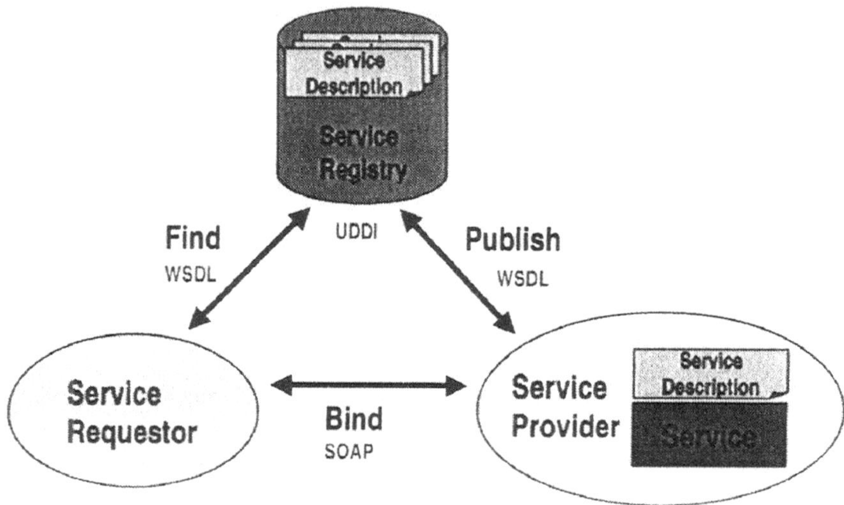

Figure 3 – Web Service Model

4. BUSINESS PROCESS MODELING

One precondition for enabling cross-enterprise business process automation is the ability to describe the public aspects of the business processes in a standard form that can be consumed by tools for process implementation and monitoring. In the following subchapters, the currently available XML-based approaches to fulfill this condition are discussed.

4.1 WSFL

The WSFL (Web Service Flow Language) is an XML language for the description of Web Services compositions as part of a business process definition. It was designed by IBM to be part of the Web Service technology framework and relies and complements existing specifications like SOAP, WSDL, and UDDI (WSFL, 2001).

WSFL considers two types of Web Service compositions:

- The first type specifies an executable business process known as a flow model.
- The second type specifies a business collaboration known as a global model.

In the first case, a composition is created by describing how to use the functionality provided by the collection of composed Web Services. This is also known as flow composition, orchestration, or choreography of Web Services. WSFL models these compositions as specifications of the execution sequence of the functionality provided by the composed Web Services. Execution orders are specified by defining the flow of control and data between Web Services. Flow models can especially be used to model business processes or workflows based on Web Services.

In the second case, no specification of an execution sequence is provided. Instead, the composition provides a description of how the composed Web Services interact with each other.

WSFL provides extensive support for the recursive composition of services: In WSFL, every Web Service composition (a flow model as well as a global model) can itself become a new Web Service, and can thus be used as a component of new compositions.

4.2 XLANG

XLANG is the XML business process language used by Microsoft's BizTalk server. The goal of XLANG is to make it possible to formally specify business processes as stateful long-running interactions. Business processes always involve more than one participant. The full description of a process must show not only the behavior of each participant, but the way these behaviors match to produce the overall process. The focus is on the publicly visible behavior in the form of message exchanged. The specific high-level feature categories that define the scope of XLANG are listed below (XLANG, 2002):

- Sequential and parallel control flow constructs
- Long running transactions with compensation
- Custom correlation of messages
- Flexible handling of internal and external exceptions
- Modular behavior description
- Dynamic service referral
- Multi-role contracts

XLANG has a close relationship with WSDL: An XLANG service description is a WSDL service description with an extension element that describes the behavior of the service as a part of a business process.

Microsoft has previously worked with IBM on both the WSDL and UDDI initiatives. And, while they have been initially creating parallel recommendations, it would not be surprising to see IBM and Microsoft jointly agree to submit a proposal to W3C that combines XLANG and WSFL in the near future.

4.3 BPML

The BPML (Business Process Modeling Language) is a meta-language for the modeling of business processes, just as XML is a meta-language for the modeling of business data (BPML, 2001). BPML provides an abstracted execution model for collaborative and transactional business processes based on the concept of a transactional finite-state machine.

The BPML specification is provided by the business process management initiative (BPMI) organization. BPMI.org is a non-profit corporation that empowers companies of all sizes, across all industries, to develop and operate business processes that span multiple applications and business partners, behind the firewall and over the Internet. The initiative's mission is to promote and develop the use of Business Process Management (BPM) through the establishment of standards for process design, deployment, execution, maintenance, and optimization.

In much the same way XML documents are usually described in a specific XML Schema layered on top of XML, BPML processes can be described in a specific business process modeling language layered on top of the extensible BPML XML Schema. BPML represents business processes as the interleaving of control flow, data flow, and event flow, while adding orthogonal design capabilities for business rules, security roles, and transaction contexts.

In addition, the BPMI is also working on a business process query language (BPQL), which will provide the interface between the application and the business process data. The idea is that BPQL will eventually be to BPML what SQL is to databases.

4.4 ebXML

To provide an open XML-based infrastructure enabling the global use of electronic business information in an interoperable, secure and consistent manner by all parties is the mission of ebXML (Electronic Business using XML). ebXML, sponsored by UN/CEFACT (United Nations body for Trade Facilitation and Electronic Business Information Standards) and OASIS (Organization for the Advancement of Structured Information Standards), is a modular suite of specifications that enables enterprises of any size and in any geographical location to conduct business over the Internet. Using ebXML, companies now have a standard method to exchange business messages, conduct trading relationships, communicate data in common terms and define and register business processes (ebXML, 2001).

The following overview introduces the concepts and underlying architecture of ebXML:

- A standard mechanism for describing a business process and its associated information model.
- A mechanism for registering and storing business process and information meta-models so they can be shared and reused.
- Discovery of information about each participant including:
    - The business processes they support.
    - The business service interfaces they offer in support of the business process.
    - The business messages that are exchanged between their respective business service interfaces.
    - The technical configuration of the supported transport, security and encoding protocols.
- A mechanism for registering the aforementioned information so that it may be discovered and retrieved.
- A mechanism for describing the execution of a mutually agreed upon business arrangement which can be derived from information provided by each participant.

- A standardized business messaging service framework that enables interoperable, secure and reliable exchange of messages between trading partners.
- A mechanism for configuration of the respective messaging services to engage in the agreed upon business process in accordance with the constraints defined in the business arrangement.

5. CONCLUSION AND FUTURE WORK

In chapter 4 the state-of-the-art in XML-based business process modeling was discussed. The future progress of standardization efforts will show if the different modeling languages will grow together to establish only one XML-based modeling language.

To realize the vision of automatically program code generation using the XML-based description of the business processes in a standardized form, the architecture shown in Figure 4 will be used.

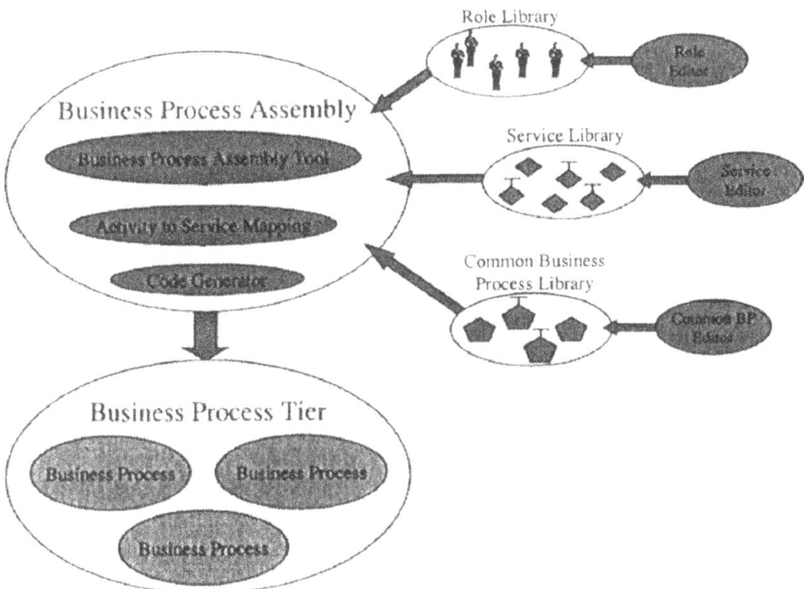

Figure 4 – Architecture for Automatically Program Code Generation

With the Business Process Assembly Tool the business processes are modeled using one of the above discussed standard language. Therefore, different libraries are used:

- Role-Library to define the participating roles
- Service-Library to define available services
- Common Business Process Library to define reusable business processes

Additional editors (Role Editor, Service Editor, and Common Business Process Editor) are necessary for the library management (e.g. create new entries, edit existing entries, etc.). Before the Code Generator is able to generate the program code for the Business Process Tier, an Activity to Service Mapping is necessary to define which service (service name, service location, etc.) is used to realize the business process activity.

The Code Generator itself can be implemented in two different ways:

- Consuming the XML-based output of the business process assembly unit shown in Figure 4, a Workflow-Engine can walk through the business processes activity by activity. Instead of program code, the executable input for a Workflow-Engine is generated.
- Using an XSLT processor to transform the XML-based description of the business processes into program code. For example, Figure 5 shows the scenario to generate Java Class Files. XSLT (XSL Transformations) is an XML-based language standardized by W3C (XSLT, 1999). There are a number of free XSLT processors available.

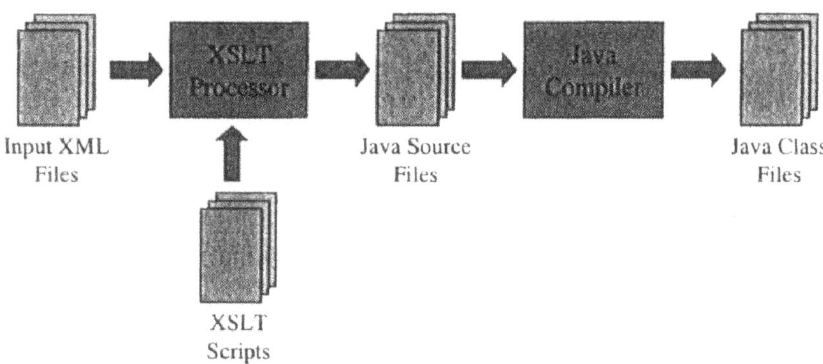

Figure 5 – Java Code Generation Using XSLT

In the near future a proof-of-concept prototype will be developed to show the usability of the proposed architecture for automatically program code generation.

6. REFERENCES

1. BPML (Business Process Modeling Language), Working Draft 0.4. Business Process Management Initiative. http://www.bpmi.org/. 8 March 2001.
2. ebXML Specifications. http://www.ebxml.org/specs/index.htm/. May 2001.
3. Fürst, Karl. „FLoCI-EE: Flexible Low-Cost Internet Extended Enterprise". E-work and E-commerce. Editor: Brian Stanford-Smith and Enrica Chiozza. IOS Press, 2001; 769-775.
4. Linthicum, David S. Enterprise Application Integration. Addison Wesley, 2000.
5. SOAP (Simple Object Access Protocol) 1.1, W3C Note. World Wide Web Consortium (W3C). http://www.w3.org/TR/SOAP/. 8 May 2000.
6. Sun Microsystems: Sun Open Net Environment (Sun ONE). http://www.sun.com/sunone/. March 2002.
7. UDDI (Universal Description, Discovery, and Integration). http://www.uddi.org. March 2002.
8. WSDL (Web Services Description Language) 1.1, W3C Note. World Wide Web Consortium (W3C). http://www.w3.org/TR/wsdl/. 15 March 2001.
9. WSFL (Web Services Flow Language) 1.0. IBM Software Group. http://www-4.ibm.com/software/solutions/webservices/pdf/WSFL.pdf. May 2001.
10. XLANG. Microsoft Corporation. http://www.gotdotnet.com/team/xml_wsspecs/xlang-c/default.htm. March 2002.
11. XSLT (XSL Transformations) 1.0, W3C Recommendation. World Wide Web Consortium (W3C). http://www.w3.org/TR/xslt/. 16 November 1999.

43

A CONCEPTUAL FRAMEWORK FOR EFFICIENT NEW PRODUCT INTRODUCTIONS

Erik Sandin[1], Mauro Onori[2]
[1] *esn@iip.kth.se*
[2] *WoxénCentrum*
Dept. of Production Engineering
The Royal Institute of Technology
Stockholm, Sweden
onori@iip.kth.se

Increasing global competition, decreasing lifecycles and outsourcing trends put new demands on product design and assembly system development. These demands call for highly flexible assembly systems, consisting of standardised, process-oriented assembly modules, offering robust processes and high equipment reuseability. To generate such a system, a new concept for cross-functional development of products and the assembly system is being developed. The concept is based on a distinct connection between product design and the assembly system. To achieve this, the Assembly Module Platform (AMP) is being developed. The AMP generates the Module Process Description (MPD), which defines the process executed by the modules. The design of the product can now be guided by the MPD, creating a process-oriented product design.

1. INTRODUCTION

The major problems incurred by companies dealing with assembly all relate to uncertainty. First of all, it is very difficult for companies to predict the type and range of products that will have to be developed. The second uncertainty regards the production volumes and lifespans reached by these future products. The overwhelming reaction to these problems has been to attempt to develop extremely flexible assembly machines that attempt to adapt themselves to different product families and production scenarios. This has led to a series of multi-purpose machines, amongst which the MarkI, MarkII and MarkIII Flexible Automatic Assembly (FAA) cells developed at our premises [1]. Another approach has been to focus on the standardisation and modularisation of high-volume manual assembly lines [2], also resulting in special robotic cells for the automatic tasks. Flexibility, instead of the actual assembly process, has been the core issue of most of these developments. This fact has been further aggravated by the fact that a firm grasp of which type of flexibility is being targeted has, until recently [3], been neglected in favour of a general description of this term. Unfortunately, this existing paradigm of highly flexible (automatic) assembly systems still prevails, resulting in expensive, highly technological solutions ([4],[5]) which cannot easily fit into existing production facilities are seldom able to assemble more than one product generation. In reality, however, 90-95% of producing companies have to deal with planned products and existing production facilities. Ideally, they would like to fit any new product into an existing assembly system with as low costs as possible. To date, this has only been a dream. The common scenario is that the existing production system principles still dictate, to a varying degree, the basic design requirements for future products, and vice versa. Basically, there is a strong dependence between product development and selected system principle (parallel flow, serial line, etc.). This entails that any new FAA, or other assembly system solution, has to fit into an existing facility. For example, as soon as a given product design leads to a potential assembly system solution, a serious analysis of the components is required to ensure that the targeted volumes, costs, etc. are attained. This often leads to a change in some system component, or product part, to enable the achievement of the goals. This is exactly where the problems arise: the maximum attainable capacity and flexibility of an assembly system are ultimately dictated by the product design and assembly equipment [6]. Therefore, if the equipment cannot easily adapt to changing market requirements and/or new products, the overall flexibility is greatly reduced. Furthermore, if the envisaged FAA solution cannot easily fit into the existing production system scenario, it will not be deemed as fully flexible by the user. Highly flexible automatic assembly cells, as developed to date, will therefore not succeed. What is required is *a solution which, being based on several re-configurable, task-specific elements (modules), allows for a continuous evolution of the assembly system.* In order for this to succeed, however, a dynamic link to the product design process must be created.

2. BACKGROUND

One of the fastest growing and knowledge intensive fields of today is the telecom market, where the annual growth has been of approximately 20-25% in the past five years (1995-2000). During this time, the trend of outsourcing of whole, or parts of, products has also increased. Consequently, sub-contracting companies are constantly gaining market shares of the total value of the production. Using the benefits of manufacturing products for a number of companies, and at the same time converting the production plants from high-wage to low-wage countries, they can keep a low manufacturing cost. The trend of outsourcing does not depend on lowering manufacturing costs alone, but also on the growing importance for the telecom companies to focus on their core-competence, which is the telecom technology and not manufacturing.

This trend of outsourcing has dramatically changed the production chain development - customer. To simplify, one can say that the traditional chain consisted of Development/Design – Manufacturing - Customer, in which both Development/Design and Manufacturing were in-house and located in the same

country as the company itself. Today, the chain consists of Development/Design - New Product Introduction (NPI)/Industrialization - High Volume Manufacturing - Customer, in which Development/Design and NPI/Industrialization are located in-house and in the same country, whilst the high volume manufacturing is outsourced and located in so called low-wage countries (see fig. 1).
Consequently, the "home" country is left with a low-volume production of many variants in the early phase of the product life cycle. Unfortunately, during such early phases, the knowledge of the product and associated assembly processes are low.

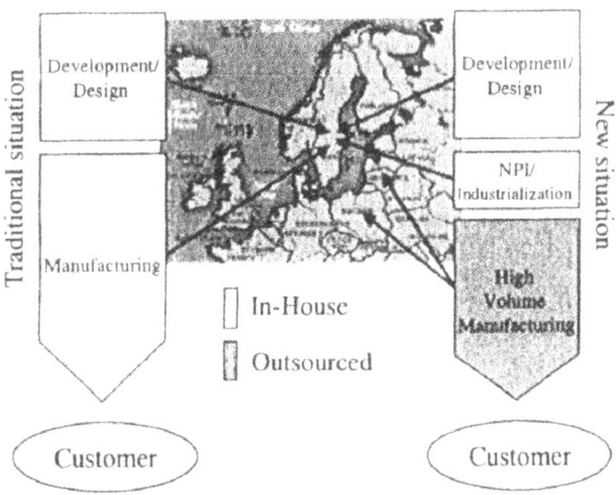

Figure 1 - TheTrend of Outsourcing

It is therefore important to analyse the functional requirements created by the outsourcing trend. This is particularly vital for final assembly systems of an NPI / Industrialization plant in the telecom market, in which the cycle NPI - volume production – Transfer Product Introduction (TPI) cycle restarts every 20 – 30 months. NPI is hereby the term used to denote all activities in a product development project, from assignment to achieved project targets (time, quality and cost), that are intended to assure production capacity, produceability and the ability to deliver market volumes at the right time, cost and minimal environmental impact (see fig. 2).

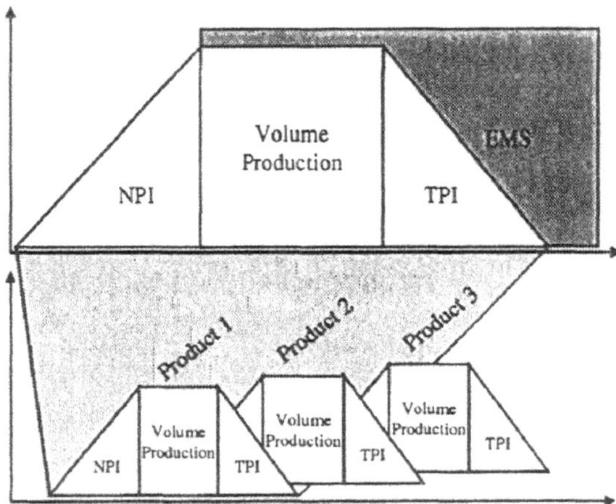

Figure 2 - NPI, Volume Production and TPI

The Assembly Module Platform (AMP) described in this article aims to create the necessary prerequisites for how to become a world-class NPI/Industrialization manufacturer.

3. THE FUNCTIONAL REQUIREMENTS

The project has defined the following production characteristics as targeted problem areas :

- *Time-To-Market (TTM)*, the time to introduce new products to the market [7]. It has been found that 80 – 90 percent of the TTM equation is absorbed in the design phase [8]. Therefore, a tool that could optimise the collaboration between designers and manufacturers is urgently needed. The tool should aim at reducing the designing time and, at the same time, render the design more process-oriented.
- *Ramp-up*, after a successful introduction of a new product, the demand of the product tends to rapidly increase and companies are often unable to close the gap between supply and demand. Therefore, it is of great importance to shorten the Time To Volume (TTV): the time it takes to reach the targeted supply capacity. Due to economical reasons, as important is obtaining a short Time To Break-even (TTB): the time taken by the product to begin generating a profit (see fig. 3).
- *Market fluctuations,* demand fluctuations that follow the economic climate, customer strategies etc. These fluctuations may vary in depth and length, and can be very irregular and unpredictable.
- *Re-useability of equipment,* The time that a product is assembled in the plant is too short to alone carry the cost of an investment in an automatic assembly system [9]. Furthermore, re-using the equipment creates a great possibility to gather process knowledge, and, as described later on, create design guidelines[10].

- *Large number of product variants,* in the early phase of the product life cycle, in which the knowledge of the product and associated assembly processes are low.

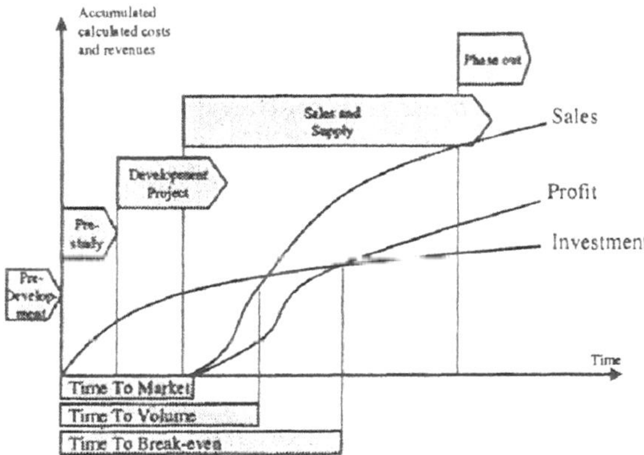

Figure 3 – The Importance of Rapid Output Increase of Production Volume

These demands call for specific assembly system properties. These properties may be summed up within the following functional requirements:

- Capacity flexibility, the ability of an assembly system to react to changing market demands in terms of the quantities asked for [11]. Vital for the adequate absorption of market fluctuations and ramp-ups.
- Capability flexibility, is the ability of an assembly system to react to changing market demands in terms of product variants asked for [11].Vital for the adequate absorption of market fluctuations and large product variant floras.
- Process robustness. Vital for true flexibility, quality levels, and the efficient re-use of equipment.

4. THE AMP APPROACH

Due to the demands and functional requirements stated above, a new approach to flexible assembly systems design and process-oriented product design, suited for the NPI-environment in the telecom market, is being developed in a long-term project that started January 2001. The project is carried out in collaboration between The Royal Institute of Technology, the WoxénCentrum, and Ericsson.

In the following section, the Assembly Module Platform (AMP) is introduced as the heart of the approach. The process-driven product design guidelines are also presented, as well as the motivations and prerequisites for standardisation.

4.1 The Architecture of the Method

A well-structured Assembly Module Platform (AMP) is currently being finalised, in which all the required assembly processes are well structured and defined, along with the specific equipment to enable the processes.
The creation of the AMP modules is based on these assembly processes. This enables a process-oriented product design since the available technological solutions are known a' priori to the start of the product design [12]. Since the design of the product is carried out on the basis of given assembly modules, one may evaluate the influence of different product designs on the assembly system and compare the different assembly system configurations which ensue, thus giving a comparative list of investment costs, assembly costs, annual production volumes, etc. For this purpose, an economical evaluation tool is also being developed for the AMP-database, in which one may select and compare different assembly system configurations and, thereby, also the product design.
The basic notion, or paradigm, in this project is the belief that extreme and long-lasting flexibility cannot be achieved without a distinct connection between product design and the assembly system, using standard process-oriented modules [13].

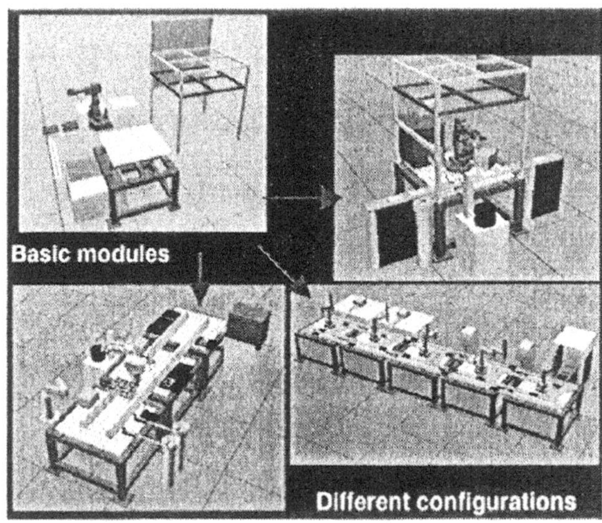

Figure 4 - The HFAA Module Concept

In order to achieve the full level of flexibility, assembly solutions must be designed to integrate any form or type of equipment: truly standardised interfacing. The equipment, in turn, must be broken down into smaller, process-oriented components. This approach [10], which allows for a stepwise automation and knowledge acquisition, requires an in-depth study, classification and structuring of the assembly process and its requirements. Once the process requirements are classified, an assembly concept which consists of small, targeted components rather than multi-purpose cells, will be attainable. This represents a shift in thinking since it implies that theoretically very flexible, multi-purpose cells will be replaced by a highly flexible concept consisting of several well-targeted but not, in themselves, highly flexible components. Hence the new project paradigm. This is in full accordance with the Hyper Flexible Automatic Assembly project (HFAA), and enables the defining of the required assembly processes a' priori to the product design. The paradigm will probably redefine some of the older focuses on flexibility. For instance, achieving product flexibility through flexible equipment has been an established goal for some time, by attempting to create equipment so flexible that it could handle almost any products or variants. However, in this project, capability flexibility is achieved through process structuring and connections to the product design.

One of the main objectives of FAA research has been the development of systems with high product flexibility ([14],[15]). The industry has, however, been very reluctant to invest in such solutions. Therefore, should the given paradigm be correct, all projects concerned with the assembly system alone, without considering the connection between the assembly processes and the product design, are assumed to fail.

5. THE ASSEMBLY MODULE PLATFORM (AMP)

The AMP is a structured platform containing standardised process-oriented modules, for use within the telecom market. The AMP consists of five levels, based on: Process-class, Cell-Module, Module, Attribute and Parameter (see fig. 5).

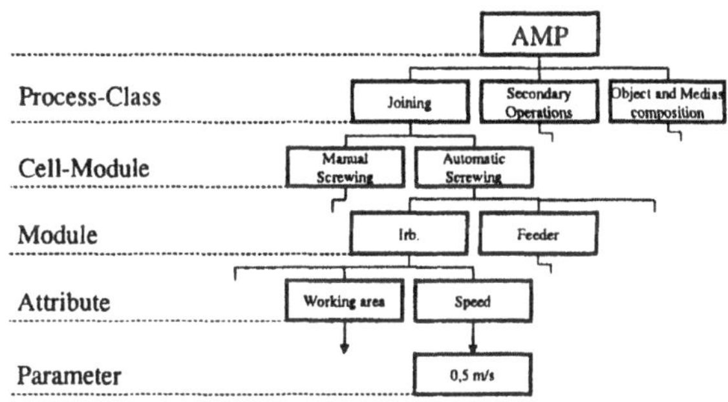

Figure 5. The AMP Structure

The definitions of the different levels are as follows:

Process-class:

A group of similar processes.

Process:

An activity that, together with other activities in the assembly system, refines parts and base-objects into a finished product. E.g. Type B soldering .

Cell-module:

A cell, or cluster of equipment, with a specific task that creates a complete building block in the assembly system. Consists of one or more modules that, through their combinability, can create a specific configuration of a cell-module. E.g. Automatic laser marking.

Module:
A combinable equipment/component that fulfils a certain functionality within the cell-module by working with other modules through standardized interfaces, then called sub-modules. E.g. Assembly robot.
Attribute:
Characteristics of a module or sub-module. E.g. Acceleration, workspace, repeatability, etc .
Parameter:
A value or range of values of an attribute. The design of the parameter should allow that the sum of the attributes, with its specific parameters, will give a complete definition of the module: the so-called Module Process Definition (MPD).

The AMP consists of three process-classes: object and media compositions, joining, and secondary operations. These are defined as follows:

Object and medias composition:
Picking, possible manipulation, and orientation of parts (in object or medium form) and base-object, whereafter insertion is performed.
Joining:
Picking, possible manipulation, and orientation of parts and base-object, whereafter fixation with one process method occurs.
Secondary operations:
Activities not in the actual value adding chain, but necessary before delivery.

Three objectives have been focused upon during the development of the AMP :

- First, the cell-modules should be at such a level that they may easily be seen as building blocks in the total assembly system, for example by performing a distinct process (e.g. an automatic soldering cell).
- Secondly, each cell-module should consist of a number of modules that, through their combinability, could create different re-configurations of the cell-module (e.g. a screwdriver or an assembly robot).
- Thirdly, each module should facilitate the complete definition of the executed assembly process. Basically, an inherent guideline for product designers and production engineers can be formed by the cell-module configuration procedure.

One can say that adding or subtracting cell-modules enables capacity flexibility, and, likewise, shifting modules in a cell-module enables capability flexibility.

6. THE GUIDELINES

In the AMP, the attributes and the parameters represent the two lowest levels. Together they generate the Module Process Definition (MPD), which fully defines each specific module's performance, geometrical abilities, etc. As the attributes can be divided into attributes affecting product design, and attributes affecting production engineering, two different guidelines can be generated:

- the product design guidelines, enabling a process-oriented product design in which the assembly process carried out by the assembly equipment is known a' priori to the product designer.
- the production engineering guidelines enabling a comparison of configuration costs, annual volumes, etc..

Since the guidelines will give a complete definition of the assembly process, the design of the product is well suited for the NPI-equipment, and can easily be introduced to the assembly system. Since the parameters are based on both today's equipment and future product demands, and are constantly updated, the guidelines create a process-oriented product design that is modern at all times and enables a long term capability flexibility.

7. THE STANDARDIZATION ASPECTS

Due to the importance of re-use of equipment and a high (re-)configuration ability of the system, all modules in the platform should be standardised, including the interfaces. Many definitions of standardisation have been given in the literature, none of which, however, fulfil the needs of this project.

Note that the standardisation being mentioned here relates to the creation of assembly equipment which has been developed out of a stringent classification and structuring of the assembly process. The solution refers to an open system into which new equipment may be brought as long as it follows the delimitations and interfacing requirements.

The benefits to be gained from a standardised solution are many, amongst which one may name the following:

- Shorter installation times.
- Lower investment costs and related risk factors.
- Simpler re-configurations of original layout.
- Second-hand market for equipment.

This entails that mechanical, electrical, pneumatic, electronic and software interfaces must be standardised, be of a common format, description, etc., and allow the transport of the particular medium (software, air, etc.) without adjustments. This also entails that the physical dimensions of the particular equipment are such that the unit may be inserted into any assembly system without requiring particular modifications.

For this purpose, standardisation guidelines have been developed, consisting of six elements that together define the standardisation levels required. The elements in the matrix are:

- Documentation
- Availability
- Recognition
- Update
- Validity
- Sector management

8. RELATED WORK

The approaches described above, including the AMP and the standardisation objectives, clearly point out that a single isolated effort will not succed. The project has therefore entered close collaboration with two other national and international projects in order to attain the intended goals.

8.1 Hyper Flexible Automatic Assembly (HFAA)/ PROPER Project

The HFAA ([9],[11]) project was initiated in order to meet the future assembly demands being posed by industry in general, and European SMEs in particular. In order to do so, a structured approach to the assembly process itself lies at the core of the project. The project is being carried out at the Royal Institute of Technology (KTH) with close industrial cooperation.
The HFAA project is being partially financed by PROPER (Programme for Production Engineering Research) and industry. The HFAA project will deal with four distinct project areas:

- Analysis of the assembly process and its interactions with product design and assembly equipment.
- Analysis of mini-assembly requirements and its requirements .
- Study of assembly factories concerned with mass customisation.
- Development of a standardised, modular, hybrid assembly system concept.

The final objective is to create a modular, HFAA system *concept* which consists of standardised assembly system components. Details may be found in the literature ([12],[15]).

8.2 Assembly Net (EC Project)

The prime aim of the Assembly Net Thematic Network [16] is to establish a well co-ordinated and effective support infrastructure throughout Europe in order to create a network in which existing national and international projects, and available solutions, are linked to urgent industrial needs.
The critical technologies to be brought into focus include assembly system component design, system design tools, control systems, assembly process analysis, mini and micro assembly developments, etc. The partners propose to set up the following activities:

- At least one conference per year.
- The distribution of a Newsletter twice a year.
- Organise workshops (defined by Special Interest Groups).
- Offer summer courses in theoretical (academia) and practical (industry) topics.
- Create and maintain an official website in which all of the above are listed, as well as links to existing projects, project partners and associated companies.

These activities are to be seen as a first stage of events. The aim is to broaden, in due time, the scope of activities to include the entire lifecycle of such products. The main objectives are:

- To analyse trends and provide a strategic vision on Assembly Automation.

- To act as a catalyst for the implementation of innovative practices by industry.
- Assist partners in finding funding sources, educational resources, etc.
- To provide a forum for developing focused initiatives and collaboration.
- To collect and present knowledge on Assembly Engineering to the industrial and academic community.
- A stimulus for the development of new initiatives, actions, and projects.
- The proposed Consortium currently consists of over 25 institutes from over 10 countries. Orchestrated by the foremost academic institutions in Europe, it intends to merge several national & international research forums and already includes a vast number of industrial members. The Assembly Net (http://www.assembly-net.org) has already succeeded in forming five specific Special Interest Groups.

9. ACKNOWLEDGEMENTS

The project has full access to state-of-the art assembly equipment for its development work. This equipment has been made available to the Woxén Centre by Ericsson.

10. REFERENCES

1. Arnström, A.; Gröndahl, P.;"Advantages of Sub-Batch Principle in Flexible Automatic Assembly as used in the IVF-KTH Concept MARK II"; Annals of the CIRP Vol.37/1/1988.
2. Fujimori;T. ;" Effectiveness of Factory Automation which Leads to Value Added Manufacturing-SONY's Case with the Super SMART System"; Proceedings of the 25th Int. Symposium on Industrial Robots (ISIR), Hannover, Germany 1995;pp.13-20.
3. Johansson, R.; "Implementation of Flexible Automatic Assembly in Small Companies"; PhD. Thesis, The Royal Institute of Technology; Sweden, Autumn 2001.
4. Meijer,B.; Jonker,P.;"The Architecture and Philosophy of the DIAC"; Proceedings of the IEEE International Conference on Robotics and Automation;Sacramento, California, USA, 1991.
5. Heilala,J., Voho,P.;"Agile and Reconfigurable Flexible Semiautomatic Assembly Systems"; Proceedings of the 30th Int.Symposium on Industrial Robots (ISR); Tokyo, Japan, 1999; pp.511-517
6. Karlsson A, Onori M.; "A New Approach to Customer-Oriented Production"; Proceedings of the 33rd CIRP International Seminar on Manufacturing Systems. Stockholm. Sweden. 5-7 June. 2000.
7. Pawar, K. S. *et.al.;* "Time to Market, Getting goods to market fast – and first", Integrated Manufacturing Systems, Vol 5 No. 1, 1994, pp 14-22
8. Charney, C.; "Time to Market. Reducing Product Lead Time", Society of Manufacturing Engimeers, Dearborn, MI, 1991
9. Alsterman, H.; Bergdahl,A.; Onori,M.; "Standardised Assembly Solutions for Secure Introduction of New Products"; Proceedings of the ISR2001, 32nd Int.Symposium on Robotics (ISR), Seoul, Korea, April 2001.
10. Tichem, M.; "Position report on flexible assembly automation", Laboratory for Production Engineering and Industrial Organisation, Delft University of Technology, Landbergsstraat 3, NL-2628 CE Delft, The Netherlands.
11. Johansson, R.; "Implementation of Flexible Automatic Assembly in Small Companies"; PhD. Thesis, The Royal Institute of Technology; Sweden, Autumn 2001.
12. Onori, M.; Alsterman, H.;"Hyper Flexible Automatic Assembly, Needs and Possibilities with Standard Assembly Solutions"; Proceedings of the 3rd World Congress on Intelligent Manufacturing Processes & Systems, June 2000, Cambridge, Ma.,USA.

13. Vos, J.A.W.M.; "Module and System Design in Flexibly Automated Assembly"; Ph.D.Thesis, TU Delft, The Netherlands, DUP Science. ISBN 90-407-2195-5
14. Sanderson, S.; Uzumeri, V.; " Managing product families: The case of the SONY Walkman"; Research Policy 24, 1995,761-782,Rensselear Polytechnic Institute, Troy,NY 12180,USA.
15. Onori, M.; Alsterman, H.; Bergdahl,A.; Johansson,R.; "The Hyper Flexible Automatic Assembly Concept Application: MarkIV"; Proceedings of the Delft Workshop on Assembly Automation, Delft, Holland, May 11-12, 2000.
16. Onori, M.; Sandin, E.; Alsterman, H.; "European Assembly: Threats and Counter-Measures"; Proceedings of the 2nd IFAC Workshop on Intelligent Assembly and Disassembly (IAD'2001), Gramado, Brazil, November 2001; Elsevier Press.

44 PRODUCT LIFE CYCLE DESIGN USING THE DFE WORKBENCH

Elena Man[1], Juan Enrique Díez[2], Camelia Chira[3], Thomas Roche[4]
National University of Ireland, Galway [1]; Galway Mayo Institute of Technology, Ireland [2,3,4]
elena.man@nuigalway.ie, juanen10@teleline.es, camelia.chira@nuigalway.ie
thomas.roche@nuigalway.ie

This paper proposes a new design framework for the development of Environmental Superior Products (ESPs) and based on this framework a new DFE methodology and tool called the DFE Workbench is presented. The DFE Workbench is a CAD integrated DFE tool developed to support the designer in the creation of ESPs. The tool has been extensively tested by multinational organisations from electronic and automotive sectors. This paper presents the testing of the latest versions of both DFE Workbench methodology and tool. Results and conclusions are drawn and future work is proposed.

1. PROBLEM STATEMENT

With the emergence of new European policies, (e.g. Integrated Product Policy), emerging legislation (e.g. WEEE and EEE) and environmental standards (e.g. ISO 14000) manufacturers are being forced to move towards the development of ESPs. According to WEEE and EOLV manufacturers are obliged to take responsibility for waste management by implementing re-use, recycle and recovery policies for their products. Design of ESPs (through DFE practices) is an effective strategy for complying with environmental drivers. Design for the Environment (DFE) is defined by Fiksel to be, ".. *the systematic consideration of design performance with respect to environmental health and safety objectives over the full product and process life cycle*"(Fiksel 1996). It is clear from this definition that DFE approaches must take a more holistic view of the life cycle than traditional design methodologies. It is therefore necessary to consider the design process and associated models when developing approaches to design for environment tools and methodologies.

The design process can be defined as an information transformation process, transforming design requirements information through a number of phases into detailed product specifications. The information transformation process is effected through a series of recurrent problem solving cycles that are used effectively to evaluate diagnose and improve the design as the design evolves (Roche 2001). It is therefore essential that DFE tools and methodologies should support this process throughout all phases. The authors' research has identified a set of requirements for the development of the methodologies and tools to support the development of ESPs. These requirements include:

- Methodologies and tools must be integrated as early as possible in the design process, as well as being integrated throughout the design process.

- All approaches must take a life cycle view for the development of ESPs as a high degree of coupling can occur between lifecycle product characteristics in the design process.
- Approaches must be developed to reduce the environmental impacts and to extend first life and post first life of products, e.g. design for reuse, remanufacture and recycling.
- CAD Integrated tools are likely to be a powerful medium through which to embed DFE tools to support the designer in the development of ESPs.
- It is important to develop web based DFE applications because of the ubiquity, standardised protocols and the need to support distributed teams in the design of environmentally superior products.

2. ESP REQUIREMENTS

Traditional models of the design process have focused on the development of tools to improve the performance of a part of the life cycle of the product, e.g. design for manufacture or design for assembly. The result is a proliferation of tools to aid the designer at individual life cycle stages (Ishii 1992, Molina 1995). As discussed in the previous section, new models must take a more holistic view, i.e. focus on the total life cycle system (see figurel), to include raw material extraction, manufacture use and end of life (Kimura 1997, Alting 1993, Alting 1997, Lee 1993, Warnecke 1996).

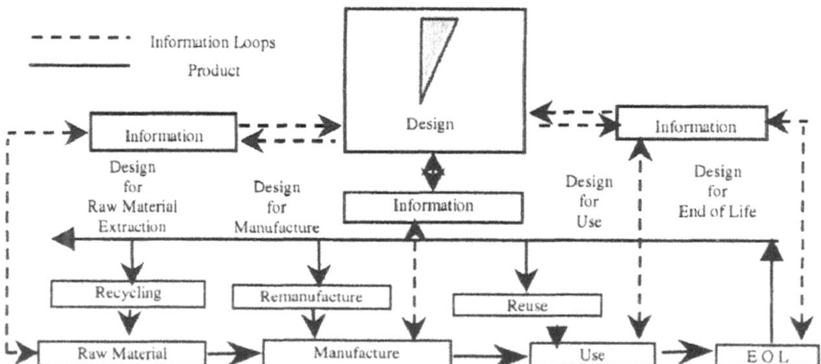

Figure 1. Design Information Loops (Roche 1999)

Four generic and interrelated strategies for the development of ESPs can be derived from the model as follows (Roche 1999):

- Select low impact materials and processes over all life cycle phases.
- Reduce life cycle resource consumption (Materials and Energy)
- Reduce life cycle waste streams (Materials and Energy).
- Resource sustainment by facilitating first life extension and post first life extension, i.e. reuse, remanufacture and recycling

In the model, shown in figure 1 life cycle information is acquired through a set of life cycle design information loops, i.e. design for raw material extraction, design for manufacture, design for use and design for end of life. The design process transforms this information into product design characteristics, which are subsequently embedded in the product. Therefore there is a need for a new design model to cater for the life cycle design information transformation loops and to support the development of new methodologies and tools to assist the designer in the creation of ESPs.

3. PAL FRAMEWORK

Roche proposed that the life cycle *design process* could be represented by a tri-axial information transformation space, i.e. design phase, activity and information axes (see figure 2) (Roche 1999). The model represents the transformation of information through four generic stages of design (namely *requirements definition, functional definition, general design* and *detailed design)*, i.e. the transformation of information from more *abstract* statements of requirements to more *concrete* details on the final design. The vertical axis is based on a synthesis of models (particularly prescriptive design process models) from the literature (Finger 1989, Cross 1994, Jones 1996, Pugh 1991, Hubka 1996, Waldron 1996, Evbuomwan 1996, Baya 1996, Pahl 1996). These phases are not discrete events within the design process, rather the designers engage in a set of decision-making cycles continuously improving the design at each level of abstraction. The problem solving cycle can be viewed as the *instrument* or *mode* of information transformation in each phase of the design process, hence a problem solving cycle is adopted to describe the *activity axis* of the design transformation space, i.e. the steps *analyse*, *synthesise* and *evaluate* (Hubka 1996, De Boer 1989, Cross 1994, Coyne 1990). The phase and activity axes define the boundaries of a design process plane. It is implicit in this plane that problem solving occurs explicitly at different levels of abstraction in the design process.

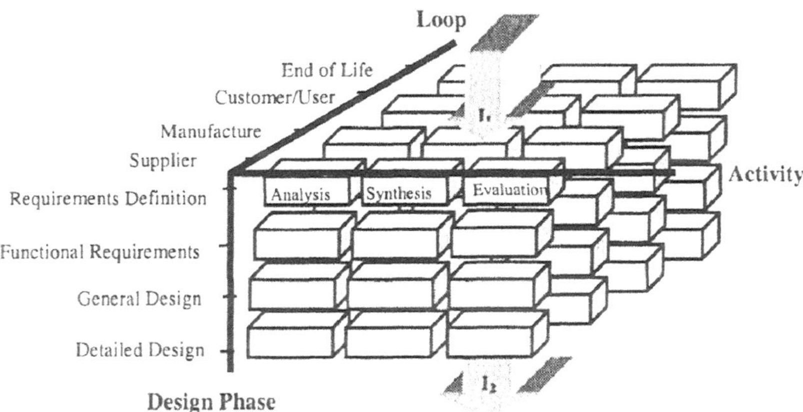

Figure 2. Tri-Axial Information Transformation Space for Life Cycle Design, (PAL) Framework, Adopted for the Design of Extended Products (Roche 2001)

This affects the types of problem solving that can occur, and hence the types of tools and methodologies used.

As defined earlier ESPs require a life cycle design view. The *design information loops* (used to describe the third axis of the transformation space) described in figure 1 represent the source of information for each life cycle phase of the product and also as a focus for life cycle methodologies and tools. The *activity* and *loop* axes bound a *life cycle problem-solving plane*. This plane ensures the analysis, synthesis and evaluation of life cycle information throughout each phase of the design process. In summary the model in figure 2, called the PAL framework, is proposed as a life cycle design framework to support the development of methods, methodologies and tools to aid life cycle design decisions. It is proposed to adopt this model for the development of information architectures, tools and methodologies to support the design of ESPs.

4. THE DFE WORKBENCH

The development of the DFE Workbench methodology (based on PAL) is focused on the analysis, synthesis, evaluation and improvement of life cycle product *General* and *Detailed* design information. The DFE Workbench exists in two forms, firstly the manual methodology, which is largely based on using special charts and reference information in a structured manner to evaluate and improve an emergent design. The second is a CAD integrated software tool, which effectively automates processes, associated with the manual methodology, as well as providing added functionality such as a WEB based report generator. There has been much iteration within the development process where the authors' have developed, tested and improved previous versions of the tool from a simple desktop CAD integrated tool to a suite of integrated tools to be delivered across the enterprise. The tool has been extensively tested in both the electronic automotive sectors influencing the evolution of the tool. The DFE Workbench currently exists in three forms that can be configured to support three levels in the global enterprise: *Desktop, Enterprise and Global* (see figure 3).

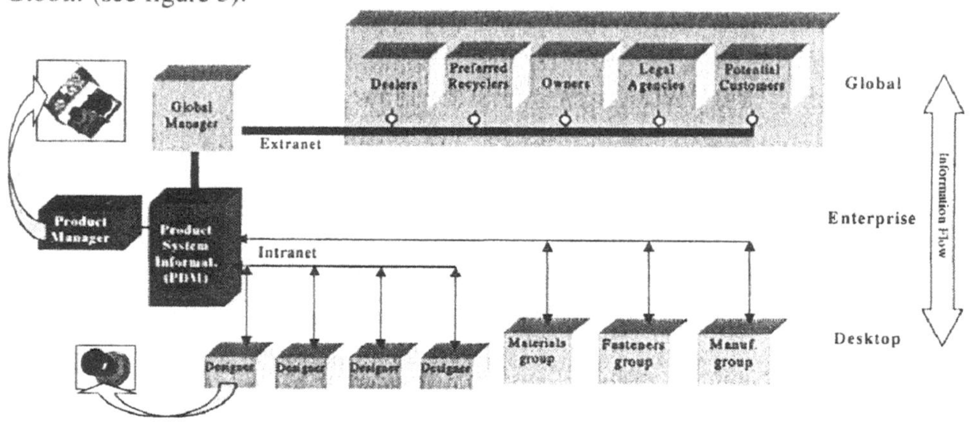

Figure 3. The DFE Workbench Structure

4.1 DFE Workbench Desktop

The DFE Workbench Desktop is a design for environment software tool integrated into a CAD environment developed to assist and advise the designer in the development of ESPs. The tool uses an intranet to connect to the main oracle databases and allows the designers to work concurrently on developing the product. The users have controlled access to the databases based on a username and a password. Currently the application has been ported to two CAD tools, namely Pro Engineer 2001 and Solid Works 2000. The appropriate data is automatically synthesised from the virtual prototype and evaluated using different DFE tools within the DFE Workbench. Each of the variables evaluated are prioritised and advice is given to the designer on alternative product or process characteristics that will enhance that variable. The designer optionally decides to accept the advice and makes the appropriate improvements. Data is then re-synthesised from the (new) model and the process begins again. The Desktop DFE Workbench consists of five modules: the Impact Assessment System (IAS), the Structure Assessment Method (SAM), the advisor agent, the knowledge agent and the dynamic report generator.

The *Impact Assessment System (IAS)* is an abridged quantitative approach to LCA, performing synthesis, evaluation, prioritisation and improvement of environmental data. It automatically extracts the appropriate data from the virtual prototype. Impact data may be calculated for each part or for the entire assembly. Improvements can be made at the part or product system levels. There are several other metrics apart from the eco indicator calculated using the LCA that are evaluated, prioritised and improved, these include: Material Types and Variety, Material Intensity of Type/s (Mass), % Recycled Material Content, % Recyclable Material and % Hazardous Material

The *Structure Assessment Method (SAM)* focuses on the structure of the emergent virtual prototype in an attempt to enhance structural characteristics of the product in the context of DFE. SAM is a complex methodology, which quantitatively measures and records data including such as material compatibility (taking into account fasteners), components serviceability, number and types of fasteners, number and types of tools required for disassembly or total standard disassembly time and part removal time. Coupling between all variables is managed and recorded by the DFE Workbench. For example if an additional fastener is added to the virtual prototype then the number and variety of fasteners and disassembly times and routes are recalculated for the product structure.

The *Advisor Agent* has two functions: firstly to prioritise variables generated by the IAS and SAM tools; secondly the advisor agent actively gives advice to the designer on alternative structural characteristics to enhance either the environmental impact or structural characterises of the emergent design.

The *Knowledge Agent* provides advice to the designer in a consultative mode. For example the designer can use the Knowledge Agent to find a material with specified mechanical and environmental properties. The designer can then use the selected material in the design process.

The *Report Generator* automatically generates reports on the product designed by the user. These reports are made available in two modes, i.e. as system reports that can be printed and viewed locally or as World Wide Web reports that can be made available via an extranet model to people who need product data. For example dismantlers may need to know the location of hazardous materials, the disassembly route and time for a specific product type. If the designer makes a change in the product structure in the design process then the data is automatically updated on the web server.

4.2 DFE Workbench Enterprise

The *DFE Workbench Enterprise* has been developed on the same principles as the DFE Workbench Desktop but it has been developed for the product system level and therefore gives a holistic view over the environmental and structural properties of the candidate design. The DFE Workbench Enterprise can work both outside and inside the CAD environment. It extracts relevant data and performs evaluation, prioritisation and improvement of the design solution. The user can focus on a subassembly structure and can drill down into component information when required. The application identifies the subassembly (or indeed the subassemblies) that has the highest environmental impacts or the undesired structural properties and will give advice on how to improve it. Functional departments within the enterprise can put 'standard' data into the DFE Workbench Databases and can synthesise data and generate reports as the design evolves. For example the materials department have access to the DFE Workbench Databases through a web-based interface that enables the addition of new materials and application advice for the designers. Additionally, they can view and generate reports and provide advice on an evolving design, e.g. product mass, hazardous material content, identify priority sub-assemblies and suggest alternatives.

4.3 DFE Workbench Global

The *DFE Workbench Global* has been developed as an Intranet/Internet tool that supports communications and reporting of the environmental and structural metrics that have been calculated, evaluated and improved using the DFE Workbench Desktop and Enterprise tools. The tool has been developed using Cold Fusion technology and works with the Oracle Databases used by the designer and the system/project engineer. It operates through a controlled environment and uses security protocols allowing various users to log in and view, upload and copy data that has been customised for their specific needs. The DFE Workbench Global may also be used via an intranet for interdepartmental reporting or information on specific issues like the preferred materials for specific components or preferred fasteners. The DFE Workbench Global has been developed as an extremely flexible application that supports a high degree of customisation.

5. DFE WORKBENCH TESTS AND RESULTS

The DFE Workbench methodology and the software tool have been extensively tested with the industrial partners from electronic and automotive industry. The tool has been developed through a number of iterations in an attempt to improve the functionality and the usability of the tool and also to ensure the compatibility of the tool with the needs of a corporate organisation. For the purpose of this paper this section describes the testing of the final versions of both manual methodology and software tool. The tests have been divided in two exercises as follows:

a) The analysis, synthesis, evaluation and improvement of an existing product using the manual method (a domestic smoke alarm).
b) The analysis, synthesis, evaluation and improvement of a virtual prototype of an automobile mirror in the design process, using the DFE Workbench software. A partner from the automotive industry provided the mirror.

The DFE Workbench methodology was tested using a protocol analysis technique involving he completion of a short designing exercise in the presence of a video camera. The subjects were provided with all the necessary materials to ensure the proper use of the manual methodology. At the end of the testing session each of the subjects were asked to fill in a set of questionnaires. The tests were carried out in the Research Lab at CIMRU, National University of Ireland Galway, and at the site of one of the industrial partners.

The objectives were twofold, i.e. to evaluate the functionality and usability of the DFE Workbench and to identify opportunities and obstacles for the customisation of the DFE Workbench to meet the requirements of a corporate organisation.

A summary of the conclusions on the DFE Workbench methodology is as follows:

- The proper application of the methodology can result in the improvement of the design irrespective of the experience of the designer. Experience combined with the correct use of the methodology is an advantage.
- The manual method takes a long time to complete. It is tedious to calculate all of the variables, particularly when having to iterate through a number of solution variants and having to recalculate every time.
- Learning was observed whilst the subjects used the manual methodology. It is also expected that learning take place in the use of Software based workbench and probably at a faster pace. It was confirmed that this learning influenced decisions made later by the designers
- With proper training on the manual methodology a non-expert user can contribute to design issues, therefore the manual methodology can act as a training medium.
- The use of standardised criteria such as; standard times, labelling, and material compatibility's, is a very positive feature of the methodology particularly for benchmarking and design comparison.
- Because of the volume of calculations and the manipulation of interdependent relationships it is considered essential to develop a software application to support the methodology.
- The methodology would benefit from the inclusion of extra tools to support different types of decisions, e.g. a cost analysis tool.
- The strong and clear linkage between the global and local indices is identified as a very positive feature of the methodology.
- The prioritisation process was found to be very useful for the search and improvement activity.
- The inclusion of an advisor was seen to essential to the operation of the methodology.

The following conclusions resulted from the testing of the DFE Workbench software:

- There are very distinct advantages for integrating the DFE Workbench in a CAD environment, not least the automation of data synthesis activity, the availability of quantitative data directly from the model, the manipulation of this data, the management of data interrelationships, the accelerated learning that takes place as a result of active experimentation and the resulting improvement in a design before it is manufactured.
- The generation of results and the manipulation of data as well as the speed of improvements made were much faster and accurate.
- It is possible to make improvements on virtual models that may not be possible in real prototypes.
- It has been viewed that the tool would increase the productivity of the design process, would reduce time to market and would support the rapid achievement of design targets.
- The attendees felt that placement of such a tool right on the designers' desktops was a key advantage
- It has been identified the need for more accurate and customised databases to cover fasteners, materials and processes that are specific for the type of industry the tool is addressing e.g. in this case the automotive industry

6. ONGOING FURTHER DEVELOPMENT

The DFE Workbench is undergoing continuous development at the authors' institution to meet the following goals:

- Construction of a Life Cycle Costing (LCC) module
- Addition of new evaluation tools apart from IAS and SAM
- Integration of a work-flow manager
- Development of new interfaces for various departments on the same organisation as for example materials department or fasteners department.
- Development of agents to handle the information management between design teams and rest of members in the organisation
- Development of a conceptual design tool to assist the decision making process associated with the development of various types of products as for example extended products, ESPs and one-use products.

7. REFERENCES

1. Alting L., Wenzel H., Hauschild M., "Environmental Assessment of Products", ChapmanHall, 1997.
2. Alting, L., "Life Cycle Design of Products: A New Opportunity for Manufacturing Enterprises", Concurrent Engineering Automation Tools and Techniques, Wiley Press, 1993, pp 1- 17.
3. Baya V., "Information Handling Behavior of Designers During Conceptual Design", Ph.D. Thesis, Stanford University, 1996.
4. Coyne R.D., Rosenman M.A., Radford M.A., Balachandran M., Gero J.S., "Knowledge based Design Systems", Addison Wesley, 1990
5. Cross N., "Engineering Design Methods", J. Wiley & Sons, 1994
6. De Boer S. J., "Decision Methods and Techniques in Methodical Engineering Design", Ph.D. Thesis, University of Twente, 1989
7. Evbuomwan N.F.O., "A Survey of Design Philosophies, Models, Methods and Systems", In Proceedings of Institution of Mechanical Engineers, Vol 210, pp301-321,1996.
8. Fiksel J, "Design for environment creating eco-efficient products and processes", McGrawHill, 1996
9. Finger S., Dixon J.R.,"A Review of Research in Mechanical Engineering Design - Part 1-Descriptive, Prescriptive and Computer Based Models of the Design Process", In Research in Engineering Design, pp 51 - 67, Springer Verlag, 1989.
10. Hubka V., Eder E., "Design Science", Springer, 1996
11. Ishii K., Hornberger L., " The Effective Use and Implementation of Computer Aids for Life Cycle Product Design", in Advances in Design Automation, Volume 1, ASME, 1992.
12. Jones J., "The Engineering Design Process", Wiley Press, 1996.
13. Kimura F., "Inverse Manufacturing: from Product to Services. Managing Enterprises-Stakeholders, Engineering, Logistics and Achievement". 1st Int. Conf. Proceed. MEP, Ltd. London UK. 1997.
14. Lee D.E., "Issues in Product Life Cycle Engineering Analysis", in Advances in Design Automation, V 65-1, ASME, 1993.
15. Molina A., Al-Ashaab A.H., Ellis T.I., Young R., Bell R., "A review of Computer-Aided Simultaneous Engineering. Systems", Research in Eng. Design, V7, Springer-Verlag, 1995.
16. Pahl G., Beitz W., "Engineering a Systematic Approach", Springer, 1996
17. Pugh s., "Total Design", Addison Wesley, 1991
18. Roche, T. Man, E. Browne, J. "Development of a CAD integrated DFE Workbench tool", IEEE 2001 International Symposium on Electronics and the Environment, Denver, 2001
19. Roche, Thomas "The Development of a DFE Workbench", Ph.D. Thesis, September 1999.
20. Tomiyama, T., "The Technical Concept of Intelligent Manufacturing Systems (IMS)", University of Tokyo, internal document. 1994.
21. Waldron M.B., Waldron K.J., "Mechanical Design Theory and Methodology", SpringerVerlag, 1996
22. Warnecke G., "A Co-Operation Model of Product Development and Recycling", Proceedings of First International Seminar on Reuse, Eindhoven 1996.

45

KNOWLEDGE MAINTENANCE IN KNOWLEDGE-BASED PRODUCT DEVELOPMENT SYSTEMS

David Guerra and Robert Young
Wolfson School of Mechanical and Manufacturing Engineering
Loughborough University, Loughborough, Leicestershire, LE11 3TU,England

Knowledge-Based Product Development Systems (KBPDS) are important tools for obtaining a competitive advantage and leverage using what the company "knows". An important characteristic of a KBPDS is providing the right knowledge to the right people at the right time in the right format, therefore structuring and maintaining knowledge within the KBPDS is critical for the future. This paper focuses on research concerned with knowledge maintenance using a manufacturing information models infrastructure in an integrated product development system.
This paper argues that the understanding of different types of knowledge, its structure and transformation in the product realisation process are key issues for product knowledge maintenance, which is important for the long-term use of a KBPDS.

1. INTRODUCTION

An important aim in human history has been to retain, transfer and improve knowledge. A country is powerful if it has the ability to take advantage of all the available knowledge and have the capability to apply this knowledge to human requirements. In this case, manufacturing companies have different systems of using knowledge to design and manufacture products. Nowadays, globalisation of the manufacturing industry and the worldwide competitive economy is forcing industrial leaders in the manufacturing and service sector to fully utilise the knowledge available. Through time, technologies have improved the knowledge used to develop products and, as a consequence, this knowledge has expanded. Under these circumstances, to improve product development decisions and to obtain a competitive advantage, industry must use up-to-date knowledge. Using KBPDS with out-of-date knowledge in the development of products can affect the competitiveness of the manufacturing company; as a consequence, these systems could fall into disrepute and no longer be used. This is one reason why the product knowledge must be readily maintained within the KBPDS.
Through time, tacit, explicit and implicit knowledge has been present in the product realisation process however, the understanding about it and its role in the design and manufacture of a product needs to be explained. Most research seems to suggest that knowledge maintenance in design and manufacture will continue to have an important role in design and manufacture. Mills and Goossenaerts (2000) stated it is

important to understand what knowledge is necessary to the product realisation process and to move towards thinking of and implementing a knowledge infrastructure and product knowledge management. Beckett (2000) suggests that intellectual assets are more important than tangible assets in effectively achieving the aims of an organisation in the 21st century. Under those circumstances, intellectual assets are developed using knowledge and learning processes emphasising knowledge value. Young *et al.* (2000) identified that although advances in the use of computer systems in product design and manufacture have been significant in recent years, the necessity to develop flexible systems that can be readily maintained with up-to-date information still exists.

The findings of studies examining the use of various forms of Knowledge Based Engineering Systems, for example Cordova and Gutierrez (2000) focus on structuring the key designs and manufacturing knowledge to support decisions. However, this key knowledge needs to be maintained. Rezayat (2000) studied methods for managing product knowledge held within KBPDS to make them more effective, emphasising that to reuse the knowledge it must be first maintained in a persistent manner and then disseminated and shared in a practical manner through the development cycle. Although much work has been done to date, more studies need to be conducted to ascertain knowledge maintenance in KBPDS.

The aim of this paper is to discuss the types of knowledge in knowledge based product development systems using machining and assembly examples, and in addition, to show research ideas about knowledge availability and its maintenance to support design and manufacture decisions.

2. MANUFACTURING KNOWLEDGE MODELS IN A PRODUCT REALISATION PROCESS

This paper is a continuation of a Manufacturing Information Model (MIM) research idea, where a Product Model (PM) and a Manufacturing Model (MM) are considered as information and knowledge repositories. A PM has an infrastructure that provides a source and repository for information concerning a product under development, in comparison a MM is a similar concept but represents the capability of the manufacturing facility and can therefore provide manufacturing related input to design decision-making. According to information models to support machining-related activities, a KBPDS was developed from various components with the ability to share knowledge and information between a PM and a MM (Zhao *et al.*, 2000).

Figure 1 depicts an information and knowledge structure with the premise that computation systems in integrated design and manufacture can provide support to engineers by offering them quality information on which to base their decisions. The current research focuses on resolving the problem of knowledge maintenance in knowledge based product development systems; therefore there is a significant link between manufacturing knowledge models and the current research. The research scope is depicted in Figure 1 using a magnifier. The authors are considering machining and assembly manufacturing processes to explore knowledge maintenance ideas, because, according to the different types of knowledge definitions, these processes are generally understood when easy manufacturing examples are used; however the knowledge maintenance ideas obtained can be applied to other manufacturing processes.

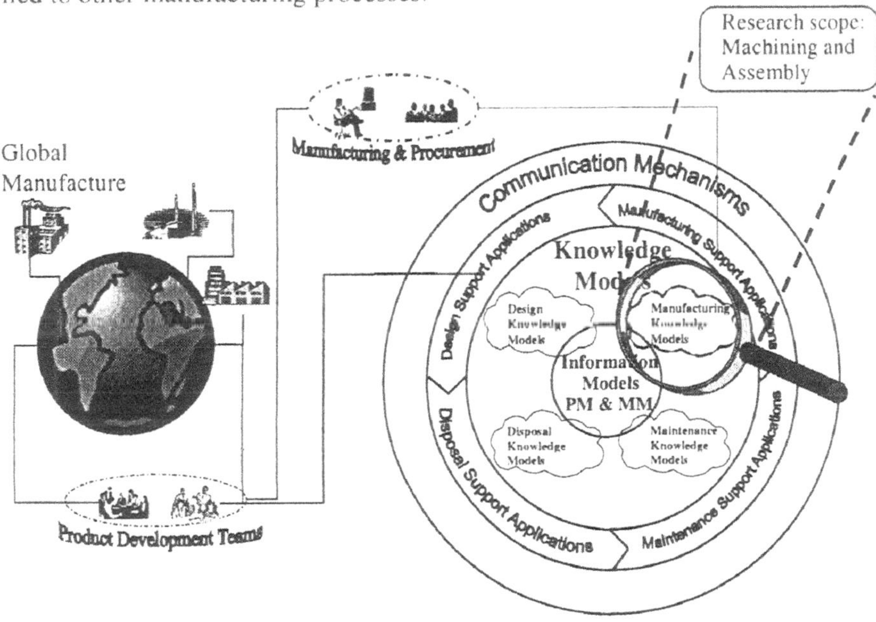

Figure 1 - Information and Knowledge Structure (Young *et al.*, 2000).

KBPDS support decisions using key knowledge related to different activities in the product realisation process, the characteristic and content of the different knowledge depends on the type of users and the purpose of the KBPDS. The product realisation process includes different activities, but according to the aim of this paper only manufacturing activities and their relation with different types of knowledge are considered in order to develop knowledge maintenance ideas. Manufacturing activities apply different types of knowledge in order to produce a product. It is relatively easy to see a product, but conversely; it is not easy to see the complete piece of manufacturing knowledge needed to produce it. In order to suggest manufacturing knowledge structures in a KBPDS, it is firstly important to emphasise differences between data, information and knowledge. Secondly, it is necessary to move towards understanding the type of knowledge as well as the relation with the users and the use of the knowledge to produce a product.

Data can be symbols, words or numbers with no context and no interrelationship. Information is data structured with a particular meaning. Knowledge is information with added detail relating to how it may be used or applied to make decisions (Mills and Goossenaerts, 2000).

Several researchers have studied the different types of knowledge that humans use to make decisions. Nonaka (1995) suggested that tacit knowledge consists of personal relationships, practical experience and shared values; and explicit knowledge consists of formal policies and procedures. In addition, Zheng *et al.* (2000) observed that in contrast to the above two extreme components; implicit knowledge has a bridge property that links together the explicit and tacit components. Mascitelli (2000) noted that tacit knowledge is the context of innovation and observed that breakthrough innovations result from the harnessing of tacit knowledge possessed by individual and project teams. On the other hand, Ackerman and Halverson (1998)

reported that there are other types of knowledge that can be managed out of the knowledge systems. However, in this paper only the different types of knowledge that can be structured and managed within KBPDS are analysed.
KBPDS use data, information and knowledge to support design and manufacturing decisions but in this paper mainly explicit, tacit and implicit machining knowledge are analysed.

3. AN APPROACH TO MANUFACTURING KNOWLEDGE MAINTENANCE

In this section a solution for the problem of knowledge maintenance in knowledge based product development systems is proposed. The identification of new knowledge and its transformation can be facilitated using suitable knowledge structures and applying a knowledge maintenance life cycle concept, as a consequence, the maintenance of current as well as new knowledge can be accomplished. In addition, knowledge expansion to other manufacturing processes can be achieved using this approach. The research work representation is depicted in figures 2, 3 and 4.

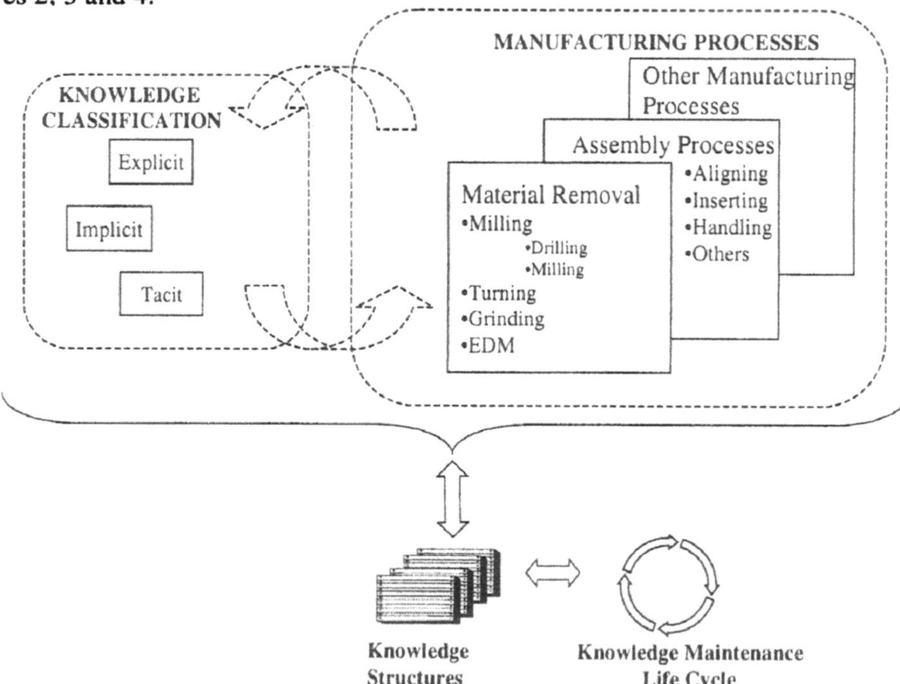

Figure 2 - Knowledge Structures and Knowledge Maintenance Life Cycle Representation.

Manufacturing knowledge related to machining processes is identified using explicit, tacit and implicit knowledge definitions. In order to manage the machining knowledge, the knowledge structures are used to up-date the different types of knowledge applying a knowledge maintenance life cycle concept. The knowledge structures suggested are explained in section 3.1 using different types of knowledge, manufacturing processes and different machining based features. In order to identify new knowledge related to the different machining processes as well as to expand to other manufacturing processes such as assembly it is necessary to have proper knowledge structures and apply a knowledge maintenance life cycle. The knowledge maintenance life cycle concept is discussed in section 3.2.

3.1 Manufacturing Knowledge Structures

Figure 3 shows the knowledge structures using different types of knowledge and manufacturing processes according to the scope of this research. The different types of machining knowledge are classified as explicit, tacit and implicit. In addition, these types of knowledge are sub-classified in different knowledge representations to make the knowledge maintenance possible.

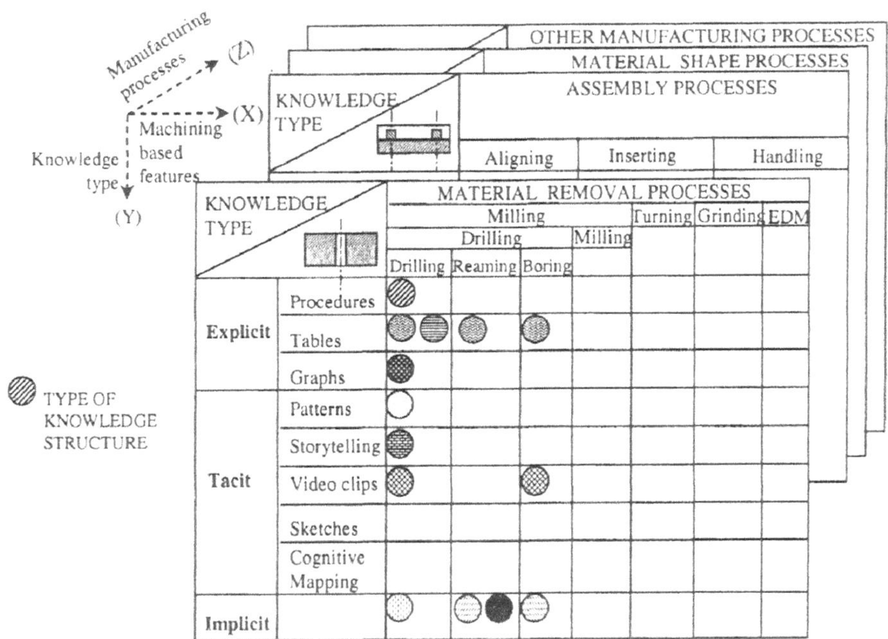

Figure 3 - Knowledge Structures and Manufacturing Processes Relationships.

Explicit knowledge is sub-classified into procedures, tables and graphs. These techniques of explicit knowledge representation are widely understood.

In the machining environment, tacit knowledge is practical experience that an expert operator develops through time whilst obtaining expertise to do machining operations. This type of knowledge is when an expert operator might use the common phrase "I know how to do this but I can't explain it". For these operators it is not easy to explain their tacit knowledge. It is necessary to use knowledge representation techniques to represent tacit knowledge and show new knowledge availability. Figure 3 also illustrates that tacit knowledge is structured in patterns, storytelling, video clips, sketches and cognitive mapping. Patterns are usually described using a format that includes a description of a problem and its solution, with additional information to support the solution of new problems. Storytelling describes a useful event in the past that can be utilised as reusable solutions to recurring problems which occurs during machining operations. Basically, storytelling can be structured as first, a strategic planner "set the stage", then "introduce the conflict", and finally a description of how the resolution to the problem was accomplished. Patterns and storytelling examples can be found in Malhotra (2000). The authors consider video clips and sketches as widely understood techniques of tacit knowledge representation. As an example of additional tacit knowledge representations, cognitive mapping will be the subject of further research.

Explicit, tacit and implicit knowledge representations can be linked together to expand the knowledge context and obtain greater knowledge availability.

The authors' hypothesis is that "Classifying the different types of manufacturing knowledge according to suitable structures helps the knowledge maintenance". At present it is possible to manage the different types of knowledge in a specific context and structure as shown in Figure 3. The marked areas in figure 3 depict the different types of machining knowledge that has been currently structured.

Three dimensions are considered in order to populate the knowledge structures.

The (x) dimension is used as a reference to develop the knowledge structure according to machining based features (ISO/IS 10303-224.2, 2000).

The (y) dimension depicts explicit, tacit and implicit knowledge and its different knowledge representation. If a new type of knowledge or sub classification is identified can be added following the same format.

The (z) dimension details the different manufacturing processes. Drilling, reaming, boring, milling, grinding and turning are considered as machining processes and aligning, inserting and handling as assembly processes.

3.2 Knowledge Maintenance Life Cycle

Figure 4 depicts the knowledge maintenance life cycle concept, it identifies the main steps in order to up-date the different types of knowledge contained in the knowledge structures discussed in section 3.1.

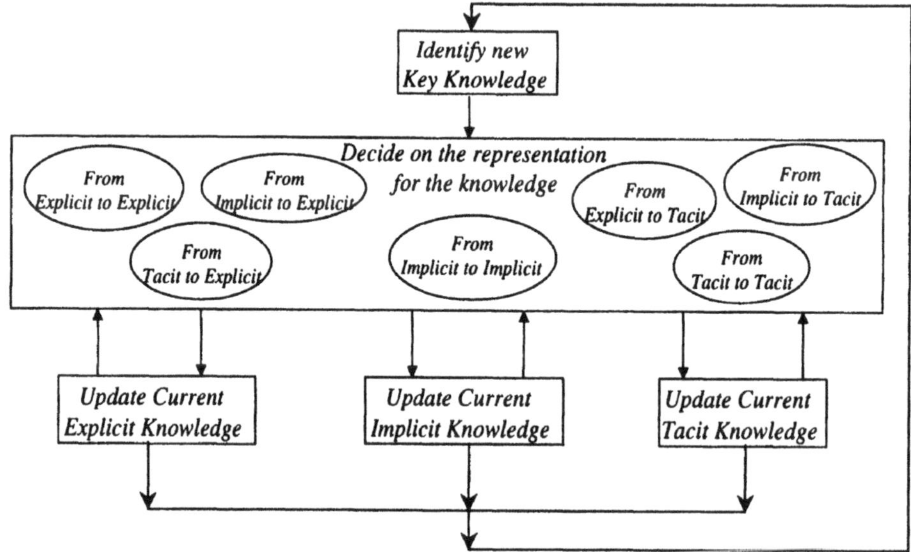

Figure 4 - Knowledge Maintenance Life cycle.

Knowledge maintenance starts when new knowledge is identified. The next step is to decide on the representation for this new knowledge. This piece of new knowledge could be expressed in different explicit, tacit and implicit knowledge representations. The premise of this transformation is that the resulting knowledge should have "richer context" and provide better knowledge availability to those which use it to make decisions. The actions to up-date the explicit, tacit and implicit knowledge is the way in which new knowledge is identified and added or substituted into the knowledge structure discussed in section 3.1. Sometimes, updating current explicit, tacit or implicit knowledge could be a change of data or a piece of information related to any knowledge representation, but in other cases it could be necessary to generate a new procedure, table, graph, pattern, storytelling, sketch or cognitive mapping in order to represent the new knowledge. Using theses knowledge structures, it is possible to store and manage the creation of new knowledge.

4. MANUFACTURING MODEL STRUCTURE

A general representation to capture a manufacturing capability of a global facility in terms of resources, processes and strategies has already been defined and reported (Molina and Bell, 2002). However the current research extends Molina's approach with a significant relationship between strategies and knowledge structures in order to update the manufacturing knowledge by applying a knowledge maintenance life cycle concept. Figure 5 shows a UML class diagram of a manufacturing data model containing a manufacturing facility in terms of its resources, processes, strategies and types of knowledge.

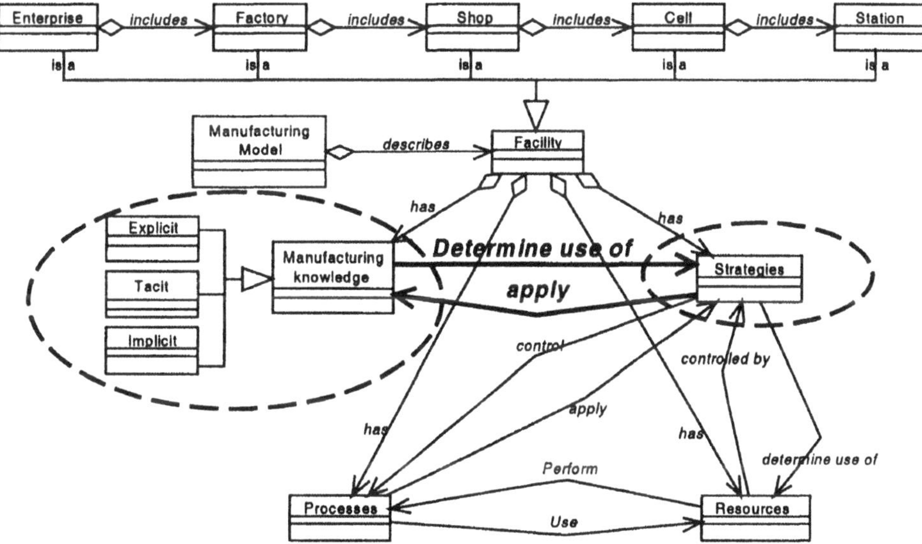

Figure 5 – A Manufacturing Data Model Representation.

5. CONCLUSIONS AND FURTHER WORK

A new approach for updating the manufacturing knowledge used in a knowledge-based product development system has been presented. The rationale behind this approach is to provide better understanding about manufacturing knowledge management. The value added up to now in this research is that even though some examples have been obtained between knowledge structures to support knowledge maintenance, additional research is needed to identify how and when manufacturing knowledge transformations happen and why a best knowledge representation take place. Future work will explore these additional research needs using machining and assembly knowledge. A manufacturing model is being constructed using UML, ObjectStore and Java to validate knowledge maintenance ideas.

7. ACKNOWLEDGEMENTS

The author acknowledges the support received by Loughborough University, and the supplementary support provided by CONACYT, MEXICO.

8. REFERENCES

1. Ackerman M. S., Halverson C., 1998, "Considering and Organisation's Memory", in: Int. Conf. on CSCW'98, pp. 39-48, ACM Press, Seattle, WA.
2. Beckett R.C., 2000, Accessing Corporate Memory – Some Knowledge structure concepts. The 4th International Conference on Design of Information Infrastructure Systems for Manufacturing 2000. 15 – 17 November, Melbourne, Australia.
3. Cordova J.L., Gutierrez A.M., 2000, Knowledge Based Engineering for Design and Manufacture of Glass Bottles, Integrated Manufacturing System Centre, Tools and methods of competitive engineering 3rd International symposium on tools and methods of competitive engineering. Horvath, I., Medland A., Vergeest J.S.M. (Editors); Delft University Press (Publisher); pp 263-274
4. ISO/IS 10303-224.2, 2000-12-01, International Organization for Standardization, Industrial Automation Systems and Integration, Product Data Representation Exchange Part 224.2, Application Protocol: Mechanical Product Definition for Process Planning using Machining Features.
5. Malhotra Y., 2000, "Knowledge Management and Virtual Organisations", Idea Group Publishing, ISBN 1-878289-73-X.
6. Mascitelli R., 2000, From Experience: Harnessing Tacit Knowledge to Achieve Breakthrough Innovation, J PROD INNOV MANAG 2000; 17: 179-193.
7. Mills J.J., Goossenaerts J., 2000, Toward information and knowledge in product realisation, The 4th International Conference on Design of Information Infrastructure Systems for Manufacturing, Melbourne, Australia. http://www.msa.cmst.csiro.au/DIISM2000
8. Molina A., Bell R., 2002, Reference Models for the Computer Aided Support of Simultaneous Engineering, International Journal of Computer Integrated Manufacturing,Vol. 15, No.3, pp 193-213.
9. Nonaka I., Takeuchi H., 1995, "The Knowledge-Creating Company," Oxford University Press, New York, Oxford.
10. Rezayat M., 2000, Knowledge-based product development using XML and KCs, Computer Aided Desing, www.elsevir.com/locate/cad
11. Young R.I.M., Dorador J.M., Zhao J., Cheung W.M., 2000, A Manufacturing Information Infrastructure to Link Team Based Design to Global Manufacture, The 4th International Conference on Design of Information Infrastructure Systems for Manufacturing, 15 – 17 November, Melbourne, Australia. http://www.msa.cmst.csiro.au/DIISM2000
12. Zhao J., Cheung W. M., Young R. I. M., 2000, The influence of manufacturing information models on product development systems, Engineering Design Conference, Brunel University, UK, 27-29th, June.
13. Zheng J., Zhou M., Mo J., 2000, Tharumarajah A., Background And Foreground Knowledge In Knowledge Management, The 4th International Conference on Design of Information Infrastructure Systems for Manufacturing, Melbourne, Australia, http://www.msa.cmst.csiro.au/DIISM2000

46

INTERNET-BASED ELECTRONIC PROCUREMENT SOLUTIONS – OPPORTUNITIES FOR SUPPORT AND RE-ENGINEERING OF DIRECT MATERIALS PROCUREMENT

Robert Alard[1], Martin Gustafsson[2]

[1] *ETH Center for Enterprise Sciences (BWI), Domain of Logistics and Information Management, Swiss Federal Institute of Technology Zurich (ETH), Zürichbergstrasse 18, CH-8028 Zurich, Switzerland, robert.alard@ethz.ch*

[2] *E-Business Competence Centre, Swiss Life Insurance and Pension Company (Rentenanstalt / Swiss Life), General-Guisan-Quai 40, P.O Box 4338, CH-8022 Zurich, Switzerland martin.gustafsson@swisslife.ch*

In businesses today, an increasingly important role is played by the procurement, taking on strategic assignments involving co-ordinating the whole supply chain. To meet the numerous challenges faced by the procurement in this context, focused organisational measures and adequate usage of Information and Communication Technology is necessary. Internet-based electronic procurement solutions (e.g. electronic procurement, electronic marketplaces, etc.) have already proved to be important. These solutions offer a wide spectra of opportunities for support and re-engineering of procurement processes. Due to the highly innovational character few frameworks for planning, implementing and operating internet-based electronic procurement solutions exist today. This paper gives an overview over existing internet-based electronic procurement solutions and highlights an approach for the planning and deployment of internet-based electronic procurement solutions.

1. INTRODUCTION

During the last decades, industrial companies have increased focus on their core competencies and reduced the vertical range of manufacture. The supplier's share of the total value addition has therefore continuously increased. As an effect of the increasing procurement volumes and the resulting increase in supplier's influence on companies' competitiveness, the cost reduction potentials and performance opportunities have shifted towards the area of procurement. The procurement as functional and organisational area has therefore experienced a considerate up-swing in appreciation and attention. The relations to suppliers and their integration in the company's value-adding processes play an increasingly important role. Only procurement concepts which are mature in terms of organisational and informational aspects will enable a modern procurement to take an active part in an integrated supply chain management approach. An approach that will provide opportunities for the producing company to create and hold sustainable competitive advantages. In the course of implementing Enterprise Resource Planning (ERP) systems, companies restructured business partner relations on the supplier side in part through Information and Communication Technology (ICT). The companies focused on improving data and information exchange with strategic partners of their business networks. During that time period, the concepts and software solutions known under the name of Supply Chain Management (SCM) were established. However, most SCM software solutions, together with the classic Electronic Data Interchange (EDI) solutions, proved to be insufficient for Small and Medium Enterprises (SME) due to the major organisational and financial efforts needed in the implementation (see Alard & Hieber, 2000; McIvor et al., 2000). Consequently, most information technology based concepts like EDI or SCM are until now implemented in large enterprises (see Buxmann, 1999). Another hurdle for acceptance is the limited variety of procurable objects supported by the majority of these software solutions. Following the breaktrough of the Internet as a high-performing and widely accepted network infrastructure, and the common use of standards (e.g. Hypertext Markup Language (HTML) or the more recently developed eXtensible Markup Language (XML)), many opportunities for usage of the modern information technologies (IT) have emerged. Most IT and organisational concepts in the Business-to-Business (B2B) area are still in development which makes the software market complex and, due to the recent developments in the "new economy", very dynamic. Consequently there are few industrial experiences made with the implementation of B2B concepts in the procurement. This is specifically true for internet-based electronic procurement solutions for direct materials. Therefore, many companies find it difficult to make strategic decisions in terms of implementation and operation of internet-based electronic procurement solutions, see figure 1.

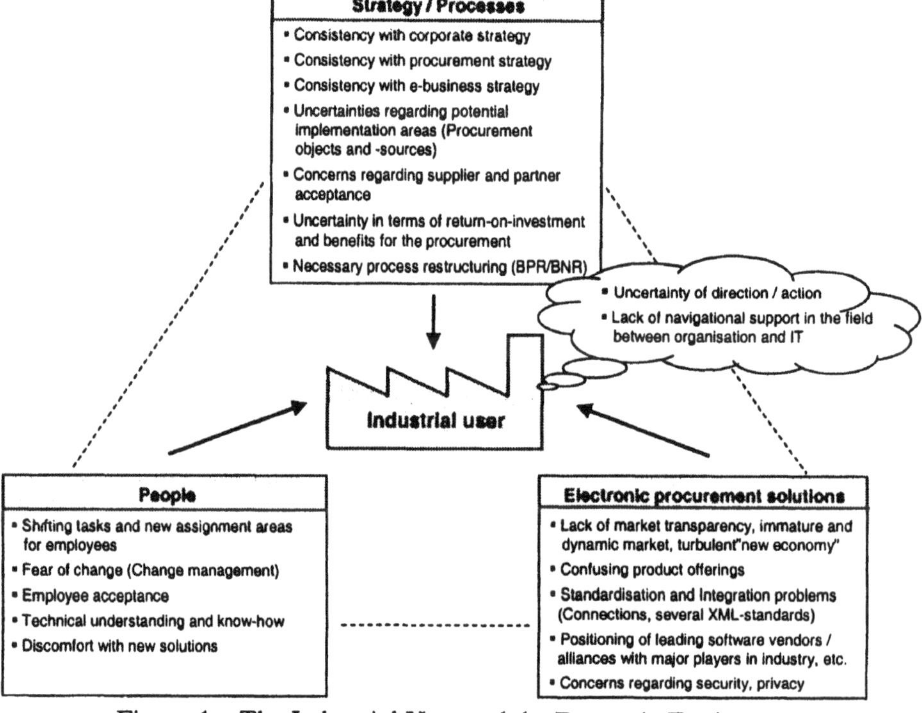

Figure 1 – The Industrial User and the Dynamic Environment

2. INTERNET-BASED ELECTRONIC PROCUREMENT SOLUTIONS

Following Arnold's definition of procurement (see Arnold, 1997), internet-based electronic procurement can be understood as electronic support, based on Internet standards, of company and/or market activities that aim to procure objects that the company requires but does not produce itself. Internet-based electronic procurement provides support for strategic and operational procurement processes and is able to adapt to the trans-corporate context and design aspects of the supplier-side of the value chain. With the emerge of electronic business, internet-based electronic procurement solutions have increased in importance. Most software solutions for the internet-based electronic procurement focus on the procurement of indirect materials (1st generation internet-based electronic procurement solutions). Indirect materials are procured, not for resale or further processing, but for the use or consumption by the company itself. Examples of indirect material are Maintenance, Repair and Operating materials (MRO) or office supplies. In fact, the general perception of internet-based electronic procurement is often focused on this particular category of materials. The reason for the initial focus on indirect materials from software vendors is the lack of organisational structure of procurement processes for this group of goods (see Aberdeen Group, 1999; Dolmetsch, 1999; Segev et al., 2000). Furthermore, the procurement of indirect materials is more easily structured and therefore more suitable to automate. The direct materials were included by the software vendors in a second phase of the applications' development (2nd generation internet-based electronic procurement solutions) (see Commerce One, 2000). Direct materials are part of the core business and thus of great importance to the company. Examples of products that are required permanently for production include raw materials, single parts/standard parts and complex components, modules or specific semi-finished items, or highly configurable products. Today, numerous solutions to support the procurement of direct materials exist on the market and the ICT implementation opportunities are equally common. They span over support of strategic procurement processes to market research and operative procurement task such as order processing and invoicing. The assessment of internet-based electronic procurement solutions is often based on the differentiation between indirect and direct goods. This situation is unsatisfying and further differentiation of direct goods is needed for a successful implementation. In chapter 4 we show an enhanced analysis approach of procurement objects. This approach enables planning and deployment of internet-based electronic procurement solutions and points out the industry usage of such solutions.

3. TYPOLOGY OF INTERNET-BASED ELECTRONIC PROCUREMENT SOLUTIONS

Internet-based electronic procurement solutions can be grouped in four basic categories according to the institutional provider (see Zbornik, 1996) and initiator of the solution: sell-side solutions, buy-side solutions, neutral electronic marketplaces and direct company-to-company links. There are no strict boundaries between the categories. In practice, there is a wide range of permutations and combinations of these fundamental categories. The four basic categories are presented below.

3.1 Sell-Side Solutions

The electronic procurement solutions in the sell-side category are provided and controlled by the supplier. In most cases, sell-side solutions offer products from one single supplier, as in Business-to-Consumer (B2C) relations (m:1 (buyer-supplier)-relation). Another form of sell-side solution is the accumulated product offering from many suppliers, e.g. a commonly used electronic distribution channel (m:n-relation). A particular form of sell-side solution is the rarely seen closed (private) electronic marketplace provided by suppliers (m:1-relation).

3.2 Buy-Side Solutions

The electronic procurement solutions in the buyer-side category are organised and controlled by buyers. The suppliers' product catalogue content is adjusted and integrated into the buying company's procurement solution. This is the classic and wide-spread form of electronic procurement (1:n-relation). This solution is typically associated with the notion of buy-side solutions. Many buyers can group to operate the procurement solution (e.g. subsidiaries group within a concern) (m:n-relation). Between buyer and supplier in the above mentioned buy-side solution, there are often intermediaries (e.g. a software vendor) who manage the catalogue etc. A particular form of buy-side solutions is the buyer-controlled electronic marketplaces. They are in practice often found in closed (private) form. These solutions are frequently used to commit strategic suppliers.

3.3 Neutral Electronic Marketplaces

In the case of neutral marketplaces, electronic procurement solutions are mainly provided and controlled by independent operators as value-adding services (m:n-relation). By restricting the number of users, neutral marketplaces can be transformed to closed (private) neutral marketplaces. Another approach is the procurement solutions controlled by several suppliers and/or buyers (m:n-relation) / consortium. Depending on market power and strength of the different players, this constellation may transform into one of the above mentioned solutions (buyer/supplier controlled marketplaces).

3.4 Direct Company-To-Company Links

Electronic procurement solutions that can be part of internal software systems (e.g. ERP) and are controlled by both suppliers and buyers belong to the category direct company-to-company links. Examples of such applications are (the non-internet-based) classic EDI-applications (based on standards like EDIFACT or ANSI X12 and a traditional EDI-architecture) and the internet-based forms of EDI such as Web-EDI and Internet-EDI as well as internet-based direct ERP-connections between buyer and supplier.

4. SUPPORTING THE PROCUREMENT THROUGH INTERNET-BASED ELECTRONIC PROCUREMENT SOLUTIONS

Internet-based electronic procurement solutions offer a wide variety of supporting functions in the procurement. However, not all strategic and operative procurement processes can be supported equally extensive. Figure 2 suggests strategic procurement processes that offer substantial potential for internet-based electronic procurement solutions.

	Type of solution		Examples
Procurement market research	Sell-Side Solutions		▪ Product catalogue ▪ Product specification and configuration
	Buy-side Solutions	Classic buy-side solution	▪ Supplier and product search in catalogue (restricted choice of products)
		Buyer controlled electronic marketplaces	▪ Offer submissions (passive supplier search)
	Neutral Electronic Marketplaces		▪ Product catalogue ▪ Supplier catalogue ▪ Register / Data bases ▪ Offer submissions (passive supplier search) ▪ Bulletin Board Services / News groups / Discussion services ("Chats") ▪ Search services / Information brokers
Supplier choice	Sell-Side Solutions		▪ Product catalogue ▪ Product specification and configuration
	Buy-Side Solutions	Classic buy-side solutions	▪ Supplier choice from catalogue (restricted number of suppliers)
		Buyer controlled electronic marketplaces	▪ Offer submissions ▪ Auctions
	Neutral Electronic Marketplaces		▪ Offer submissions ▪ Auctions
Contracting	Sell-Side Solutions		▪ Auction ▪ Preparation of contracts
	Buy-Side Solutions	Buyercontroled elektronic marketplaces	▪ Auction ▪ Preparation of contracts
	Neutral Electronic Marketplaces		▪ Auction ▪ Contract preparations

Figure 2 – Aspects of Strategic Procurement and the Potentials for Support Through Internet-Based Electronic Procurement Solutions/Examples

Beside the support of strategic procurement processes, the operative procurement processes provide numerous opportunities for the support and /or restructuring through internet-based electronic procurement solutions. These appear mainly in the procurement process phases ordering, order tracking/controlling and invoicing. Other procurement solutions are found in classic IT-solutions e.g. logistics software (ERP), purchasing informations systems, workflow management and communication systems (see Monczka et al., 2002; Schönsleben, 2000; Schönsleben, 2001). To evaluate and guarantee an adequate usage of internet-based electronic procurement solutions, an extensive analysis of the initial procurement situation is necessary. The main task is to analyse the procurement items, sources and processes. There have been various efforts to structure the decision field to provide the buying company with an overview of the main aspects and features of procurement items and sources and to ensure an appropriate basis for the strategic decision-making (see Hütte, 1996). In procurement theory and practice, the portfolio technique has proved to be a particularly promising method (see Syson, 1992; Wildemann, 2001). Combining the well-known materials-approach by Kraljic (see Kraljic, 1977) with ABC/XYZ analysis (see Schönsleben, 2000), a three-dimensional framework for analysis can be built (see Baumgarten & Bodelschwingh, 1996; Hamm, 1997) that captures significant parameters of the procurement situation and allows the strategic procurement units and procurement items to be categorised, as shown in figure 3. To each strategic procurement unit or procurement item, one of five "reference" procurement processes is assigned, depending on the position of the procurement items and strategic procurement units within the framework. Our research project in co-operation with partner companies in the machine and plant industry have identified the following five characteristic reference procurement processes: partnership processes, supply-dominated processes, buyer-dominated processes, market-oriented processes and usage-driven processes. These processes state different organisational demands and determine the feasibility of varying options of support through internet-based electronic procurement solutions.

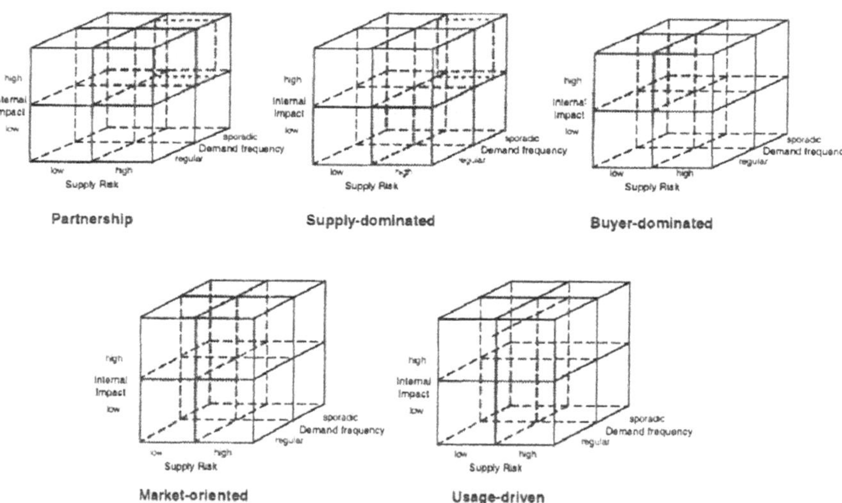

Figure 3 – Analysis Framework for Structuring Procurement Items and Strategic Procurement Units and Characteristic Procurement Reference Processes

The support provided by internet-based electronic procurement solutions in the case of partnership processes is outlined below. The procurement objects and units that are positioned in the partnership category are characterised through a high market-related procurement risk. Frequently these objects and units are complex semi-finished products or integrated sub-systems. The objects are highly specified according to customer specifications and are of considerate importance for the buying company. By building relationships between buyer and supplier and thereby creating interdependencies, the market complexity of the procurement is reduced. One or two suppliers are typically designated per procurement object (single/dual sourcing) and long-term partnerships are developed in the direction of value added partnerships. In the case of strategic partnership procurement processes, most of the in figure 2 shown internet-based electronic procurement solutions are suitable for the support of the strategic procurement processes, with exception of the classic buy-side solutions. These are not suitable for the support of partner strategic procurement process, due to their static structure with pre-configured catalogues (e.g. standard components) with no new suppliers entering the supplier pool. The operative partnership procurement process can also be supported in numerous ways by different internet-based electronic procurement solutions. In this context, the implementation of buyer-controlled electronic marketplaces or direct company-to-company links are suitable. A research project partner company was able to support "order placement" (placement of order, order confirming) and "invoicing" (controlling and acceptance) in partnership procurement processes through a buyer-controlled electronic marketplace and could thereby reach significant process and cost advantages. The binding of strategic suppliers was strengthened and the solution was continuously extended with more suppliers. Direct company-to company links also offer a considerate potential for the support of operative partnership procurement processes. The direct company-to-company links require a substantial organisational and financial effort in the implementation. However, this can be justified through the substantial potential for optimisation (e.g. cost, process quality, delivery time/time to market, etc.) in the long-term character of the buyer-supplier relations in these procurement processes. In general the support potential through internet-based electronic procurement solutions must be evaluated by inter-disciplinary teams from procurement, IT, logistics, production and finance in the company-specific context and for procurement units, objects and sources. In this process, leading questions focus on company strategy consistency and technical and personnel consequences. In the context of the evaluation, "best-practice"-examples, reference projects or innovative case studies from other companies should be considered and particularly the connection to legacy IT (back-end systems) should be secured.

5. CONCLUSIONS

This paper introduced an enhanced framework for the structuring of internet-based electronic procurement solutions which, besides the normal three sub-groups (sell-side, buy-side and neutral marketplaces), defined a fourth group of applications. The institutional providers of these applications are buyers as well as suppliers and can be implemented through EDI-applications (e.g. Web-EDI, Internet-EDI) as well as direct inter-company ERP connections. Internet-based electronic procurement solutions offer a multitude of opportunities for the support of different phases in the procurement process. Depending on the type of procurement object / unit and the (following) procurement reference process, different organisational and IT-structure considerations are to be made to achieve a differentiated view on buyer-supplier-relations (see Bensaou, 1999). The procurement of standard components (indirect materials, standard items, commodities) e.g. in the usage-driven and market-oriented procurement reference processes are since some time supported through internet-based electronic procurement solutions whereas in the case of strategically important components, such as semi-finished products or highly configurable products, that are typically procured with partnership buyer-supplier-relations, internet-based electronic procurement solutions are mainly yet to be developed and implemented. The dynamic and fast growth of the internet-based electronic solutions produces challenges to the companies to formulate strategies with flexible and extensive procurement focus. In the dynamic environment and immature market of internet-based electronic procurement solutions, companies find it difficult to make decisions as far as which solution to choose. The hurdles do not end with the availability of technologies, business models and standard (e.g. XML) but also include lack of user experience with such solutions. In the planning and implementation of internet-based electronic procurement solutions for support of inter-company co-operations the different aspects of technology, organisation and people need to be considered. In doing this, the organisational and personnel implications have priority and not, as is frequently the case, IT issues. More specific, these issues include material flow structure, information exchange, supplier development and co-operation management. The presented approach offers the procurement a well-founded and powerful tool for the planning and implementation of internet-based electronic procurement solutions by structuring procurement objects and object groups and based on this structure evaluate and suggest the deployment of internet-based electronic procurement solutions.

6. REFERENCES

1. Aberdeen Group: Internet Procurement: The Importance of Maintenance and Repair. AberdeenGroup, Inc. An Executive White Paper, June 1999.
2. Alard, R.; Hieber, R.: Lösungen für unternehmensübergreifende Kooperationen - Supply Chain Management und Business-to-Business Commerce. PPS Management 5 (2000) 2, pp. 10-14.
3. Arnold, U.: Beschaffungsmanagement. Stuttgart: Schäffer-Poeschel, 1997.
4. Baumgarten, H.; Bodelschwingh, K. v.: Logistikorientierte Beschaffungsstrategien; Kostenreduzierung durch gestraffte Abläufe. Beschaffung aktuell (1996) 2, pp. 35-38.
5. Bensaou, M.: Portfolios of Buyer-Supplier Relationships. MIT Sloan Management, 40 (1999) 4, pp. 35-44.
6. Buxmann, P.: Die Zukunft von EDI - XML als Grundlage für den Aufbau zwischenbetrieblicher Geschäftsprozesse. Industrie Management 15 (1999) 1, pp. 61-64.
7. Commerce One: Direct Materials E-Commerce Via Multi-Enterprise Trading Exchanges. White Paper; Commerce One, Februar 2000.
8. Dolmetsch, R.: Desktop Purchasing - IP-Netzwerkapplikationen in der Beschaffung. Dissertation Universität St. Gallen; Bamberg: Difo-Druck OHG, 1999.
9. Hamm, V.: Informationstechnikbasierte Referenzprozesse: prozeßorientierte Gestaltung des industriellen Einkaufs. Wiesbaden: dt. Univ.-Verl.; Wiesbaden: Gabler, 1997. Zugl.: Freiberg, Techn. Univ., Diss., 1997.
10. Hütte: Produktion und Management - Hütte. Akademischer Verein Hütte e.V. (Ed.); Eversheim, W.; Schuh, G. (Hrsg.). Berlin u.a.: Springer, 1996.
11. Kraljic, P.: Neue Wege im Beschaffungsmarketing. Manager Magazin (1977) 11, pp. 72-80.
12. McIvor, R.; Humphreys P.; Huang, G.: Electronic commerce: re-engineering the buyer-supplier interface. Business Process Management Journal; 6 (2000) 2; pp.122-138.
13. Monczka, R.; Trent, R.; Handfield, R.: Purchasing and Supply Chain Management. South-Western; Thomson Learning, 2002.
14. SAP: SAP Business-to-Business Procurement - Funktionen im Detail. SAP AG, March 1999.
15. Schönsleben, P.: Integral Logistics Management. (St. Lucie Press/APICS Series on Resource Management). Boca Raton, London, New York, Washington: St. Lucie Press, 2000.
16. Schönsleben, P.: Integrales Informationsmanagement: Informationssysteme für Geschäftsprozesse; Management, Modellierung, Lebenszyklus und Technologie. Berlin u.a.: Springer, 2001.
17. Segev, A.; Gebauer, J.; Färber, F.: The Market for Internet-based Procurement Systems - Part I: The Context of Procurement Transformation. Fisher Center for Information Technology and Marketplace Transformation, Haas School of Business, University of California, Berkeley. CTM Research Report, WP1040; Part I, Februar 2000.
18. Syson, R.: Improving Purchase Performance. London: Pitman Publishing, 1992.
19. Wildemann, H.: Logistik Prozeßmanagement. München: TCW Transfer-Centrum, 2001.
20. Zbornik, S.: Elektronische Märkte, elektronische Hierarchien und elektronische Netzwerke. UVK – Universitätsverlage Konstanz, 1996. Zugl.: Dissertation, Univ. Konstanz, 1995.

47

USING REJECTION METHODS IN A DSS FOR PRODUCTION STRATEGIES

Massimiliano Caramia[1], Pasquale Carotenuto[2]
Stefano Giordani[3,4], Antonio Iovanella[4]
[1]I.A.C. – C.N.R., Viale del Policlinico, 137, I-00161 Rome, Italy
caramia@iac.rm.cnr.it
[2]I.T.I.A. – C.N.R., Via del Politecnico 1, I-00133 Rome, Italy
carotenuto@disp.uniroma2.it
[3]Centro Interdip. "Vito Volterra" – Univ. of Rome "Tor Vergata",
Via di Tor Vergata, I-00133 Rome, Italy, giordani@disp.uniroma2.it
[4]Dip. Informatica Sistemi e Produzione – Univ. of Rome "Tor Vergata",
Via del Politecnico 1, I-00133 Rome, Italy, iovanella@disp.uniroma2.it

In this paper we face the problem arising in an enterprise that must decide whether and when scheduling production orders in order to maximize the production efficiency. In particular we developed an on-line scheduling algorithm able to manage such decisions. Computational results are provided to show the performance of the algorithm.

1. INTRODUCTION

Today an increasing number of manufacturing enterprises must collaborate and communicate with a large number of suppliers spread in large areas to design and produce their products. The Information and Communication Technology gives an effectiveness support to this activity, but a well suited decision support system is also necessary to manage the supply chain with the final goal to increase the enterprise production efficiency [6].

The problem we study is the following. Suppose that an enterprise receives production orders continuously from the customers in an on-line fashion with the over time paradigm [5], that means that the enterprise does not know anything in advance about the requested orders until they arrive. Moreover, suppose that all the orders must be dispatched before a deadline and have a time length equal to their production time.

To produce what is ordered, the enterprise needs production resources (say machines) to be allocated to orders for certain times. In particular, we suppose that the machines are linearly ordered and each order requires a certain number of consecutive machines for a certain production time. Moreover, once an order is scheduled it can not be preempted.

However, it is not sure that all the incoming orders can be scheduled. In fact, we are in a twofold scenario: either the order can be scheduled within the deadline, or it must be rejected as there is not enough space in the schedule.

In this paper we developed an on-line scheduling algorithm able to manage decisions maximizing the production efficiency. Computational results are provided to show the performance of the algorithm.

The remainder of the paper is organized as follows. Section 2 contains the model; in Section 3 we sketch the on-line algorithm and in Section 4 computational results are provided. Section 5 concludes the paper with some final remarks.

2. THE MODEL

We are given a set of H parallel identical machines arranged in a linear order, a time limit W and a set of orders (requests) J, with $n = |J|$. Each request $j \in J$ requires h_j consecutive machines for a certain time w_j , and can not be preempted. This is a special case of multiprocessor task scheduling problem with parallel identical processors (see [1-4]).

The requests are presented one by one, and the requirement of each request becomes available only when the request is presented. Each time a new request j is presented we have to decide to reject it or to accept it. In the latter case, we have to assign a subset of h_j consecutive machines for the entire request duration w_j to j; this is the same as assigning to j a free rectangular area X_j (of height h_j and width w_j) contained in the area A of height H and width W. Clearly, the areas assigned to accepted requests have to be mutually disjoint.

Our objective is the maximization of the production efficiency index ρ, measured as the ratio between the resources assigned to accepted orders and the maximum assignable production capacity. In terms of the proposed model ρ is the ratio between the size of the total assigned area and the minimum between the size of A and the total size of the area required by the set of requests. Of course, ρ is in between 0 and 1.

3. THE ON-LINE ALGORITHM

Without loss of generality, we consider the requests indexed according to the order in which they are presented. Given a list L={1, 2,..., n} of such requests, an algorithm A considering L is said to be on-line if [2, 5]:

1. A considers requests in the order given by the list L;
2. A considers each request i without knowledge of any request j, with $j > i$;
3. A never reconsiders a request already considered.

The algorithm operates in $n = |J|$ iterations, and during iteration (j) the request j is considered (accepted or rejected) and a new (eventually empty) free sub-area A_{j+1} of A is defined.

Let us consider iteration (j). Let $A^{(j-1)}$ be the non-assigned (free) area of A, and $\{A_1^{(j-1)}, \ldots, A_j^{(j-1)}\}$ a partition of $A^{(j-1)}$, that is $A_p^{(j-1)} \cap A_q^{(j-1)} = \varnothing$, for $p \neq q \in \{1, \ldots, j\}$ and $\cup_{s=1}^{j} A_s^{(j-1)} = A^{(j-1)}$, where each $A_s^{(j-1)}$ is a free rectangular area of A. See for example Figure 1. Clearly, at the beginning, we have $A_1^{(0)} = A^{(0)} = A$.

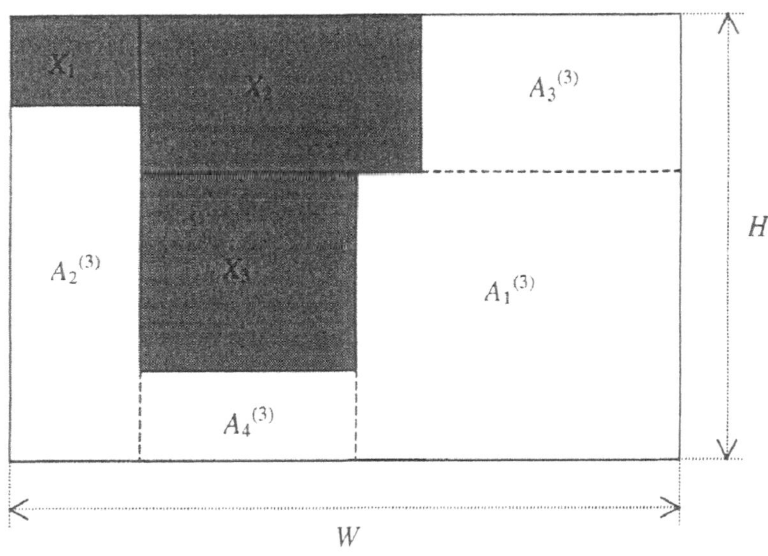

Figure 1 – Assigned and Free Rectangular Areas at the Beginning of Iteration (4)

The request j is accepted if there is a free area $A_k^{(j-1)} \in \{A_1^{(j-1)}, \ldots, A_j^{(j-1)}\}$ that may satisfy the requirement of j, that is both $W_k^{(j-1)} \geq w_j$ and $H_k^{(j-1)} \geq h_j$, with $W_k^{(j-1)}$ being the width and $H_k^{(j-1)}$ the height of $A_k^{(j-1)}$, respectively, otherwise j is rejected. In particular, if j is accepted let $A_k^{(j-1)}$ be the smaller (in terms of size) free area satisfying the requirement of j.

When j is accepted (see Figure 2), a sub-area X_j (of height h_j and width w_j) in the north-west corner of $A_k^{(j-1)}$ is assigned to j, leaving two free rectangular sub-areas, namely $A_k^{(j)}$ and $A_{j+1}^{(j)}$, of $A_k^{(j-1)}$.

In particular, let $A_k^{(j)} = A_k^{(j-1)} \setminus M_k^{(j)}$ and $A_{j+1}^{(j)} = M_k^{(j)} \setminus X_j$, with $M_k^{(j)}$ of size $m_k^{(j)} = \min\{w_j H_k^{(j-1)},\ h_j W_k^{(j-1)}\}$ be the rectangular sub-area of $A_k^{(j-1)}$ located on the west side of $A_k^{(j-1)}$ if $m_k^{(j)} = w_j H_k^{(j-1)}$ otherwise in the north side; with this choice we have $A_k^{(j)} \geq A_{j+1}^{(j)}$, and the k-th free rectangular area A_k area is reduced by a minimal amount. If j is rejected, we consider $A_k^{(j)} = A_k^{(j-1)}$ and $A_{j+1}^{(j)} = \varnothing$.

The value of the solution found by the on-line algorithm is

$$\rho = \frac{W H - \sum_{s=1}^{n} (W_s^{(n)} H_s^{(n)})}{\min\{WH, \sum_{j=1}^{n} w_j h_j\}}$$

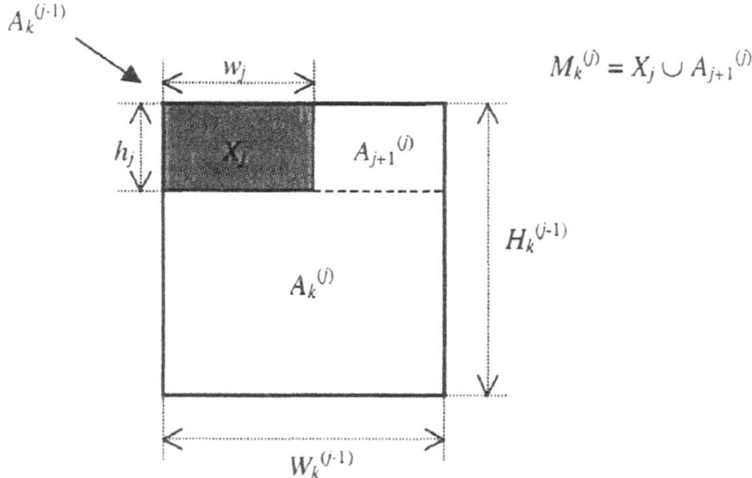

Figure 2 – Accepting Request *j*.

4. COMPUTATIONAL RESULTS

4.1 General

The algorithm was tested on randomly generated instances with n = 10, 20, 50 and 100 order requests getting a total number of 4 classes of test cases. For each class we have considered different test cases according to different choices of two parameters, say w_{max} and h_{max}, being the maximum time that can be associated with a request, and the maximum number of parallel contiguous machines for a request, respectively, and different areas A; in particular, we have considered h_{max} = 5, 10, 15 and w_{max} = 5, 10, 15, and 3 different areas A with the following value for the height H and the width W: (H, W) = {(15, 20), (20, 30), (25, 50)}, for a total number of 27 test cases for each class. For each one of the 108 different test cases we randomly generated ten instances where the request time w_j and number of machines h_j required by a request j are uniformly distributed in the intervals [1, w_{max}] and [1, h_{max}], respectively.

The algorithm and the instance generator have been implemented in the C language, compiled with the GNU CC 2.8.0 with the -o3 option and tested on a PC Pentium 600 MHz with Linux OS.

4.2 The Data Comparisons

In Figures 3-5 we summarize average results of the efficiency index ρ. It can be noted that if we have a small number of requests but with the longest duration and highest resource requirements the algorithm performs the lower values. As soon as the requests are small in the sense of the duration and/or number of resources required the efficiency reach a value almost one. This is due to the chance the algorithm has to allocate resources to "small" requests.

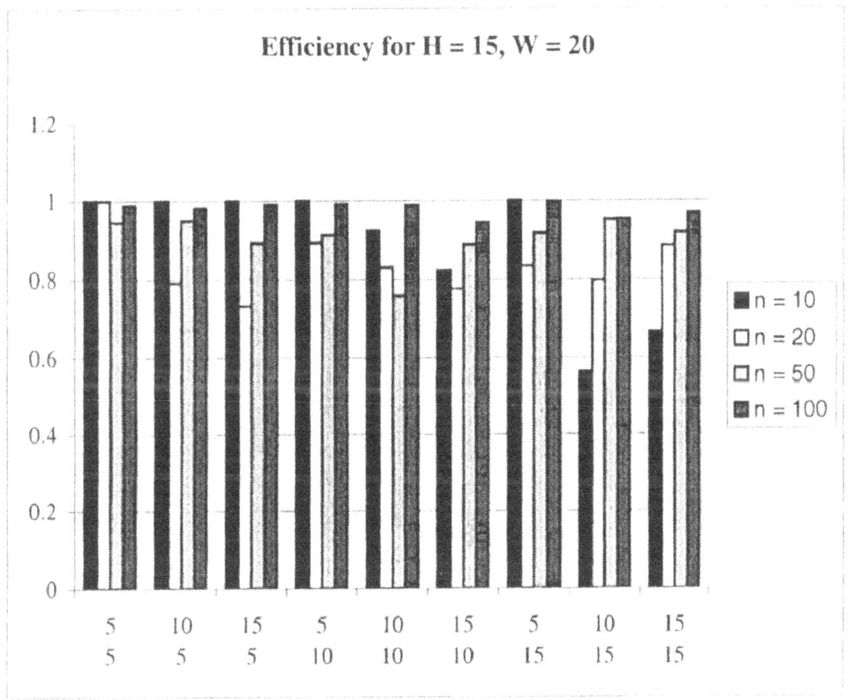

Figure 3 – Efficiency for $H = 15$ and $W = 20$.

For the sake of completeness, we report also in Tables 1 and 2 the complete results for the cases (W = 15, H = 20, n = 10) and (W = 15, H = 20, n = 20), respectively, which are the cases where we obtained the worst results. In those tables, the first column is the maximum number of resources required by a request, the second column is the maximum time, the third the number of the average rejected requests, and the last three columns are the minimum value of ρ, say ρ_{min}, the average values of ρ, say ρ_{ave}, and the maximum value of ρ, say ρ_{max}, respectively, taken over ten different instances.

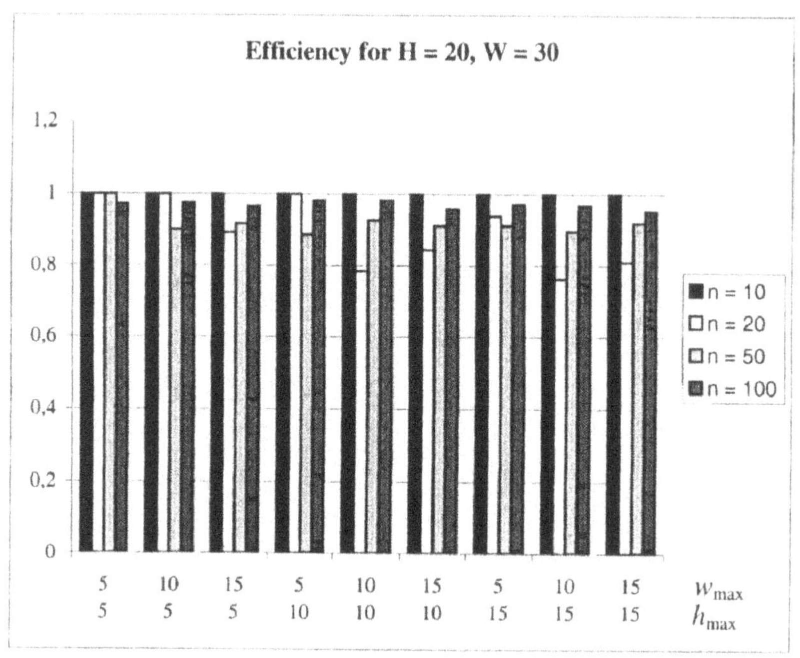

Figure 4 – Efficiency for $H = 20$ and $W = 30$.

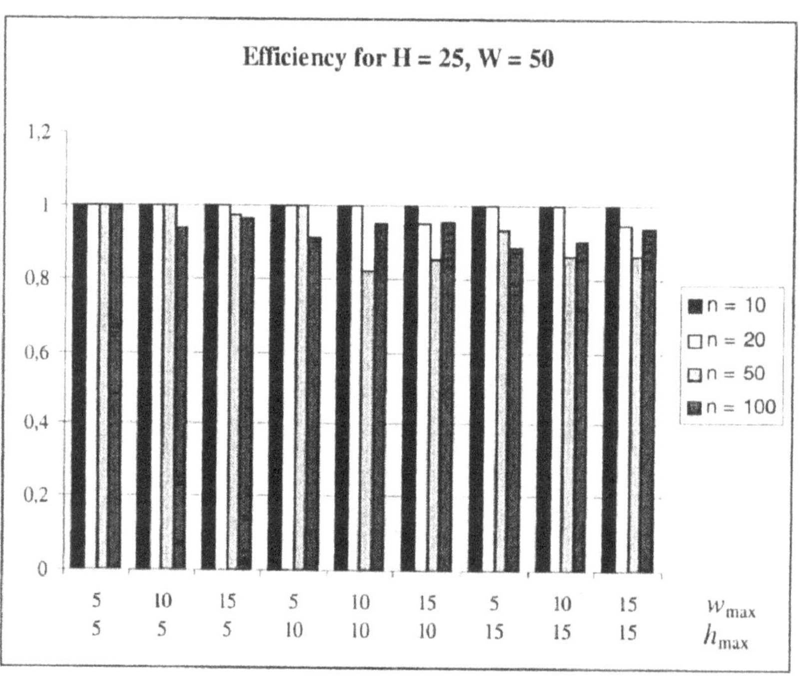

Figure 5 – Efficiency for $H = 20$ and $W = 30$

Table 1 – Results for $W = 15$, $H = 20$ and $n = 10$

h_{max}	w_{max}	*Rejected*	ρ_{min}	ρ_{ave}	ρ_{max}
5	5	0.0	1.000	1.000	1.000
5	10	0.0	1.000	1.000	1.000
5	15	1.0	0.911	1.000	1.000
10	5	0.0	1.000	1.000	1.000
10	10	1.5	0.623	0.923	1.000
10	15	3.0	0.731	0.822	0.913
15	5	0.5	0.935	1.000	1.000
15	10	3.4	0.547	0.561	0.570
15	15	6.4	0.637	0.665	0.780

Table 2 – Results for $W = 15$, $H = 20$ and $n = 20$

h_{max}	w_{max}	*Rejected*	ρ_{min}	ρ_{ave}	ρ_{max}
5	5	0.0	1.000	1.000	1.000
5	10	2.7	0.680	0.790	1.000
5	15	5.8	0.687	0.731	0.767
10	5	2.3	0.833	0.891	0.937
10	10	6.0	0.783	0.829	0.937
10	15	9.2	0.763	0.776	0.807
15	5	7.2	0.797	0.832	0.840
15	10	12.6	0.643	0.797	0.940
15	15	14.5	0.863	0.884	0.947

The worst results are obtained for the cases ($h_{max} = 15$, $w_{max} = 10$, $n = 10$) and ($h_{max} = 15$, $w_{max} = 15$, $n = 10$), both in terms of number of rejected requests and efficiency. This is due to the fact that in these cases we have to process requests requiring almost the whole production capacity. A similar situation occurs for the cases ($h_{max} = 10$, $w_{max} = 15$, $n = 20$) and ($h_{max} = 15$, $w_{max} = 15$, $n = 20$), even though the efficiency is higher with respect to the previous two cases with $n = 10$; this can be justified because with $n = 20$ we have more chances to efficiently use the whole production capacity. As one can expect the worst cases to deal with are those ones with h_{max} and/or w_{max} values close to H and W, respectively; indeed, in this cases we could have a very small chance to fit a request whose size is very close to the size of the whole (available) area A, especially if small requests have been accepted before implying a reduction on the size of the available areas. Nevertheless, the algorithm seems to perform well providing almost always solutions with efficiency value ρ greater than 0.8.

5. CONCLUSIONS

In this paper, we present a very simple on-line algorithm for scheduling production requests able to accept or reject incoming requests to maximize production efficiency. We performed a wide computational analysis showing the behavior of the proposed algorithm. Performance results show that the on-line algorithm provides good solutions in almost all the tested cases.

6. REFERENCES

1. Brucker P. Scheduling Algorithms, Springer-Verlag, Berlin, 1995.
2. Caramia M., Dell'Olmo P., Iovanella A. On Line Algorithms for Multiprocessor Task Scheduling. Foundations of Computing and Decision Science, 2001, 26 (3), 197-214.
3. Dell'Olmo P., Giordani S., Speranza MG. An Approximation Result for a Duo-processor Task Scheduling Problem. Information Processing Letters, 1997, 61, 195-200.
4. Drozdowsky M. Scheduling Multiprocessor Task. An Overview. European Journal of Operations Research 1996, 94: 215-230.
5. Fiat A., Woeginger GJ. Online Algorithms. LNCS State of the Art Survey, Springer-Verlag, Berlin,1998.
6. Shapiro JF. Modeling the Supply Chain. Duxbury Press, 2000.

48

INTRODUCTION TO THE PROTOTYPING OF AN INTELLIGENT SUPERVISION SYSTEM

Samuel Bassetto[1, 2], Ali Siadat [1], Patrick Martin [1]
[1] *LGIPM-ENSAM, 4 rue Augustin Fresnel, 57050 Metz, France*
[2] *SYNLOG, 16 Chemin de Malacher, ZIRST 4402, 38944 Grenoble, France*
samuel.bassetto, {ali.siadat, patrick.martin}@metz.ensam.fr

This paper introduces the prototyping of an intelligent supervision system, intended to become an advanced manufacturing process control system, and is a summary of its conceptual framework. Constraints linked to each development on an industrial field let emerge new concepts and in our case the two parts of this framework: the structure of the advanced manufacturing process control system and the advanced application development methodology. Their instantiations to our industrial study-case let us prove their validity by solving environmental constraints and exploiting industrial and scientific issues.

1. INTRODUCTION

Industrial development areas are rich of scientific issues and potential innovations, but they contain a lot of barriers for this richness exploitation. Among others, the acceptability constraint must not be underestimated, so as being able to explore industrial and scientific issues. A balance between knowledge and technology must be at the heart of industrial scientific developments so as exploring industrial potential and reasoning on impacts of such exploitations. In accordance with such an argument, we followed an innovation process explained in [PEUGEOT PSA CITROEN, 1999], which led us to the development of a conceptual framework for the construction of an advanced manufacturing process control system. Its declination to our scenario application, allowed us to exceed some industrial constraints and build a prototype of an intelligent process supervision system. The scope of this paper is to give in the first chapter a summary of this conceptual framework and in the second chapter to introduce the prototyping of the intelligent process supervision system through its development and its results.

2. CONCEPTUAL FRAMEWORK SUMMARY AND ITS DISPLAYS

While taking as a starting point [Avenier, 1989] our research can be viewed as an intervention and an integration research. The conceptual framework aims to fulfill the need of an advanced manufacturing process control system, its usability and acceptability in an industrial context.

2.1 Conceptual Framework Summary

To answer at those requirements, we make the distinction in the framework between "What is to do?" which explains basis concepts to be implemented to achieve this goal and "How to do it?" which explains the implementation process.

The conceptualization operations used for the development of this framework means shed light on concepts, their articulations and the study of their feasibility. This feasibility is studied either a-priori with a full bibliography or a-posteriori with tests implementing concepts and their articulations.

The conceptual framework is composed of two main parts: the architecture of an advanced manufacturing process control system and the advanced iterative collaborative prototyping.

2.1.1 Conceptualization of the advanced process control system

The framework, shown Figure1, underlines the four main parts which are the heart of the advanced manufacturing process control system. This system is built in the following order: the transmitting and collecting data module, the analysis and case base module, the control learning module, and the knowledge retroaction module. It is plugged over the production system, from which it retrieves data and to which it gives orders or advices. At the end of the instantiation process users can access to a set of off line tools and to a set of on line tools.

2.1.2 Conceptualization of processes used to exceed industrial usability and acceptability constraints

The incremental methodology proposed by [Jacqueson and al., 2001] combined with the collaborative prototyping approach explained in [Terwiesch and Loch, 2002] helped us in the conceptualization of a methodology used to answer at the "how to do it ?" question.

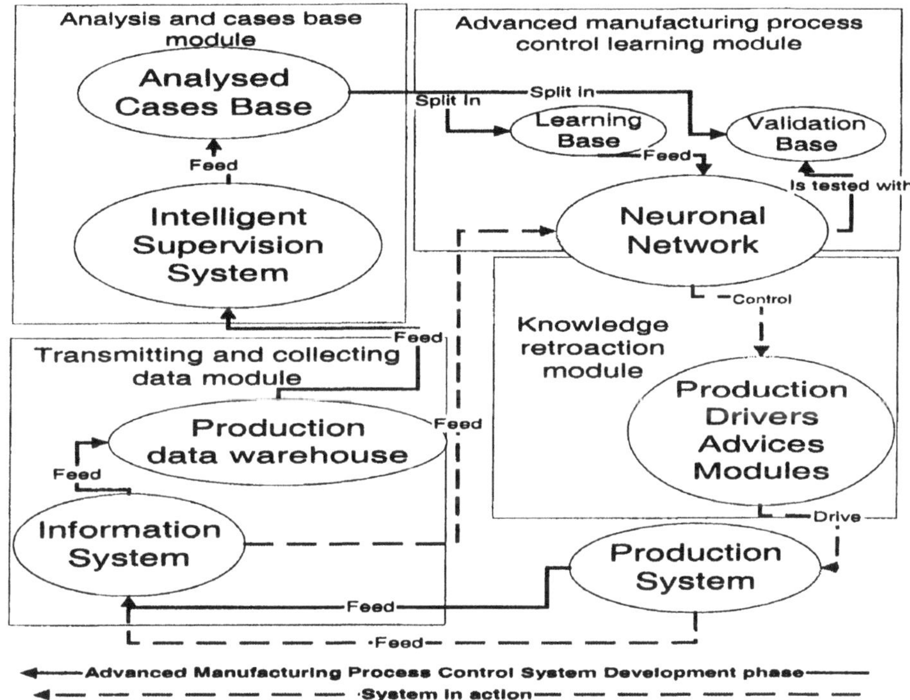

Figure 1- Advanced Manufacturing Process Control System Conceptualization

Detailed Figure 2, two approaches are used which look at the industrial problem in different manners in order to be able to emphasize users needs easily. A development phase follows the discovering of functionalities. The iteration of this circuit leads to the rapid development of a prototype containing a large part of the functionalities needed by users.

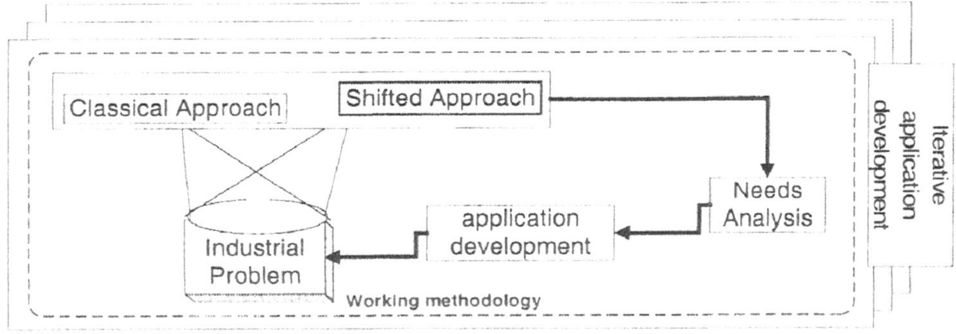

Figure 2 - Advanced Collaborative Prototyping Conceptualization

2.2 Declination of this Conceptual Framework to our Study Case

Once the conceptual framework has been created, its feasibility must be tested. This is done by a-priori and a-posteriori ways. This framework is instantiated to a particular industrial case. We pay a particular attention to the intelligent supervision system. We identify four major constraints to solve with the advanced collaborative prototyping approach:

- *A resource constraint:* a little programming background is required and each development is done using basic tools.
- *A fixed development time:* seven months have been allocated for the specific system development. This constraint was not extendable.
- *A goal constraint:* software, which is stable when you follow the procedure, must answer user's specifications at the end of the development time (USABILITY CONSTRAINT).
- *Utility goal:* We focus our approach on the important point of acceptability and the fixed goal of building an accepted tool (UTILITY CONSTRAINT).

The classical approach is the user's specifications analysis while the shifted approach is a knowledge management one, MKSM[1], detailed in [Ermines, 1996] and [Ermine & al. 1996]. This emphasized approach is, explained at and chosen with, the final user. Other shifted approach could have been chosen. In particular, the CIM-OSA[2] methodology [Vernadat, 1996] could have been used as a guideline into the complex world, in the sense of [Morin, 1990], of enterprise and specifications understanding. The reason for choosing the MKSM approach is explained further in the text.

3. PROTOTYPING AND RESULTS

The prototyping of the intelligent supervision system is, as mentioned before, a crucial piece of the advanced process control system. It hangs on an existing process datawarehouse. It is built in a continuous flow production.

3.1 Aspects of the Prototyping Steps

The prototype, Figure 3, is composed of five modules which each provide different functionalities. The intelligent supervision system finds its data into a process data warehouse, built for collecting and organizing process sampled signals. This construction comes from industrial goals and groundwork.

---

[1] Methodology for Knowledge System Management
[2] Computer Integrated Methodology - Open System Architecture

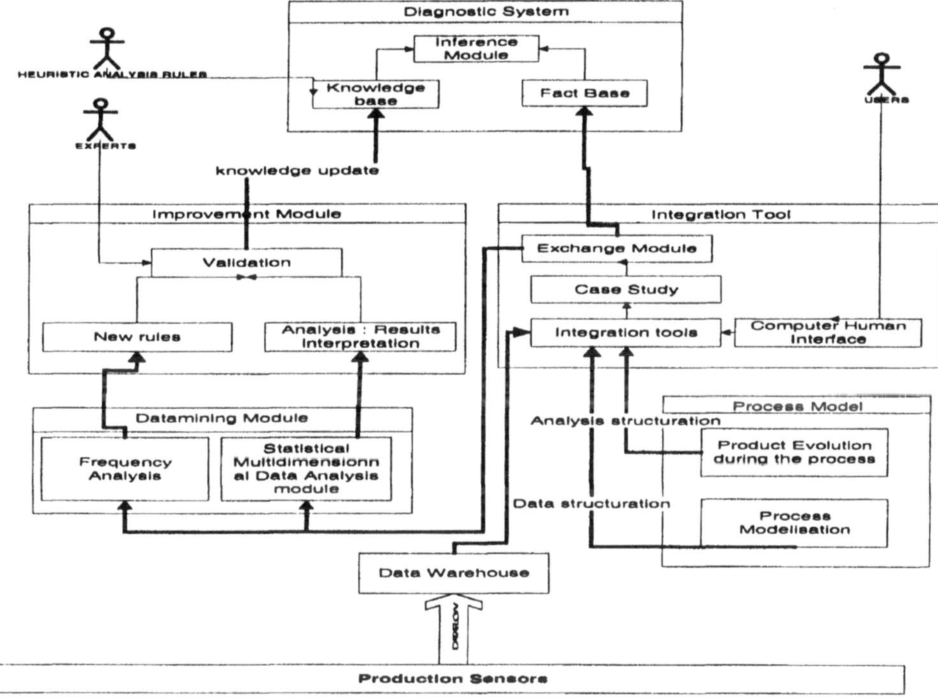

Figure 3 - Intelligent Supervision System for a Manufacture Process Default Analysis Prototype

3.1.1 Industrial Scenario and Groundwork

On one hand a data warehouse was still built and there wasn't any powerful exploitation of it. On the other hand, process experts possess a precise knowledge of the manufacture but without a formalization of it. Moreover, no express knowledge management methodology was used to capitalize on projects and individual experiences. [Faure & Bisson, 2000] and [Ermine & al.1996] the MKSM knowledge management approach for the shifted view.

An important problem is that data warehouse exploration algorithms like those explain in [Szymkowiak & al., 2001] or in [Agrawal & Srikant, 2000] and knowledge reuse system like classical expert system as CLIPS[3], JESS[4], CLASSIC[5] etc are really incompatible. PCA[6], clustering algorithms [Sudipto, G. and al. 1998] and frequency analysis requires a wide range of data to discover some relevant information and knowledge. At the opposite, cases based systems and rules systems require a small amount of filtered data and a large scale of formalized knowledge as explained in [CLIPS, 1998] and [Napoli, 1997]. Algorithms used for mining data and those used for knowledge manipulation are different and can not be swapped. However those systems are useful for solving industrial needs (for example): capitalizing on process knowledge and discovering new process rules. The

[3] C Language Integrated Production System
[4] Java Expert System Shell
[5] CLASSIC is a Knowledge Representation language.
[6] Principal Component Analysis

intelligent supervision system fills in this lack by providing a solution able to use expert system and to find and reuse the new rules as shown in 3.2.

The intelligent supervision system prototyping hangs on an existing process data warehouse which aims to store all sampled process variables able to be retrieve through the information system. Its design is similar than those explained in [Lefébure & al., 2001]. Before being stored in the data warehouse, data are rudimentary compressed, in order to reduce their size. With this technique one day of data is a ~200MB sized base. This rudimentary compression can be improved. Therefore the goal of this data warehouse is to be implemented in an elementary manner on very simple and inexpensive tools in order to be quickly operational and to save the larger amount of process data. We find again the necessity of solving industrial constraints underlined above. This data warehouse is done to store pairs (Time, Value) of each process variable able to be retrieved through the information system. Each table containing those couples, contain also the date of their recording, the correspondent variable, its dimension, and commentaries on this variable. Tables are indexed by a unique table name correlated to the measurement name. A table can be represented by the vector (VariableName; Measuresdimension; Date;Commentary;(Time1,Value1);...;($Time_{LimitOfTheTableLength}$,$Value_{LimitOfTheTableLength}$)

3.1.2 Prototyping the Integration Tool

The integration tool module is the heart of the prototype. We can see its importance throughout its development phases.

- In the first construction step, it retrieves basically user's relevant data from the data warehouse and shows them to users.
- In the second development step, it integrates a physical process model to analyze basically some of the user's relevant data and deliver its analysis. This entity-relationship model leads to the formalization of process variables and their physical implantation.
- In the third step, it integrates a model of the product evolution during its manufacture, which allows the tool to make a complete case study with the user's relevant data. This model, combined with the use of a data warehouse, bring some innovations detailed in the next paragraph. At this level the integration tool possess an advanced Computer Human Interface.
- In the last development cycle, exchange modules are conceived in order to build an integrated system with other modules.

The integration is done by exchanging, between modules, well known information transformed or created for this purpose from data. Four validation steps enroll users for using the developed tool and achieving the software acceptability goal. This acceptation process is fully discussed in [Beauvois & al., 1987]. The main part of usability constraint is achieved; this module answers basic users' questions. Its construction is detailed in [Bassetto, 2001].

3.2 Prototype Main Contributions and Limitations

3.2.1 Integration Tool

Implemented in VB, using the limited, but fully spread into the firm, database engine ACCESS® and following some specific models, the integration tool disconnects the data warehouse from data preprocessing steps and data treatment parts. With its models, the integration tool, picks data up from the data warehouse and applies different algorithms on retrieved data. Either data can be preprocessed for a wider analysis, with some statistical algorithms as detailed below, or data can be filtered with particular production models to obtain users relevant information and feed an expert system. So, the integration tool allows the coexistence of those two ways of thinking.

3.2.2 Product/Process Model

Product quality tests are provided at the end of the manufacturing process. If a particular failure is detected, process experts have to find the position where the default occurs for the first time. This is empirically done by process experts who follow the product in the inverse sense of its manufacture evolution. Each sensor encountered during this evolution is tested. However experts look at sensors' values during a fixed temporal window of M minutes before the event measurement. Let note: t_{event} is the time where the default is measured and X is a number of seconds, $\mu_{Measurement}$ is the mean of a specific measurement and $\sigma_{Measurement}$ its standard deviation. In order to find the default origin process experts look at the variation of each sensor during the $[t_{event} - X; t_{event}]$ period. They infer that the focused sensor "sees" something if some outsider measures are detected. An outsider is a measure which is not into the interval $[\mu_{Measurement} - 3\,\sigma_{Measurement}\,;\,\mu_{Measurement} + 3\,\sigma_{Measurement}]$. This way of analyzing signals is not satisfactory. The product evolves in the plant during its production. If we want to find the default origin, we must look at each sensor value at the time when the part of the product analyzed containing the default was in front of the sensor. Only at this time, if an outsider is detected, we can infer a probable source of default as shown Figure 4., where no outsiders are detected!

The process can be modelized by Figure5., and the follwing equations: the product speed between Xe & Xs, which is : $Vx = V(x) = a * x + b$, where a & b are determined by the line geometry and product Velocity. We measure, $V_{Xs}=V_{out}$, $V_{Xe}=V_{in}$. Xe, Xs, X_{obs}, $\forall$ i $Xsensor^i$ is known with industrial plans, then if a default is detected at t_{event}, then it was in front of $sensor^i$ at $t_{sensor}^{\ i}$:

1 If $X_s < X_{sensor}^i < X_{obs}$, then $t_{sensor}^i = t_{event} - (X_{obs} - X_{sensor}^i)/V_{out}$

2 If $X_e < X_{sensor}^i < X_s$, then $t_{sensor}^i = t_{event} - (X_{obs} - X_s)/V_{out} - (a^{-1} * \ln(((X_s - X_{sensor}^i) - ((X_s - O) - Vs/a)) * a/V_{Xs}))$, where $a = (V_{Xs} - V_{Xe})/(X_s - X_e)$

3 If $X_{sensor}^i < X_e$, then $t_{sensor}^i = t_{event} - (X_{obs} - X_s)/V_{out} - (a^{-1} * \ln(((X_s - X_e) - ((X_s - O) - Vs/a)) * a/V_{Xs})) - (X_e - X_{sensor}^i)/V_{in}$.

This is the model use to analyze accurately data. It is implemented in the integration tool. This operation of retrieving important signals can be a form of filtering. Analyzing the process by this way, noises around relevant process experts information are heavily reduced and only important information are coming out this filter. The case study operation is done more quickly with this model embedded, than without. This operation is more accurate than its correspondent realized by process experts with their analysis method. They are not able to determine exactly if a noised signal contain or not outsiders.

This basic Product/Process model is used here to achieve concepts validation. It could be developed in order be more accurate in the process analysis and to allow a kind of process simulation.

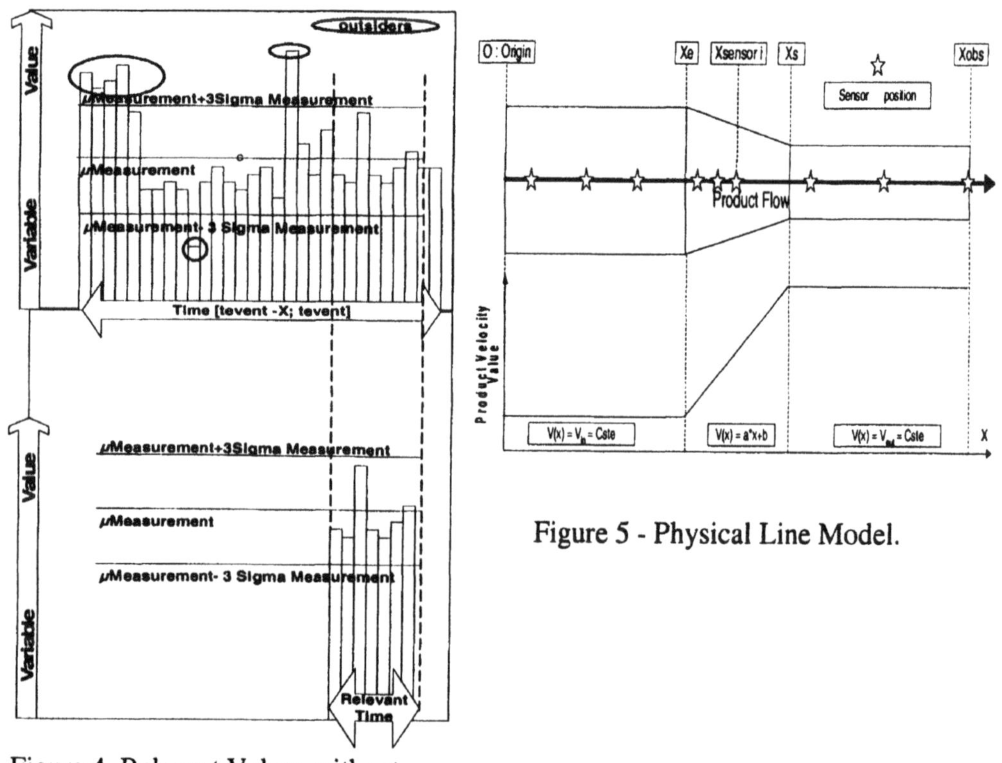

Figure 4. Relevant Values without Outsiders

Figure 5 - Physical Line Model.

3.2.3 Datamining and Its Integration

To underline the contribution of the datamining module, the following example is considered. Starting with 150 variables for a relevant part of the process with a sampling rate of 1 sample per second, we apply a PCA algorithm and reduce the dimension space from 150 to 8, we project all data onto the two more significant variables and a result among others, as shown in Figure 6, underlines that no trend can be observed from a stationary zone to an unstable one.

Before this analysis the knowledge base contains, among others, the following rule: *If* A DEFAULT IS MEASURED *then* LOOK AT ALL PROCESS TRENDS. This process rule was based on expert routine experiences to looking at any sensors trends. By our analysis we found that the default occurs too quickly to be measured and no trend can be observed. The rule emphasized before has been revised. The new knowledge has been validated by an expert committee and the knowledge base has been modified. This process of rule validation is more challenging than generating rules with the datamining module. The next step of this prototype development is to better prepare data sets to find new relevant rules.

Being based on classical multivariate data statistical analysis algorithms, the data mining module must be fed with "good" data. This ensures users to discover new phenomena. For example, we can imagine that for some data sets, a process trend can be observed and for other data set, no trend can be observed. The main problem is then to master the domain range of data and to link it with information inferred by datamining algorithms.

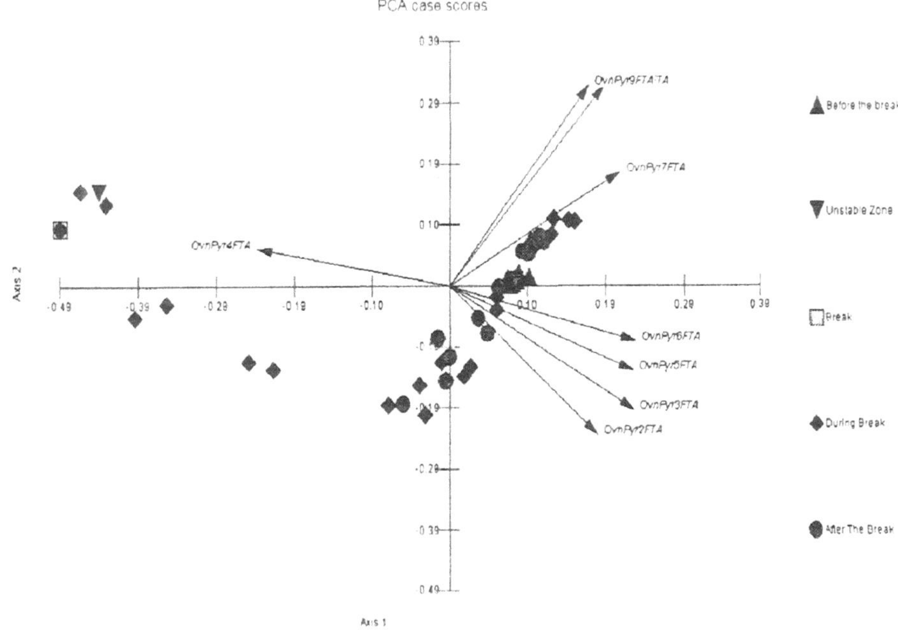

Figure 6 - The PCA of a Process Variable Set and its Correspondent Clusters Analysis.

4. CONCLUSION

We achieve our goal of conceptualization and open the way for building a full featured product in a particular industrial area, with the manufacturing intelligent supervision system prototype and the advanced application development process. Connecting different concepts, this work approach can be called "research integration". This prototyping allows us to apply "basic" and "basis" concepts detailed during the conceptualization work. The conceptual framework, applying a balance between knowledge, technology and human management approach, allows us to exceed constraints linked to industrial developments and therefore allows us to exploit some scientific issues and richness of a specific industrial field.

5. REFERENCES

[Agrawal & Srikant, 2000] Agrawal R, Srikant R, Fast Algorithms for Mining Association Rules, IBM Almaden Research Center, 2000

[Bassetto 2001], Bassetto S. Master thesis dissertation, 2001 ©®ENSAM

[Beauvois & al. 1987] Beauvois J.-L, Joule R.-V. Petit traité de manipulation à l'usage des honnêtes gens. PUG publishing, 7rd Ed, 1987.

[CLIPS, 1998], CLIPS 6.10 beginner and advanced Programming Guide, NASA, 1998.

[Ermine & al. 1996], Ermine, JL., Chaillot, M., Bigeon P., Charreton B, Malavieille, D. La méthodologie MKSM, Cahier de lecture du MCX/APC n°8 , 1996

[Ermine, 1996] Ermine J.-L. : Les systèmes de connaissances, Hermès Publishing , Paris, 1996.

[Faure & Bisson, 2000] Faure, A. Bisson, G. Gérer les retours d'expériences pour maintenir une mémoire métier, étude chez PSA Peugeot Citroën, INRIA & PSA Peugeot Citroën 2000

[PEUGEOT PSA CITROEN, 1999] PEUGEOT PSA CITROEN Direction de la qualité et de l'innovation, Guide de créativité, 1999

[Jacqueson & al. 2001] Jacqueson, D. Millet, S. Minel, A. Aoussat, Dynamique des connaissances en conception : acquisition, capitalisation et réutilisation, CPNI, PRIMECA 2001.

[Lefébure & al, 2001] Lefébure R. and Venturi G., Datamining, Gestion de la relation client, personnalisation de sites web, Eyrolles publishing, 2nd Ed. 2001.

[Morin, 1990] Morin, E. Introduction à la pensée complexe, Paris, ESF Publishing, 1990.

[Napoli, 1997], Napoli, A. une introduction aux logiques de description, RR 3314 INRIA, 1997

[Sudipto, G. and al. 1998], Sudipo Guha, Rajeev Rastogi, Kyuseok Shim, CURE an efficient Clustering Algorithm for Large Databases, Stanford University & Bell Laboratories, 1998

[Szymkowiak & al., 2001], Szymkowiak, A. Larsen J., Hansen L.K. Hierarchical Clustering for Datamining , Technical University of Denmark, 2001.

[Terwiesch and Loch, 2002], Terwiesch C., Lock, C.H. Collaborative Prototyping and the pricing of customized products, The Warton School, R&D INSEAD, 2002.

[Vernadat, 1996] Vernadat, F. Entreprise Modelling and Integration, Chapman & Hall Publishing, 1996

49

BUSINESS INTELLIGENCE SUPPORT FOR SUPPLY CHAIN MANAGEMENT

Ricardo J. Rabelo, Alexandra A. Pereira-Klen
Federal University of Santa Catarina, Brazil
{rabelo; klen}@gsigma-grucon.ufsc.br

This paper presents a system called SC^2, which has been developed based on the business intelligence paradigm in order to better support the management of dynamic supply chains. SC^2 is a multi-agent decision support system that offers an integrated environment for dealing with the production, distribution and sales chains. Via a lean interface based on XML and CORBA, SC^2 can obtain reliable, timely and interoperable information from the supply chain members, comprising a number of heterogeneous information sources and legacy systems. Results are presented and discussed at the end of the paper.

1. INTRODUCTION

This paper presents how the management of the supply chain (SC) can be more effective and transparent making use of the business intelligence paradigm.

With the advent of the globalization, the companies have invested a lot in ways to improve its business (processes) as well as to know more about their clients and their suppliers in order to be more competitive. E-commerce sites, integration of legacy systems, more powerful communication infrastructures, etc., are examples of actions companies have taken in order to improve competitiveness. No matter the topology of the virtual organization the companies are used, all these actions have provided the companies with a basis for receiving and sending plenty of information. However, the more the companies use information, the more tough is the task to treat it in an efficient and smart way. In practice, the managers have been plunged into so many information that, in opposite to the core objective, it has brought even more difficulties for taking smart and agile decisions.

Within this scenario, the paradigm of business intelligence (BI) comes in. In general, BI can be defined as the process to get (digital) information about the company's entire business so that it can be used to provide the so-called competitive advantage (Malhotra, 00). Following this trend, systems to support BI have been put into the market in the past recent years, aiming to offer an integrated and global decision-making environment to the managers. These systems normally make use of information generated by other (legacy) subsystems, especially the Data Warehouses, i.e. typically "passive" information. In spite of the importance of this kind of systems, they fail in the sense that they do not consider real-time data from the SCs in the course of their BI analysis. This is critical as consistent decision-making is a must nowadays, particularly in dynamic SCs. Therefore, there is a need to provide a more balanced basis for adequate decision-making (Levi et al., 00).

This work presents a system called SC^2, which offers to a SC manager a wider, integrated and user-friendly environment based on the BI paradigm as a support for the supply chain management. SC^2 is one result of the IST DAMASCOS project (DAMASCOS), whose ultimate goal was to develop an open and low cost platform and management services for SMEs in the fashion industry.

The paper is organized as follows: Chapter 2 gives an overview of the difficulty to manage the supply chain. Chapter 3 provides a general description of the DAMASCOS and SC^2 approaches. Chapter 4 shows some implemented results of SC^2. Chapter 5 discusses the results achieved and the next steps.

2. PROBLEM DESCRIPTION

One significant problem the enterprise has to manage SCs is to handle the enormous amount of information about and from its members (pre-suppliers, suppliers, the main producer itself, distributors, sales agents, retailers, and so on) and hence to coordinate the current (distributed) business they all are involved in. Demand, production capacities, stocks, material flow are some of the information data that should be quickly analyzed to attend an even more and more demanding market.

In more dynamic SCs, the core partners do not remain the same for a long period of time, and each one of the partners uses to participate in several SCs simultaneously. Thus, the SC management is being driven by the information related to each business, where the various relationships between the business processes can be coordinated as well as the material and the product flows can be constantly monitored. Figure 1 shows how complex this task can be even for a relatively small scenario. It is composed of ten SC members (1 pre-supplier, 4 suppliers, 1 principal producer, 1 sales agent and 3 retailers) and only five end-products. The thickest arrows indicate the information flow and the material flow.

As it can be noted, the complexity in the management increases "exponentially" with the number of supply chain members and end-products (and the quantity of its sub-components). The SC^2 (*Supply Chain Smart Co-ordination* system) (Rabelo et al., 02) has been developed to collect, to analyze, and to organize the information about the SCs, as well as to supervise the operational phase of the business and to support the SC Coordinator in decision-making.

3. THE SC^2 APPROACH

SC^2 is a typical "information consumer" system. In order to support the BI concept, SC^2 assumes that each node (member) of the SC is able to provide selected data through the Internet. It assumes that each enterprise has a sufficient communication infrastructure and integrated services to support the inter-enterprises cooperation.

The DAMASCOS suite (Ferreira et al., 00), for instance, corresponds to a set of cooperation services, which are carried out by specific software modules. This suite is added and integrated on the top of the enterprises' legacy systems. Within the DAMASCOS suite – and from the SC co-ordination and BI perspective – SC^2 is on the top of the hierarchical architecture of DAMASCOS. On the bottom, there are the modules *SALSA* (for sales support), D_3S_2 (for forecasting purposes), *IDLS* (support for individual logistics), and *IPO* (support for some level of production management). At the middle level, there is the *WfBB* (a workflow system, which controls the inter-modules and inter-enterprises information exchange). Therefore, all these modules act as an intelligent front-end between the SC^2 and the legacy systems. Figure 2 illustrates the global SC^2 / DAMASCOS framework.

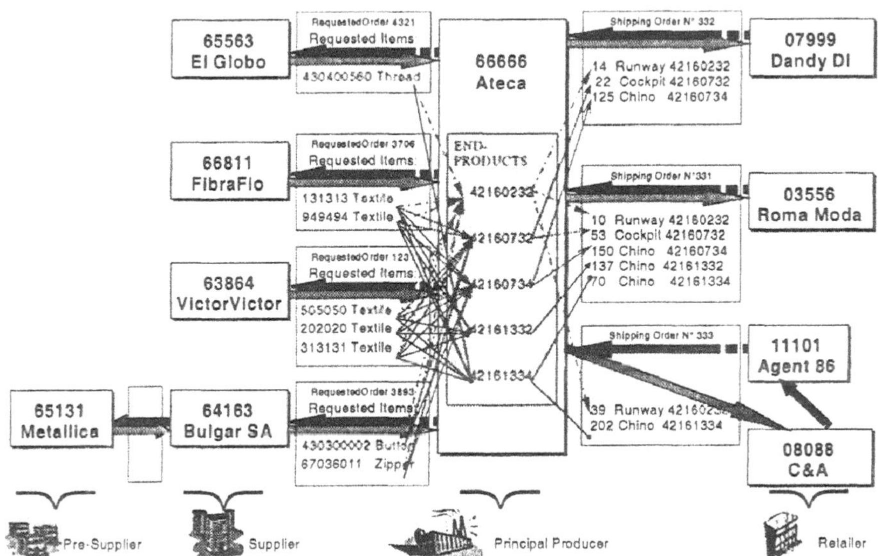

Figure 1 – Material and Information Flow of a Supply Chain

In this sense, SC² manages heterogeneous data provided by the heterogeneous legacy systems from each heterogeneous different SC members. Each of the DAMASCOS modules has its local database. The modules are integrated to the enterprise's database, which in turn is fed by its internal systems [1]. Besides that, some modules offer ASP services (to the other modules) so that some selected data from the enterprise's database can be accessed via a browser.

The DAMASCOS suite is to be installed at each SC member, regarding that its composition is configurable according to the enterprises' characteristics and needs. For instance, if a given enterprise do not manufacture anything, then the IPO module is not used. In the case of SC², it is presented in all the SC members. However, there are two "levels" of the SC² system. The full set of the SC² services are only enabled when the SC member acts as the SC coordinator / main producer. A small subset of its services is then enabled when they are not coordinators, i.e. they act as suppliers, distributors, etc. (this issue is stressed in more details in the next chapter).

3.1 SC² System as a Business Intelligent Support

According to (Levi et al., 00), a number of features can characterize a system for BI support, such as: extraction and integration of data from multiples / heterogeneous sources; usage of experience and knowledge; analysis of data by multiple views; work with simulation and hypothesis; searching for cause-effects relations; transformation of passive data into useful knowledge.

The essential objectives of the SC² is to offer to the manager/principal producer an integrated environment that provides reliable and timely information about the production, distribution and sales perspectives of these chains for smart and agile decision-making – an important key to improve the enterprise competitiveness.

A complete BI system for dealing with SCs should support functionalities to comprise the SC life cycle, i.e. the activities involved in the SC creation, configuration, operation and dissolution (Camarinha-Matos et al., 00). At the current stage of developments, the SC^2 system is more concentrated in the second and third phases, reflected into the following macro inter-related / integrated functionalities:

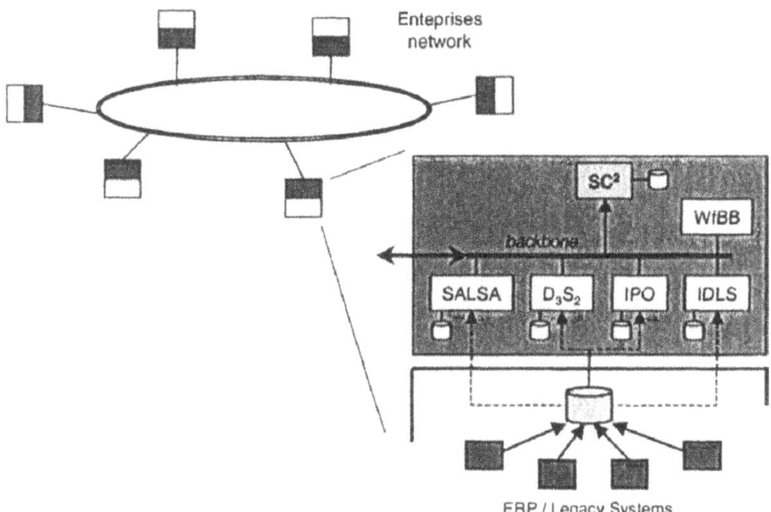

Figure 2 – SC^2 Framework for Business Intelligence Support

- *Supply Chain Configurator*
  Graphical and interactive specification of the "actors" of the SC, comprising their roles and inter-relations. It is the kick-off action to activate the other functionalities after the SC is created.. Figure 3 shows an example of its graphical interfaces, semi-automatically created after each member of a given SC sends some predefined information.
- *Supply Chain Smart Map*
  Once the SC is started, this functionality aims to offer to the SC coordinator a graphical and easy-to-use possibility of seeing the production, distribution and sales stages and their main characteristics. Its main graphical interface is quite similar to the one showed in the figure 3. However, here it is possible to get information about the SC as a whole as well as about the SC members.
- *Ad Hoc Report*
  It aims to provide the SC coordinator with detailed information on specific areas of performance for consistent decision-making. There are two types of reports:
  - *Diagnostic report*: it provides "real-time" information about the SC so that the SC coordinator can feel more confident in the decision-making. It comprises the sales, the production and the distribution chains. These information are organized in several "views", such as the end-products involved, the business processes, the SC Members per products and sub-components, etc. (Figure 4). In the case the coordinator wishes to go into the legacy systems' database, "WWW doors" to their ASP functions are automatically instantiated (previously configured) in the interfaces.
  - *Position paper*: it is triggered when a problem is identified during the SC operation. Alternative courses of actions (such as rescheduling) and probable consequences are drawn up based on decisional protocols (previously) modeled from the SC principal producer.

- *Demand Driven*
  The distribution and sales chains are an independent environment where uncertain customer demand determines independent inventory requirements. This functionality allows a faster reaction to conflicts observed in the end product's inventory.
- *Distributed Business Process Management*
  It is a decision-support functionality that helps the manager in solving problems from the production perspective (Pereira-Klen et al., 01). By means of an intensive information gathering from the SC, a periodic follow up of orders is made as well a set of alternatives schedules are suggested in the presence of problems in the SC schedule (Figure 5).

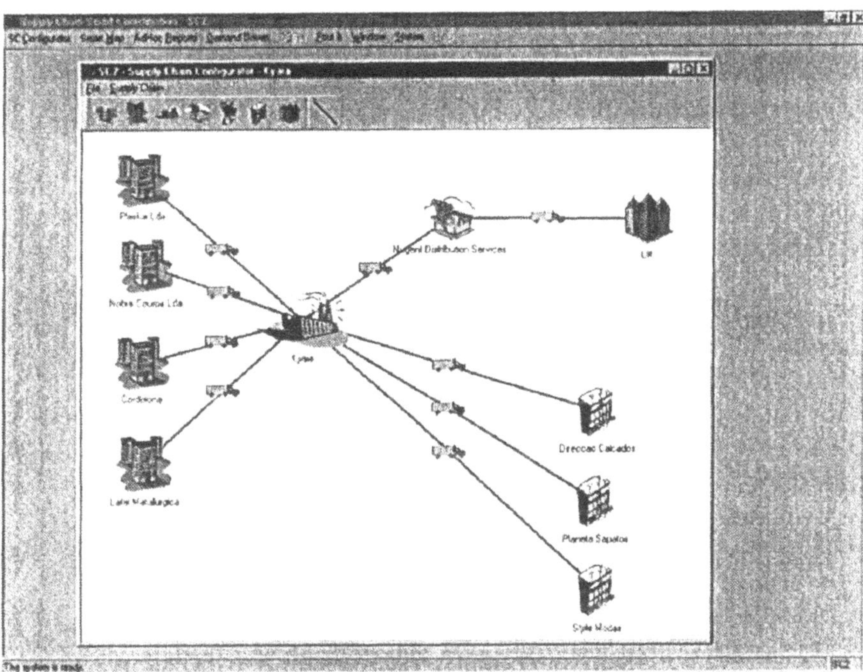

Figure 3 – Example of the SC Configuration Phase

According to the functionalities described above, the BI concept is "inserted" in the SC^2 in different levels offering support for SC management. The synergy between the BI paradigm and the SC^2 can be better understood if one consider that – in different levels – in the following sense: i) support of orders along the SC; ii) collaborative decision-making in the production chain; iii) lean integration of heterogeneous and distributed systems; iv) support for inventory planning and forecasting at the SC level; v) flexible SC (re)configuration; vi) simulation and analysis of problems; vii) global and unified environment for decision-making, and viii) storing of organized historical data.

4. SC^2 ARCHITECURE AND IMPLEMENTATION ISSUES

SC^2 is a decision support system that manages the distributed business process of a dynamic supply network by means of real-time monitoring and supervision activities. It facilitates the conflict analysis and its resolution supported by decisional protocols, providing a human-centered smart coordination of the SC.

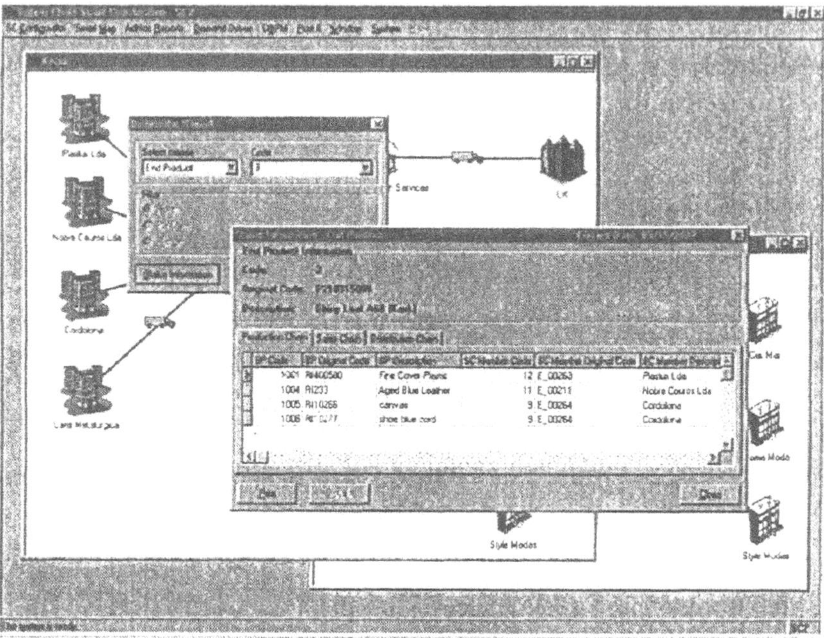

Figure 4 – Example of an AdHoc Report

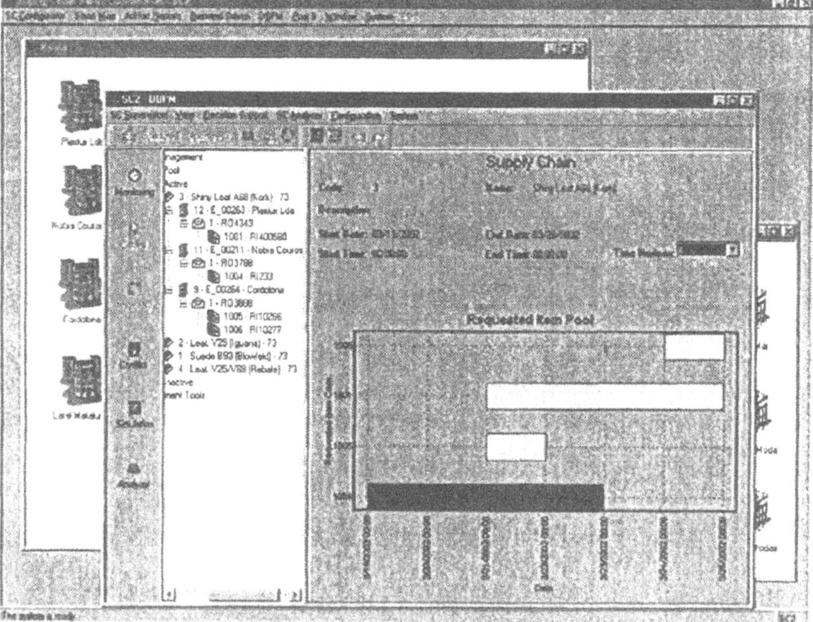

Figure 5 – Example of the Orders Follow Up & Simulation of Alternatives

SC^2 is multi-agent system. This technology has been used because it supports the main SC^2 requirements, namely: (i) the SC^2 agents can be launched in distributed PCs; ii) as problems use to occur along the SC operation, the agents can work based on flexible constraints relaxation; iii) new knowledge can emerge from the agents cooperation hence providing smarter decisions; iv) other agents / supply chain perspectives can be added into the SC² without altering its control architecture; and v) each perspective of the chain is managed in/by an autonomous way/agent.

The SC² system is composed of five agents (figure 6): *Smart Agent* (responsible for the global SC management), *Production Agent*, *Sales Agent* and *Distribution Agent* (responsible for dealing with the production, sales and distribution individual chains, respectively), and the *XML Agent* (responsible for dealing with the communication among the agents and with the "external environment"). All the functionalities addressed in the previous section are carried out by these agents. However, this is totally transparent to the end-user.

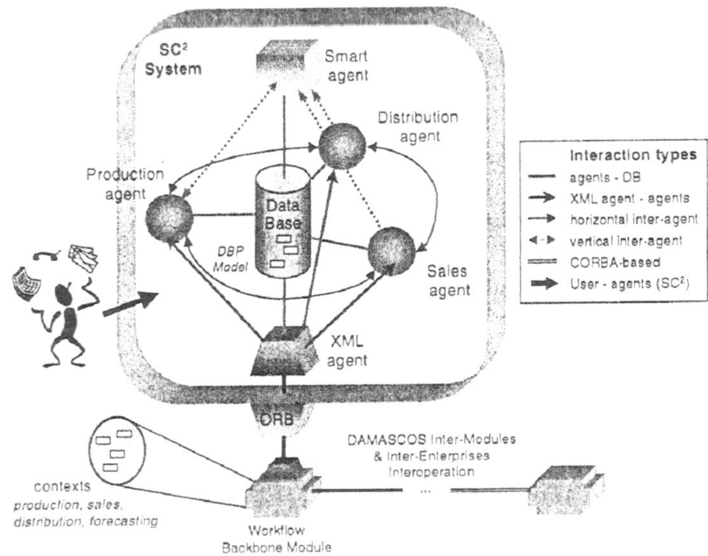

Figure 6 – The SC² Architecture

The SC² implementation model combines multi-agent systems, CORBA, XML, databases, and decision support systems. SC² receives the required information from the IPO, IDLS and SALSA modules via the WfBB module, regarding the "contexts". Each of these contexts corresponds to a XML DTD, accessed by a SC²'s ORB specific service. Once the information is obtained, it is sent and managed by the *XML agent*, which parsers the XML message received and makes a matching with the DTD "reference". After this pre-processing, the information is encapsulated as an object and sent to the SC² database. The involved DBMS stores it in a reference data model called *Distributed Business Process* (DBP) Model (Pereira-Klen et al, 01). In parallel, the XML agent sends a message to the Production, Sales and Distribution agents so that they can be aware about the arrival of updated information. Thus, the agents access the information only when they need.

SC² has been developed in a low cost platform: *PC / Windows-NT / C++*. Free software and standards have been used as much as possible, regarding systems efficiency, configurability and interoperability. The C++ CORBA ORB *TAO* (TAO) has been chosen, and the system is modeled in *UML*. The multi-agent infrastructure has used the MASSYVE KIT (MASSYVE). The (*shareware*) *Interbase* database has been utilized, with a simple object-oriented layer to allow the agents to have access to the database as objects and not as table structures.

5. CONCLUSIONS AND NEXT STEPS

This paper presented the SC^2 (*Supply Chain Smart Coordination*) system, a system to manage dynamic supply chains making use the business intelligence paradigm.

This work has been developed in the scope of the IST DAMASCOS project, evaluating the market trends, as well as based on an extensive research of related projects and the end-users' requirements. Besides that, it was conceived taking into account the supply chain life cycle, hence prepared for further extensions.

SC^2 is a widely integrated system. It manages heterogeneous data provided by the heterogeneous legacy systems from each heterogeneous supply chain members, basically supported by a workflow-driven module and the use of XML and CORBA. The system offers some innovations concerning current BI systems, such as global integration of the whole supply chain as well as the involvement of several non-passive information sources. The real-time information obtained from the supply chain members is properly modeled/selected and presented in graphical interfaces so that the manager can take decisions in an easier, smarter and more agile way.

Additionally to the results already achieved, there are some new improvements planned to be done in a short new future: integration of a partners' search and selection functionality into the SC^2; the replacement of the sockets-based internal communication among the SC^2 agents by a CORBA platform; introduction of more sophisticated heuristics to support global inventory planning; access rights configuration upon the smart map; and finally, the evaluation a more sophisticated information management system for dealing with the whole information of the supply chain and systems, without centralization or information redundancy.

6. ACKNOWLEDGMENTS

This work has been supported by CNPq – The Brazilian Council for R&D – project n.480101/00-0. Thanks to M.Sc. Edmilson Rampazzo Klen, Mr. André Jacomino, Mr. Fabiano Baldo, and Mr. Rui Tramontin Jr. for the system implementation.

7. REFERENCES

1. Camarinha-Matos, L.M.; Afsarmanesh, H.; Rabelo, R. J., *Supporting Agility in Virtual Enterprises*, in E-Business and Virtual Enterprises, Eds. L. M. Camarinha-Matos, H. Afsarmanesh, and R. J. Rabelo, Kluwer Academics, pp. 145-156, 2000.
2. DAMASCOS, http://bart.inescn.pt/~damascos.
3. Levi, D.S.; Kaminsky, P.; Levi, E.S., *Design. and Managing the Supply Chain*, McGraw-Hill, 2000.
4. Ferreira D., Ferreira H., Ferreira J. J., Goletz T., Levin B., Holst A., Gillblad D., Ferraz R., Lopes F., Antunes N., Pereira Klen A., Rabelo R., *A Workflow-Based Approach to the Integration of Enterprise Networks*, Proceedings CARS & FOF 2000, Port of Spain, Trinidad, 2000.
5. MASSYVE, http://www.gsigma-grucon.ufsc.br/massyve.
6. Pereira-Klen, A.; Rabelo, R. J.; Ferreira, A. C.; Spinosa, L. M., *Managing Distributed Business Processes in the Virtual Enterprise*, Journal of Int. Manuf., ISSN 09565515, V12, April 2001.
7. Rabelo, R. J.; Pereira-Klen, A.; Klen; E. R., *A Multi-agent System for Smart Coordination of Dynamic Supply Chains*, to be presented in the PRO-VE'2002 3rd IFIP Working Conference on Infrastructures for Virtual Enterprises, Portugal, May 2002.
8. TAO, http://www.cs.wustl.edu/~schmidt/ACE.html.
9. Malhotra, Yogesh, *Knowledge Management and Virtual Organizations*, Idea Group Publishing, USA, 2000.

---

[1] This integration approach with the legacy systems corresponds to the one implemented in the pilots of the project.

50

A COORDINATION LEVEL IN SUPPLY CHAIN SIMULATOR

Marcius Fabius Henriques Carvalho [1]
Carlos MACHADO [2]
[1] *CENPRA/UNICAMP - marcius.carvalho@cenpra.gov.br*
[2] UNICAMP - cmachado@fem.unicamp.br

This paper suggests a two level simulation tool for supporting the planning decision of a supply chain. The first level coordinates the business process among enterprises through decision rules while the second level analyzes the behavior of each enterprise subjected to the targets established by the coordination level.

1. INTRODUCTION

A Supply Chain can be defined as a network of autonomous or semi-autonomous business entities (department, plant, enterprise) collectively responsible for the procurement, manufacturing and distribution activities associated with one or more families of related products. Supply Chain Management is a process-oriented, integrated approach, which crosses the enterprise boundaries, to manage the above system in procuring and producing activities, delivering products and services to customers. It has a broad scope including sub-suppliers, suppliers, internal operations, trade customers, retail customers, and end-users. To execute an effective management, looking for the best design or operation point in the supply chain, is necessary to model the information, production and control flow inside each participant and among partners. But the participants might not be enthusiastic to share their strong and weak points or operation secrets with all other partner enterprises. Moreover financial data, cost data, client data and others would be kept inside the enterprise but, to get better results for the integrated system, targets data of these items would be shared. Then the group of enterprises should share information to reach the corporation objectives through a model of the entire system, but due to strategic reasons, this policy would be restrict to some information level.

The design, planning and operation of this integrated system, considering the conflicting objectives, are difficult tasks needing to be supported by computational tools. Analytical models are too complex to solve this class of problem and simulation tools have gained considerable attention (Lee and Billington, 1993) as a vehicle for an organizational decision-making process. The system simulation has evolved fast since the 80s and many commercial tools have emerged (Davis, W. J., 1998). Once Supply Chain models demand a specific requirement, commercial tool is not suitable to build a supply chain simulation models efficiently (Vernadat, 1999).

This work proposes a two level distributed modeling and simulation technique as supporting technology that allows a group of enterprises to construct a simulation model and to conduct a supply chain business process through a precise representation of the enterprises as well as business process among them. In the lower level, the enterprise level, each enterprise models and runs its own simulation model at its own site. The detailed model (application codes and data) information is encapsulated within the corporation and the external integration of this corporation occurs thought essential information exchange following a predefined business process structure. The second level coordinates the integration of the business process models according to the Supply Chain structure and management rules.

2. DECISION LEVELS FOR A SUPPLY CHAIN

To understand how the system works is important for the development of a precise simulation model. This section describes the material and information flow in an assembly sub-chain considering mainly two points: 1) in a large production system, a dozen changes occur in a short period of time. However, many of them turn out to be self-canceling or can be accommodated within a system slack. Then, at the enterprise business process level, the significant changes can be taken into account through the consideration of a fixed time interval in which all changes are accumulated and the final effect of them considered for the decision making process among enterprises. The time interval length can have different length for each pair of partner enterprises. 2) These changes are important at the enterprise level since they describe the dynamic behavior of the production system and the ability of an enterprise to meet the supply chain objectives. At this level is necessary a precise description of the events only possible through a discrete event representation.

Two decision levels are identified of the above consideration: The level for coordination of the business process among enterprises and the level to represent the dynamics of the enterprises. The coordination decision level considers the business process among enterprises. Events representing these decisions as new information or new material flow among enterprises (sending product, order, order confirmation, etc.) occur at a discrete time interval (daily, weekly) driving by business process rules and agreements previously established.

The discrete time business process can be described as: at the end of each period, there is a final event, representing the accumulated changes that every enterprise sends to the coordination level. In general, these events are goods been shipped, planned capacity for the next period, orders been requested and unpredictable events. Upstream partners send goods while downstream enterprises send requests according to their internal rules (new order, product shipped, warning of machine breakdown, etc.). After receiving the events of every enterprise, the coordination level use decisions rules to establish production target to be pursued for every supply chain member.

The information and material flow between enterprises occur at discrete time period and represent the supply chain dynamics, as shown in the Figure 1. The production of supplier 1 and supplier 2, during the interval T=1▲, are shipped to be assembled at time T=2▲ (taking the delay period equal to 1) and to be delivered to the warehouse at time T=3▲. Also during the time T=1▲, the assembly enterprise plans its future activities, based on the warehouse requests sent at the end of time T=0▲, and places orders to the suppliers S1 and S2 to be produced during the time T= 2▲.

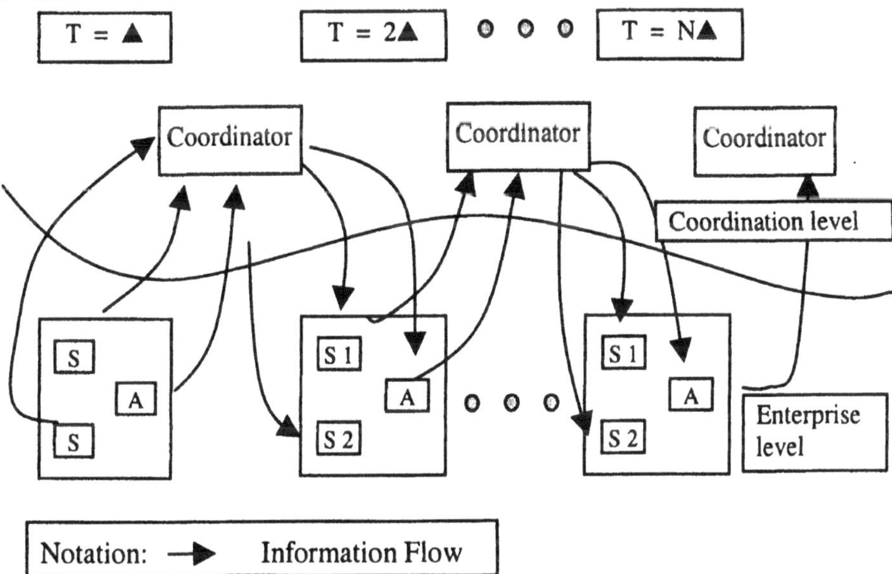

Figure 1. Supply Chain and Enterprise Information Exchange

3. THE TWO LEVEL SIMULATOR

A two-level simulation hierarchy is suggested for supporting the designing and planning activities within a supply chain, Figure 2. In this hierarchy every enterprise processes its discrete event simulation in the time interval (t▲, (t+1)▲) and, at the end of this interval, sends its final state (through vector of events) to the supply chain coordination level, as shown in the Figure 1.

At each time interval, the coordination model receives the vectors of the enterprise's state and starts its simulation, while the enterprise simulator clocks are *stopped*. The decisions at the coordination level are based on the enterprises states and rules agreed among enterprises and are taken in a sequence of discrete time intervals (0, ▲, 2▲, ...). This level generates new targets to every enterprise. At the enterprise level the discrete event simulation occurs in the time interval (t▲, (t+1) ▲). The results of these simulations, represented by a vector of enterprise state, are sent to the coordination level that generates production/orders targets to be pursued by the enterprises in the next time interval ((t+1)▲, (t+2)▲). A three-stage supply chain, shown in the Figure 3, is taken as reference to analyze the influence of two different information management policies in the bullwhip effect.

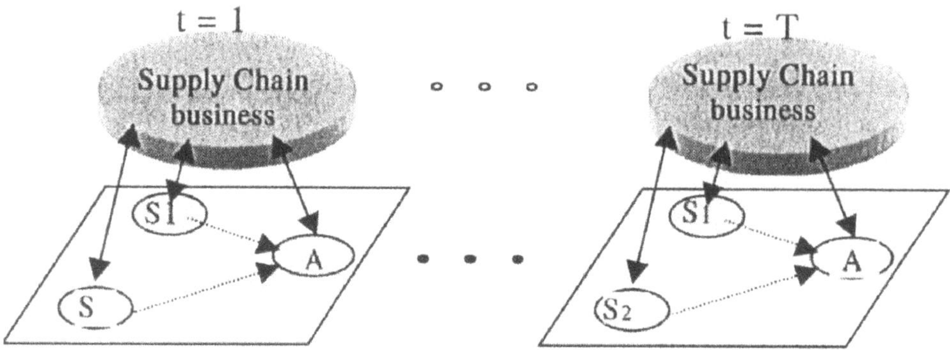

Figure 2. Two Level Simulator

These policies are: Decentralized Information Management System (DIMS) and Centralized Information Management System (CIMS). In the DIMS, the demand information flows upstream of the Supply Chain enterprise by enterprise. In the CIMS the demand is communicated immediately to every supply chain members as shown by dashed line in the Figure 3.

In the traditional management policy, scenario one, each supply chain participant performs its role and then passes product and/or information to the next enterprise in the line. That implies linear flow of information and processes up and down the supply chain and limited information about the end customer behavior for the upstream supply chain components. This approach causes demand distortion, known as bullwhip effect (Lee, Padmanabhan and Wahng, 1997), as it is interpreted, processed and propagated upstream in the chain. This distortion produces several operational inefficiencies as: excessive inventory, poor production forecast and customer service, misguided capacity plans, ineffective transportation, etc.

The integration and coordination of the information is the way to overcome these distortions in the supply chain. Integration means to consider both, business process among enterprises defined by predefined rules and at the same time the internal business process of the enterprises. The evaluation of the implementation of this scenario is possible through the simulation of a Centralized Information Management System where each enterprise is considered as an autonomous agent and its messages are equivalent to events that will start the actions of others agents in the next period of time coordinated by the supply chain management level.

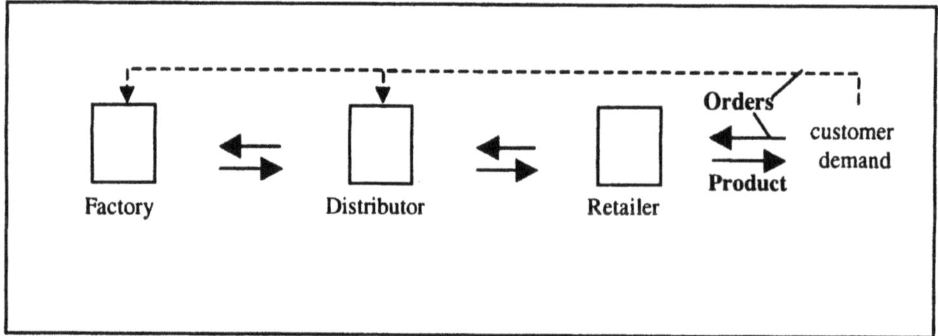

Figure 3 - The Supply Chain Management Models

The simulation schema above suggested is defined as distributed simulation, with spatially decomposition of the simulation model through enterprises (corporation, departments). The objective of distribution is to maintain the encapsulation of each partner enterprise model preserving their secrets, but allowing the coordination of enterprises operations by the coordination level. In this schema, it is not necessary to encode an explicit synchronization strategy in a distributed simulation program since the simulation of the coordination level evolves in a discrete time interval. This strategy considerably simplifies the implementation of the synchronization mechanism as described in the next section.

4. THE COORDINATION PROCESS

The simulation environment for the coordination level represents sales forecasting, as well as inventory management, dispatching and procurement polices modeled by *rules* and *equations*. The supply chain manager can customize its model by choosing from a specific template the rule or equation that describes the enterprises agreement or enterprise behavior. For instance, in the sales forecasting template provides the following techniques: moving average, exponential smoothing, linear regression and time series.

Both management polices of Figure 3 are modeled by choosing correctly rules and parameters to describe the business process among enterprises. The templates for the factory/assembler and distributor/retailer, shown in the Figures 4 and 5, model the DIMS scenario. The Factory demand forecast is defined as a ten period moving average based on the distribution's orders, Figure 4. The inventory policy is chosen as reorder point with demand uncertainty. Some predefined order rules are available to be chosen. The expression to calculate the reorder point has attributes defined by the manager. The fields "Buyers" and "Suppliers" specify the buyer and the supplies of this Factory. Other attributes to model the Factory are listed in the field "Attributes:" The variable AVG, calculated by the AVERAGE function is defined as: mean of the last ten orders received from the distributor.

The coordinator template, Figure 5, coordinates the interrelation among enterprises in the DIMS scenario. Also, this template describes the interaction of external elements with the supply chain (clients and the supplier of the factory). In this example, there are two external elements: "CLIENTS" and "SUPPLIER". The CLIENT has its demand generated from a random variable that follows normal distribution function with mean equals to 40 and variance equals to 4. The SUPPLIER supplies material to the Factory with 97% of service level. The coordinator template allows the manager to specify some indicator functions for evaluating the performance of each supply chain member. In this example, the inventory turnover is defined as a performance indicator.

In the CIMS scenario, the sales forecast, the inventory and the production rules as well as demand sharing are defined at the coordinator template. In the Figure 6 representing the Factory template, is specified who sends and what kind of information is sent and the policies that drive the process. The coordinator template, Figure 7, defines the contract between the Factory and the Distributor and the configuration of the information flow. This Figure shows that the Distributor and the Factory share demand information.

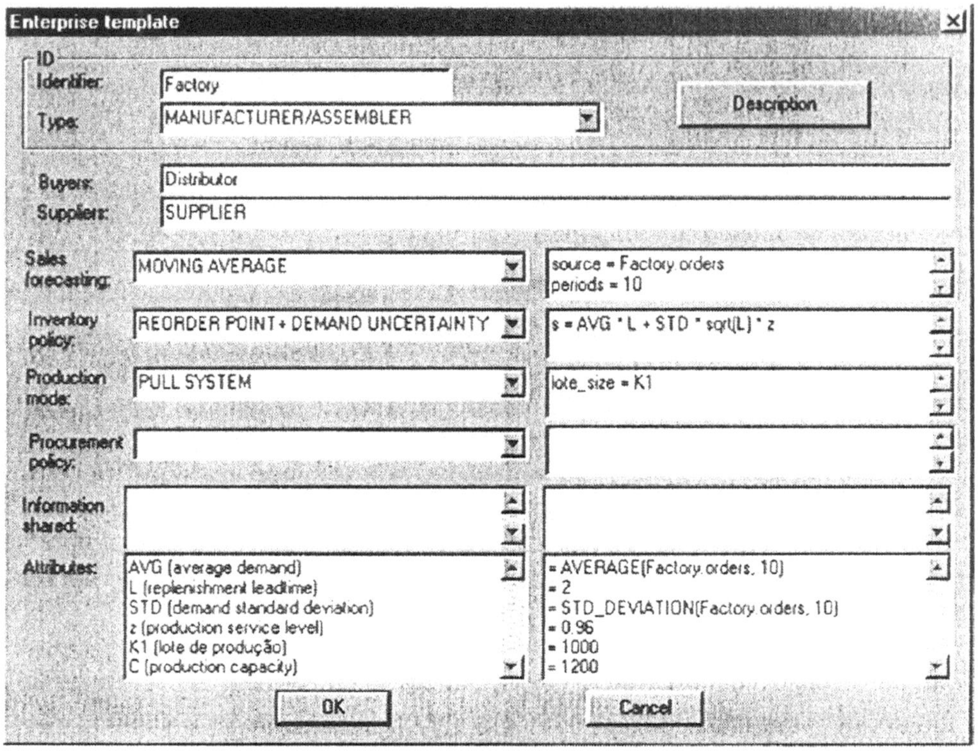

Enterprise template

ID
Identifier: Factory
Type: MANUFACTURER/ASSEMBLER
Description
Buyers: Distributor
Suppliers: SUPPLIER
Sales forecasting: MOVING AVERAGE | source = Factory.orders; periods = 10
Inventory policy: REORDER POINT + DEMAND UNCERTAINTY | s = AVG * L + STD * sqrt(L) * z
Production mode: PULL SYSTEM | lote_size = K1
Procurement policy:
Information shared:
Attributes:
AVG (average demand) = AVERAGE(Factory.orders, 10)
L (replenishment leadtime) = 2
STD (demand standard deviation) = STD_DEVIATION(Factory.orders, 10)
z (production service level) = 0.96
K1 (lote de produção) = 1000
C (production capacity) = 1200
OK Cancel

Figure 4 – Factory Template

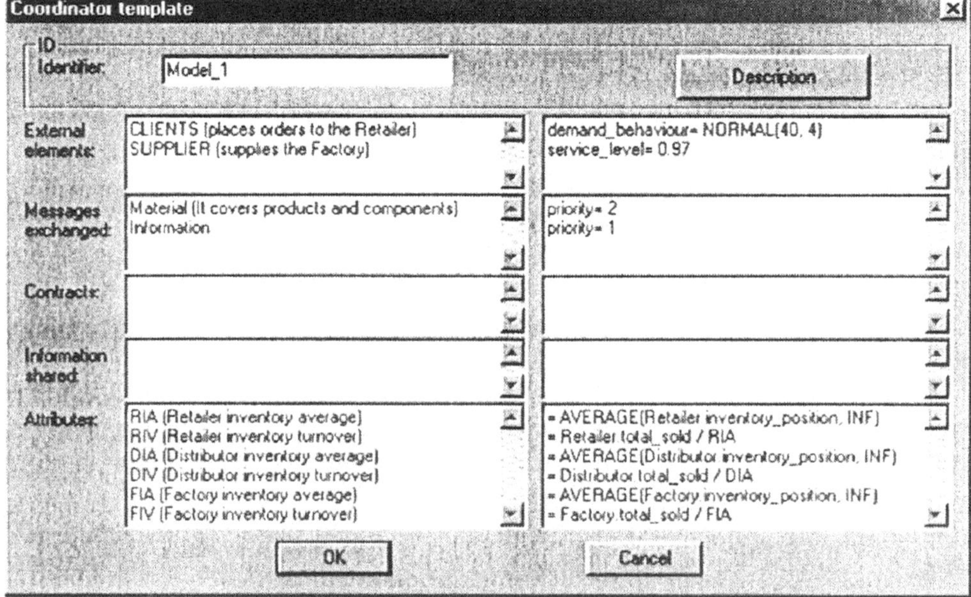

Figure 5 – Coordinator Template

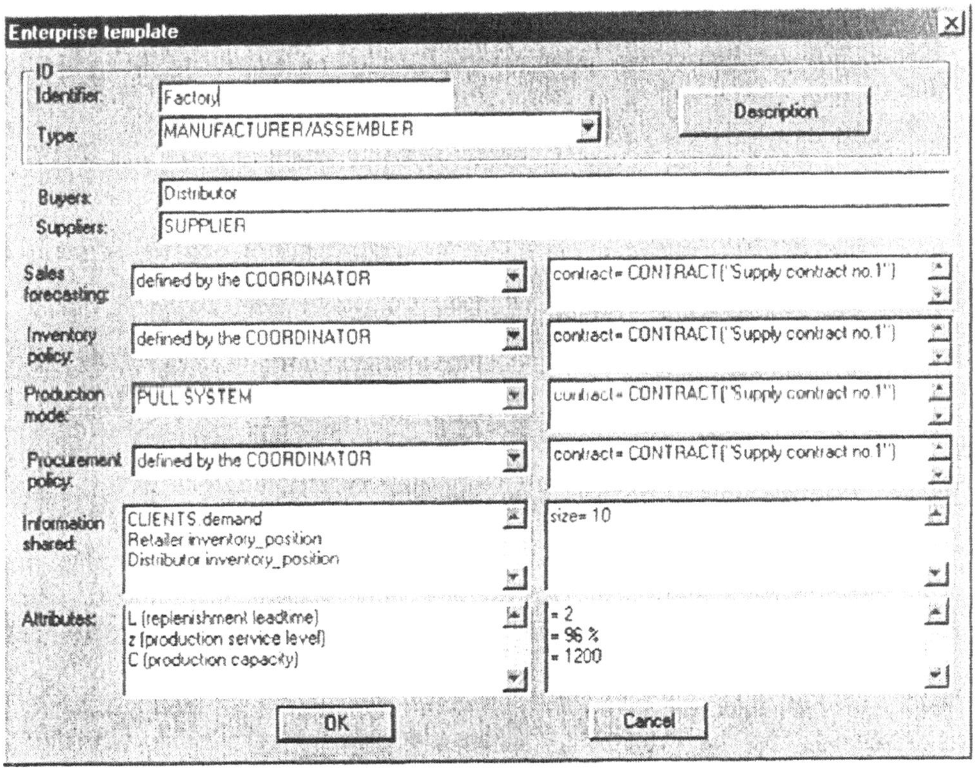

Enterprise template

ID
Identifier: Factory
Type: MANUFACTURER/ASSEMBLER
Description

Buyers: Distributor
Suppliers: SUPPLIER

Sales forecasting: defined by the COORDINATOR | contract= CONTRACT('Supply contract no.1')
Inventory policy: defined by the COORDINATOR | contract= CONTRACT('Supply contract no.1')
Production mode: PULL SYSTEM | contract= CONTRACT('Supply contract no.1')
Procurement policy: defined by the COORDINATOR | contract= CONTRACT('Supply contract no.1')
Information shared: CLIENTS.demand, Retailer.inventory_position, Distributor.inventory_position | size= 10
Attributes: L (replenishment leadtime) = 2; z (production service level) = 96 %; C (production capacity) = 1200

OK Cancel

Figure 6 – Enterprise Template

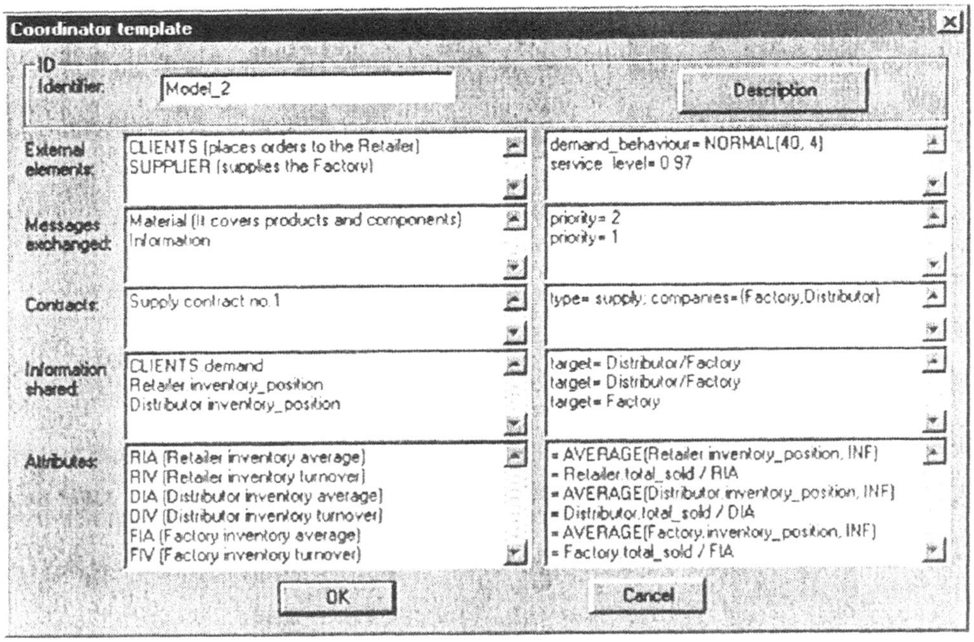

Coordinator template

ID
Identifier: Model_2
Description

External elements: CLIENTS (places orders to the Retailer) | demand_behaviour= NORMAL(40, 4); SUPPLIER (supplies the Factory) | service_level= 0.97
Messages exchanged: Material (It covers products and components) | priority= 2; Information | priority= 1
Contracts: Supply contract no.1 | type= supply; companies= (Factory,Distributor)
Information shared: CLIENTS.demand | target= Distributor/Factory; Retailer.inventory_position | target= Distributor/Factory; Distributor.inventory_position | target= Factory
Attributes:
RIA (Retailer inventory average) = AVERAGE(Retailer.inventory_position, INF)
RIV (Retailer inventory turnover) = Retailer.total_sold / RIA
DIA (Distributor inventory average) = AVERAGE(Distributor.inventory_position, INF)
DIV (Distributor inventory turnover) = Distributor.total_sold / DIA
FIA (Factory inventory average) = AVERAGE(Factory.inventory_position, INF)
FIV (Factory inventory turnover) = Factory.total_sold / FIA

OK Cancel

Figure 7 – Coordinator template

The figure 8 shows the Factory, the Distributor and the Retailer inventory dynamics during 100 periods of time for each one of the two above management scenarios. The largest inventory level, in the scenario CIMS, occurs at the retail and is half of in the DIMS scenario. Also in the CIMS scenario the inventory has better behavior than in the DIMS approach.

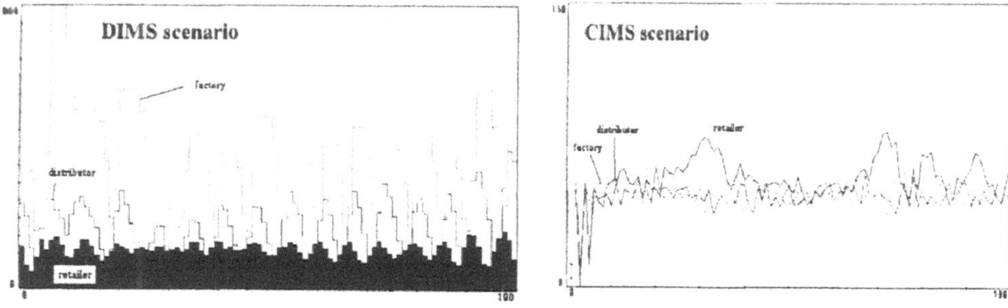

Figure 8 – Inventory Dynamics

6. CONCLUSIONS

New Supply Chain strategies are necessary to provide the market with high-mix, low volume, fast response at low costs products. These challenges require customer-oriented Supply Chain operations through re-engineering the business processes among partner enterprises. System simulation is an important decision support tool that can contribute to re-think these processes. A specialized simulation tool is necessary to consider a distributed modeling and simulation environment oriented to business process rules.

7. ACKNOWLEDGMENTS

The research reported in this paper was supported by FAPESP (Fundação de Amparo à Pesquisa do Estado de São Paulo) through a scholarship to Carlos Machado and CNPq through a research project.

8. REFERENCES

1. Al-Ahmari, A.M. and Ridgway, K. "An integrated modeling method to support manufacturing systems analysis and design", *Computer in Industry*. Vol. 38 (1999).
2. Bruno, G., Agarwal, R. "Modeling the Enterprise Engineering Environment", *IEEE Transactions on Engineering Management*. Vol. 44, No. 1 (1997).
3. Davis, Wayne J. "Looking into the Future of Simulation", *IEEE Solutions*, May (1998).
4. Kellert, P., Tchernev, N., Force, C. "Object Oriented Methodology for FMS modelling and simulation", *International Journal of CIM*. Vol. 10, No. 6 (1997).
5. Lee, H.L., Billington, C. "Material Management in Decentralized Supply Chains", *Operations Research*. Vol. 41, No. 5 (1993).
6. Lee, H.L., Padmanabhan, V. and Whang, S. "Information distortion in a supply chain: the bullwhip effect", *Management Science*. Vol. 43, 546-558 (1997).
7. Simchi-Levi, D., Kaminsky, P. and Simchi-Levi, E. (2000) Designing and Managing the Supply Chain: Concepts, Strategies, and Cases. McGraw-Hill.
8. Vernadat, F. "Requirements for Simulation Tools in Enterprise Engineering". *CAR&FOF'99*, August, MT5/19-23 (1999).
9. Whitman, L., Huff, B. and Presley, A. (1997). "Structured Models and Dynamic Systems Analysis: The Integration of the IDEF0/IDEF3 Modeling Methods and Discrete Event Simulation". *Winter Simulation Conference* (1997).

51

REFERENCE CONFIGURATIONS TO SUPPORT THE IMPLEMENTATION OF THE PRODUCT RECOVERY SUPPLY CHAIN

Aysin Rahimifard, Stephen T. Newman and Shahin Rahimifard
Wolfson School of Mechanical and Manufacturing Engineering
Loughborough University, United Kingdom
A.Rahimifard@lboro.ac.uk

Increased public awareness towards the global environmental problems together with government regulations has forced current manufacturing companies to be more conscious of the effect of their activities on the natural environment. One of the many efforts to combat these environmental problems is to recover products at the end of their life in order to conserve natural resources, minimise energy consumption and reduce waste disposal problems. Recently an increasing number of manufacturing enterprises aim or are forced by legislation to adapt product recovery into their existing business practices. This has highlighted a need for a systematic approach for enhancement of information, business and production management systems to deal with additional activities and processes related to the recovery of products. The research reported in this paper aims to provide a clear understanding of such product recovery activities by extending the traditional manufacturing supply chain through the definition of a product recovery implementation methodology an its application via two reference Configurations.

1. INTRODUCTION

The mass industrialisation over the last century has had a negative impact on the natural environment, contributing towards serious problems such as global warming, ozone depletion, acid rains and natural resource depletion. As a result, there is an increasing demand by customers, suppliers and the public from manufacturing industry in general to minimise any negative impact of their products and operations on the natural environment, i.e. being environmentally conscious. As a result, the recent research in this area has led to the development of Environmentally Conscious Manufacturing (ECM) concepts, which are concerned with developing equipment, methods and procedures for manufacturing activities from conceptual design to final disposal (including re-use and recycling) such that the environmental standards and requirements are satisfied. Two of the major research areas in ECM is the End-Of-Life (EOL) management and Product Recovery (PR) which is the transformation of the used and discarded products into useful condition through re-manufacture, re-use and recycling. The main motivations for PR are economic gains, complying with legislation, improving the public image and personal ethical initiatives. However, complying with legislation related to PR will become more crucial in the near future because national and international directives will make take-back and recovery of used products obligatory for the Original Equipment Manufacturer (OEM) instead of being an option. In Europe, Waste from Electric and Electronic Equipment (WEEE) directive is in the preparation stage and expected to be in law by the end of year 2002. This directive will require one hundred percent take-back and a high percentage of PR of used products from electric and electronic goods producers. As a result, this puts extra pressure on such companies to establish take-back and PR as a part of their business activities.

In this paper the issues related to product recovery activities within an extended manufacturing supply chain are discussed and a number of reference configurations for such supply chain are defined. The initial part of this paper provides a review of relevant literature, and the major sections discuss the new concept of the product recovery chain and analyses the implication of extension of the existing manufacturing supply chain through product recovery adaptation. Furthermore, a PR implementation methodology together with a number of reference configurations has been presented to support the realisation of various product recovery supply chain scenarios within different manufacturing applications.

2. REVIEW OF RELEVANT RESEARCH

The increasing significance of product recovery within manufacturing activities has brought a corresponding influence in the research covering the production life cycle stages from product design to final disposal. In the design stage, new concepts have emerged such as design for disassembly, re-manufacturing, re-use, and recycling, which incorporate end-of-life decision considerations as design objectives (Alting and Legarth 1995, Harjula *et al.* 1996). Within the production stage, operational management issues related to product recovery include disassembly and re-manufacturing planning and control (Gupta and Taleb 1994, Gungor and Gupta 1999, Lambert *et al.* 2000). The important issue is to find a balance between the cost of disassembly and re-manufacturing and the returned benefits, as explored by Lambert (1997) and Navin-Chandra (1994). There are also a number of studies exploring the use and suitability of a Material Requirement Planning (MRP) based approach with some modifications for scheduling in recovery environments (Gupta and Taleb 1994, Guide *et al.* 1997). Other researchers propose and investigate the use of alternative approaches for scheduling and control at the shop floor such as the drum-buffer-rope concept (Guide 1996), flexible KANBAN (Kizilkaya and Gupta 1998), "Push" and "Pull" control strategies (Van der Laan *et al.* 1999). Other issues investigated in this area relate to inventory control requirements within recovery systems which differ from traditional manufacturing systems due to a high degree of uncertainty in timing, quantity and quality of returned products and the demand for recovered parts (Fleischmann *et al.* 1997, Guide *et al.* 1999, Richter and Sombrutzki 2000).

One of the critical decision making tasks relates to end-of-life (EOL) management, namely the selection of options among the recovery of the used product as a whole, component or part recovery, material recovery (recycling) or disposal. The objective is to maintain the profitability and not to violate the technical feasibility constraints (Johnson and Wang 1998, Krikke *et al.* 1998, Low *et al.* 1998,

Jung and Bartel 1999, Goggin and Browne 2000). Finally, a significant body of research has explored the new material flows within PR applications from the user to the producer, which includes the collection and transportation processes and is referred to as reverse distribution (Spengler *et al.* 1997, Jung and Bartel 1999, Klausner and Hendrickson 2000).

3. PRODUCT RECOVERY SUPPLY CHAIN

In product recovery applications, the traditional view of the manufacturing supply chain has been extended to include the activities, actors and the structures required to accomplish recovery at the end of products' life. This has resulted in the emergence of the new supply chain concept, referred to as 'product recovery supply chain'. The original manufacturing supply chain concepts supports a one-way economy, which transforms raw material into useful products. However the recovery of products, parts, material and energy within the product recovery supply chain is ultimately resulting in a bi-directional physical flow within what the authors defined as a complete 'manufacturing loop' (see Figure 1).

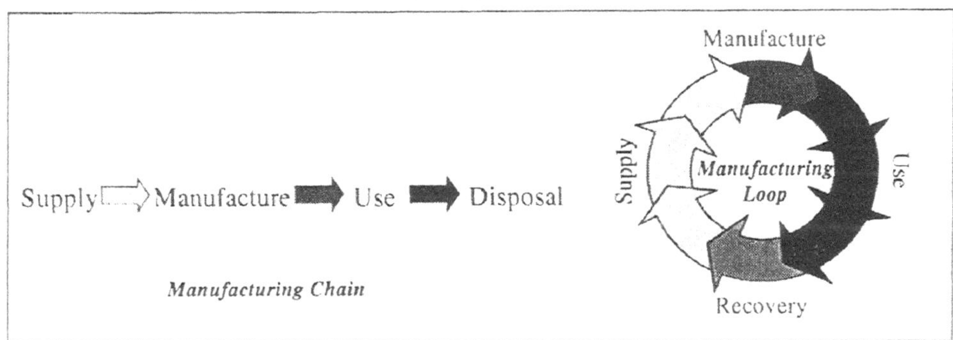

Figure 1 - Manufacturing Chain vs. Manufacturing Loop

The additional activities in the product recovery supply chain as opposed to the traditional manufacturing supply chain are the collection, assessing, sorting, and re-processing redistribution and disposal of waste. There are new actors associated with each of these activities and the new bi-directional workflow structures to represent not only the traditional flow of products from the manufacturer to customer, but also the flow of used products back from the customer to be recovered. This recovery of used products can be classified into a number of levels as illustrated in Figure 2 and outlined below :-

- *Product recovery* is the reintroduction of used product back into the market through a series of processes such as inspection, disassembly, replacing or repairing bad components and re-assembling (often referred to as re-manufacturing).
- *Module & part recovery* where a subset of parts and components of used products can be recovered, repaired or re-conditioned for re-use in production of new products.
- *Material recovery* is retrieving the material content of the whole or a subset of the components of used products through a range of processes at the end of

which the identity of the product is completely lost (often referred to as recyclying), and finally,

- *Energy recovery* where in limited applications some of the material not recovered through one of aforementioned process is used to generate energy (often in the form of heat and electricity).

It should be noted that in most applications due to the economical and environmental implications such as cost, effort, time, and energy associated with re-production, the most preferred approach to recovery in the first place should be directed at the recovery of the product, followed by modules and parts. The latter two options, namely material and energy recovery should be considered in industries that are characterised by short technology cycles and high technological obsolescence.

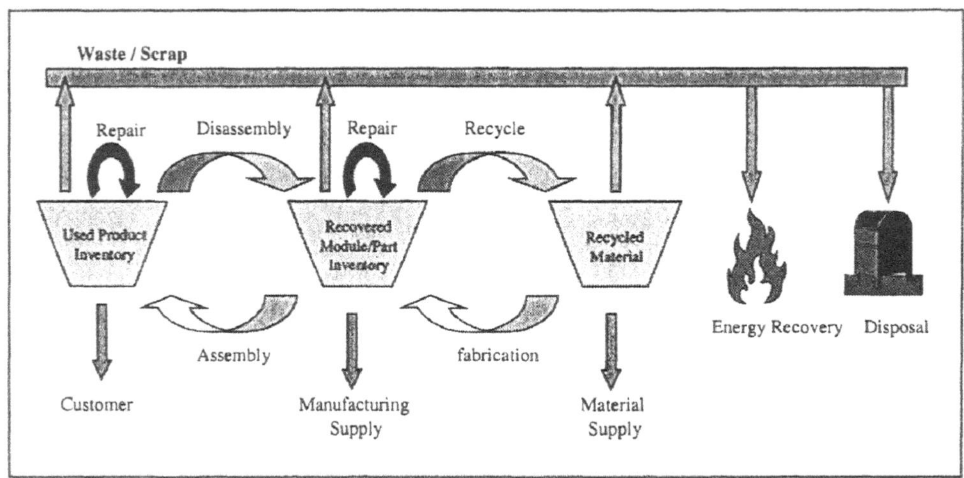

Figure 2 - Product Recovery Operations and Their Relationships.

4. REFERENCE CONFIGURATIONS FOR PRODUCT RECOVERY

The adoption of PR procedures within manufacturing enterprises requires a major alteration on both the internal and external business and operational structures. Clearly, there should be an in-depth understanding of such implications on the existing manufacturing activities before considering any major modification of business and operational processes. It is crucial to assess and evaluate alternative approaches in product take-back and recovery before final decisions are made. In order to develop reference configurations for product recovery, the research reported in this paper has generated a novel systematic five-stage methodology, referred to as the 'Product Recovery Implementation MEthodology' (PRIME). The various stages of PRIME are illustrated in Figure 3 and outlined below :-

i) *Technological Assessment*: the evaluation of available technologies in various applications to identify the most appropriate PR procedures for a specific product, resulting in adoption of a re-manufacturing, re-use or recycling approach.

ii) *Business and Economical Evaluation*: this includes a cost-benefit analysis, investigation of relevant national and international legislation, identification of marketing implications for both the original and recovered products, and business process planning to include new processes and actors.

iii) *Resource Assessment*: the evaluation of various required resources including the internal and external hardware, software and human resources.

iv) *Logistic and Operation Planning*: Product take-back logistics, planning and control of recovery processes, inventory control of new and recovered product.

v) *Information Specification*: identification of product and manufacturing information related to additional activities included in a product recovery supply chain.

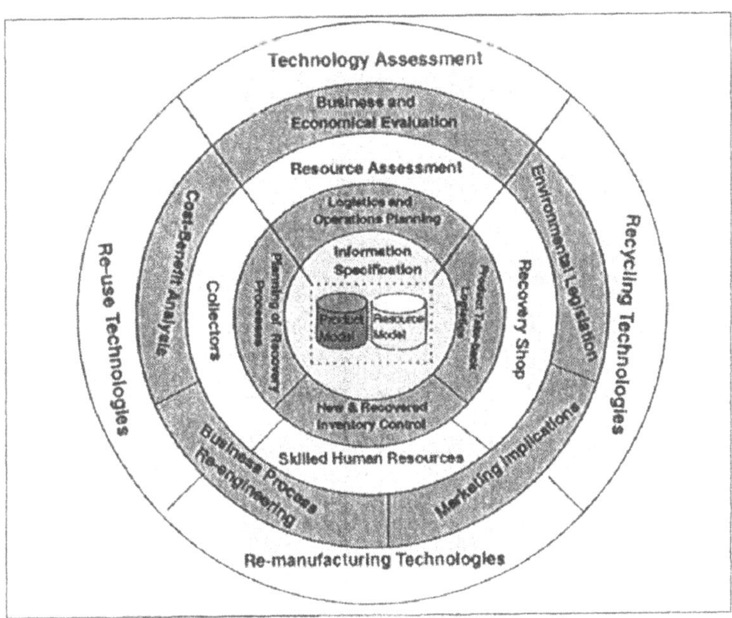

Figure 3 – Product Recovery Implementation Methodology

There are basically two possible business solutions for the realisation of product recovery within manufacturing applications, namely (a) through addition of recovery capabilities to Original Equipment Manufacturer (OEM) activities or (b) by third party independent recovery companies whose sole business is to re-process used products. This correspondingly highlights two possible reference configurations for the realisation of PR procedures within a manufacturing enterprise, namely

- *Reference Configuration 1 - Recovery by Manufacturer* : in this reference configuration the original manufacturer of the product takes the products back at the end of its life and carries out the recovery processes in-house, as illustrated in Figure 4a. This is often achieved by the expansion of the business and manufacturing facilities to include the required resources to undertake the recovery processes. This reference configuration provides more control over the secondary market for the OEM, and the information required for disassembly and remanufacturing is readily available within the company which makes the implementation of product recovery procedures easier.
- *Reference Configuration 2 – Recovery by Independent Recoverer* : in the second reference configuration, an independent recovery company undertakes

PR on behalf of one or more OEMs (see Figure 4b). The recoverer receives the product(s) from the collectors at the end of their life and carries out the required recovery processes, and supplies them back to the original manufacturer or sells them on to a secondary customer. Clearly, in this reference configuration a particular OEM has less control over the secondary market, and issues related to product confidentiality and EOL information management is much more complex. The independent recoverer often has access to a vast amount of information supplied by a number of OEMs, and has the additional advantage of supplying the recovered products to a much larger market.

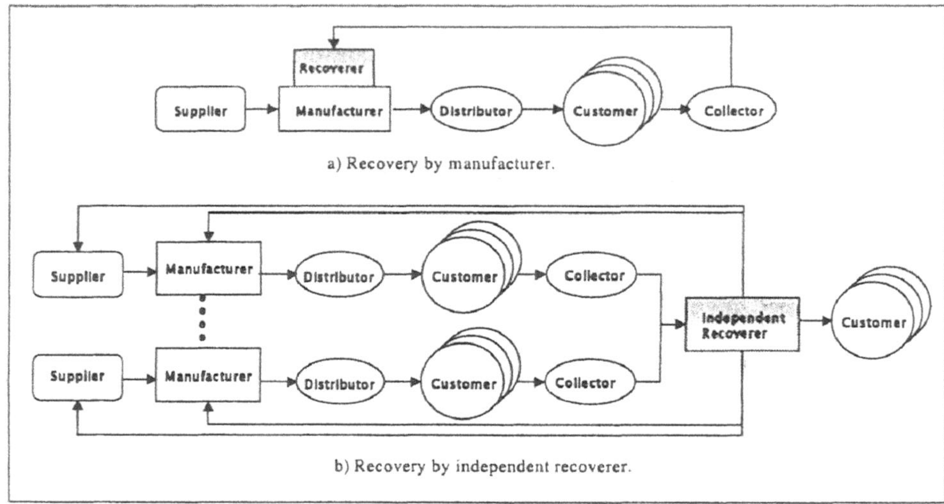

Figure 4 - Product Recovery Realisations.

There are a large number of factors influencing the suitability of one of these reference configurations for a particular manufacturing company, including product size and type, process complexity, production capacity, geography of the initial distribution, and relevant legislation. These factors should be carefully analysed and assessed before establishing the suitability of one of these recovery reference configurations. For example, within a company where manufacturing activities are mainly consists of assembly of large and specially designed products in small batches, the first reference configuration is considered to be more attractive than within a high volume components manufacturing company. One of the other key decision issues is the geographical distribution of customers and effort involved in the collection of used products which may make the first reference configuration infeasible. Furthermore, the PR processes such as disassembly, repair and reassembly will require additional planning, control and co-ordination which could result in undesirable complexity and higher product costs.

The second reference configuration provides OEMs with the advantage of outsourcing the recovery processes thus not needing a major alteration in their production facilities. Such a shared recovery approach may significantly reduce the cost of recovery processes. However, due to complexity of recovery technologies and unfamiliarity of such re-manufacturing business concepts, in many industrial sectors these independent recoverers may not exist at present.

5. CONCLUDING DISCUSSION

The frequent emergence of a large number of national and international legislations are necessitating the adoption of PR procedures in an increasing number of industrial sectors and placing the responsibility of recovery and final disposal of used products firmly on the original manufacturer. Furthermore, the significant attention paid to the environmental impact of manufacturing activities in recent years, highlights the paramount importance and inevitability of the inclusion of product recovery procedures within an increasing number of manufacturing applications in the near future. This has also resulted in emergence of new customer and manufacturer relationships such as the ever increasing popularity of 'product leasing' in electronic and automotive industries.

At present the recovery of products may not be economically viable in many industrial sectors. In addition the adoption of PR may or may not have a positive marketing impact. For example, the use of a recycled product with a complex disposal requirement (e.g plastic bottles) provides a positive image and marketing implications, whereas the use of recycled or reconditioned parts within the automotive industry may not encourage an increase in sales. This has resulted in a lack of significant and a consistent desire by the manufacturing companies and in particular the small to medium enterprises (SMEs) to adopt the PR procedures. SMEs represent the largest proportion of the manufacturing sector, generating more than half of the total production output in every industrial country, and therefore the required and desired levels of reduction in negative impacts of manufacturing activities on environment can only be achieved through development of simple, economical and systematic approach for the adoption of PR within SMEs.

The review of literature has shown that the previous PR research work has concentrated on isolated topics rather than developing a holistic view linking and integrating all aspects of product recovery procedures. The research reported in this paper has defined reference configurations based on a systematical methodology for the implementation of PR procedures. These reference configurations encapsulate the results from the assessment and definition generated by each stage of the methodology and provide a clear view of a possible approach to realisation of PR procedures. Future research will aim to generate a CASE software tool to support the various stages of the PRIME methodology for each reference configuration. This CASE tool includes a knowledge based advisory system for PR legislations and technologies, a business model, a planning model, supported by the product and resource information models which are enhanced to include the PR related information.

6. REFERENCES

1. Alting L, Legarth JB, 1995, Life cycle engineering and design, *Annals CIRP*, **44** (2), 569-580.
2. Fleischmann M, Boemhof-Ruwaard JM, Dekker R, van der Laan E, van Nunen JAEE, van Vasenhove LN, 1997, Quantitive models for reverse logistics: a review, *European Journal of Operational Research*, **103**, 1-17.

3. Goggin K, Browne J, 2000, The resource recovery level decision for end-of-life products, Production Planning and Control, **11** (7), 628-640.
4. Guide VDR, 1996, Scheduling using drum-buffer-rope in a remanufacturing environment, International Journal of Production Research, **34** (4), 1081-1091.
5. Guide VDR, Jayaraman V, Srivastava R, 1999, Production planning and control for remanufacturing: a state-of-art survey, Robotics and Computer Integrated Manufacturing, **15**(3), 221-230.
6. Guide VDR, Kraus ME, Srivastava R, 1997, Scheduling policies for remanufacturing, International Journal of Production Economics, **48** (2), 187-204.
7. Gungor A, Gupta SM, 1999, Issues in environmentally conscious manufacturing and product recovery: a survey, Computers and Industrial Engineering, **36**(4), 811-853.
8. Gupta P, 1995, A management overview of ISO 14000, Circuits Assembly, **5**(12), 36, 38.
9. Gupta SM, Taleb KN, 1994, Scheduling disassembly, International Journal of Production Research, **32** (8), 1857-1866.
10. Harjula T, Rapoza B, Knight WA, Boothroyd G, 1996, Design for disassembly and the environment, Annals CIRP, **45**(1), 109-114.
11. Johnson MR, Wang MH, 1998, Economical evaluation of disassembly operations for recycling, remanufacturing and reuse, International Journal of Production Research, **36** (12), 3227-3252.
12. Jung LB, Bartel TJ, 1999, Computer take-back and recycling: an economic analysis for used consumer equipment, Journal of Electronics Manufacturing, **9** (1), 67-77.
13. Kizilkaya E, Gupta SM, 1998, Material flow control and scheduling in a disassembly environment, Computers and Industrial Engineering, **35** (1-2), 93-96.
14. Klausner M, Hendrickson CT, 2000, Reverse-logistics strategy for product take-back, Interfaces, **30** (3), 156-165.
15. Krikke HR, van Harten A, Schuur PC, 1998, On a medium term product recovery and disposal strategy for durable assembly products, International Journal of Production Research, **36** (1), 111-139.
16. Lambert AJD, 1997, Optimal disassembly of complex products, International Journal of Production Research, **35**(9), 2509-2523.
17. Lambert AJD, Jansen MH, Splinter MAM, 2000, Environmental information systems based on enterprise resource planning, Integrated Manufacturing Systems, **11**(2), 105-112.
18. Low MK, Williams DJ, Dixon C, 1998, Manufacturing products with end-of-life considerations: an economic assessment to the routes of revenue generation from mature products, IEEE Transactions on Components, Packaging and Manufacturing Technology-C, **21** (1), 4-10.
19. Navin-Chandra D, 1994, The recovery problem in product design, Journal of Engineering Design, **5**(1), 65-86.
20. Richter K, Sombrutzki M, 2000, Remanufacturing planning for the reverse Wagner/Whitin models, European Journal of Operational Research, **121** (2), 304-315.
21. Spengler T, Puckert H, Penkuhn T, Rentz O, 1997, Environmental integrated production and recycling management, European Journal of Operational Research 97, 308-326.
22. The European Parliament and the Council of the European Union, 2000, Proposal for a Directive of the European Parliament and of the Council on waste electrical and electronic equipment (WEEE), http://www.compliance-club.com/WEEE.htm, date accessed: November 2001.
23. Van der Laan E, Salomon M, Dekker R, 1999, An investigation of lead-time effects in manufacturing/remanufacturing systems under simple PUSH and PULL control strategies, European Journal of Operational Research, **115** (1), 195-214.

52

ON THE VALUE OF INDUSTRIAL SERVICE

Pontus Johansson
Department of Production Economics
Linköping Institute of Technology
SE-581 83 Linköping, Sweden
pontus.johansson@ipe.liu.se

This paper deals with the value of industrial services, i.e. the supply of after sales services to industrial users of capital goods. A tool is proposed that measure the monetary value of future industrial service activities, and that considers non-monetary values as well. The paper further highlights the need for an increased strategic focus on manufacturing firms' industrial service business.

1. INTRODUCTION

Kotler (1997, p. 52) defines a profitable customer as one "...that over time yields a revenue stream that exceeds by an acceptable amount the company's cost stream of attracting, selling, and servicing that customer". Profits are measured monetarily and presented through accounting statements, *value* on the other hand is a bit trickier; what is for example the value of a good customer relation?

Manufacturing firms are traditionally viewed upon as producing and selling goods and that through the transaction of goods for money the customer takes over the produced item. For strategic planning of manufacturing activities a strong theoretical foundation has been laid (see Skinner, 1969, Hayes and Wheelwright 1979a and 1979b, Hill, 2000). With manufacturers delivering an increasing amount of services, more and/or new strategic tools are required. Turning away from goods production and looking at "pure" services, they come in many variations and several attempts to categorize them has been made, see for example Schmenner (1986), Silvestro *et al.* (1992), Kellogg and Nie (1995), Lele (1997), Cohen *et al.* (2000), and Buzacott (2000). This paper deals with an intersection of goods and services which here is called Industrial Service, and defined as *the supply of after sales services, such as spare parts, consumables, education, repair services, and upgrades, related to the maintenance of industrial goods.*

The focus of this paper is the monetary value of supplying industrial service, and the purpose is to develop a decision tool which adjusts for interest rates, inflation, and uncertainty, to be used by after sales managers. Furthermore, a discussion is held on how to assess non-monetary customer value, which could be translated into revenue potential for the industrial service provider.

Although the results are aimed at ultimately finding a use in industrial applications, this paper as it is should be seen as theory generating. Empirical testing and evaluation is still to be carried out, and could lead to corrections of the proposed decision tools. The theory used in this paper is taken from numerous research fields, including manufacturing strategy, service management, corporate finance, and marketing.

This paper first looks at after sales characteristics, especially in monetary terms and in a consideration of the outlook for this kind of business. The first part also discusses good/service aspects of various products. Secondly, a summary is made on the use and application of net present value (NPV). Next follows an analysis of the value of industrial services, focused on methods to measure monetary value. Then comes a section containing the conclusions to be drawn from the analysis, and finally there is a discussion on the managerial impact of the conclusions, including ideas for future research.

2. AFTER SALES CHARACTERISTICS

A building ground for the coming discussion is that a product can consist of a good, a service, or both. After sales service and thereby also industrial service, which is a subset of the former, is considered to be a product, thus capable of having both good and service characteristics. It is also of importance to note that after sales service goes by many names, according to Goffin and New (2001) these include customer support, product support, technical support, and service.

Knecht et al. (1993) consider the after sale market as a largely unexplored opportunity for industrial companies. Their investigations state that after sales business accounts for 10-20 % of revenue in their four company types, but at the same time 20-40 % of profit contribution. Wise and Baumgartner (1999) also point to after sale activities as one part of their conclusion that many manufacturing companies could profit by expanding down the value chain. Marsh (1999) point out that most engineering companies already have after sales divisions, and that these are increasingly becoming the focus of operations.

Looking at the customers who purchase the industrial service also reveal how large the business potential is. The major Swedish rail company, SJ, is a large customer of various after sales services. Comparing their expenses for vehicle maintenance (i.e., after sales service) to their expenses for acquiring new rolling stock exposes that the company spends roughly twice as much on vehicle maintenance as on new acquires (SJ, 2001).

Levitt, in the 1983 article "After the sale is over...", considered how products were, and would be, valued. He claimed that goods (*items* using Levitt's term) had gone from being just a simple product to being an augmented product, and in the future would transform to system contracts. He further said that service would increase in value from modest in the past to important in 1983 to vital in the future. It is difficult to argue against these claims, and today we are in what Levitt in 1983 called the future. So, what is next?

A very logical reasoning for the changing strategies in after sales service is made by Lele (1997). The alterations predicted by Lele are (i) Service contracts will become an endangered species, (ii) Support services will be unbundled, and (iii)

Profits will be squeezed. Thus the conclusions to draw from Lele's paper is that manufacturers will find their profitability shrunk not only from new sales competition but also in the previously so successful after sales business, and to remain overall competitive companies must include after sales activities into their strategic planning. However, based on the possibilities to increase revenues from service activities - albeit at lower profitability - an increased importance of services in general and after sales services in particular is to be expected. (Wise and Baumgartner, 1999, Cohen et al., 2000, Mathieu, 2001).

In providing after sales services, the original equipment manufacturer (OEM) has numerous advantages. Among these are product knowledge, access to drawings, existing customer relations, and market knowledge. The possibilities for 3rd party companies to compete with their own industrial service products must however be seen as increasing. Powerful computers and CNC-machinery make fast reengineering of goods a realistic option, and modern information technology greatly increases market access. This reasoning supports the conclusion that after sales competition will be tougher in the future.

3. NET PRESENT VALUE

There is a considerable difference between cash flow and the accounting income statement. For the purpose of finding a capital investment's value cash flows should be, and normally is, used (see for example Ross et al., 1996). To explain the difference, let us consider a firm buying a building for € 500,000. The entire sum is an immediate cash flow (cost), but from an accounting perspective with a 50 years straight depreciation the cost, or earnings reduction, is only € 10,000. There is however no doubt that the company needs to fully finance the cash outflow of € 500,000.

The net present value (NPV) of a project is found by considering all *future* cash flows stemming from the project at hand. Furthermore, only incremental cash flows are considered, that is, we look at the difference in the company's cash flow with or without the project.

Mathematically, there are two basic ways to determine an NPV, both giving correct answers (at least as correct as the input) but useful for different applications. Firstly, cash flows are considered as time-discrete events, which are discounted to a net present value in time zero as shown by:

$$NPV = \sum_{i=0}^{N} a_i (1+r)^{-i} \qquad \text{Formula (1)}$$

where a_i is the discrete cash flow (annuity) a at time i, discounted with the interest rate r.

Secondly, cash flows can be considered as a continuous stream, giving that net present value is found through integration:

$$NPV = \int_0^T a(\tau) e^{-\rho\tau} d\tau \qquad \text{Formula (2)}$$

with $a(\tau)$ being the cash flow stream at time τ discounted with the continuous interest rate $\rho = ln(1+r)$ when one year is used as the time base.

The use of NPV as a tool has become quite simple compared to earlier. Strong analytical skills that were once required to solve difficult sums and integrations have now been replaced (or at least greatly facilitated) by the now common use of computers and spreadsheet programs. For more details on the use of NPV, see Ross et al. (1996), or basically any other textbook on corporate finance/capital budgeting.

4. THE VALUE OF INDUSTRIAL SERVICES

In chapter 2 it was found that after sales services, and thus industrial services, are normally profitable. Here methods for finding the value, beyond accounting principles, of such products are investigated. The last subsection of this chapter contains a summary of the presented methods.

4.1 Bottom Line

In a steady state condition the ratio between new sales and after sales would remain constant. Both contribute with revenue and profits (or losses), and over time not much change is expected. To increase company value it is thus enough to focus on increasing this year's bottom line, for example by investigating the effect of changing margins, sales volume, market share, costs, price, etc., and efforts are concentrated on the area with would give the best yield.

The presumption made about no change over time is in "the real world" very unlikely. The practice of focusing on the present year's bottom line is however a viable method in attempts to maximize profits and increase shareholder value. When valuing a company, it is simple to use historical data; future cash flows are harder to estimate. Many analytical methods for valuing a company therefore put a strong emphasis on the latest financial reports, and thus motivate companies to focus on the bottom line.

It is easy to criticize a bottom line focus as being to shortsighted and possibly even destroying potential future value. But, since shareholder value is undeniably important to many companies, the bottom line effect of industrial service activities is one method to use.

4.2 Single Project

Company A has just signed a contract to supply company B with a new production facility. The price is 10000 monetary units (monetary unit = FMU), and due to tough competition in the bidding process, the profit for A is only FMU 200 (or 2%). However, company A expects to provide industrial services the coming years, but this has not been included in the sales calculation. What is the present value of providing these services?

In calculating the value, future cash flows are discounted with respect to interest rates, inflation and uncertainty. If prices change in line with general inflation, a real interest rate is preferably used, if not it is often easier to use a nominal interest rate. The relation between the two is (r_n/r_r = nominal/real interest rate, h = inflation):

$$1 + r_n = (1 + r_r) \times (1 + h)$$ Formulae (3)

Assuming that real prices are viable, the forecasted real cash flow of the industrial service supply is shown with striped columns in Figure 1. Only the net cash flow is presented, calculated as 20% profit on an order size that annually is 5% of the initial order. Year 1 is covered by warranties, and in year 9 a major retrofit is sold, increasing the final years' cash flow as well. The gray columns show the discounted value of each year's cash flow, which is summarized into an NPV. Tax is assumed to be 30%.

The calculation is done using formulae (1) with an interest rate of 25%. The discount interest rate is derived from a company cost of capital of 12,5% (interest rate required on investments) and adjusted for risk up to 25%. In the end this calculation increases the value of the contract with FMU 325, to be added to the initial FMU 325.

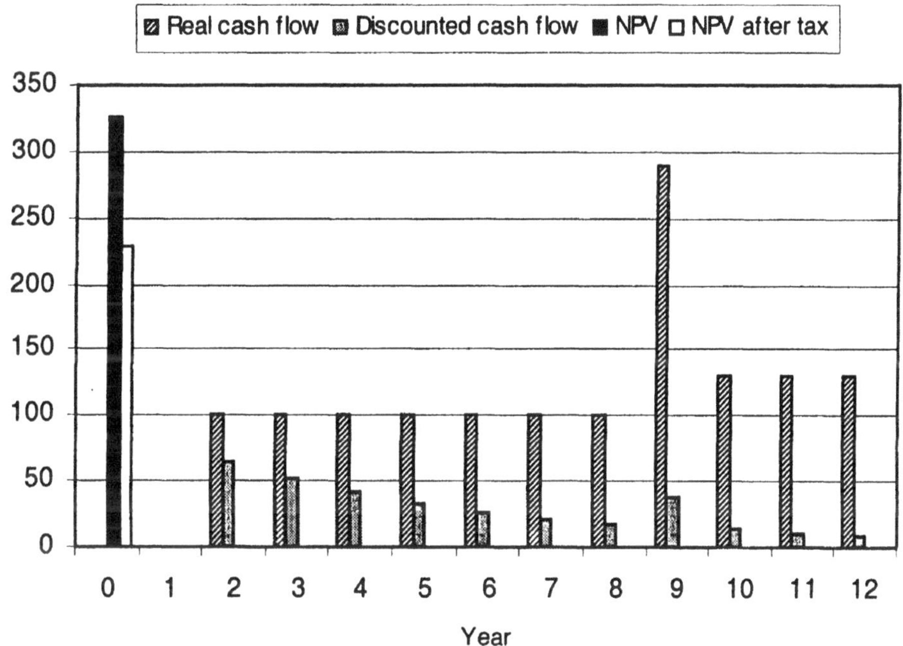

Figure 1 – Net present Value of a Forecasted Industrial Service Supply

4.3 High Volume

When valuating the life cycle cost/profit/income of industrial service, the continuous NPV calculation has some strong sides. A basic requirement however is that future cash flows can be described as a function of time.

Armistead and Clark (1991) shed some light on how a product's life cycle affect after sales activities. The authors suggest strategies for dealing with the various stages of the life cycle, but without measuring the value. If the life cycle can be described mathematically, formula (2) is quite easily used to discount, with adjustment for risk, inflation, and interest rates, the life cycle into a NPV.

When performing an NPV as described here, it is important to consider where in the life cycle the calculation is made. Any economic activity, whether resulting in positive or negative cash flow, that has already taken place is not included in the NPV, but is considered a "sunk costs". *Only future cash flows shall be included.*

4.4 Non-Monetary

Cohen et al. (2000) use Saturn Corporation as a case example on how to build the link between after sales service and customer loyalty. This link is considered to be critical, and the authors claim that a supply-chain strategy targeted at service is one key to achieve customer satisfaction. Taking into account the potential value from returning customers, careful management of the service supply-chain is one way to find value through industrial service.

Outsourcing, core competence, and other management theories changes the way maintenance activities are carried out at the industrial service customers (Sherwin, 2001). Sherwin criticizes how maintenance is commonly measured "against artificial targets fixed according to MBO [management by objectives] principles" (p. 163), and instead advocates contributions to life cycle profit as superior to shortsighted "bottom line" management. Thus it should be the industrial service supplier's task to deliver such life cycle profit in what could hopefully be a win-win situation.

Industrial service can also be considered as an I/O condition for a manufacturing company. Using the concepts of order winner and order qualifier (Hill, 2000), being able to provide the right industrial service can be what wins (or qualifies) a company orders in the market.

4.5 Choosing a Valuation Method

Sections 4.1 – 4.4 propose four different methods to think about the value of industrial service. The names given to these four methods say some about when they are applicable, but for clarification and easy overview Table 1 lists the pros and cons of each method.

Table 1 – How to Value Industrial Service

Method	Pros	Cons
Bottom line	- Increase stock value - Profit maximization	- Effect on long term value creation
Single project	- Intuitive, ease of use - Considers interest rate, inflation and uncertainty	- False reliability through "exact" numbers
High volume	- Analytical solution - Considers interest rate, inflation and uncertainty	- Non-intuitive - Only practical for simple flows
Non-monetary	- Considers uncertainty to a chosen extent - For strategic planning	- Hard to measure profit contribution

5. CONCLUSIONS

This paper shows how traditional methods from financial theory can be applied to estimate the present value of future industrial service activities. It is further shown that depending on the conditions different methods are better suited than others.

When considering all of the methods suggested here, they form a tool that can evaluate the importance of industrial service activities in a company.

One conclusion, which has been drawn by others as well, is that the increased merger of goods and services offers revenue and profit opportunities for manufacturing companies able to expand downstream by supplying industrial services. The tools provided in this paper can be used to highlight the strategic value of increasing a company's focus on this industrial service product.

Apart from the purely monetary valuation, the analysis also covers "softer" values of industrial services. When industrial service becomes a requirement to get orders at all, it is no longer a question of adding value, but of survival. This stresses the need for strategic thinking on manufacturing firms' after sales activities. Or, maybe better put:

"Rarely is customer service discretionary. It is a requisite of getting and holding business, just like the generic product itself." (Levitt, 1972, p. 10)

6. MANAGERIAL IMPLICATIONS

Increased competition (as discussed in section 2) means that an increased focus on industrial service is required to maintain or improve competitiveness. This paper hopefully highlights this problem (or opportunity, if thought of more positively). Apart from NPV calculations, decision theory is very likely a tool that could find use in strategic thinking regarding industrial service. In future work on industrial service such a tool ought to be investigated. Empirical testing of the proposed tool is another "next step".

Owning a tangible good is, in these days of core competency and outsourcing strategies, not central to many manufacturers. It is therefore likely that that the blending of new sales and after sales into *functional sales* is a phenomenon on the rising. At least it is a phenomenon worth to consider by managers of B2B manufacturers. The tool described in this paper should find use in most companies who are considering functional sales approaches. When ownership of a good is not transferred to the user, the future cash flows around the good become critical to measure.

What the supplier calls industrial service is often called maintenance by the customer. In an overview if maintenance management models by Sherwin (2001), one of the conclusions is that the use of modern IT should make it possible to manage maintenance activities in way that net contribution to life-cycle profit is maximized. An after sales manager that understands how to contribute to his/her customer's maintenance needs is in the right position to create value for both parties.

Your company provides a product, and to do that that a certain cost arises. For the costumer this product has a certain value, which should be higher than the production cost. This gap is divided between seller and buyer. In a competitive market there should be more than one supplier, and given two suppliers delivering products with identical value, the company with the lower cost will be the most profitable one. Thus the tendency among manufacturing companies to lower costs, and the opportunity to gain profits by increasing the created value is often overlooked.

Risk adjustments in NPV calculation is likely based on gut feeling, requiring experienced managers for good results. The same can be said about forecasting industrial service cash flows, and as is valid for all calculations; output will not be more accurate than input.

7. REFERENCES

1. Armistead C, Clark G. A framework for formulating after-sales support strategy. International Journal of Operations & Production Management 1991; **11**(3): 111-124.
2. Buzacott, John A. Service system structure. International Journal of Production Economics 2000; **68**(1): 15-27.
3. Cohen MA, Cull C, Lee HL, Willen D. Saturn's supply-chain innovation: high value in after-sales service. Sloan Management Review 2000; **41**(4): 93-101.
4. Goffin K, New C. Customer support and new product development. International Journal of Operations & Production Management 2001; **21**(3): 275-301.
5. Hayes RH, Wheelwright SC. Link manufacturing processes and product life cycles. Harvard Business Review 1979a; January-February: 133-140.
6. Hayes RH, Wheelwright SC. The dynamics of process-product life cycles. Harvard Business Review 1979b; March-April: 127-136.
7. Hill, Terry. Manufacturing Strategy – Text and Cases, 2nd edition. Houndsmills, Hampshire: Palgrave, 2000.
8. Kellogg DL, Nie W. A framework for strategic service management. Journal of Operations Management 1995; **13**(4); 323-337.
9. Knecht T, Leszinski R, Webe FA. Making profits after the sale. The McKinsey Quarterly 1993; 4: 79-86.
10. Kotler, P. Marketing management – analysis, planning, implementation, and control, 9th edition. Upper Saddle River, New Jersey: Prentice-Hall, 1997.
11. Lele, MM. After-sales service – necessary evil or strategic opportunity?. Managing Service Quality 1997; **7**(3): 141-145.
12. Levitt, T. Production-line approach to service. Harvard Business Review 1972; September-October: Reprint 72505.
13. Levitt, T. After the sale is over... . Harvard Business Review 1983; September-October: Reprint 83511.
14. Marsh, P. At your service. Financial Times 1999; May 12.
15. Mathieu, V. Service strategies within the manufacturing sector: benefits, costs and partnership. International Journal of Service Industry Management 2001; **12**(5): 451-475.
16. Ross SA, Westerfield RW, Jaffe J. Corporate finance, 4th edition, International student edition. Irwin, 1996.
17. Schmenner, RW. How can service business survive and prosper?. Sloan Management Review 1986; **27**(3): 21-32.
18. Sherwin, D. A review of overall models for maintenance management. Journal of Quality in Maintenance Engineering 2000; **6**(3): 138-164.
19. Silvestro R, Fitzgerald L, Johnston R, Voss C. Towards a classification of service processes. International Journal of Service Industry Management 1992; **3**(3): 62-75.
20. SJ. SJ Årsredovisning 2000. 2001. (Swedish railways, Annual report 2000).
21. Skinner, W. Manufacturing – missing link in corporate strategy. Harvard Business Review 1969; May-June: 136-145.
22. Wise R, Baumgartner P. Go downstream – the new profit imperative in manufacturing. Harvard Business Review 1999; September-October: 133-141.

53

ON-LINE ANALYSIS OF UTILITY NETWORKS

Zdeněk Kouba, Kamil Matoušek, Petr Mikšovský
Department of Cybernetics, Czech Technical University in Prague
Technická 2, 166 27 Prague 6, Czech Republic
{kouba, matousek, miksovsp}@labe.felk.cvut.cz

Geographical information systems (GIS) are often used as visualization and analytical means for utility networks applications, because they enable to store information on geographical objects together with their topological and geographical relations. They handle large amounts of geographical data and provide spatial query evaluation on this data. The computationally expensive spatial queries may be improved thanks to the development of on-line analytical processing systems (OLAP) speeding-up the analysis of huge amounts of data stored in large databases. An integration of data warehouse and GIS technologies is the way to enable on-line analysis of geographical information and present its results in geographical contents by native means of the GIS system.

1. INTRODUCTION

Current geographical information systems (GIS) handle large amounts of geographical data that are usually stored in relational databases. From their nature, GIS systems store information on geographical objects together with their topological and geographical relations and they enable spatial query evaluation. As spatial queries are usually very expensive form the computational point of view, major database vendors developed special plug-ins in order to make retrieval of geographical data more efficient. For example, Oracle offers their Spatial Cartridge based on quad-tress, Informix offers the Spatial Data Blade based on R-trees, etc. (Gavrila, 1994, Guttman, 1984). This approach is suitable for those spatial queries, which select objects in certain user-defined area. It does not help so much in the case of analytical queries.

On the other hand we can observe a fast development of so called OLAP systems, i.e. on-line analytical processing systems. The development of such systems has been originally motivated by the need to speed-up the process of analysis of huge amount of data stored in very large databases (Kurz, 1999).

The idea of integration a data warehouse and GIS technologies (Kouba et al., 2000) promises to be the way of enabling on-line analysis of geographical information and present its results in geographical contents by native means of the

GIS system. The data warehouse contains materialized views on geographical data. Instead of running a complicated and time consuming spatial query each time when some information is required, the on-line analysis is run on pre-aggregated data. Such integration enables top executives to carry out on-line analytical processing of data originated in a geographical information system. Moreover, it makes possible to present the analysis' results in corresponding geographical context by the native graphical means of the respective geographical information system.

From this perspective the integration is not just a one-way connection. GIS plays a two-fold role in the integrated system. It is not only the data source, from which the data is extracted and pumped into data warehouse. It is also the presentation platform for presenting results of the analyses.

The concept has been tested in a test-bed application oriented on prediction of water consumption in particular nodes of a water supply network.

2. DATA WAREHOUSE

Even a user without special education on data modeling is able to run prepared on-line analysis on a data warehouse. Data warehouse provides him by a transparent concept of a multidimensional abstraction of the data stored in the data warehouse (Kimball, 1996). He understands very well the semantics of data stored in the data cube and the semantics of the corresponding axes (dimensions) of the cube.

He is allowed to carry out very natural analytical operations like slicing the cube, pivoting it, drilling inside the cube etc. These operations are called OLAP (on-line analytical processing) operations.

However, implementing the data cube directly by means of a multidimensional database (MOLAP) is quite rare case. In practice the population of the data cube is rather sparse and therefore the straightforward multidimensional implementation would be inefficient. MOLAP is used for implementation of data marts, i.e. excerpts from the data warehouse with low number of dimensions.

Usually, the data warehouse itself is implemented by means of relational database technology (ROLAP) and is built on the top of a relational database management system. Current state of the art in relational database technology makes possible to process huge amount of data efficiently by means of massive parallel processing.

In relational implementation the OLAP subsystem makes possible to translate the multidimensional queries into SQL.

3. DATA WAREHOUSE MODELING

The data warehouse model is built on several basic concepts. Let us mention shortly and informally some of them.

Any elementary data cell in the above mentioned data cube represent a value of a given fact in context of corresponding positions along the particular axes of the data cube. Each axis represents a dimension of the data warehouse. There is defined a number of aggregation levels for each dimension. It means, each dimension of the data cube can be viewed from different levels of detail. E.g. the fact turnover in a retail company can be observed from a perspective of weekly turnover in particular district. In this case week is a selected aggregation level of the time dimension, whereas district is the selected aggregation level of the location dimension. By changing the aggregation levels along particular dimensions we change the granularity of the observed data.

Not any two aggregation levels of given dimension may be comparable. For example the aggregation levels month and week of the time dimension are not comparable, as there exists instances of the week aggregation level, which belong to two instances of the month aggregation level. It means that there exists a partial ordering on the set of all aggregation levels of any dimension. This partial ordering may be represented by so-called aggregation graph of given dimension.

The location dimension is the basic concept of GIS – data warehouse integration. It represents the common context of data both in GIS and the data warehouse.

4. INTEGRATION MODULE

The core component of the designed approach is the integration module.

The integration module (IM) has three main functions:

- IM enables the extraction, transformation and load process (ETL) (Kouba et al., 1998) populating the data warehouse by data originating in GIS – see the data stream labeled by (1) in Figure 1.
- IM makes possible to synchronize the status of the GIS with the current status of the data warehouse – see arrow labeled (2) in Figure 1.
- GIS participates in formulation of the multidimensional OLAP query – see arrow labeled (3) in Figure 1.

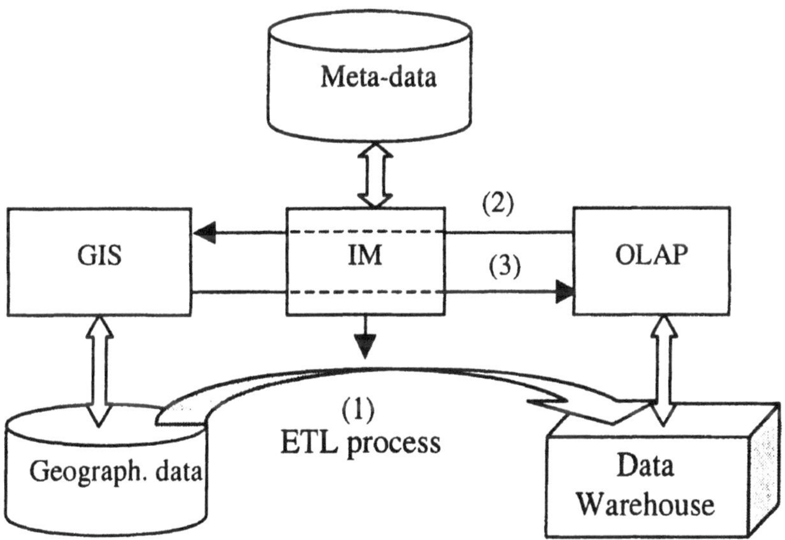

Figure 1 – The Overall Architecture

The integration module is built around the meta-data repository (described bellow), which contains mainly the following types of meta-data:

- Data model of the data warehouse
- Data model of the GIS data source
- Data transformation scripts
- GIS – data warehouse class and instance correspondence
- Definition of data security policies

Purpose of these individual types of information will be described in following paragraphs.

4.1 Meta-Data Repository

Meta-data repository consists of an abstract syntax tree (an internal meta-data representation, which serves as a vehicle for keeping all the meta-data for the system in one place), parser, and methods for meta-data access and maintenance.

ETL operations form an inseparable part of integration module. Thus, the meta-data concept has been enriched by a part related to these ETL operations.

A parser of the meta-data language has been developed. The parser is based on object-oriented version of the PCCTS toolkit by Purdue University. During the parsing process the basic syntax check is performed. The parser builds an internal representation in a form of an abstract syntax tree (AST). All the meta-data is kept in the only tree, which starts from the artificial root. Particular meta-data files are mounted into this tree the size of which is almost unlimited.

Currently, the core of an object-oriented toolkit for the AST manipulation has been finished. It enables the access to the meta-data repository, navigation in the AST, export to text file as well as its parsing into AST. The toolkit is designed as a modular system making possible to add additional modules in future. An interactive graphical editor enabling visualization and maintenance of the AST has been developed as well.

4.2 Extraction, Transformation and Load Process

The extraction, transformation and load process (ETL) is responsible for population the data warehouse from multiple data sources. The designed solution handles unification of data coming from heterogeneous data sources with not fully compatible data models.

Two types of scripts stored in the meta-data repository define the ETL process.

- The transformation scripts extract data from data sources, aggregate them and store the result in the data warehouse.
- The other type of scripts enables evaluation of data validity. Under certain circumstances it is possible to reconstruct wrong or missing data, provided that the data contains some redundancies.

4.3 Class and Instance Correspondence

For purposes of the system integration we consider an object GIS model distinguishing these basic elements:

- *GIS objects* represent individual data items (points, lines, areas etc. with attached sets of data values).
- *GIS classes* are abstract groups of objects of the same level (region, district, building, etc.).

These GIS classes relate to respective aggregation levels of *location* dimension on the data warehouse side. Similarly, the GIS objects correspond to instances of respective aggregation levels on the data warehouse side. Such a correspondence is set up by means of geographical meta-data class defined in the meta-data repository.

It is not necessary to map each internal GIS class to geographical meta-data class and vice-versa. In general, the GIS system should be able to manipulate with the whole geographical data under examination. For example, the GIS system need not be aware of the details about the aggregation graph of the *location* dimension of the data warehouse.

In most cases we expect the GIS system to be a geographical data source providing the rest of the system with geographical data. A subset of this data is then retrieved and offered to the data warehouse.

The binding elements between GIS and data warehouse are the elements of the data warehouse *location* dimension and the GIS taxonomy objects. The task of the integration is to provide three kinds of necessary dynamic correspondences:

1. *Class correspondence* maps particular aggregation levels of the location dimension to the corresponding GIS taxonomy levels and vice versa. This is relatively long-time static pre-defined information stored in integration meta-data.
2. *Instance correspondence* maps particular instances of aggregation levels to the instances of the "classes" in sense of the previous item and vice versa. This is a more dynamic part of the integration information and it guaranties the run-time data integrity. Integration module should keep track of the instance changes in both GIS and DWH and propagate them to the second sub-system.
3. *Action correspondence* is the most dynamic correspondence, which ensures navigation consistency. E.g. after changing aggregation level using particular front-end tool, level information has to be changed in meta-data, data warehouse and GIS. Another example: When performing a GIS selection, just particular sub-cube should be considered for calculation, i.e. corresponding filter should be applied in the data warehouse and the front end tool should show it.

Meta-data objects support all of the three correspondences.

Taxonomy structure of GIS objects is coupled with aggregation levels of a data warehouse via class correspondence. Correct mapping of particular objects is guarded by class correspondence (GIS object "Czech Republic" is related to the instance "Czech Republic" of an aggregation level *country* of the *location* dimension of the data warehouse).

4.4 Data Security Aspects

The issues of authorization and access control concepts relating security concepts to data warehouse technology have been studied. In contrast to record-oriented access policy in typical database systems, in case of coupling both data warehouses and GIS the access rights should be related to the data granularity.

A user may exist, for which the data on very detailed level of granularity are not accessible. Such data may have private nature and therefore it has a restricted access. On the other hand, some data on very general granularity level may not be available to the user, as the data is of strategic nature.

The new cell-level security developments are useful for the needs of GIS-DWH interoperability.

5. APPLICATIONS

A pilot project: "Drinking water distribution system in western Bohemia" use the designed approach. It runs on commercial GIS and Data Warehousing systems to assure the concept, its usefulness and its extensibility by other commercial or non-commercial information systems. Examples of these applications are presented here.

Extensible Markup Language (XML) was determined as a meta-language for data transfer. Selected XML documents contain the particular information that is necessary for inter-system communication and synchronization. Various data models have to be mapped to each other using both static and dynamic portions of such meta-data. Document Object Model (XML-DOM) enables easy document and data transformation among different software platforms. The implementation of the Integration Module (Matoušek et al., 2001) was designed using modern technologies like Component Object Model (COM), Office Web Components (PivotTable Service) and ActiveX Data Objects (ADO). End users can use a broad variety of front-end tools to manipulate and analyze the geographical and dimensional data of their interest. The applicable user interfaces include Dimensional Navigator Snap-In for GIS, Microsoft Excel Pivot Table and others. The tested GIS system is ArcView 3.2.

5.1 Drinking Water Distribution System in Western Bohemia

This pilot application concerns drinking water distribution and consumption. The distribution network begins in the manufacturing part, where the natural water quality is improved for the water to become drinkable and then water is pumped to the primary water supply. Water is distributed to customers indirectly via storage reservoirs. The best quality of water and most efficient production is achieved by constant amount of water produced per time unit. Therefore the consumption peaks must be foreseen and the reservoirs must be pre-filled to contain enough water for the following peak. However, keeping non-necessarily high level of water in water reservoirs is bad, as the water quality is affected by slow exchange of reservoir contents.

The GIS and data warehouse models correspond to each other in following "classes" (levels) of geographical dimension:

- *Reservoir* - represents a water reservoir containing one or more tanks
- *Pipe line* - corresponds to a pipe line connecting several reservoirs
- *Region* - defines an administrative region.

A dimensional data model of the drinking water distribution application, which covers all user requirements, is shown in Figure 2. The model consists of one fact table, two dimensions (i.e. time and geography), and three look-up tables (weather, area, and pipe line).

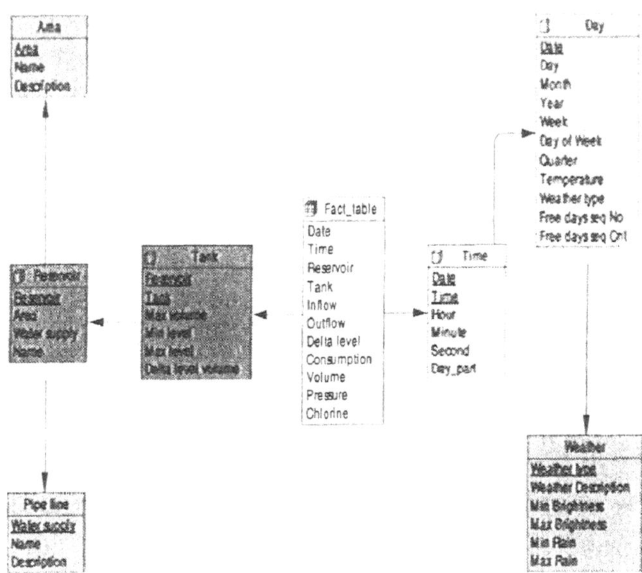

Figure 2 – Water Distribution Data Model

7. CONCLUSIONS

The basic principles for integration of geographical information systems with data warehouses using integration module were formulated. The two integration prototypes concerning two pilot applications were described.

Data warehouses represent a technology, which is able to analyze huge amounts of data in relatively short time. The OLAP engine is optimized for fast query evaluation. Data warehouse principle is based on a specific multidimensional data model, which is powerful in performance and easily understandable. This power is augmented by pre-calculated aggregations of some subsets of the data on various dimensional levels that radically increase the performance.

On the other hand, geographical information systems are designed for storage of structured and spatial information with all the spatial data specific features and functionality. Its drawbacks are the spatial queries that are computationally very demanding.

Therefore GIS integrated together with a data warehouse technologies profit from each other. For example data warehouses can store the pre-calculated results of spatial queries posed within GIS. The conventional OLAP and GIS coupling is capable to analyze on-line pre-defined geographical areas.

The concepts can be used on different system platforms, are extensible and open for further research activities.

8. ACKNOWLEDGMENTS

The work related to this paper has been carried out with support of the INCO-COPERNICUS No. 977091 research project *GOAL – Geographical Information On-line Analysis* and the research grant of the Czech Ministry of Education, Youth and Sport: "Decision Making and Control for Industrial Practice", No. 212300013.

The authors want to express thanks to their colleagues from the *Gerstner Laboratory for Intelligent Decision Making and Control* for creating a friendly environment.

9. REFERENCES

1. Gavrila, DM. R-tree Index Optimization, CAR-TR-718, Comp. Vision Laboratory Center for Automation Research, University of Maryland, 1994
2. Guttman, A. "R-trees: a dynamic index structure for spatial indexing", In Proc. of SIGMOD Int. Conf. on Management of Data, 1984
3. Kimball R. The Data Warehouse Toolkit. Practical Techniques for Building Dimensional Data Warehouses, John Willey & Sons Inc., 1996
4. Kouba Z, Mařík V, Mikšovský P, Tjoa AM. "Data Warehousing and Geographical Information", In Proc. of 4th World Multiconference on Systemics, Cybernetics and Informatics - SCI 2000, 2000
5. Kouba Z, Matoušek K, Mikšovský P, Štěpánková O. "On Updating the Data Warehouse from Multiple Data Sources". In DEXA '98, Vienna, Springer-Verlag, 1998
6. Kurz A. Data Warehousing – Enabling Technology, (in German), MITP-Verlag GmbH, 1999
7. Matoušek K, Mordačík J, Janků L. "On Implementing the Data Warehouse – GIS Integration". In Proc. of World Multiconference on Systemics, Cybernetics and Informatics - SCI 2001

54

DATA MINING AND RESOURCE ALLOCATION: A CASE STUDY

Olga Štěpánková[1], Jiří Kléma[1]
Štěpán Lauryn[2], Petr Mikšovský[1], Lenka Nováková[1]

[1]*Department of Cybernetics, CTU Prague,*
Technicka 2, 166 27 Prague 6, Czech Republic
{step,klema,miksovsp}@labe.felk.cvut.cz
[2]*Lauryn, v.s.o., Pražská 255, 530 06 Pardubice 6,*
{stepanl@lauryn.cz}

This paper presents a case study concerning scheduling and resource allocation issues in a spa. The paper is data-mining oriented. It discusses and describes how the history data can be used as a source for data-mining leading to discovery of rules or algorithms useful for prediction of resources requirements. In particular, we focused to identify groups of patients which appear frequently in the training set and which exhibit characteristic behavior or requirements of spa utilities. Then we predicted a set of health procedures to be passed for each member of such group. This approach resulted in a health procedure prediction algorithm satisfactory for early and convenient scheduling.

1. INTRODUCTION

In industry, everybody understands that scheduling influences efficiency of any serious industrial activity significantly. Due to good scheduling the customers can get their ordered goods in time and for reasonable price which is not increased due to extra fee for storage of the intermediate product. But industry is not the only domain where scheduling has clear economic impact. Scheduling is important in those types of complex services, which have to be ensured e.g. through cooperation of several persons using restricted number of resources. Such a situation appears often in medical environment. Nurses' rostering belongs to well-known cases frequently referred to when describing applications of various techniques for scheduling. But similar problems appear e.g. in a typical health farm or a spa.

Spa offers a set of various health procedures to heal medical problems of the patients who are arriving into the health farm for a restricted period. Obviously each patient obtains an individual treatment, i.e. a set of procedures assigned to the patient by the spa physician, who makes his recommendation after careful inspection of the patient upon his arrival. But recommendation of the spa physician is not enough to ensure that the patient gets those procedures he is supposed to get. To reach such a goal it is important to ensure that necessary resources are available in appropriate quantity. Two basic types of resources – human resources (appropriate skilled personal) and technical equipment (e.g. a bath tube or diathermia) - have to be combined while there has to be met a number of diverse local constraints, e.g.

- Each member of the personal has several skills and can operate several types of equipment. On one hand, a single person cannot exercise all the day one type of a physically demanding job. On the other hand, he/she cannot switch among his/her skills every now and then as the adjustment can be time consuming, etc.
- Sometimes several pieces of equipment are situated in a single room but they cannot be used simultaneously.
- There is a minimal amount of patients for which certain type of equipment can be opened (e.g. a sauna for 10 persons).

All over the fact that the groups of patients occupying the spa are changing frequently, the spa aims to provide the appropriate individual treatment for each of its patients. How can such a goal be achieved? It is vital for the spa administration to know in advance (before the group of patients arrives) what will be the total requirements for all procedures offered by the spa. This knowledge can point to the fact that special precautions should be taken for the considered limited period of time, e.g. extra day off can be offered to some professions or on the contrary extra personal has to be hired or a long day introduced for certain wards ensuring specific procedures. Such decisions have to be planned several days or even weeks in advance. That is why timely prediction of resources requirements is a vital task.

Administration gets the basic information (including rough anamnesis) about the patients to come several weeks in advance. Moreover, the administration owns all the data about the treatment of patients from the last years. Can the history data be used as a source for data-mining leading to discovery of rules or algorithms useful for prediction of resources requirements? In the rest of the paper we will describe a data-mining case-study providing a positive answer to the considered question. This case study is based on real life data.

2. CASE STUDY DESCRIPTION

2.1 Data Exploration and Determination of Data-Mining Goals

Our intention is to predict spa resources requirements given all available information about the group of patients to be present in the spa in the considered week. There are three premises to such a data-mining exercise:

1. Information available about each patient before his/her arrival is a significant factor in determining the schedule of procedures that will be prescribed by the spa physician to the considered person.
2. Treatment schedules prescribed by different spa physicians are consistent.
3. The full set of procedures offered by the spa is fixed, no procedures are added or removed.

If all the premises are true, the history data from the last period (1 or 2 years) could be used to search for prediction rules. Our considered history data-set, referred to as training data, is based on real life data about all 17 953 patients attending one specific spa resort during the years 1999, 2000 and their treatment schedules (protection of patient's personal data has been ensured by the administration of the spa). Data from the same facility covering the year 2001 are used as a test set.

The method to solve the prediction task has to be chosen with respect to the complexity of the treated problem. First, what is known about a single patient before he/she arrives into the health farm? Each person is described using 7 discrete attributes (Sex / 2 values, Cure_type / 8, Disorder / 12, Motility / 8, Stay_length / 33, Accommodation / 5 and Age). These attributes differ in their domain sizes and frequency of the individual attribute values (e.g., for Cure_type, the most often value covers 59% of patients, Stay_length can be from 3 to 35 days, but the patients mostly stay for 21 (60%) or 28 days (28%), etc.).

Suppose each value of each attribute has the same weight from the point of view of the considered prediction task. How many different types of patients we would have to take into account? First, let us ignore the attribute with the most extensive domain, the age. Even excluding the age we would have to distinguish 2 x 8 x 12 x 8 x 33 x 5 = 253 440 different types of patients. But our training data cover less then 1/10 of this amount only. It is clear we have to suggest simplification of the task.

The first step towards simplification is the change of granularity in the used domains – design of the restricted domains. Domains of some attributes are rather extensive (e.g. Stay_length), but what really counts is the frequency with which individual values appear in the considered training data. Obviously, the most frequent values have to be represented even in the restricted domain (the original domain has finer granularity than the restricted one). If we introduce appropriate segmentation (e.g. age approx. in decades), we can distinguish 2 x 4 x 8 x 2 x 5 x 8 = 5120 different types of patients. Even under this simplification, given data of less than 18 000 patients only we are not ready to learn to answer a question "Will the considered patient be prescribed procedure No. A?" The attempt to use ID3 for this purpose failed both in the original and in the simplified case. But this question is too specific. The spa administration does not want to replace their physicians by a SW system. All they need is an estimate of resources necessary in the coming weeks. That is why the final goal for the data-mining was rephrased as follows:

- Use the original attributes (with restricted domains) to identify groups of patients which appear frequently in the training set and which exhibit characteristic behavior or requirements of spa utilities.
- For each such group predict a set of procedures to be passed by a typical patient during a typical week. Consequently calculate sums of procedures for the specific week according to the actual number of patients in the spa and their distribution among the groups.

2.2 Data Aggregation

Each data entry in the original dataset describes one specific allocation of a single procedure for a specific patient. These entries have to be aggregated to make explicitly available necessary information about full week of a stay for each patient. This task was approached as a time-series problem leading to significant amount of preprocessing. SumatraTT (Aubrecht, 2001a, 2001b) proved to be very useful for all the applied DM tools by ensuring the following tasks:

- Data aggregation – counting the total of procedures wrt. patient, week, etc.

- Data transformation – new dataset was generated so that n-records of the original table become n-columns of one record in the new set (matrix transposition).
- Export of the dataset into specific formats required by various DM tools applied.

2.3 New Table CTU_GWEEKS

Data exploration (using SQL) identified some mistakes or misprints. Consequently appropriate cleaning (standardization of considered cases) was designed and the size of domains of some these attributes was restricted (e.g. the minor and rare cases are neglected). The new attributes (modified by a change in the domain of values) can be identified in the sequel easily by the prefix CTU.

Suppose the solution of the considered task is based only on the attributes Sex (2), CTU_Gdisorder (6), CTU_Gage (6) and CTU_Gcompany (2) - the size of the corresponding restricted domain is given in brackets. This restriction leads to introduction of 144 = 2 x 6 x 6 x 2 different groups corresponding to the Cartesian product of the relevant domains. Is it possible to neglect information e.g. about the Cure_type? What is the reasonable amount of groups to consider?

The time unit we are going to work with is a week. We know that there is about 500 of patients staying in the spa each week. In an extreme case, it can happen that all the considered groups of patients appear among the 500 spa visitors in a single week. Moreover, the domain expert claims that 1 or 2 patients more or less does not make a difference in spa resources requirements. Thus a single group has to contain 5-10 patients at least to become significant for the considered prediction task. Consequently, it makes little sense to introduce more than 100 different patients' groups. These groups have to be derived from 144 upper mentioned groups, which are further split due to the value of the attribute Cure_type. Is this feasible at all? This seemingly intractable problem can be solved using similar type of data analysis as that used when restricting the domains of considered attributes. For the present task, there will be necessary to analyze the training data wrt. the size of groups of patients defined by combinations of values of considered attributes. This simple approach points to the fact that some combinations are rare or absent in the training data. This is most decisive for the combination Disorder x Cure_type and that is why this combination is replaced by a new combined attribute Disorder_CureType having 8 possible values only. Occurrence analysis in the training data entitles us to define new types of groups as the Cartesian product combining the attributes SEX (2 values), AGE_DIS (5 values), Disorder_CureType (8 possible values). Consequently, we have 2 x 5 x 8 = 80 disjunctive groups plus 1 additional one covering the rest of the patients.

A new table CTU_GWEEKS generated with a heavy support of SumatraTT consists of 81 attributes (Gr1, ..., Gr81) corresponding to the upper mentioned groups and 35 additional attributes representing the procedures (Pr1, ..., Pr40 – five of procedures are never prescribed). One record summarizes data concerning all patients present in the spa during a single week. Let us specify the contents of the table for the week *n*:

- Gr_{ik} is the number of days spent by patients belonging to the k-th group during the i-th week.

- Pr_{ij} is the total number of all prescriptions of the j-th procedure during the i-th week.

The final table CTU_GWEEKS contains 147 records corresponding to all the weeks in the period 1999-2001 (126 records in the training set, 21 records in the test set).

3. PREDICTIVE MODELING

3.1 General Overview, Score Function

As defined above, for the effective resource allocation it is critical to know (predict) how many individual health procedures are going to be prescribed for the following time period. This chapter focuses on construction of predictive models estimating the total number of prescriptions of different types of procedures in a particular week according to the actual number of patients in the spa and their distribution among the patient groups.

All the presented models use the same scoring function frequently applied in regression tasks. The model fitting is evaluated in terms of mean absolute percentage error (MAPE) and its standard deviation (STDEV). This error measure is defined as follows:

$$MAPE(M_j) = \frac{100}{n} \sum_{i=1}^{n} \frac{\left|Pr_{ij}^{pred} - Pr_{ij}^{real}\right|}{Pr_{ij}^{real}} \quad [\%]$$

where M_j is the predictive model designed for the j-th procedure,
n is the number of predicted weeks,
Pr_{ij}^{real} is the real number of prescriptions of the j-th procedure in the i-th week,
Pr_{ij}^{pred} is the predicted number of prescriptions of the j-th procedure in the i-th week.

3.2 Simple Regression

A simple regression approach represents the most straightforward solution of the given predictive task in terms of the selected representation. The model is most simplified as it assigns all the patients to the same group while ignoring any patient specific information. It utilizes the overall number of patient-days in the predicted week only:

$$Pr_{ij}^{pred} = a_j GrAll_i$$

where $GrAll_i$ is the number of days spent by all the patients during the i-th week $(GrAll_i = Gr_{i1} + \ldots + Gr_{i81})$,
a_j is the regression coefficient learnt for the j-th procedure on the training data (average number of the j-th procedures prescribed per patient and day).

Apparently, this non-informed prediction represents the worst case prediction result and when compared with well-informed models it can give a basic outline of utility of patient description. When averaged over all the procedures, the simple regression model gives MAPE about 17.5%.

3.3 Regression by Patient Groups

The regression by patient groups tries to put in use differences among the individual patient groups. Instead of learning the single regression coefficient a_j it learns separate coefficients for all the considered groups. The total in the predicted week is then the sum of predictions obtained for the considered groups (Novakova, 2002):

$$Pr_{ij}^{pred} = \sum_{k=1}^{81} a_{jk} Gr_{ik}$$

where a_{jk} is the regression coefficient learnt on the training data for the j-th procedure and the k-th group.

When averaged over all the procedures, the regression by patient groups gives MAPE about 14.5% (further dented as the general MAPE), i.e., it brings general improvement as compared with the simple regression (17.5%). When regarding the individual health procedures, two different points of view have been considered: the above-mentioned MAPE and ability to follow the real trends. Considering these criteria, the regression by groups is significantly better for 6 procedures (see Figure 1), on the other hand it does not show any significant difference in the other 29 procedures (see Figure 2).

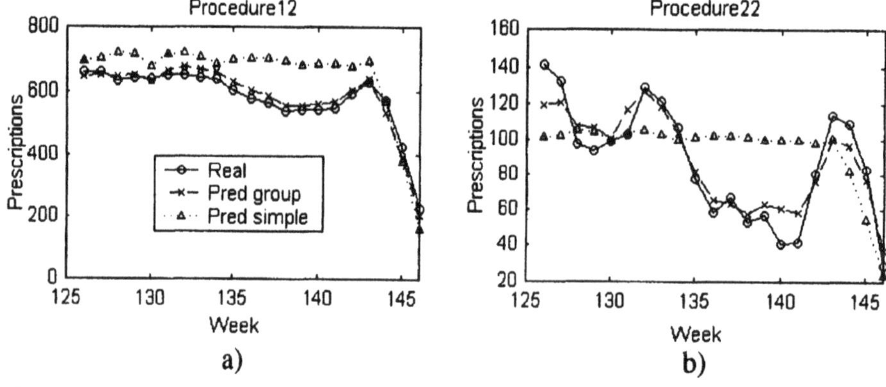

Figure 1 – Examples of Health Procedures for Which the Regression by Groups (Pred Group) Significantly Outperforms the Simple Regression (Pred Simple).

This diversity confirms that some procedures show little sensitivity to patient characteristics and they are prescribed with a nearly uniform distribution over the patient set. For these procedures, the simple regression either represents the competent solution immediately (see Figure 2a) or it can be a good solution having reduced a systematic prediction error, i.e., regarding long-term changes of a_j (see Figure 2b). This issue can be solved by a heuristic approach presented in 3.4.

The last minority of procedures might ask for a different group definition. These procedures can be predicted on bases of the procedure specific group definition that can be precisely tuned regarding the target procedure. We have applied the LISp-Miner system (Rauch, Simunek, 2000) to derive specific association rules describing the strong groups relevant to the critical procedures. The group segmentations can be surprisingly simple. For example, application of the single association rule resulting into two-group segmentation improves the prediction ability to follow the real trends of Pr37:

Cure_type(1, ..., 6) and Sex(Woman) → "Pr37 is likely to be prescribed"

The given rule splits the patient set between two almost equal sized sub-groups. For the first group, the frequency of Pr37 prescriptions is about twice higher than in the original set. On the contrary, the second group shows almost zero frequency of Pr37 prescriptions.

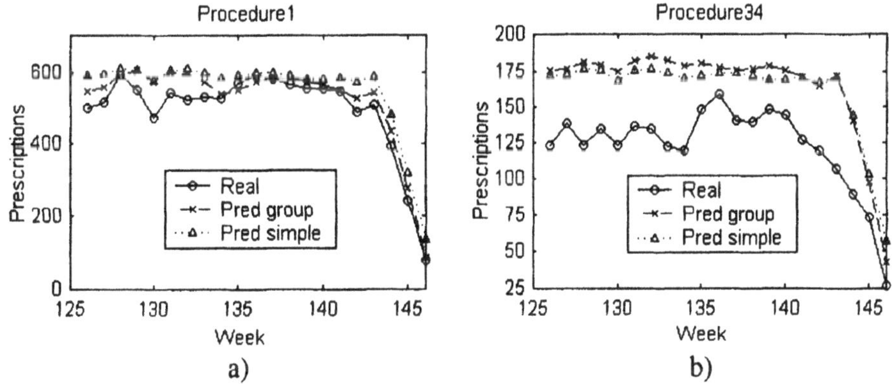

Figure 2 – Examples of Health Procedures for which both the Regression Approaches Show Similar Performance, either Working Well (a) or Having High MAPE (b).

3.4 Heuristic Approaches

Another simple predictive algorithm is based on a pure copy of the number of prescriptions in the last week. The simple regression is used if and only if $GrAll_i$ changes rapidly from one week to the other one. This approach gives the general MAPE 12%, i.e., it clearly outperforms more sophisticated methods. However, the predictions have to be often available several weeks in advance. This demand asks for utilization of the precedent weeks which decreases the prediction accuracy – 15.3% / 1 (when available 1 week in advance), 17.3% / 2, 18.7% / 3. Utility of the previous weeks is obvious, the major part of patients stays for 3 or 4 weeks. It follows that not more that one third of the patients changes each week.

Although this history approach cannot be applied for longer-term predictions directly, it brings forward time equability of most procedures. It can be utilized in correction of the systematic error observed in both regression approaches. For certain part of procedures, the prediction can be improved by subtracting the error of the same predictor taken from the last evaluated week.

4. CONCLUSION

The approach described in this paper results in the general mean absolute prediction error which is approximately 12%. This error is reached by the simple regression or the regression by groups with the heuristic correction. Most of procedures (32) are predicted using the group definition given in 2.3. The prediction of the remaining procedures (3) is based on the specific groups derived by the LispMiner.

The spa administration requested 20% precision only. This request is satisfied for 31 of 35 predicted health procedures. It is hoped that the spa management can benefit from the prediction (information about the amount of necessary procedures available few weeks in advance). How can it be applied and what its main contributions? Prediction of reasonable accuracy can have significant impact on the activity of the spa complex in the following aspects:

- It will be possible to plan full use of capacity of workers operating the balneo services (some can be moved to the overloaded procedures, new people can be temporarily hired, planning of vacations, ...).
- The operating regime of various balneo services will be tuned according to the actual needs (restriction of operating costs for electricity, water, ...). Procedures, which are not necessary for patients staying in the spa, can be offered to the general public.

The developed method is easily re-usable for other similar facilities. According to the domain experts, every spa facility has a different structure of patients, even if they offer almost the same procedures. It means that a new segmentation of patients has to be designed for every spa facility. Currently, it is the only step where SumatraTT cannot help. This will be improved when current development of a new statistical template for SumatraTT is finished. On the other hand, the other steps of data pre-processing and analysis remain the same. In this context, SumatraTT proves to be an indispensable tool for the considered DM tasks as it can replace lot of tedious and demanding data processing. There have been developed appropriate data processing templates to do the job. Each template takes groups' description stored in a table and generates and executes SQL commands that calculate aggregated values. Finally, the data is exported into a text file. There is being prepared a script ensuring export of the data into the WEKA format. This opens possibility to apply any algorithm provided by the rich WEKA ML package including the regression, too.

5. ACKNOWLEDGMENTS

This research was supported by the EU project Sol-Eu-Net IST-1999-11495 *Data Mining and Decision Support for business competitiveness: A European virtual enterprise.*

5. REFERENCES

1. Aubrecht, P. (2001a). Specification of SumatraTT. Technical Report K333-2/01, CTU, Dept.of Cybernetics, Technická 2, 166 27 Prague 6, www: http://krizik.felk.cvut.cz:8080/SumatraReg/.
2. Aubrecht, P. and Kouba, Z. (2001b). Metadata Driven Data Transformation. In SCI 2001, volume I, pages 332-336. International Institute of Informatics and Systemics and IEEE Computer Society.
3. Chapman, P., Clinton, J., Kerber, R., Khabaza, T., Reinartz, T., Shearer, C. and Wirth, R.: CRISP-DM 1.0: Step-by-step data mining guide. CRISP-DM consortium, 2000.
4. Data Mining and Decision Support for Business Competitiveness: A European Virtual Enterprise, SolEuNet pages available at http://soleunet.ijs.si/.
5. Novakova, L.(2002): Prakticke aplikace metod strojového uceni. In Czech, Diploma thesis K333, FEE CTU, Prague, January 2002.
6. Rauch, J., Simunek, M. (2000): Mining for 4ft Association Rules. In Discovery Science 2000. Red. Arikawa, S. – Morishita S. Springer Verlag 2000, pp. 268 – 272.
7. Witten,I., Frank,E.: Data Mining - Practical Machine Learning Tools and Techniques with Java Implementations. Morgan Kaufmann, 1999.

55 A METHOD TO OPTIMIZE SCHEDULING IN SMALL BATCH MANUFACTURING

Adrián Guillermo Lucero[1], Abelardo Alves de Queiroz[2]

[1] *Dep. of Mechanical Eng., UFSC, CEP 88040-900. CP N°476, Florianópolis, SC, Brazil*
aglucero@grucon.ufsc.br

[2] *Dep. of Mechanical Eng, UFSC, CEP 88040-900. CP N°476, Florianópolis, SC, Brazil.*
abelardo@emc.ufsc.br

This paper reports on research into the development of a procedure that improves the way to arrange job shop schedules. The principal components of the method are a) Remove early restrictions to the schedule process; and b) Decide the manufacturing routes as late as possible. A complete method description is presented, including the conceptual model and the method development with the application of Bellman's dynamic programming technique. The tool has been programmed and made available in software for integration into production planning and scheduling systems such as MRP and ERP.

1. INTRODUCTION

The manufacturing process underwent dramatic changes in concepts and methods in the early 1980's, and worldwide markets along with the objectives of manufacturing systems demanded change. The new manufacturing process is a chain of activities directed toward meeting a set of objectives defined by management. These objectives such as non-engineering functions of the organization including sales, marketing and finance, together with engineering functions such as product development, part production, assembly of products, customer production design, etc, changed to give more emphasis on competitiveness.

Modern production no longer can rely on general methods and procedures. Focused transformation and management processes lead to progressively more specialized technology in order to achieve better performance. In the past management methods were applied across the board for the whole manufacturing arena, but nowadays they are developed for different size plants, types of industry and types of production. The focused approach leads to more specialized and optimized solutions. The trend for the future certainly will be a different solution for each company.

Small-batch manufacturing is a very particular type of production which has been well described by Rantakyro (2000) as follows: "Production is very difficult to plan, because there are many customers and a lot of different products are fabricated. The companies bid on all jobs, and products are produced in very small batches, sometimes a lot size of one. Generally they fabricate parts for the manufacturing industry or provide services for large companies like mines, steel, mills, paper mills, and the wood industry. There have been changes in the relationship with bigger corporations during the last decade. The manufacturing industry no longer has long-term contracts, and they want parts delivered just-in-time, in small batches, or only a couple of weeks' or days' production.".

This type of production in which a great variety of products are manufactured in a specific short time period and the material flow for producing each of these products is not similar and often complicated, can be characterized as follows (HITOMI, 1979):

- Variety of product items - With diverse production volumes and due dates;
- Variety of manufacturing processes - Frequently complicated;
- Complexity of productive capacity - Because of the dynamic nature of demand;
- Uncertainty of outside conditions - There are frequent changes in product specification, due dates and volumes;
- Difficulty of production planning and scheduling - Because of topics described above;
- Dynamic implementation conditions and control of production - Due to the uncertainty of outside conditions.

Examples of this type of manufacturing are the aeronautical industry and all its supply chain, the naval chain sector and part of the measurement instruments industry. All shop floors have process layouts and the principal planning characteristic that the product must be scheduled in order to fulfill the customer delivery promise, because the customers are as interested in delivery time as product price.

2. THE SCHEDULING METHOD

The method has a general philosophy: the decisions on manufacturing routes must be taken at the last possible moment in order to avoid other early restrictions, which may compromise both delivery time and cost.

Commonly the process planners choose the manufacturing routes based on their experience. A decision is taken at the beginning, so process planners details and schedulers view routes as a restriction.

The present model analyzes all alternative machines for each operation, develops process plans, defines the criterion for the optimization (time, cost or profit) and defines the best route for each manufacturing task. After taking into considering resource restrictions it defines the best schedule. A schematic presentation of the method model follows (Fig.1):

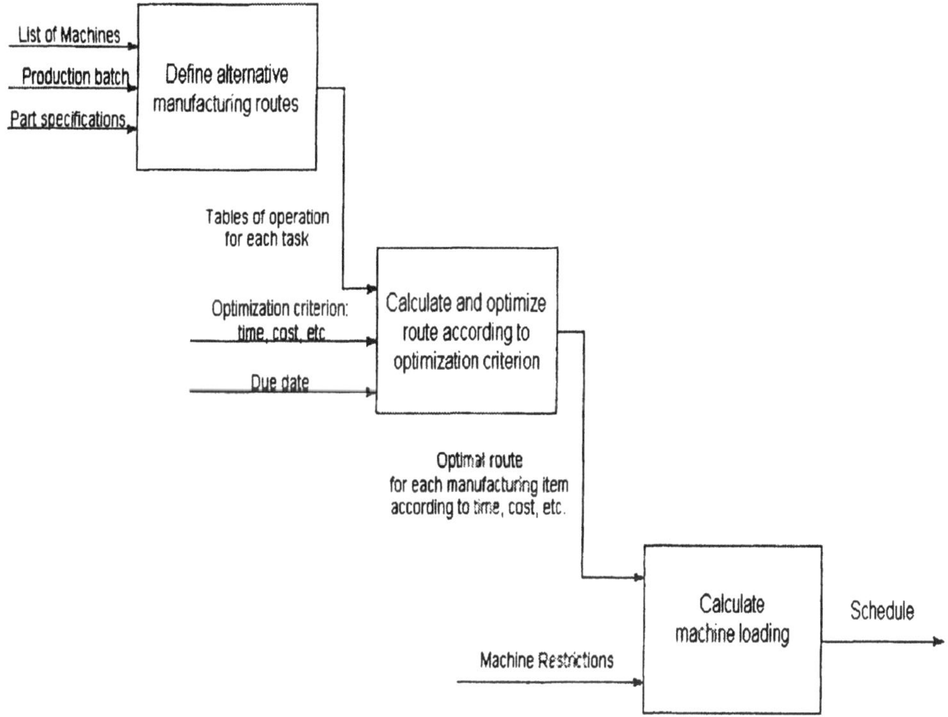

Figure 1 – Conceptual Scheduling Model

So, the steps necessary to schedule the manufacturing process according to the method are:

i. STEP 1: Define alternative manufacturing routes;
ii. STEP 2: Calculate and optimize route according to criterion;
iii. STEP 3: Calculate machine loading taking alternative machines into consideration;

2.1 STEP 1: Define Alternative Manufacturing Routes

The method begins by collecting specifications of the part design; including the production batch and the list of machines that comprise the shop. The process planners supply the necessary information for the process plan after dividing the job into operations. In this step all the alternative machines for each operation are considered in order to avoid early decisions that cause unnecessary constraints to planning the workflow.

The data collection is presented in three matrices that give information about Operation Time T(o,m), Setup Time S(o,m) and Transfer Time R(i,j). The Operation Time matrix is arranged in lines that represent operation numbers, which establish the precedent relation among operations; and columns of machines. The matrix is filled with operation times for single items T_{om} defined in the process planning. When a time/machine combination for the operation does not make sense for technological reasons a number 99 is placed in the position.

The second matrix expresses the Setup Time S(o,m) and each position on the matrix is constructed in the same fashion as the Operation Time table.

The third matrix expresses the Transfer Time R(i,j) between each of the two machines.

2.2 STEP 2: Calculate and Optimize Route According to Criterion

The calculation of optimal manufacturing route for each task uses, as input, the data inserted in the matrices from STEP 1 and the optimization criterion chosen following strategic policies.

The Operation Time matrix and the Setup Time matrix for a previously defined batch are combined in a single table (Table 1), because both are related to the operation itself. The Transfer Time matrix (Table 2) and the optimal criterion complete the data needs for the calculation of optimal manufacturing routes in this step.

Table 1 – Times of T(o,m) and S(o,m) Combined for Single Item Production

	T(o,m) + S(o,m) – Times					
Operation	Machine1	Machine2	Machine3	Machine4	Machine5	Machine6
1	0.8	0.67	1.28	99	1.62	1.18
2	0.52	0.48	0.88	99	1.22	0.59
3	0.61	0.81	0.97	99	0.46	99
4	2.58	2.04	1.99	99	99	2.14
5	0.55	0.8	0.99	99	1.32	0.74
6	4.38	4.51	4.82	99	99	4.41
7	0.48	0.49	0.69	0.69	1.03	0.1
8	0.37	0.38	0.88	0.88	1.22	0.47

Table 2 - Transfer Time Table R(i,j)

Mach/Mach	Machine1	Machine2	Machine3	Machine4	Machine5	Machine6
Mach.1	0	3.0	2.6	4.7	3.2	2.9
Mach.2	3.0	0	2.4	3.1	2.8	4.0
Mach.3	2.6	2.4	0	2.5	3.4	2.2
Mach.4	4.7	3.1	2.5	0	4.1	5
Mach.5	3.2	2.8	3.4	4.1	0	2.9
Mach.6	2.9	4.0	2.2	5	2.9	0

The method uses the Dynamic Programming technique (Bellman, 1957) and the procedure called the Halevi Matrix (Halevi, 1993 and 1999), an adaptation of Dynamic Programming for this kind of problem.

The optimal manufacturing route is arrived at through the calculation of the minimum Cumulative Time table or Z table. Eq. 1 gives the general equation for the elements of Z:

$$Z_{i,j} = \min_{k=1 \to m} \left\lfloor T_{i,j} + Z_{i+1,k} + R_{j,k} \right\rfloor \quad \text{where } i = o\text{-1 to 1} \qquad \text{Eq. (1)}$$

$$j = 1 \text{ to } m$$

and o: operations number
m: machines number

With the initial condition

$$Z_{o,j} = T_{o,j} \qquad \text{where } j = 1 \text{ to } m \qquad \text{Eq. (2)}$$

The numeric example shows the calculation of the two tables with data from Tables 1 and 2. The analysis of the two tables leads to the minimum cumulative lead-time and the manufacturing route necessary to obtain this value as shown in Tables 3 and 4.

Table 3 – Table of Minimum Cumulative Time Z(i,j)

Operations	Machine1	Machine2	Machine3	Machine4	Machine5	Machine6
1	9.74	9.57	10.27	108.02	10.63	10.19
2	8.94	8.9	9.32	107.47	9.52	9.012
3	8.42	8.58	8.68	106.81	8.30	106.8
4	8.19	7.77	7.71	104.80	104.74	7.86
5	5.61	5.94	6.06	104.18	6.41	5.72
6	5.06	5.24	5.48	99.77	99.68	4.98
7	0.85	0.87	1.16	1.194	1.52	0.57
8	0.37	0.38	0.88	0.88	1.22	0.47

The Route Pointers table P(i,j) is constructed in order to store the values correspondent to the machine that offers the best partial minimum cumulative time (Table 3). The calculation process used to define the manufacturing route begins by ascertaining the position corresponding to the total minimum time of Z(1,j), for this example Operation 1 and Machine 2. To continue the route the P_{ij} element indicates the transfer to the next machine and so on up to the end.

Table 4 – Routes Pointers Table P(i,j)

Transfer	Machine1	Machine2	Machine3	Machine4	Machine5	Machine6
1→2	1	2	2	2	2	6
2→3	5	5	5	5	5	5
3→4	3	2	3	3	3	3
4→5	1	1	1	1	1	6
5→6	1	6	6	6	6	6
6→7	6	6	6	6	6	6
7→8	1	2	1	1	1	6

2.3 STEP 3: Calculate the Schedule

In small batch manufacturing shops most machines are multipurpose in order to provide the flexibility for this type of production. Another characteristic is the delivery time reliability because most of these shops function as suppliers for other companies in the supply chain. So, the due date is the start point for calculating the schedule.

The machining load is calculated using the following strategy:

a) Calculate the lead-time for all products required to be manufactured in the period to be scheduled. The calculation for each product is the addition of the optimal times for the tasks, obtained in STEP 2, which comprise product structure (bill of materials). Here the approach is: infinite resource.
b) The critical product, indicated by the optimized criterion and demonstrated by the lead-time, is chosen as the first to be loaded. At this point all the resources required by the process plan for the work period are reserved (made unavailable for other products). Here the finite resource approach is established.
c) The following products are loaded in order of the priority established in the same way to that used in the definition of critical order.

The computer calculation produces a Gantt like chart to illustrate the product structure; Fig. 2 shows an example of two products where the critical one is that assigned as *ORDEM* 2. The assembly of product order n°2 is treated first. It is scheduled from a set of tasks, each one defined in STEP 2. Task #5 is the final assembly for 9 items that finish on day 13, the length of the box indicates the time span.

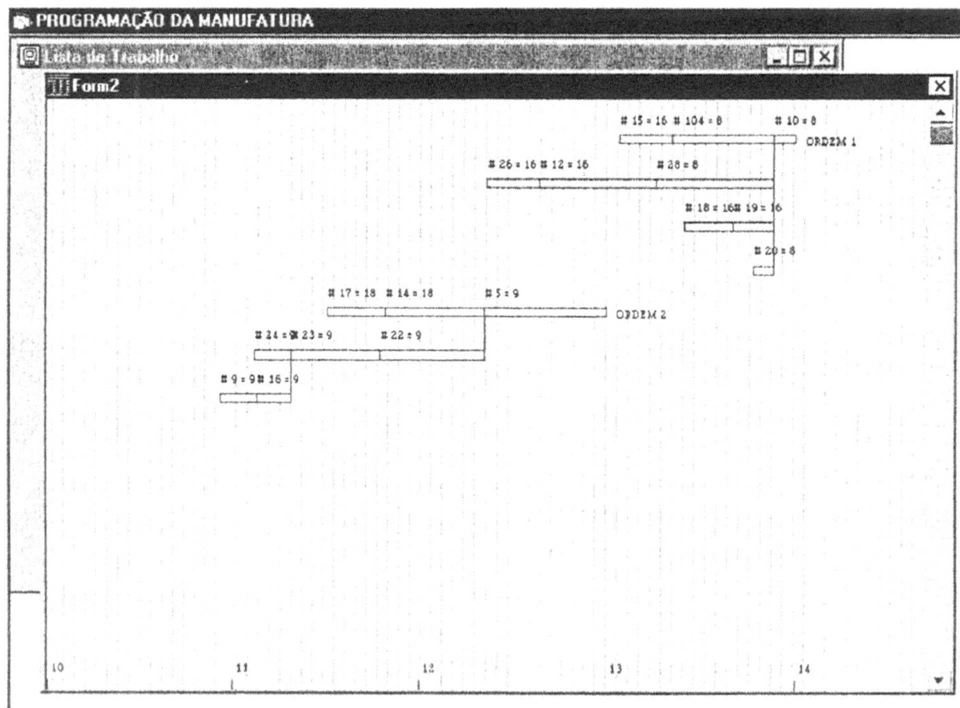

Figure 2 – Product Structure and Lead-Time for Two Orders

At this point the availability of resources, mainly machines, should be considered so, the computer automatically verifies this restriction. When a resource is unavailable STEP 2 is called in and another manufacturing route (the next best option to attend the restriction) is assigned.

The resource chart of Fig.3 shows the allocation of each machine where the order number/task number in the scheduling (hours) is assigned. For example a code 02009 indicates that machine n°7 is loaded during the first hour with task n°9 (009) of order nº2 (02). The manufacturing route of a part can be followed as it progresses through the time (lines) and the various machines are allocated (columns).

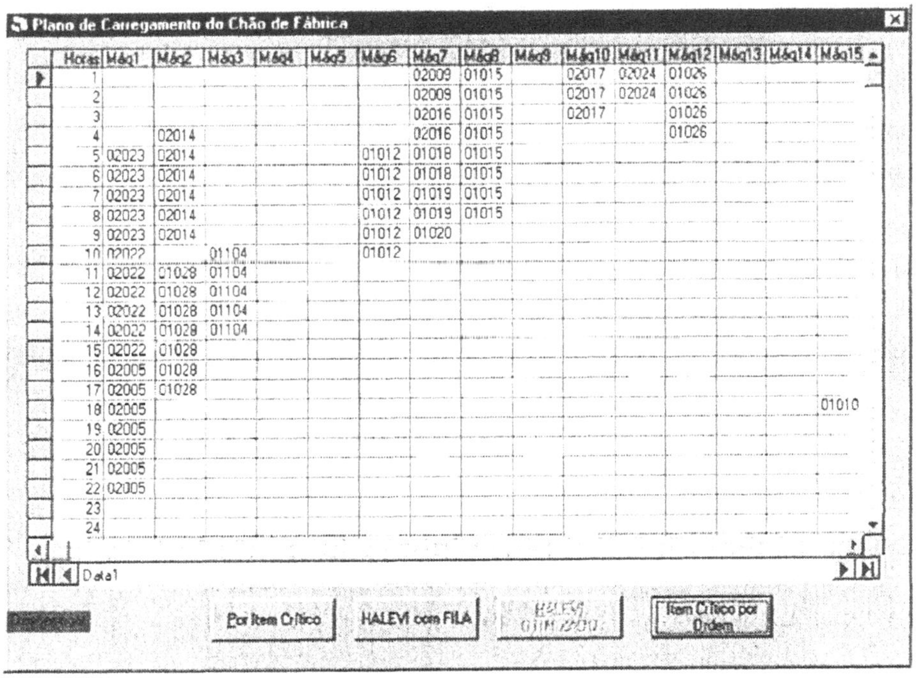

Plano de Carregamento do Chão de Fábrica

Horas	Máq1	Máq2	Máq3	Máq4	Máq5	Máq6	Máq7	Máq8	Máq9	Máq10	Máq11	Máq12	Máq13	Máq14	Máq15
1							02009	01015		02017	02024	01026			
2							02009	01015		02017	02024	01026			
3							02016	01015		02017		01026			
4		02014					02016	01015				01026			
5	02023	02014				01012	01018	01015							
6	02023	02014				01012	01018	01015							
7	02023	02014				01012	01019	01015							
8	02023	02014				01012	01019	01015							
9	02023	02014				01012	01020								
10	02022		01104			01012									
11	02022	01028	01104												
12	02022	01028	01104												
13	02022	01028	01104												
14	02022	01028	01104												
15	02022	01028													
16	02005	01028													
17	02005	01028													
18	02005														01010
19	02005														
20	02005														
21	02005														
22	02005														
23															
24															

Data1

Por Item Crítico | HALEVI com FILA | Item Crítico por Ordem

Figure 3 – Machines Scheduling Allocation

3. CONCLUSIONS

An improved and focused method of scheduling is the result of this work. Small batch manufacturing with its multiple difficulties and inefficiencies can benefit from decisions on process routes being taken at the last possible moment.

The method begins with some simple work on process planning (STEP 1) and the optimal route at the level of task (STEP 2). The work on scheduling begins with the infinite resource approach considering all products and then choosing the critical product. The finite resource approach begins from the critical product followed by the next critical up to the complete demand, considering all availability of resources. When the calculation is completed the operator can analyze it and, if necessary, make changes and submit again the data to be reprocessed by the system.

This method can be operated in standalone mode or integrated into MRP/ERP systems for pre-process scheduling. The balance between computing data processing and human intervention makes the method a good tool to cope with the extreme flexibility required for the jobbing process in small batch manufacturing. The initial test in manufacturing environments brought very good results.

4. ACKNOWLEDGMENTS

To WEG Máquinas S/A, a Company of the Group WEG Motores – Jaragua do Sul / SC – Brazil where this work was developed in cooperation.

To FINEP and CNPq for the financial support.

5. REFERENCES

Bellman R. Dynamic Programming. Princenton: Princenton Univ. Press, 1957.

Halevi, G. The Magic Matrix: the smart scheduler, Computers in Industry, vol. 21, 1993, pp. 245-253.

Halevi, G. Restructuring the manufacturing process, Boca Raton: The St. Lucie Press/APICS Series on resource management, 1999.

Hitomi, K. Manufacturing Systems Engineering. London: Taylor & Francis Ltd., 1979.

Rantakyro, L. Strategic management in small metal job shops in Sweden and the U. S. Engineering Management Journal, vol. 12. n. 2, 2000, pp. 15-23.

56

LAYOUT PROBLEM OPTIMIZATION USING GENETIC ALGORITHMS

Jiří Kubalík, Jiří Lažanský, Petr Zikl
Department of Cybernetics, CTU Prague,
Technicka 2, 166 27 Prague 6, Czech Republic
{kubalik, lazan, zikl}@labe.felk.cvut.cz

This paper presents an application of genetic algorithm to a problem of finding of an optimal layout of objects on a material strip with the aim to reduce the total length of material used. In order to reduce the total search space the problem was solved as an ordering problem. This paper focuses on the representation issues of the problem and on designing of such a crossover operator that would allow building blocks formation and facilitate their mixing. Different implementations of the genetic algorithm were experimentally evaluated on a number of test cases. Some interesting results which illustrate a performance of the genetic algorithm are presented here.

1. INTRODUCTION

This paper presents an application of a genetic algorithm (GA) to a hard optimization problem of layout planning. GAs are probabilistic search and optimisation techniques, which operate on a population of chromosomes, each representing a potential solution of the given problem, with aim to breed some high quality solution [1]. They are operationally simple and represent a good choice for solving problems with large search space, where only little is known about its characteristics and even for solving black-box problems. As such they have been applied to many problems from the field of parameter optimizations, planning and scheduling, design, etc. [2].

The problem addressed in this paper is defined so that we want to find an optimal layout of a set of two-dimensional objects such that (*i*) the objects cannot mutually overlap and (*ii*) the length of the used piece of the material is minimal. The material strip has defined its length L and width W. For the sake of simple representation and manipulation of the objects we consider only rectangular shapes, which use the same grid structure.

The first and the most important step of a design of the genetic algorithm is to choose the representation of the problem to be solved. This is a crucial point since on the representation other features of the algorithm depend. These are the size of the search space, efficiency of the genetic operators, etc.

The most natural way of representing solutions of this problem would be a sequence of genes, each coding the actual position of individual object. On the other hand there is a considerable drawback of such an approach which is the size of the search space. Note that we are seeking the optimal solution among all possible combinations of N objects' positions. Since each object can happen to be anywhere on the stripe, defined by dimensions L and W, the total number of possible layouts configurations of objects would be $L^N \cdot W^N$. Thus, if we used for example L=200 and W=50 the total size of the search space would be $200^{20} \cdot 50^{20}$, which is too much for any technique not using explicit knowledge on the problem.

That is why we focused on solving the problem as an ordering one; the implementation is described in next section.

2. IMPLEMENTATION ISSUES

The original layout planning problem as defined above can be seen as an ordering problem so that the algorithm generates sequences of objects and uses some localization algorithm according to which the objects are properly[1] placed on the grid in the given order. So the goal is to find an optimal order in which the objects will be laid on the stripe making the most compact layout. The size of the search space is of order $N!$ now. The same approach has been already proposed in [3]. The core of that paper was just the layout determining algorithm used to find a position of individual objects.

In this paper we are focusing on analyzing of the problem from the point of view of the genetic algorithm as the main concern is to facilitate the building block formation, propagation and mixing.

2.1 Localization Algorithm

The localization algorithm used in this work searches the partially covered grid for a free space, where the next object can be placed. Algorithm starts at the top left corner of the grid and moves the object down till it either finds the available space or it reaches the bottom of the grid. If it finds the place the object will be put there.

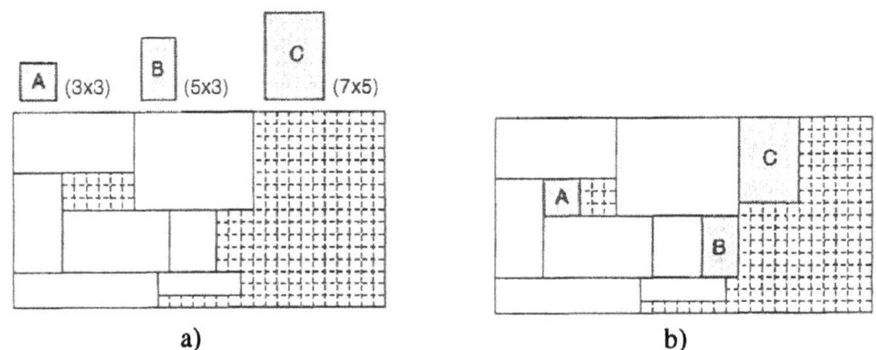

Figure 1 – Localization Algorithm

Otherwise the algorithm returns the object back on the top edge of the grid, shifts to the right and tries to find the free space within that new column. The search goes

[1] Properly means that each shape is placed on the grid so that it does not overlap with any other already located shapes and the length of the used material is minimal.

on until any legal position for the objects is found. In the same way all objects are processed in the order as they appear in the chromosome.

The function of the algorithm is illustrated for three different objects in Figure 1. The left picture depicts the initial situation on the grid. The right picture shows simultaneously the final states after inserting object A, B or C. On the example of object A we can see the situation when it is possible to place the object at position which is surrounded by other objects. Object B did not fit into that place even that its absolute dimensions does not exceed the size of the place, which is 3×6 units, due to its actual rotation. Another place had to be found for it. The last object C was too large for any blank space in the current layout so it was placed on the first available position after all the objects.

In order to reduce the computational time spent by the localization algorithm the size of steps by which the search moves down and right is optimized. While the object is moving down across the grid the column of cells, wide as the width of the object, is checked and a distance from the left most free cell is recorded. This value is then used to set the size of the step to the right if needed. In the same way vertical *stepping stones* are determined.

2.2 Fitness

In this case the candidate layouts are assessed according to the following fitness measure, which incorporates the requirements on maximal compactness of layouts and non-overlapping of objects

$$f = (L_{max} - L) + 1/(1+S),$$

where L_{max} stands for the maximal length of the material stripe that can be used, L is the actual length of the layout and S is the amount of the residual scrap particles that lie idle among the objects. The measure is a compound of two components. The first part expresses the length of the layout in terms of the unused part of the stripe. This is defined so in order to have bigger fitness for shorter layouts. The second part represents a compactness of the layout so that it is larger for more compact layouts with less scrap. Its value ranges between 0 and 1 so it can only distinguish between the layouts of the same length. Note that the primary goal is to find the shortest possible layout with the least inside scrap.

2.3 Genetic Operators

A very important role in genetic algorithm applications plays the recombination operator. This is the only means to generate new candidate solutions. The basic idea behind the crossover is that given two promising solutions[2] their offspring could hopefully inherit the best parts of each. Optimally the crossover should be designed in order to allow for any useful inheritance. On the other hand, this is very difficult to achieve in practice. The reason is that we do not know much about the decomposition of the solutions into parts that might represent important features of solutions or the information to be inherited is known but hard to capture within the used representation. For instance, when solving a classical ordering traveling

[2] Parents are selected on the basis the better solutions have the bigger chance to be selected.

salesman problem it turned out that the most important information that should be inherited from the parents to the offspring is the individual connections between cities. New tours are then generated by maximally utilizing the links that appeared in the original tours; the operator is known as the edge-recombination [4].

Unfortunately this is not the approach we could adopt here. The adjacency of two objects in the chromosome does not have to mean the actual spatial adjacency of the objects on the grid. For example see the links between objects in pairs J-B and P-N in the first parent in Figure 2. Objects J and B are neighbors in the chromosome while they are far away from each other on the grid. On the other hand P and N lie close together on the grid even though they are not directly linked in the chromosome. This happens because the spatial position of each object does not depend on the links between objects in the chromosome. Instead it is determined by the partial layout to which the object is added with use of the localization algorithm. Apparently, focusing on utilization of links from parents is not worth in this case.

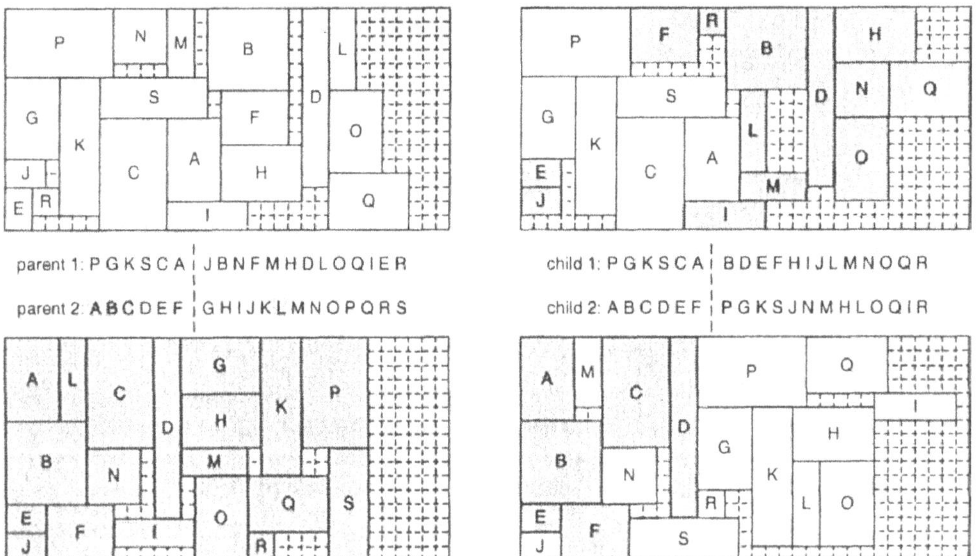

Figure 2 – Simple 1-Point Crossover

1-point crossover. Due to the reasons described above we decided to use a type of a simple 1-point crossover and its modifications. Simple 1-point crossover works so that first a crossing point is chosen randomly. The new chromosomes get the head part from the parental chromosomes and then are completed with the remaining objects in the order as they appear in the other parent. Obviously any chromosome generated this way must represent a feasible solution since all the objects will be present just once in it.

Let us take a look at what happens with layouts when they are crossed over, especially what of the parents passes on to the offspring. An example of the crossover action is shown in Figure 2. The two chromosomes are crossed over after the sixth position. As can be seen the effect of the operation is rather destructive. The children do not have much in common with their parents. This is not surprising in the case of the tale parts taken from the parents. It is natural that the sequence of objects from the tail part of one chromosome will be represented by completely different layout when appended to the head sequence taken from the other parent. This is because the position of each object strongly depends on the actual state of the layout into which it is added. In other words, as the context of objects, determined by the antecedent sequence of objects, changes the spatial position and links of the objects change as well.

However, even the head sequence of objects does not represent fully compact part of the whole layout. This is due to the fact that objects, which are neighbors in a chromosome, are not adjacent to each other on the grid and vice versa. There are many gaps that are filled by objects that appear later in a chromosome. Simply because they are placed on the grid on position found by the localization algorithm. That is why we can observe for instance object L surrounded by objects A, B and C in first parent although its position in the chromosome is quite far away from the triple A, B, C. When simply crossing the chromosomes the head parts does not map onto compact block of objects as the parental chromosomes did. Instead the head sequence generates just a partially compact skeleton structure with possibly many gaps. Since the remaining objects are then added in a different order, determined by the other parent, the gaps might not be filled as optimally as in the original layout.

Reordering algorithm. The situation described above can be improved to some extent when using an adjusted ordering of objects, which takes into account the right order of objects as they appear on the grid. The original chromosome is reordered according to the following algorithm:

1. create an ordered list L of objects, the objects are ordered according to their actual position on the grid – the more left and up the better - in a descending manner.
2. use an auxiliary empty grid, $j = 0$
3. $i = 1, j = j + 1$
4. take i-th object of list L
5. find a position for the given object
6. if position is different from its actual position in the original encoding
   then $i = i + 1$ and goto step 4
7. insert the object into the new chromosome at j-th position
8. if j < *number_of_objects*
   then goto step 2
   else stop

The performance of the algorithm is illustrated in Figure 3. The main goal is to order the objects in such a way that the compact parts of a layout will correspond to a compact group of objects within the chromosome. Note that the position of any object cannot be changed by just reordering the chromosome since it could cause changes in the compactness of the overall layout. This is guaranteed by checking each object's position made in step 6. If the positions were not checked the following situation might happen. Let us assume example from Figure 3 where we have already placed first eight objects into the new chromosome. The next candidate is the object I since it is the left-most unused object of the original layout. The localization algorithm will find the available position for it, which is by one row higher on the grid than it was in the original layout. This would cause that object D would be placed by three columns to the right of its original position and position of other objects will be influenced as well. When the step 6 is used, first object D and then object I will be inserted into the new chromosome and the layout does not change.

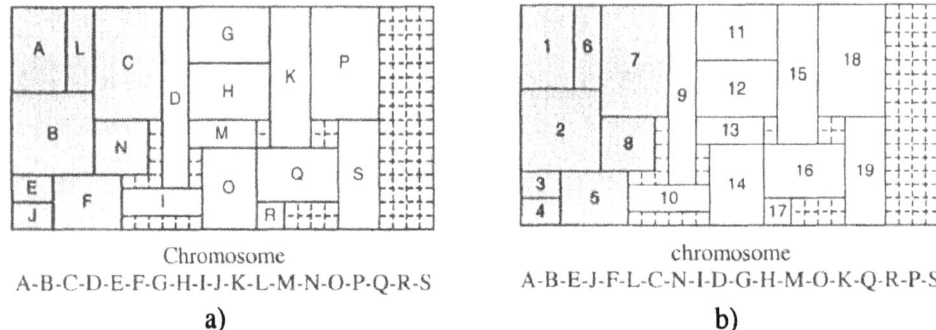

Figure 3 – Original vs. Adjusted Ordering of Objects in Chromosome

Let us now explore the ability of the genetic algorithm with the simple 1-point crossover to form and propagate useful building blocks to subsequent populations. As described above the crossover operator uses the head part of one parental chromosome to begin a new layout, which is then completed with objects taken in order defined by the other parent. So the first part of the offspring represents something that is more or less[3] inherited from one of the parents. The second part of offspring is created in rather random manner, where only little can be inherited from parents. Thus the most influencing part of chromosome is its very beginning. This is also the best candidate for possible forming of building blocks that can be preferred and propagated during the evolution. This means that once some good-looking beginning sequence shows up in the population it is hard to replace it with anything else. In some sense the process of evolution of the best solution can be seen as that it starts with competition among the candidate solutions to find the best beginning of the layout, and then the search gradually proceeds towards the end of the layout.

In order to further boost the exploration abilities of the algorithm following modification of the crossover operators was proposed. The operators are based on the idea of so called *hot-spots* as crossing points that are likely to generate some improvement. Here the hot-spots represent objects that are bound to the top edge of the material sheet; for instance objects L, C, D, G, K, and P in Figure 3. The basic idea behind the operators is that there might be some group of objects somewhere in the middle of chromosome that could better fit at the beginning of the layout.

1-point crossover with hot-spots (1-point HS). This operator does not strictly inherit the beginning of parental chromosome (layouts). It differs from the simple 1-point crossover in such a way that the randomly chosen crossing point (any top-most object of the layout) determines a starting object of the generated layout. From this object till the end of chromosome, i.e. the end of the parental layout, all objects are inserted to the offspring. Then the new chromosome is completed with remaining objects in the order as they appear in second parent.

2-point crossover with hot-spots (2-point HS). This operator is an extension of the previous one. It cuts out a "reasonable" part of one layout, uses it as a beginning of a new layout, and completes it with the objects from the other parent in a standard

[3] Depending on whether the adjusted ordering of chromosomes is used or not.

way. Here the reasonable part means a group of objects, which are chained in a *column* from the top to the bottom edge of the area. The algorithm of cutting out the parts from inside of parental layout starts with an arbitrary object that subtends right below the upper edge of the area. Let us denote the object as O. Object O is inserted at the first position of the new chromosome and the algorithm proceeds as follows:

1. $i = 2$ // position of object in new chromosome
2. find unused object such that it lies under O on the grid, and is close to the bottom edge of O
3. if such an object exists
   then insert the object into new chromosome at position i
   denote the object as O
   $i = i + 1$
   goto step 2
   else choose an arbitrary end-object E out of the objects lying behind O on the grid and add them in that order into the new chromosome

The operator described above works so that from one parent it extracts group of objects that represents a compact block on the grid. Such a block should start with a complete column of objects if possible, see step 3 of the algorithm. For example in Figure 3b we can find the following columns {1, 2, 3, 4}, {6, 2, 5}, {7, 8, 5}, {9, 10}, {11, 12, 13, 14}, {15, 16, 17}, and {18, 19}. Thus any of the columns can become a beginning of new layout. This makes the algorithm more explorative and may increase the possibility of finding better solutions.

2.4 Configuration of Genetic Algorithm

The genetic algorithm used in our experiments belongs to the class of generational genetic algorithms with overlapping populations of size *PopSize*=50. This means that every generation $P_{cross} \times PopSize$ new individuals are created by crossover and the remaining individuals are added by replication operator. Probability of crossover was chosen $P_{cross} = 0.8$. A mutation changing position of randomly chosen object was used. Selection method was the simple roulette wheel with linear scaling.

3. EXPERIMENTS

This section presents experiments carried out (1) to evaluate capabilities of the genetic algorithm to solve the layout problem and (2) to investigate an effect of proposed reordering algorithm and hot-spots. All results are averaged over 20 runs.

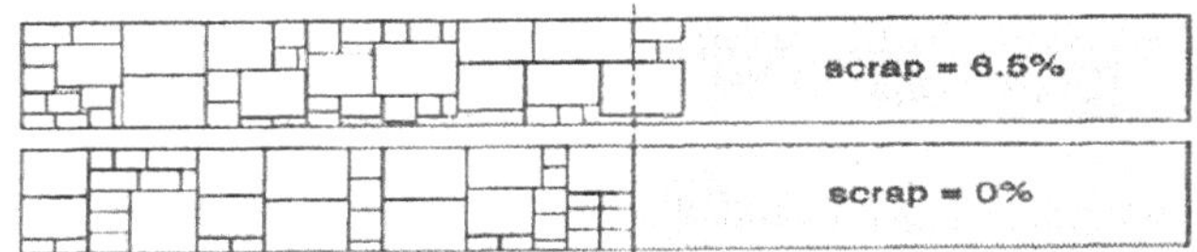

Figure 4 – The best layout of the initial population and the final optimal layout

Two problems with 40 and 42 objects were used in the experiments. Figure 4 shows a successful resolving of the later problem that was achieved with 1-point HS crossover. The same good solution was found also with 2-point HS crossover.

Convergence curves are shown in Figure 5. Figure 5 a) compares simple 1-point crossover (dashed line) with 2-point HS crossover (solid line) on the first problem.

Figure 5 b) compares simple 1-point crossover (dashed line) with 1-point HS crossover (solid line) on the second problem. Both figures as well as the results in Table 1 show the improvement achieved when crossovers use the hot-spots. On the other hand the effect of the reordering algorithm was not as big as we had expected. A significant improvement was observed only when the first problem was solved using the 1-point HS crossover.

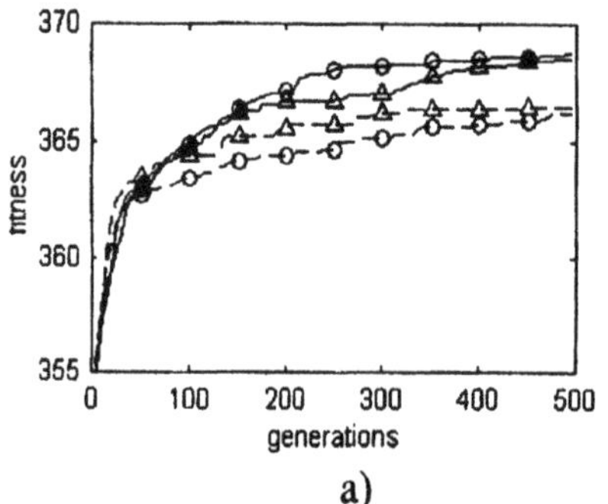

a)

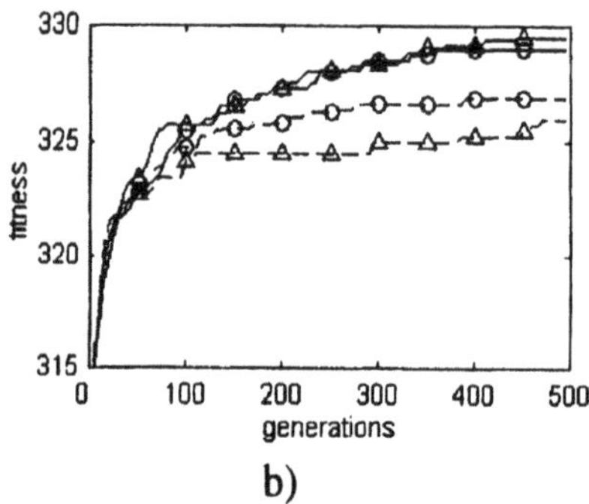

b)

Figure 5 – Convergence Characteristics with the Three Crossover Operators

Table 1 – Results Obtained with the Three Tested Crossover Operators

	simple 1-point		1-point hot-spots		2-point hot-spots	
Problem (objects)	sort on	sort off	sort on	sort off	sort on	sort off
1 (40)	366.5	366.2	369.8	367.5	368.3	368.8
2 (42)	326.0	327.0	329.5	329.0	328.8	328.2

4. CONCLUSIONS

This paper presents an application of genetic algorithm to the problem of finding an optimal layout. The problem was solved as an ordering problem with the main focus on the representation issues and recombination operators. First experiments have shown the applicability of the presented ideas. However more comprehensive analysis should be carried out yet.

5. ACKNOWLEDGMENTS

The research was supported by the State Department of Education within the frame of the project MSM 212300014.

6. REFERENCES

1. Goldberg D. E.: *Genetic Algorithms in Search, Optimization and Machine Learning*. Addison-Wesley, Reading, MA, 1989
2. Dasgupta, D., Michalewicz, Z.: *Evolutionary Algorithms in Engineering Applications*. Springer-Verlag, Germany, ISBN 3-540-62021-4, 1997
3. Ono, T., Watanabe, G.: Genetic Algorithms for Optimal Cutting, in [2], pp. 515-530
4. Whitley D., Starkweather T., Fuguay D.: Scheduling Problems and Traveling Salesman. The Genetic Edge Recombination Operator. In Proceedings of the Third ICGA, San Mateo, CA, Morgan Kaufmann Publishers, pp. 133-140, 1989

57

FORMAL METHODS IN PLC CONTROL DEMONSTRATED AT A FLEXIBLE MANUFACTURING LINE

Georg Frey
Institute of Automatic Control
University of Kaiserslautern, Germany
frey@eit.uni-kl.de

This paper presents various formal approaches in the development of logic control algorithms. Programmable Logic Controllers (PLCs) are commonly used in automation and the algorithms running on them tend to be quite complex. This motivates the application of formal approaches to PLC programming. The approaches range from completely formalized design methods on the one end over the verification and validation (V&V) of formally described controllers to V&V of existing algorithms (developed in some industrially used PLC programming language) on the other end. This paper contains an overview and comparison of various design and verification approaches applied to a common example – the model of a flexible manufacturing line – presented at a session organized by the author at the American Control Conference 2002.

1. INTRODUCTION

Programmable Logic Controllers (PLCs) are the primary workhorse of industrial automation. Due to the growing complexity of control algorithms, and the growing power of formal approaches, there is a lot of interest in applying formal methods to PLC programming. In recent years, a lot of interdisciplinary work was aimed in this direction. This work results in the formalization of different steps in the control design process depending on what problems are to be solved (Frey 2000):

(1) The demand for reduced development times, and the possible reuse of existing software modules result in the need for a formal approach in the development of the PLC programs.

(2) The demand for high quality solutions and especially the application of PLC in safety-critical processes result in the need of validation procedures, i.e. formal methods to prove specific static and dynamic properties of the programs.

(3) The large numbers of already installed PLC programs together with the high expense of programming, leads to the search for verification and validation methods that can be applied directly to programs written in PLC specific programming languages like Ladder Diagram.

This paper contains a summary and comparison of various design and verification approaches applied to a common example presented at a session organized by the author at the American Control Conference 2002. The idea is not to do a benchmark, which isn't even possible, due to the varying nature of the presented approaches but to give the reader an impression on how a reasonably simple logic control problem is viewed from quite different angles.

The paper is organized as follows: In the next Section the fischertechnik manufacturing line that serves as common example in all the presented approaches is introduced. Section 3 presents the various formal approaches in detail and Section 4 compares them. The paper is concluded by a summary and an outlook on further work in this area.

2. FISCHERTECHNIK MANUFACTURING LINE

The flexible manufacturing line used as example is a fischertechnik model consisting of three machines (drill, vertical mill with tool charger, horizontal mill) and three conveyors connecting the machines. There are 15 binary input signals and as many binary output signals. Several production scenarios for the line are possible. The model serves as Logic Control Testbed at the ERC/RMS at the University of Michigan (cf. Figure 1). A second model is installed at the University of Kaiserslautern, Germany (cf. Figure 2).

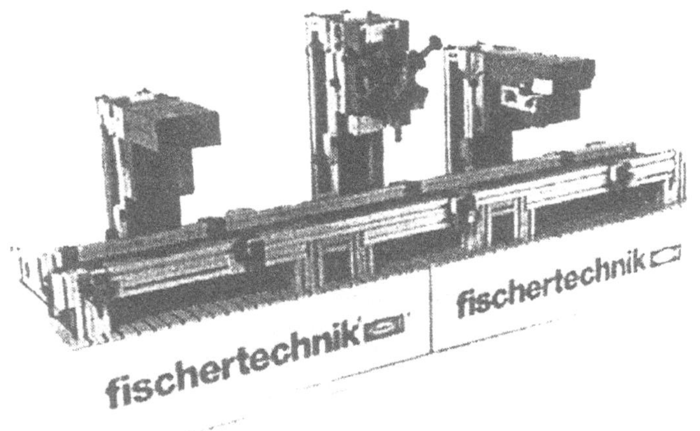

Figure 1 – FMS at the ERC in Michigan (Tilbury 2001)

Although the plants at the Universities of Michigan and Kaiserslautern are very similar there are a few reasons why neither the software nor the controllers are directly interchangeable. First of all, the Michigan line is controlled via a PC and programmed in C++ language – generated from finite state machines, whereas the Kaiserslautern line is controlled either by a PLC programmed with Siemens STEP7 or an IPC with a proprietary real-time system that is programmable via standard IEC 61131-3 languages (John 2001) – generated from Petri nets (Frey 2000). Hence, the programs are not compatible. The controllers are not compatible with the other plant either because the plants use different voltage levels.

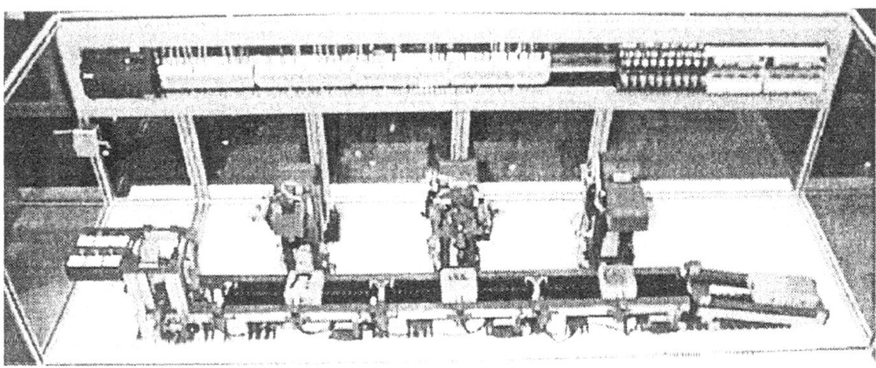

Figure 2 – FMS at the University of Kaiserslautern (Maas 2001)

The programs cannot be translated one-to-one into the language the other institute uses because the input and output tables are different as well. At the ERC in Michigan all the inputs are low active. On the Kaiserslautern plant either low active or high active inputs can be found. Below all the differences in hardware are listed sorted by the hardware units.

Table 1 – Differences in the Mechanical Setup of the Two Plants

Units	**FMS at Kaiserslautern**	**FMS at Ann Arbor**
User I/O	Six push buttons with LEDs	One switch for on/off
Feeder	One motor to push the parts out of the feeder; a reed sensor for the position of the chain; one infrared one way photoelectric relay to see when the feeder is empty; two reed sensors to distinguish the parts	No feeder
Conveyors	Six inductive position sensors in total; one at the entrance of each conveyor and one in front of each machine	Four infrared sensors in total, one at the entrance of the first conveyor and one in front of each machine
Machines (Vertical Mill)	One limit switch at the tool changer of the vertical mill to recognize the working position of one tool.	An additional switch to recognize when the changer is rotating
Storage	At the entrance of the storage for the finished parts is a two way photoelectric relay that is triggered when a part is directly above the sensor	No storage
Parts	There are four different types of workpieces	No distinction between the workpieces possible

3. FORMAL APPROACHES

3.1 Design of a Controller for a FMS with SIPN and SFC, Validation and Verification of both Descriptions via Model-Checking

In (Klein 2002) Stephane Klein, Xiying Weng, Georg Frey, Jean-Jaques Lesage, and Lothar Litz present the results of a joint project done at the ENS Cachan, France and the University of Kaiserslautern, Germany. The aim of this project is to assess the interest of performing formal validation on both the behavioral model and the implementation program of the same controller.

First, a formal model of the controller of the Flexible Manufacturing System is designed using Signal Interpreted Petri Nets (Frey 2002). This formal description is validated via model-checking (Klein 2001, Weng 2001). and then translated into a programming language of the IEC61131. Due to its graphical representation, Sequential Function Chart has been chosen. This program has been validated anew to make sure that the former validated behavior has not been modified during the translation phase. The second validation, again using model-checking with the same properties, shows that, even if the SFC is a simple translation of the former validated SIPN, errors can occur because of the different dynamics of the models.

This example shows that formal methods like validation are well suited for the design of control algorithms. But due to the different languages, and therefore the different semantics, used along the design process, a new step of validation has to be performed after each translation of the controller. None of these validation steps can be omitted if we want to be sure that *What You Prove is What You Get.*

3.2 Verification of a Controller for a Flexible Manufacturing Line Written in Ladder Diagram

In (De Smet 2002) Olivier de Smet and Olivier Rossi from the ENS in Cachan, France show how verification can work under real-life conditions. Rather than building a model of a controller and then analyzing it, they take a given controller written in Ladder Diagram as a starting point. The controller is supplied with the reference example in (Tilbury 2001).

In a first step the controller is translated in to a transition system. To do so, each primitive of the LD language and the LD execution rules are mathematically defined. Furthermore, a model of the PLCs execution behavior is build. The execution cycle of a PLC consists of the three steps: reading of the input image, processing of the algorithm, and writing of the output image (cf. Figure 3).

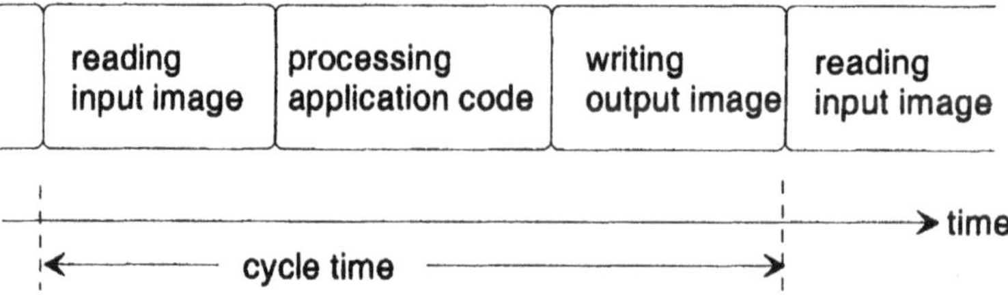

Figure 3 – Program Execution in a PLC

With these definitions a parser was programmed that automatically generates the transition system from a given LD program. The resulting transition system is used as input for a model-checker.

To verify the system 90 properties are generated. The verification is done two times with different general approaches (Frey 2000). In the first run non-model-based (i.e. without any model of the plant) and in the second run constrained-based (i.e. using very restricted knowledge about the plant as for example that the drill cannot be in the upper and lower end-position at the same time).

Using 4 constraints about the switches in the model all properties could be verified in less than a minute on a BDD of about 30000 nodes. In the non-model-based approach the state space is several orders larger. Therefore the check of some properties needed several hours of computation time. Furthermore some properties were shown to be false. This is due to the fact, that "impossible behavior" of the plant is considered in the verification process. However it has to be pointed out that even physically impossible system states may be reported to the controller whenever there is a damaged sensor or a communication problem.

Therefore, De Smet and Rossi conclude that finding out whether a falsified property is caused by an error in the design or by abnormal system behavior is an open problem in model-checking approaches. Furthermore, they find model-checking of LD programs to be effective for small to medium sized industrial systems but not feasible for large systems.

3.3 Application of Specification Language SOL and Its Verification Method to A Flexible Manufacturing Line

In (Ikkai 2002), Y. Ikkai, T. Nakashiba, and N. Komoda from Osaka University, Japan, show that conventional temporal logic descriptions of properties could be quite lengthy and error prone especially if exceptional processes in distributed control systems are described. An example for exceptional processes in the manufacturing line model is the unexpected entering of a new part. In this case the behavior of the line is different from the standard processing in the form that the unexpected part is moved to the end of the line without any machining operations. If the properties of the line are described in temporal logic formulae, most of them have to be rewritten to account for a special case like this. To avoid this problem, the Sequence Oriented Language (SOL), which is the intelligible language to describe specifications for distributed sequential control systems is proposed. SOL allows to describe the order of processes *and exceptions* from this order.

Verification using SOL is performed by a supporting tool that takes a model of the plant (described by finite state machines), the controller described by Function Blocks according to IEC61131 (translated into finite sate machines) and the SOL properties.

The presented tool not only allows verification but can also be used for the graphical design of the controller and the plant model. The application to the flexible manufacturing line shows the feasibility of the presented approach.

3.4 Reconfigurable Logic Control Using Modular FSMs: Design, Verification, Implementation, and Integrated Error Handling

In (Shaw 2002) S. S. Shah form the University of California and E. W. Endsley, M. R. Lucas, and D. M. Tilbury from the University of Michigan describe the implementation and reconfiguration of controllers for the reference example.

They present an algorithm for the design of a modular controller that proceeds in six steps from the determination of the modular structure of the system under control to the implementation of the controller on the hardware.

The single modules of the logic control code are written using modular finite state machines and are verified to be internally correct before they are combined. After the combination of the resulting single finite state machine is verified before it is converted to C code for implementation.

The strength of this formalized modular development approach lies in the easy reconfiguration of the controller. Using the fischertechnik line it is shown how additional functionality can be integrated into the controller without writing it anew. This is a clear improvement to standard PLC programming languages where changes in the functionality of a controller are very hard to program and often a completely new controller is programmed instead.

3.5 Quantitative and Qualitative Comparison of PLC for a Small Testbed with a Focus on Usability Issues

In (Lucas 2002) M. R. Lucas and D. M. Tilbury from the University of Michigan describe similar programs written for the control of the fischertechnik manufacturing line in three languages: Ladder Diagram, Modular Finite State Machines, and Petri nets.

The aim of their work is to compare different programming languages or description formalisms from a users viewpoint. To do so they define some complexity metrics that are applicable to all the used languages. Furthermore the effort in writing and modifying the programs is measured. Finally the accessibility of the code, i.e. the ease of understanding the control logic, is compared.

There is no best formalism resulting from this multi-dimensional comparison. However the proposed framework for evaluating and comparing different formalisms can be used to find out whether new formalisms bring any advantages from a users point of view. Therefore it is a further step towards the integration of software quality concepts into logic controller development.

4. COMPARISON OF THE PRESENTED APPROACHES

4.1 Verification and Validation

In all of the presented approaches verification and validation of PLC programs is a main topic. Common to them is that they all use model-checking techniques. This clearly shows the importance of this V&V method. The main difference lies in the formalism used to describe the control algorithm and the way in which the behavior of the plant is included.

For the control algorithms there are, on the one side, formal descriptions from academics as Petri Nets used in (Klein 2002) and Finite State Machines in (Shah 2002). On the other side, there are approaches that start from standard industrial descriptions as Ladder Diagram (De Smet 2002), Function Block Diagram (Ikkai 2002) or Sequential Function Chart (Klein 2002).

The behavior of the plant is either ignored (non-model-based V&V) as done in (Klein 2002), abstracted by some constraints (constrained-based V&V) which showed to dramatically reduce the state-space during model-checking in (De Smet 2002) or completely described by a formal model (model-based V&V) as presented in (Ikkai 2002).

A common problem in all approaches is the generation of formal properties to be verified on the system and the correct interpretation of the model-checking results. Furthermore it turns out that model-checking reaches its limits even for small controllers if there is no additional information on the plants behavior.

4.2 Formal Design Approaches

(Shaw 2002) propose a completely formalized design approach for reconfigurable controllers using modular finite state machines. Using this approach the reconfiguration of a controller is made much easier and faster as with conventional techniques.

In a comparative study (Lucas 2002) Ladder Diagrams, Petri Nets, and Modular Finite State Machines are used to develop a controller for the fischertechnik testbed. After the design the effort for writing the controller, the effort for changing the controller and the ease of understanding of the controller are evaluated. Further development of the presented metrics and the inclusion of even more formalisms could lead to a decision table that assists a user in finding the best language for the application at hand.

5. CONCLUSIONS AND OUTLOOK

In this paper several formal approaches to PLC programming are presented. All of them have been applied to the same control problem. The comparison of the approaches shows that verification and validation (V&V) of controllers is the main aim of formal methods in this area. However, new methods that try to improve the development process as a whole also begin to emerge. These development approaches try to avoid errors by formalized development procedures instead of finding them afterwards by V&V.

Open problems to be addressed are the complexity of real-life controllers that are still out of range for the presented methods and the difficulties in finding the error if during V&V properties turn out to be false.

To conclude, the application of more and more techniques from Software Engineering to PLC programming is the only way to cope with the increasing complexities in this application driven area.

This survey should also be seen as a step to promoting the use of reference examples like the fischertechnik line in the presentation of new methods. A reference example allows the author and the reader to get to the relevant new points of the work rather fast, because the application is already known.

6. ACKNOWLEDGEMENTS

This paper would not have been written without Jim Christensen who had the idea of summarizing the results of the ACC session and invited me to present them at the BASYS conference. The paper would not have been possible without the valuable input from all the authors of the invited session on *Formal methods in PLC control demonstrated at a flexible manufacturing line* at the American Control Conference 2002.

7. REFERENCES

1. De Smet O, Rossi O. Verification of a Controller for a flexible manufacturing line written in Ladder Diagram. Proceedings of the American Control Conference ACC2002, Anchorage, Alaska, pp.4147-4152, May 2002.
2. Frey G, Litz L. Formal methods in PLC programming. Proceedings of the IEEE Conference on Systems Man and Cybernetics SMC 2000, pp. 2431-2436, Nashville, Tennessee (USA), Oct. 8-11, 2000.
3. Frey, Georg. Automatic Implementation of Petri Net based Control Algorithms on PLC. Proceedings of the American Control Conference, ACC 2000, Chicago (IL), pp. 2819-3823, June 2000.
4. Frey, Georg. Design and formal Analysis of Petri Net based Logic Control Algorithms. Dissertation University of Kaiserslautern, Aachen: Shaker Verlag, 2002.
5. John KH, Tiegelkamp M. IEC 61131-3: Programming Industrial Automation Systems. Berlin, New York: Springer, 2001.
6. Klein S, Weng X, Frey G, Lesage JJ, Litz L. Design of a controller for a FMS with SIPN and SFC. Validation and verification of both descriptions via model-checking. Proceedings of the American Control Conference ACC2002, Anchorage, Alaska, pp.4141-4146, May 2002.
7. Klein, Stéphane. A case study in design and formal verification of control algorithms using interpreted Petri Nets and SFC. D.E.A. de Production Automatisée, Ecole Normale Supérieure Cachan, June 2001.
8. Lucas MR, Tilbury DM. Quantitative and Qualitative Comparison of PLC programs for a small testbed with a focus on usability issues. Proceedings of the American Control Conference ACC2002, Anchorage, Alaska, pp.4165-4171, May 2002.
9. Maas H, Frey G. Documentation and Control Scenarios for a Flexible Manufacturing Line. Technical Report I17/2001, Institute of Automatic Control, University of Kaiserslautern, Dec 2001.
10. Shah SS, Endsley EW, Lucas MR, Tilbury DM. Reconfigurable Logic Control using Modular FSMs: Design, Verification, Implementation, and Integrated Error Handling. Proceedings of the American Control Conference ACC2002, Anchorage, Alaska, pp.4153-4158, May 2002.
11. Tilbury, Dawn. Logic Control Testbed 2001 http://www-personal.engin.umich.edu/~tilbury/testbed/
12. Weng X, Litz L. Model checking of Signal Interpreted Petri Nets. Proceedings of the IEEE international Conference on Systems Man and Cybernetics, SMC 2001, Tucson (AZ), USA, pp. 2748-2752, Oct. 2001.
13. Y. Ikkai Y, Nakashiba T, Komoda N. Application of Specification Language SOL and its Verification Method to a Flexible Manufacturing Line. Proceedings of the American Control Conference ACC2002, Anchorage, Alaska, pp.4159-4164, May 2002.

58

TOWARDS ENVIRONMENT MODELING BY AUTONOMOUS MOBILE SYSTEMS

Libor Přeučil, Petr Štěpán, Miroslav Kulich [1], Roman Mázl
The Gertsner Laboratory for Intelligent Decision Making and Control
[1] *Center for Applied Cybernetics*
Czech Technical University in Prague
{preucil,stepan,kulich,mazl}@labe.felk.cvut.cz

The process of how to acquire knowledge about the operating environment is one of the most challenging problems that autonomous mobile robots must solve. The quality of the model depends on a number and the kind of sensors used and upon the precision the robot recovers its position. This paper introduces two crucial components of the map building procedure: the position localization based on data gathered from laser rangefinders and the dead-reckoning system together with a novel method for map-building through data fusion from a monocular camera and a laser range-finder.

1. INTRODUCTION

In order to explore a working environment and to build a model of the environment a robot has to fulfill two fundamental tasks: (1) *localize its position from observations* and (2) *recover the environment shape and structure.* Both tasks are complementary and cannot be solved alone.

Local navigation systems of mobile robots typically provide sufficient accuracy only in a short-term periods, therefore independent localization technique has to be applied. The localization methods relying on range-measurements of the environment can be split into the following basic categories:

The main idea of *landmark localization* is to detect and match characteristic features (artificial or natural) in the environment from sensory inputs. (Leonard et al. 1991). The *Markov localization* evaluates a probability distribution over the space of possible robot states that represent positions (Fox et al. 1999).

The most promising *sensor matching* techniques compare raw or pre-processed sets of range-data obtained from sensors (actual scan) with a map or previously obtained sensor range-measurements (reference scan). These can be distinguished into *point-to-point*, *point-to-line* or *line-to-line* methods which compare particular types of measurements - or from these recovered point-based features as corners, line segments, etc. The comparison is done in a two-step process: building point-pair or feature-pair correspondences followed by translations and rotations to fit the actual and the reference scan.

A critical part of the *point-to-point* approach is retrieval of the corresponding pairs of points what leads to preference of the *point-to-line* algorithms. The main idea is to approximate the reference scan by a list of lines or to match the actual scan with visible lines of the map (Gutmann et al. 1998). Similarly, method extension to *line-to-line* approach is straightforward and has been applied in the following (Chmelař et al. 2000).

Having solved the localization task, other sensors (which do not provide direct range measurements) can be incorporated to improve the robot navigation performance. Major attention is devoted in particular to integration of a monocular camera into the navigation process and world model build-up procedure. The task setup is thoroughly constrained to situations in which the robot operates on a plane and which covers a significant class of problems. The typical situations alike appear in indoor environments or even outdoors, where this condition is satisfied on the roads (Broggi, 1998).

Fusion of the camera data with the rangefinder data seems to be possible by applying occupancy grids (Elfes, 1989), (Menezes et al., 1994), the central part of the method introduced in the following. Similarly, knowing the robot position the range-finder data can be used to calibrate the probability profiles for the camera. The combination of diverse sensors like range-finders and monocular camera in the introduced approach leads to building more accurate 2-D maps of the environment.

2. SYSTEM LOCALIZATION

The localization problem, as mentioned above, is invoked by the need of knowing position and heading of the robot in the global coordinate system. This information determines correspondences between subsequent sensor measurements from different positions during robot mission and therefore enables us to create and efficiently update internal models (in this case maps – occupancy grids) of the environment.

2.1 Range-Data Segmentation

As range-finder measurements are in a form of distances to rigid obstacles in selected discrete directions, the processing of obstacle boundaries requires segmentation into point sets creating a particular boundary segment.

For the segmentation a recursive interval-splitting approach (Chmelař et al., 2000) selecting the candidate points for a straight-line boundary segment has been developed. The algorithm takes advantage of naturally angle-ordered points obtained from a laser range-finder. Evaluation of the maximum segment curvature criterion followed by application of a LSQ provides sets of points that optimally split the original boundary into particular segments.

The less important and possibly missegmented elements are discarded in a post-processing filtration using heuristic rules (Chmelař et al., 2000), (Mázl et al., 2001).

2.2 Correspondence Line Search

A crucial part of the method is to find for each line from the actual scan a corresponding line from the reference scan (if exists). We say, that two lines correspond if and only if differences of their directions and positions are sufficiently small. To specify this, lets denote x and y lengths of the lines, a, b, c, d distances between their vertices, and ϕ stands for the angle between lines, all satisfying the following expressions (the Φ_{MAX} and K are preselected thresholds for the desired level of line similarity).

$$\phi < \Phi_{MAX} \qquad \frac{\min(a,b)+\min(c,d)}{x+y} < K,$$

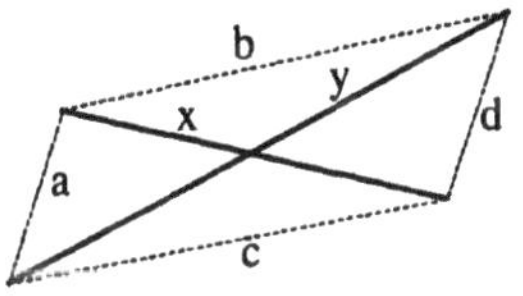

Figure 1 - Distance definition for evaluation of line-to-line similarity.

2.3 Heading and Position Correction

In this step, the heading correction is determined as the angular declination α between two scans. The leading idea is to evaluate a weighted sum of angular differences of each corresponding lines as:

$$\alpha = \frac{\sum_{i=1}^{n} \phi_i w_i}{\sum_{i=1}^{n} w_i}$$

where n is a number of corresponding line pairs, ϕ_i is an angle between lines of the i-th pair, and w_i is the weight of the i-th pair. The weight is defined as a product of the lines' lengths, which prefers pairs containing long lines to pairs of short lines.

In order to correct shifts in the position, we express each line of the reference scan in a standard form:

$$a_i x + b_i y + c_i = 0$$

and each line of the actual scan is represented by its outer points $([x_i^1, y_i^1], [x_i^2, y_i^2])$, so that the shift $[p_x, p_y]$ of the actual scan can be determined by minimizing the following penalty function. The minimization problem itself can be solved via Nelder-Mead type simplex search.

$$\min_{p_x, p_y} \sum_{i=1}^{n} \sum_{j=1}^{2} (a_i (x_i^j + p_x) + b_i (y_i^j + p_y) + c_i)^2 .$$

Illustrative results of position and heading correction based on processing of subsequent range-scan data are illustrated in the following figures.

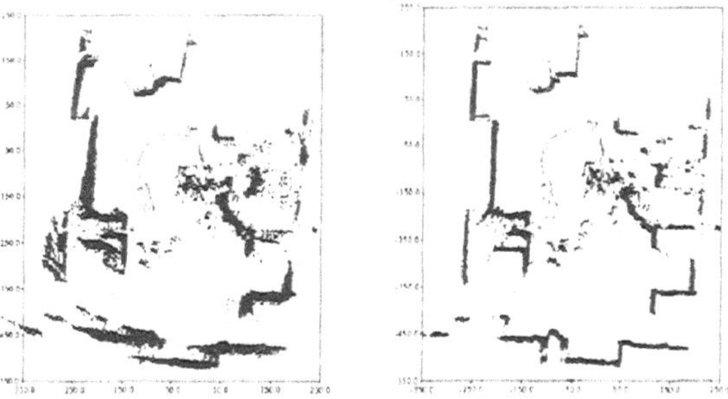

Figure 2 - Original Range-Data (Accumulated) with Errors in Heading and Shift (Left) and after Correction Using the Line-To-Line Approach (Right).

3. OCCUPANCY GRID FROM MONOCULAR CAMERA

The occupancy grids belong to the most common low-level and sensor-based type model of the environment in robotics. The occupancy grid approach is very robust for fusion of noisy data and its application field has previously been limited to exclusive use with range sensors (originally designed for sonar data fusion).

The following shows, that under certain but reasonable circumstances the occupancy grid concept can also be used for fusion of monocular camera sensor.

A central assumption guaranteeing admissibility of the method is a robot operation on a flat ground-plane (floor). This assumption enables to determine all parameters of the robotics system. The parameters of the camera system can be calibrated on special images and afterwards used to detect obstacles in the robot surrounding.

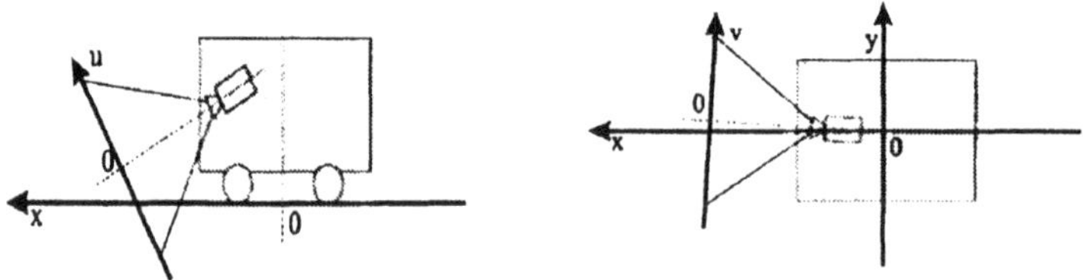

Figure 3 - Coordinate Systems for the Mobile Robot Onboard Camera

Our goal is to obtain 2-D map of the robot operating environment. It is necessary to find parameters of the robotic system to evaluate the transformation from the image coordinate system *(u, v)* into the robot coordinate system *(x, y)* - see figure 3. It means to determine the projection function $f(u, v) = (x, y)$ (Šonka et al., 1998). The first step is a reduction of the radial distortion and decentering. The constants u_c, v_c and p_1, p_2, p_3 can be determined from a calibration pattern according to the following equations:

$$dist = (u - u_c)^2 + (v - v_c)^2$$

$$u' = (u - u_c)(1 + p_1 dist + p_2 dist^2 + p_3 dist^3)$$

$$v' = (v - v_c)(1 + p_1 dist + p_2 dist^2 + p_3 dist^3)$$

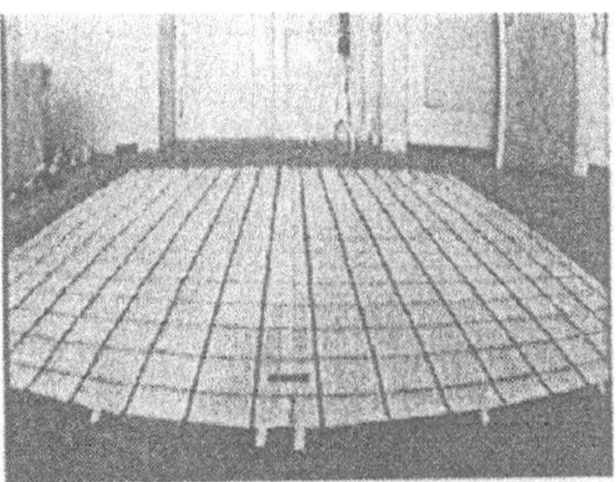

Figure 4 – The Calibration Pattern

To set the parameters of radial distortion and decentering the pattern in the Figure 4 was used. The image serves to detect the points from lines and the minimization of the square distance of these points to corresponding line was done. The results of this minimization are the u_c, v_c and p_1, p_2, p_3 parameters.

The double (u', v') determines the coordinates of the image after correction of the radial distortion. The next step is to detect the shift of the camera from the center of the robot x_{cam}, y_{cam}, and parameters of the plane that describes the floor of the environment, so Δu, Δv, X and Y. The following equations describe the projective transformation:

$$x_0 = -\frac{(u' - \Delta u)X}{v' - \Delta v} + x_{cam} \qquad y_0 = -\frac{Y}{v' - \Delta v} + y_{cam}$$

A complete transformation is desired to correct the angular difference of the camera axis and the robot axis α as well as to obtain the coordinates in the robot world. Assume the robot position is x_{rob} , y_{rob}, ω_{rob}, the complete transformation can be described as:

$$x = x_{rob} + x_0 \cos(\alpha + \omega_{rob}) - y_0 \sin(\alpha + \omega_{rob})$$
$$y = y_{rob} + x_0 \sin(\alpha + \omega_{rob}) + y_0 \cos(\alpha + \omega_{rob}),$$

Eleven measurements of a reference box were done by camera and laser range finder to determine the above mentioned parameters. Each camera measurement represents four points (the borders of the box and two points on the front side) and the laser range finder provides the real position of this box. Minimization of the square distance from the real to the computed position in the camera image produces x_{cam}, y_{cam}, Δu, Δv, X, Y, α for the robot system.

3.1 Definition of the Probability Profiles

Detection of the free space is done making-use of the color of the floor. Suppose that the color is different from the obstacle surface color. If the color of the floor is known the probability distribution of a free space can be defined. The occupancy grid (Elfes, 1989) is built using the Bayes' update formula:

$$P(Occ \mid R) = \frac{P(R \mid Occ)P(Occ)}{P(R \mid Occ)P(Occ) + P(R \mid Emp)P(Emp)}$$

where: $P(Emp) = 1 - P(Occ)$ $\qquad$ $P(R \mid Emp) = 1 - P(R \mid Occ)$

The preceding formula defines new conditional probability, that the cell is occupied given measured color reading $R = (h,s,v)$. The probability depends on the old value $P(Occ)$ and the probability distribution $P(R|Occ)$. The probability distribution $P(R|Occ)$ can be represented as a difference of the measured color R and the reference color of the floor in the hsv-space. The following can be used to compute the conditional probability depending on the reference color of the floor (h_r, s_r, v_r):

$$dif(x) = e^{-\frac{x^2}{2\sigma^2}}$$
$$P(R \mid Occ) = dif(h - h_r)dif(s - s_r)dif(v - v_r),$$

where σ represents sensitivity of the difference function.

3.2 Calibration of the Probability Profiles with Range-Data

If the color of the floor is similar to the color of the obstacles, the previous method fails. Another approach deriving the probability profiles uses definition of the profiles $P(R|Occ)$ with help of additional information about environment.

The additional information can be map of a training environment or combination of a sonar and laser data which can correctly measure the training environment. The probability profiles can be then calculated directly from the camera images. The free space and the border of the obstacle is determined from the range finder data or from the map of the environment in this case.

The matrices *free* and *occ* can be computed for a discrete hsv-space and they denote a number of cells with concrete color that are free or occupied, respectively. In our example, 10 images with different lighting conditions were used to create the matrixes *free* and *occ* with dimension 20 x 20 x 20. For each pixel of the camera image, the occupancy of this pixel in the robot coordinate system was calculated. If the pixel with color $(h,s,v) \in \langle 0,1 \rangle^3$ represents a free space then the matrix value $free([20h],[20s],[20v])$ is increased. If the pixel belongs to the occupied space, the matrix value $occ([20h],[20s],[20v])$ is increased. The probability profile $P(R|Occ)$ for reading $R = (h,s,v)$ is defined by the following formula:

$$\text{if } \; free(h',s',v') + occ(h',s',v') > 0 \; \text{ then}$$

$$P(R \mid Occ) = \frac{occ(h',s',v')}{free(h',s',v') + occ(h',s',v')},$$

$$\text{otherwise: } P(R \mid Occ) = 1, \text{ where: } h'=[20h],\ s'=[20s],\ v'=[20v]$$

The figure 5 shows original image from the onboard camera, the same image after coordinate transformation, where each pixel determines 5 x 5 cm cell of the robot environment and finally the created occupancy grid using a probability profile matrix of dimension 20 x 20 x 20.

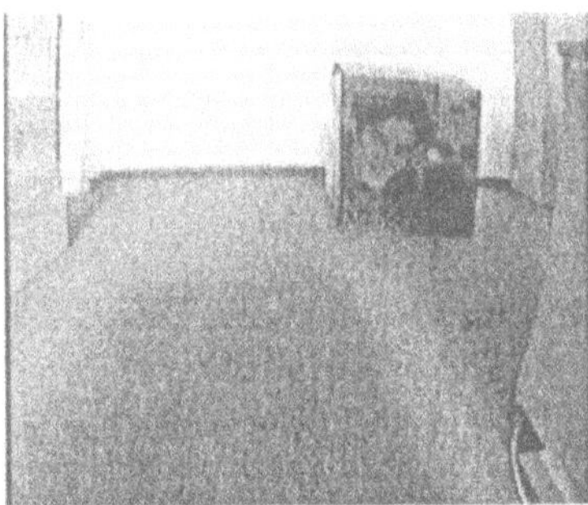
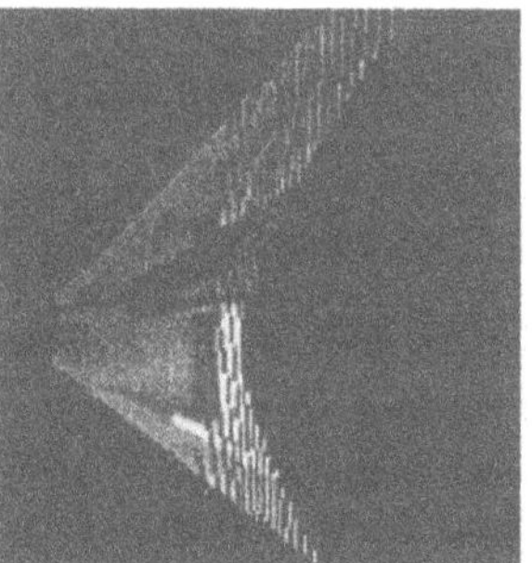
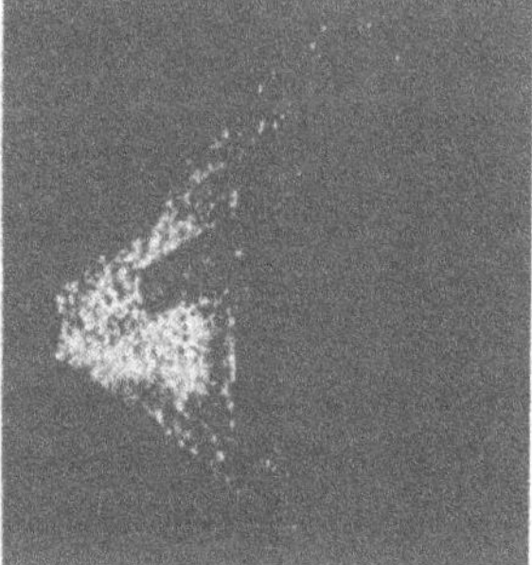

Figure 5 -The Original Onboard Camera Image (Left); after Transformation into the Floor Coordinate System (Middle) and the Final Occupancy Grid (Right).

The robot position is located on the left side of the picture a the camera aspect is oriented to the right in this case. White color stands for a free space as detected by the color probability profile of the floor plane.

3.3 Building the Final 2-D Map

The final occupancy grid construction originates from the information about visibility. Unfortunately, it can often happen, that the color of the floor can appear at the obstacle too, even when the border of the obstacle is detected very well. Therefore, the final computation of the grid is done only within the interval from the position of the robot to the border of the grid. The accumulated probability is computed applying the following formula:

$$P_{new}(Occ) = P(Occ)P_{Acc}(Occ)$$

There are two possibilities how the accumulated probability $P_{Acc}(Occ)$ can be defined. The first one is simply the multiplication of the probabilities of all cells from the viewpoint. The second approach uses the Bayes formula for a recursive definition of this probability.

$$P_{Acc'}(Occ) = \frac{P(Occ)P_{Acc}(Occ)}{P(Occ)P_{Acc}(Occ) + (1 - P(Occ))(1 - P_{Acc}(Occ))}$$

The result of the Bayes update formula for the visibility occupancy grid is shown in the following figures.

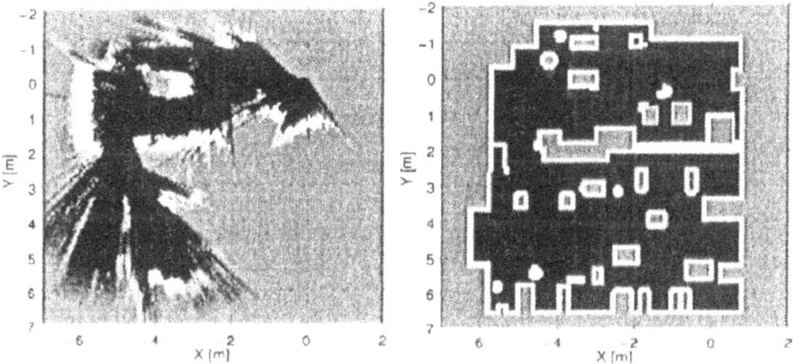

Figure 6– Final Occupancy Grid (Left) Created from Camera Data and the Obtained Environment Map after Segmentation (right).

The preceding figure illustrates an occupancy map created exclusively from camera data. The color model of the floor was created in a free space and the final map of a typical office environment can be obtained via image segmentation process (Šonka et al. 1998).

4. CONCLUSION

The problem of environment modeling for autonomous mobile systems – robots lasts still for a challenging field of many opened problems. The environment model recovery stands hand in hand with the localization problem. As there still does not exist any unified approach to reliable recovery of the environment models, the robustness is typically improved through data and model fusion from multiple sources.

The introduced novel method combines improved localization approach based on range-data from a LIDAR with a brand new usage of the occupancy grid approach. It has been illustrated, that under assumption that the robot operates in a 3D environment with a more or less uniform and flat ground-plane (e.g. floor, road, etc.), the occupancy grids can be extended towards data fusion from monocular camera. The introduced extension opens new possibilities in fusion in sensor–based models from more diverse sources like range-finder and monocular camera. This is expected to enable further improvement of the robustness and accuracy while building environment models in mobile robotics.

The early achievements of the described approach were experimentally verified with real data in real indoor environments. Respecting the limited space of this contribution, selected results were briefly illustrated in the running text above.

5. ACKNOWLEDGMENT

The work was supported by the Ministry of Education of the Czech Republic within the frame of the project "Decision-Making and Control for Manufacturing" number MSM 212300013, FRVŠ 2156/2002 and the Grant Agency of the Czech Republic 102/02/0641/A grants. The support of the Ministry of Education of the Czech Republic, under the Project No. LN00B096 to Miroslav Kulich, is also gratefully acknowledged.

6. REFERENCES

1. Broggi A, Bertozzi M, Fascioli A. An Extension to the Inverse Perspective Mapping to Handle Non-flat Roads. In: Proceedings of the IEEE International Conference on Intelligent Vehicles, Stuttgart, Germany, pp.305-309,1998.
2. Chmelař B, Přeučil L, Štěpán P. Range-data Based Position Localization and Refinement for a Mobile Robot. Proceedings of the 6th IFAC Symposium on Robot Control, Austria, Vienna, pp. 364-379, 2000.
3. Elfes A. Occupancy Grids: A Probabilistic Framework fo Robot Perception and Navigation. PhD thesis. Electrical and Computer Engineering Department/Robotics Institute. Carnegie-Mellon University, 1989.
4. Fox D, Burgard W, Thrun S. Markov Localization for Mobile Robots in Dynamic Environments. Journal of Artificial Intelligence, 11, pages 391-427, 1999.
5. Gutmann JS, Burgard W, Fox D, Konolige K. Experimental Comparison of Localization Methods. International Conference on Intelligent Robots and Systems, Victoria, B.C. , 1998.
6. Leonard JJ, Cox IJ, Durrant-Whyte HF. Dynamic Map Building for an Autonomous Mobile Robot. In Proc. IEEE Int. Workshop on Intelligent Robots and Systems, pages 89-96, July 1990. Also published in Autonomous Mobile Robots, edited by S. Iyengar and A. Elfes, Los Alamitos, CA: IEEE Computer Society Press, 1991.
7. Mázl R, Kulich M, Přeučil L. Range Scan-based Localization Methods for Mobile Robots in Complex Environments. In: Proceedings: Intelligent Transportation Systems. IEEE Computer Society Press, New York, 2001, vol. 1, p. 280-285. ISBN 0-7803-7195-X
8. Menezes P, Arujo H, Dias J, Ribeiro MI. Obstacle Detection in Mobile Robots Using Sonar Data. In: Associacao Portuguesa de Controlo Automatico, Int. Conf. - Controlo 94, I.S.T., Lisbon, 1994.
9. Šonka M, Hlaváč V, Boyle R. Image Processing, Analysis, and Machine Vision. Brooks/Cole Publishing Co., Boston, 1999, 800 p. ISBN 0-534-95393-X.

59

NOVEL ADAPTIVE CONTROL OF MECHANICAL SYSTEMS DRIVEN BY ELECTROMECHANICAL HYDRAULIC DRIVES

János F. Bitó, József K. Tar, Imre J. Rudas
Budapest Polytechnic
H-1081 Budapest, Népszínház utca 8, Hungary
jbito@zeus.banki.hu, jktar@donat.banki.hu, rudas@zeus.banki.hu

Electric servo systems have superior performance in comparison with hydraulic drives in the small and medium applications they are comparatively expensive and may be dissipation-sensitive. In contrast to the DC motor driven systems hydraulic differential cylinders are very intricate, non-linear, strongly coupled multivariable electromechanical engines of significant parameters, which are very difficult to control or even to measure. Traditional controllers require a relatively accurate information on these parameters. In this paper a novel adaptive control is presented which evades the problem of the incomplete and inaccurate information of these parameters as well as their time-dependence. The method is promising in other fields of application where the behavior of a complex system under unknown environmental interaction is to be predicted

1. INTRODUCTION

In spite of the definite virtues of electric DC drives, due to several practical reasons alternative solutions are widely searched, e.g. the possibility of developing pneumatic servo systems (e.g. Drakunov et al, 1997). Traditional PID control of robots driven by hydraulic differential cylinders have to cope with the problem of instabilities, too. The desirable values of the appropriate feedback parameters may significantly depend on the actual pose of the robot arm. Two different control approaches were recently proposed for such robots (Bröcker and Lemmen, 2001). One of them is based on disturbance rejection, the other one on the partial flatness principle, respectively. In each case it is necessary to measure the disturbance force and its time-derivative as well as to know the exact model of the hydraulic cylinder.

However, it is very difficult to keep these parameters under perfect control or to measure them in real-time. The viscosity of the hydraulic oil is very sensitive to the temperature normally increasing due to its circulation in the pipe system. Oil compressibility depends on the amount of air or other gases solved in it, therefore it also is temperature-dependent. Other phenomena related to friction as the adhesion of the piston at the cylinder introduce rough non-linearity into the behavior of the system. Combined with other dynamical properties of the physical system to be driven by such drives as well as with not always measurable external disturbances normally very complex control tasks may arise.

In general it seems to be expedient to apply adaptive control instead of trying to measure the ample set of unknown and time-varying parameters. On the other hand this adaptive control need not to be too intricate, actually shouldn't be much more complicated than an industrial PID controller. Normally, their improvement via the traditional self-tuning essentially remains within the realm of linear control and doesn't anticipate too much success. A particular branch of soft computing has recently been proposed (e.g. Tar and Rontó, 2000). In the development of the method at first certain symmetry properties of Classical Mechanics were taken into account, later the Modified Renormalization Transformation was applied for SISO systems, finally satisfactory convergence criteria were given to its extension to MIMO systems (Pátkai et al, 2002). In the meantime the method was further simplified by the introduction of the Partially Stretched Orthogonal Transformations (El Hini, 2001).

The above cited methods were tested in the control of DC motor driven electromechanical systems. In the present paper their applicability is illustrated in the case of hydraulic differential cylinders under external perturbation unknown by the controller. Modeling errors and external perturbations reveal themselves in the actual behavior of the system in comparison with that of a very simple and approximate model.

2. OPERATION OF THE DIFFERENTIAL HYDRAULIC CYLINDER

The operation of the differential hydraulic cylinder is described in details by Bröcker and Lemmen (Bröcker and Lemmen 2001). Let x denote the linear position of the piston in m units. The acceleration of the piston is described by (1) as

$$\ddot{x} = \frac{1}{m}\left[\left(p_A - \frac{1}{\varphi} p_B\right)A_A - F_f(\dot{x}) - F_d\right] \tag{1}$$

in which p_A and p_B denotes the pressures in chamber A and B of the piston in bar, $\varphi = A_A/A_B$, that is the ratio of the "active" surfaces of the appropriate sides of the piston, m is the mass of the piston in kg, F_f denotes the internal friction between the piston and the cylinder, F_d denotes the external disturbance forces. The pressure of the oil in the chambers also depends on the piston position as

$$\dot{p}_A = \frac{E_{oil}}{V_A(x)}\left(-A_A\dot{x} + B_v K_v a_1(p_A, U)U\right) \tag{2}$$

$$\dot{p}_B = \frac{E_{oil}}{V_B(x)}\left(\frac{A_A}{\varphi}\dot{x} - B_v K_v a_2(p_B, U)U\right) \tag{3}$$

where B_v denotes the flow resistance, K_v is the valve amplification, U is the normalized valve voltage. E_{oil} means the oil's compressibility. The oil volume in the pipes and the chambers are expressed as

$$V_A(x) = V_{pipeA} + A_A x,$$
$$V_B(x) = V_{pipeB} + A_B(H - x) \tag{4}$$

(H is the cylinder stroke.) The hydraulic drive has two stabilized pressure values, the *pump pressure* p_0, and the *tank pressure* p_t. Under normal operating conditions (that is when no shock waves travel in the pipe line) these pressures set the upper and the lower bound to p_A and p_B. The functions a_1 and a_2 are defined in (5).

$$a_1(p_A, U) = \begin{cases} sign(p_0 - p_A)\sqrt{|p_0 - p_A|} \\ if \quad U \geq 0, \\ sign(p_A - p_t)\sqrt{|p_A - p_t|} \\ if \quad U < 0 \end{cases}$$
$$a_2(p_B, U) = \begin{cases} sign(p_B - p_t)\sqrt{|p_B - p_t|} \\ if \quad U \geq 0, \\ sign(p_0 - p_B)\sqrt{|p_0 - p_B|} \\ if \quad U < 0 \end{cases} \tag{5}$$

Under "normal conditions" $sign(a_1) \geq 0$, and $sign(a_2) \geq 0$, too, according to the limiting role of the pump and tank pressures. The *disturbance rejection approach* (Bröcker and Lemmen 2001) is based on creating the time-derivative of (1) resulting in the appearance of the time-derivative of the disturbance force in the equations. In the sequel a control approach not needing measurement of the disturbance force and exact knowledge of the system parameters will be presented.

3. THE ADAPTIVE CONTROL APPROACH

Supposing the need for a desired piston acceleration determined via kinematic considerations, on the basis of the available system model a *desired value* can be prescribed to $(p_A - p_B/\varphi)$. (In this model the piston friction and disturbance force can be omitted.) If at least p_A, p_B, x, and dp_A/dt, dp_B/dt, dx/dt are measurable in real-time it is possible to know the *actual value* of this quantity and its time-derivative. Therefore a *desired time-derivative* can be prescribed to this quantity. By using the approximate system model via combination (2) and (3) an appropriate control signal U can be proposed for this purpose. (Taking into account the inconvenient behavior of the piston's friction, it is expedient to apply a PI-type controller for $(p_A - p_B/\varphi)$, and for the desired trajectory tracking.) The adaptive controller compares with each other the *realized* and the *desired* value of $y \equiv d(p_A - p_B/\varphi)/dt$. Via the application of a *dummy parameter D* of no direct physical interpretation either a symplectic matrix or a two-dimensional vector is created as

$$\mathbf{S} \equiv \begin{bmatrix} 0 & 0 & -y/s & D/s \\ 0 & 0 & -D/s & -y/s \\ y & -D & 0 & 0 \\ D & y & 0 & 0 \end{bmatrix}, s = y^2 + D^2, \mathbf{v} \equiv \begin{bmatrix} y \\ D \end{bmatrix} \tag{6}$$

This matrix/vector can be constructed for the *desired* and the *actual* value of y. Taking into account the definition and the group properties of the *symplectic matrices* it is very easy to construct a symplectic matrix **T**, which transforms the actual value into the desired one as

$$\mathfrak{I} \equiv \left[\begin{array}{c|c} \mathbf{0} & -\mathbf{I} \\ \hline \mathbf{I} & \mathbf{0} \end{array}\right], \quad \mathbf{S}^T \mathfrak{I} \mathbf{S} = \mathfrak{I}, \quad \mathbf{S}^{-1} = \mathfrak{I}^T \mathbf{S}^T \mathfrak{I}, \quad \mathbf{T} = [Des][Act]^{-1} \tag{7}$$

or, following El Hini, construct an orthogonal matrix rotating the actual vector **v** into the desired one and leaves their orthogonal sub-spaces unchanged and making the appropriate shrink/dilatation only in the direction of the transformed actual vector (this means the creation of the appropriate *Partially Stretched Orthogonal Transformation*). Each mapping can be created in a computationally very inexpensive manner, and they can be regarded as a kind of *experimental identification of the actual system on the basis of its rough model and experimentally observed behavior.*

From purely mathematical point of view this kind of *system-identification* can be formulated as follows: there is given some *imperfect model of the system* on the basis of which some *excitation* is calculated for a desired input $\mathbf{i}^d$ as $\mathbf{e}=\varphi(\mathbf{i}^d)$. The system has its *inverse dynamics* described by the *unknown function* $\mathbf{i}^r=\psi(\varphi(\mathbf{i}^d),\mathbf{p})=\mathbf{f}(\mathbf{i}^d)$ and resulting in a realized $\mathbf{i}^r$ instead of the desired one, $\mathbf{i}^d$. The parameter vector **p** symbolizes the parameters of the actual system not taken into account in its rough model, as well as the unknown external perturbations. They may be slowly varying function of time, too. Normally only the "net" function **f**() can be observed, but there is no possibility to directly "manipulate" it. [Only the nature of the *model function* $\varphi()$ can be modified.] It is rather possible only to *deform* its actual input $\mathbf{i}^{d*}$ in order to achieve and maintain the $\mathbf{i}^d=\mathbf{f}(\mathbf{i}^{d*})$ situation. The Modified Renormalization Algorithm invented by Tar (e.g. in Pátkai et al, 2002) consists in creating a series of linear transformations defined as follows

$$\begin{gathered} \mathbf{i}_0; \quad \mathbf{S}_1\mathbf{f}(\mathbf{i}_0)=\mathbf{i}_0; \quad \mathbf{i}_1=\mathbf{S}_1\mathbf{i}_0;\ldots;\mathbf{S}_n\mathbf{f}(\mathbf{i}_{n-1})=\mathbf{i}_0; \\ \mathbf{i}_{n+1}=\mathbf{S}_{n+1}\mathbf{i}_n; \quad \mathbf{S}_n \xrightarrow[n\to\infty]{} \mathbf{I} \end{gathered} \tag{8}$$

It was proved by Tar that if **f**() is flat, that is has a small gradient according to its variables, and that if the $\mathbf{S}_n$ matrices are close to the identity operator, the above algorithm converges to the proper deformation of the desired input. The *dummy parameter D* has the following role: in general it avoids the occurrence of the identification from two near-zero vectors, and in particular if $|y| \ll D$, the appropriate transformations will be very close to the identity operator, which is needed for the proper convergence. For guaranteeing the other condition especially at the beginning of the identification a simple linear transformation is applied depending on the estimated "extent" of the necessary transformation as

$$\xi = \frac{\left\|\mathbf{i}^d - \mathbf{f}\right\|}{1 + \max\left(\left\|\mathbf{i}^d\right\|, \left\|\mathbf{f}\right\|\right)}, \quad \lambda = \lambda(\xi), \quad \hat{\mathbf{i}}^d = \mathbf{f} + \lambda\left(\mathbf{i}^d - \mathbf{f}\right) \tag{9}$$

and the original input $\mathbf{i}^d$ is replaced by $\hat{\mathbf{i}}^d$. The function $\lambda(\xi) \rightarrow 1$ if $\xi \rightarrow 0$ and it can be constructed in many various ways via applying certain parameters in it.

4. SIMULATON RESULTS

In the simulations 20% error was applied in modeling oil compressibility. The piston's friction was taken into account in simulating the real system only, but it was unknown for the controller. The disturbance force had an exponentially damped sinusoidal component of the initial amplitude of 200 N and a constant component of 500 N.

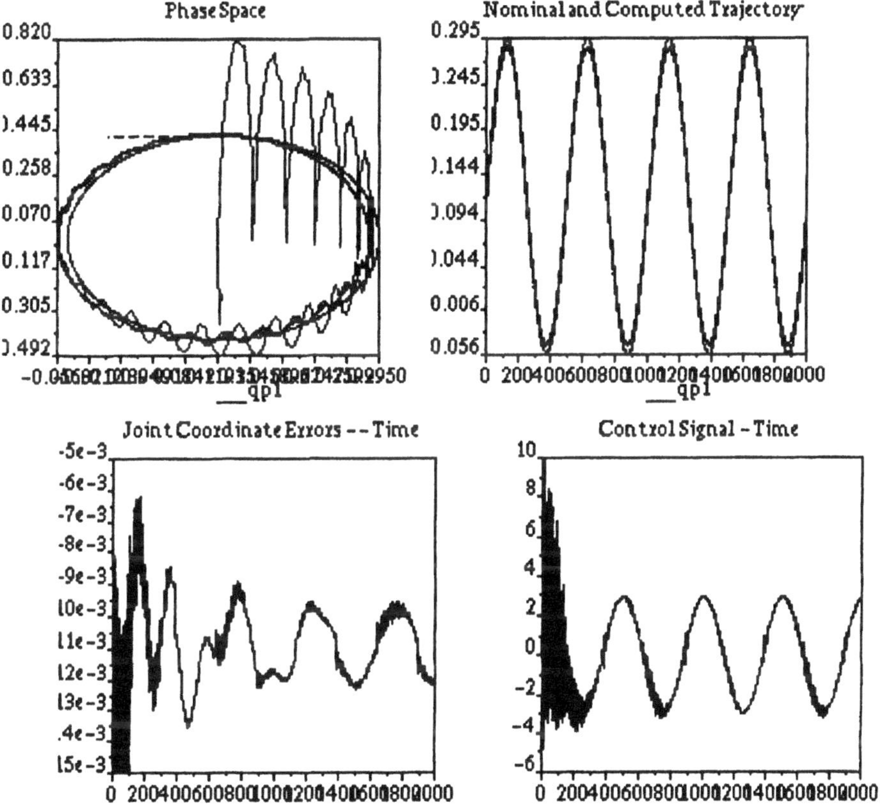

Figure 1 – The phase space [*m* and *m/s* units], the nominal and the simulated trajectory [coordinate in *m*, and time in 5 *ms* units], the trajectory reproduction error versus time [in *m*], and the not control signal of the valve (not normalized)

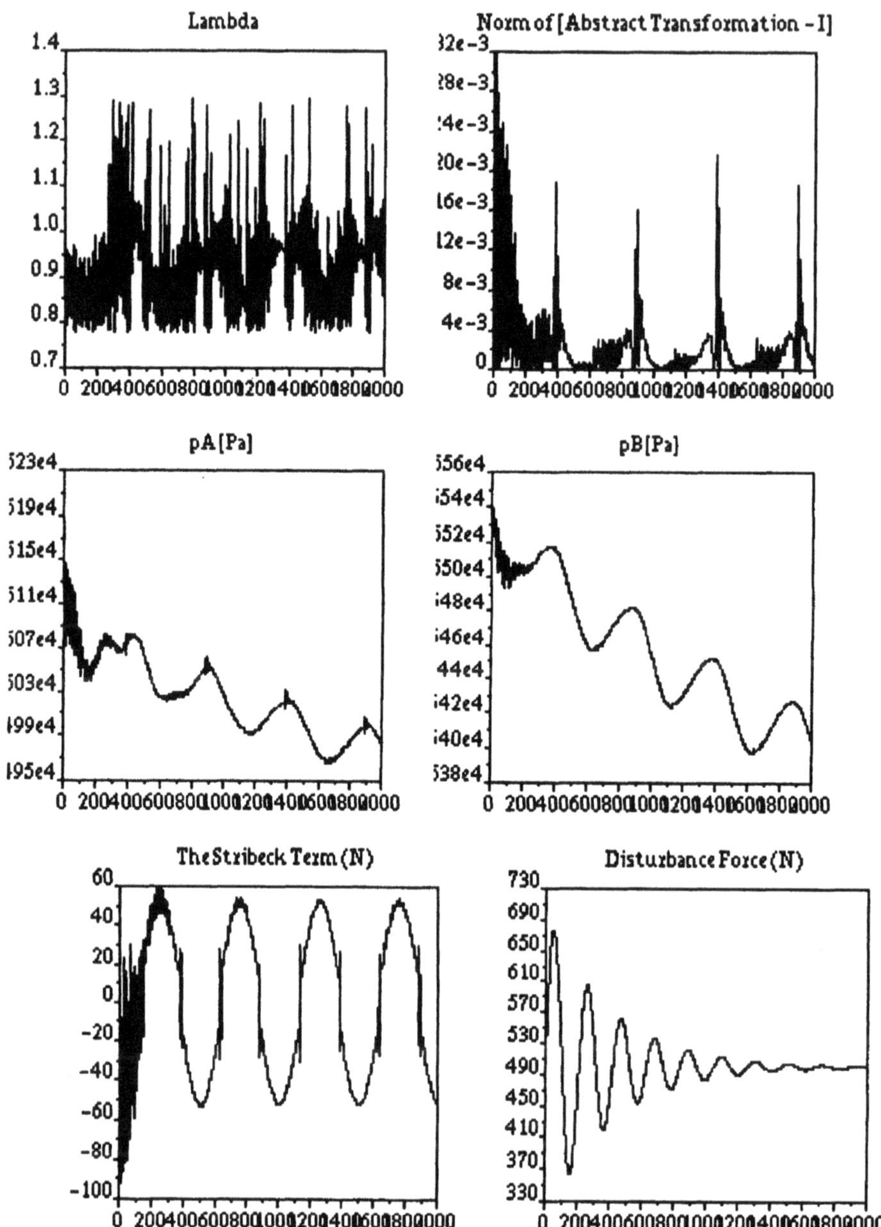

Figure 2 – The factor of the linear interpolation (λ), the norm of the (**T-I**) matrices, the variation of the pressure in the chambers of the pistons [*Pa*], the friction force [*N*] calculated according to the Stribeck model, and the external disturbance force [*N*] are described.

At first the special symplectic matrices were applied for adaptation. In Fig. 1 the phase space, the trajectory of the nominal and the simulated motion, the trajectory tracking error, and the control signal of the hydraulic cylinder are described. It can well be seen from the figures that in spite of the considerable perturbations not taken into account in the rough model the adaptive control successfully learns the observable properties of the system and results in smooth variation of the pressure in the chambers of the cylinder.

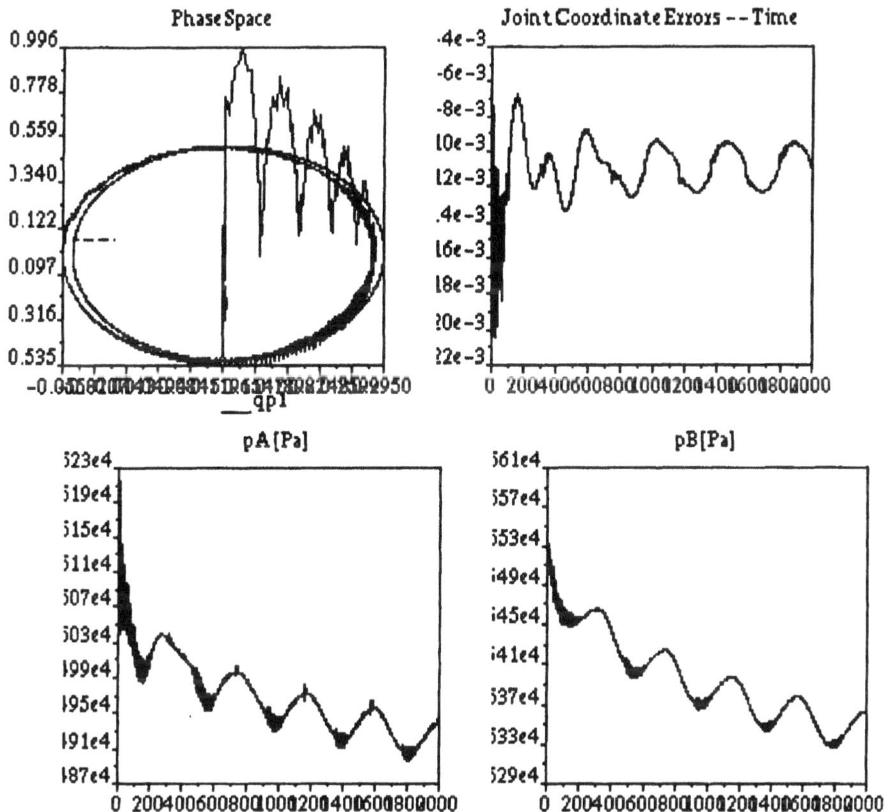

Figure 3 – The Counterparts of Certain Characteristics of the Symplectic Transformations Based Control in the Case of the Application of the Partially Stretched Orthogonal Transformations

In Fig. 3 the operation of the Partially Stretched Orthogonal Transformations based control are given for the same nominal trajectory and external perturbations. This latter approach seems to be a little bit more noisy. Fig. 4 reveals that the non-adaptive control under the same circumstances operates as a noisy bang-bang controller.

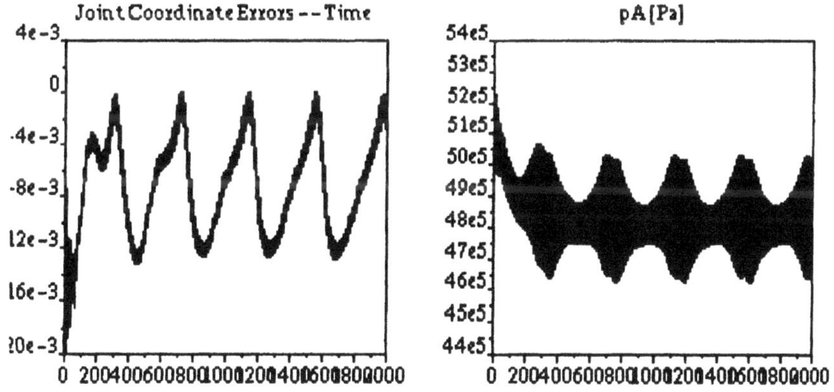

Figure 4 – The Behavior of the Non-Adaptive Control under the Same Circumstances

5. CONCLUSIONS

In this paper a recently developed adaptive controller based on the "Modified Renormalization Algorithm", the "Partially Stretched Orthogonal Transformations", specially constructed "Symplectic Transformations", and a simple linear interpolation technique was applied to the control of a differential hydraulic cylinder under external disturbances not modeled by the controller. The simulation results well illustrate that such an adaptive technique can well improve the simple linear PI controller's operation. The information need of this adaptive controller is far much less than that of the traditional disturbance rejection controller needing the measurement of the disturbance force and its time-derivative. The simulation results well testify the fruitful co-operation of the linear interpolation part and the application of the symplectic / partially stretched orthogonal matrices. The method is promising in other fields of application where the behavior of a complex system under unknown environmental interaction is to be predicted: in appropriate column vectors several properties of time-dependent quantities (0th, 1st, n^{th} order time-derivatives) can be placed and mapped wit the convenient algebraic technique here presented.

6. ACKNOWLEDGMENTS

The authors thankfully acknowledge the support by the Hungarian National Research Fund in the program OTKA T 034651.

7. REFERENCES

1. Bröcker, M., Lemmen, M. Nonlinear Control Methods for Disturbance Rejection on a Hydraulically Driven Flexible Robot. Proc. of the 2nd Intl. Workshop On Robot Motion And Control, RoMoCo'001, October 18-20, 2001, Bukowy Dworek, Poland, pp. 213-217, ISBN: 83-7143-515-0, IEEE catalog Number: 01EX535.
2. Drakunov, S., Hanchin, G.D., Su, W.C. and Ozguner U. Nonlinear Control of a Rodless Pneumatic Servoactuator, or Sliding Modes versus Coulomb Friction, Automatica, 1997, Vol. 33, no. 7, pp. 1401-1408.
3. El Hini, Yahya. Comparison of the Application of the Symplectic and the Partially Stretched Orthogonal Transformations in a New Branch of Adaptive Control for Mechanical Devices. Proc. of the 10th Intl. Conference on Advanced Robotics, August 22-25, Budapest, Hungary, pp. 701-706, ISBN 963 7154 05 1.
4. Pátkai, B., Tar, J.K., Rudas, I.J., Bitó, J.F. Convergence Properties of the Modified Renormalization Algorithm Based Adaptive Control Supported by Ancillary Methods, under for publication in the 2002 IEEE Intl. Symp. on Industrial Electronics (ISIE 2002), July 8-11, 2002 L' Aquila, Italy.
5. Tar, J.K., Rontó M. Adaptive Control Based on the Application of Simplified Uniform Structures and Learning Procedures. Zbornik Radova, Vol. 24 No. 2, 2000, pp. 174-194. (ISSN: 0351-1804).

60

LOW COST EDUCATIONAL TECHNOLOGY BASED ON OPEN SYSTEM REFERENCE ARCHITECTURE FOR ENGINEERING COURSES

Miguel de Jesús Ramírez Cadena
CSIM-ITESM
Ave. Eugenio Garza Sada 2501 Sur
Monterrey, N.L. 64849 Mexico
mdramire@campus.mty.itesm.mx

This paper describes a software-based control reference architecture based on the open systems concept use it as a development tool to building common system by a group of users working individually on separated parts of the system. An application of the architecture in engineering courses is showed. In this case, the author had developed an educational frame in computer science, electronic, electrical, mechanic and others related engineering courses where the professor can organize the course in sections in order to be developed by each student or team of students. The concept can be brought to collaborative environments to support virtual organizations where need it multidisciplinary teams.

1. INTRODUCTION

Open Systems is a concept used to development control systems. The IEEE define open system as follow: "An open system provides capabilities that enable properly implemented applications to run on a variety of platforms from multiple vendors, interoperate with other systems applications and present a consistent style of interaction with the user." (IEEE 1003.0).

The main goals for open system architecture are interoperability, portability, scalability and inter-changeability. Interoperability will only be guaranteed by using standardized data semantics and behavioral models, communication and interaction mechanisms. Portability allows operate the system components on different platforms without any changes. Scalability is a feature to enables the customer to increase or decrease the functionality of a system by upgrading or downgrading specific components. Inter-changeability allows the interchanging of one component per another due to its specific capabilities, reliability or performance. Also open system architecture concept is related to internal openness and external openness. The first one refers to openness concerning the internal control functions and the second cover all external interfaces. (Ramírez et al., 2001).

A lot of efforts had been realized in order to create controls based on open systems (Pritschow et al., 2001) :

- Japan. OSEC (Open System Environment for Manufacturing).
- USA. OMAC (Open Modular Architecture Controllers).
- Europe. OSACA (Open System Architecture for Controls within Automation Systems).
- USA-NIST. EMC (Enhanced Machine Controller).

The Manufacturing Integrated Systems Center (CSIM) of the Monterrey Institute of Technology (ITESM) had developed the concept of Universal Numerical Control (CNU) based on open system concept. The rationale of CNU project is related with the fact that in countries like Mexico, small and medium metal-working industry rarely have access to computer numerical control (CNC) machine tools and then they work with conventional machine tools. On the other hand, only well established companies have access to automated machine tools due to its cost. Also the research group has pointed out that Mexican small and medium metal-working industry has been facing major problems in international markets due to lack CNC technology which is the basis for competition in this sector (Phillips et al., 1997).

Therefore an area of opportunity has been identified to develop national technology in the area of CNC using low cost PCs, object oriented programming technologies and software based open system architecture implemented with real-time operating systems. The research group had developed a control prototype used to retrofitted an outdated machine-tool. Actually, five small metalworking enterprises of Mexico had expressed their wish to implement the CNU project on their outdated machines.

The CNU project had created reference architecture based on open systems theory. A reference architecture is a conceptual model that establish rules and methods of integration and standard interfaces between its components in order to reach a structure to let developers build systems with the characteristics established by the architecture (Ramírez (5), 2001).

With the reference architecture is possible design and implement systems formed with different combinations of software modules that can plug and play on the architecture to reach the needed functionality.

Because of the success of the CNU project, an opportunity had been viewed by the author with regards to the open system reference architecture on the scope of real-time systems. The reference architecture really can provide an educational frame in computer science, electronic, electrical, mechanic and others related engineering courses. The professor can organize the course in sections or software modules in order to be developed by each student or team of students. Each team needs to follow the specifications of the reference architecture so get communication with the others parts. Each team can do their particular work with independence of the other teams because the reference architecture establishes the communications rules between all parts of the system. Previously, the professor need design the communication rules related with the control system to implement.

The development of low cost educational technology for engineering courses let meeting students with many technical profiles.

2. EDUCATIONAL REFERENCE ARCHITECTURE

The proposal to use open system reference architecture to organize engineering courses let the follow:

- Planning build a system by a group of users working individually on separated pieces.
- Using ready-to-use libraries of software in order to development systems.
- Work on the scope of real-time operating systems.
- Prepare the course by the teacher focus on the functionality of each part and the integration of the system.

The real-time item is a key concept of the architecture and let to system respond to internal or external events with an appropriated answer time. The main differences between real-time and standard programming are (Everett, 1995):

- The real-time systems are compacts but complex.
- The real-time make sure the good performance of the systems.
- The real-time programming drive the interrupts scheduler of the systems resources.

The figure 1 show the concept reached by the architecture in order to be use on engineering courses with different profiles of students, this concept get a library of software modules developed by the students which can be integrated to common reference architecture designed by the professor.

This concept of reference architecture is like a "Black Box", where the professor designs the "Black Box" and the students full the box with the necessary modules to reach the functionality designed by the professor. Before starting the course, the professor must to design the interfaces between the different software modules establishing the communications among themselves.

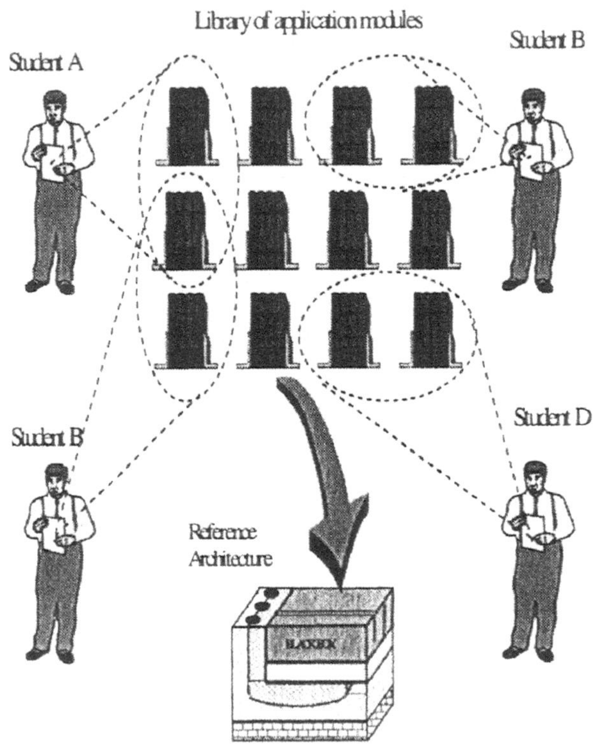

Figure 1. The Reference Architecture Application Concept

The reference architecture offers system software layers to serve as link between applications software modules and hardware. It offer an exactly specified application interface which will provide standard services in the fields of communication, data storage, graphics, dialogue management, configuration and operating system (Ramírez(4), 2001).

The system software layer hide the specific characteristics of processes, operating systems or communication media which are used within the architecture, so that the student always finds the same application interface and just will dedicate effort to develop his part.

3. APPLICATION ON ENGINEERING COURSES

The next section shows the organization of electronic engineering course gave in Monterrey Institute of Technology last year. The objective was development a Computer Numerical Control for retrofit a conventional machine-tool (lathe) using the reference architecture. Previously, the professor established the application software modules and designed the communications in the architecture. The professor established the architecture with five software modules (see figure 2): External communications module, movement control module, axis control module, auxiliary process module and sensor-actuator module.

The professor must to program three modules belong to the reference architecture: Man-machine module, Configuration system module and Database management module. These modules have the information to manage the application software modules mentioned before.

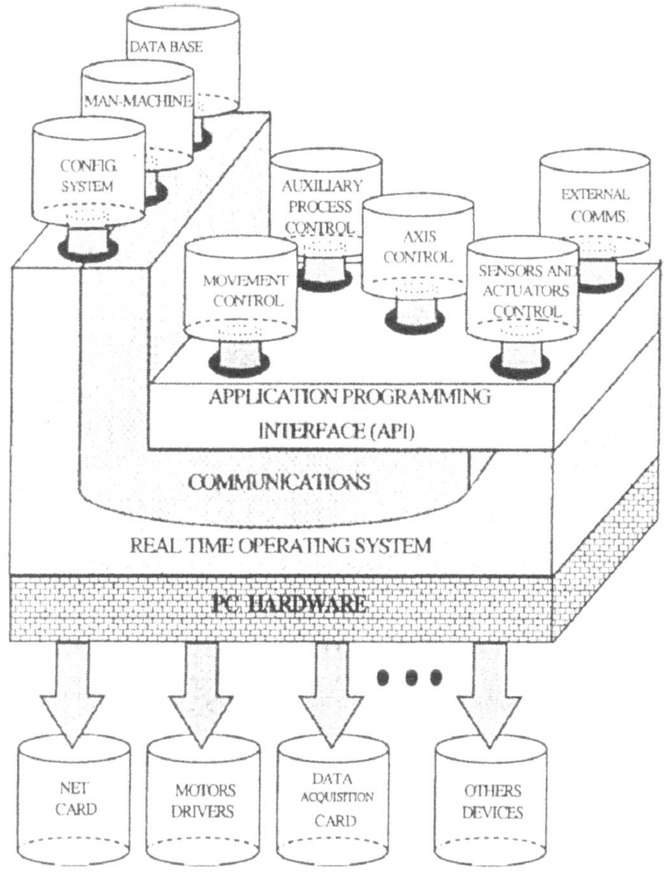

Figure 2. The Reference Architecture of CNU

Ten students of electronic and computer science careers developed the software modules, two students developed each module. In addition, participated three mechanical career students so that help in machining process concepts, mounting equipment on the lathe and machining test pieces.

The information flow for a CNC program is show in figure 3. The flow begins when the user introduce a CNC program in the man-machine interface. The CNC code is driven by movement control module to get the basic length unit table. The axis control module processes the basic length unit table to get the signal table for each axis. The auxiliary process module drive the information related with M codes. The sensors and actuators module converts this information in electrical signals send to machine motors and receive the retrofeed signal of the sensors in the machine-tool.

The professor developed a object oriented model using FUSION method and gave, to each development group of module, the document with specific messages that receive and send from/to others modules of the architecture. All modules were programming in C++ using parametric classes (Ramírez et al., 2001).

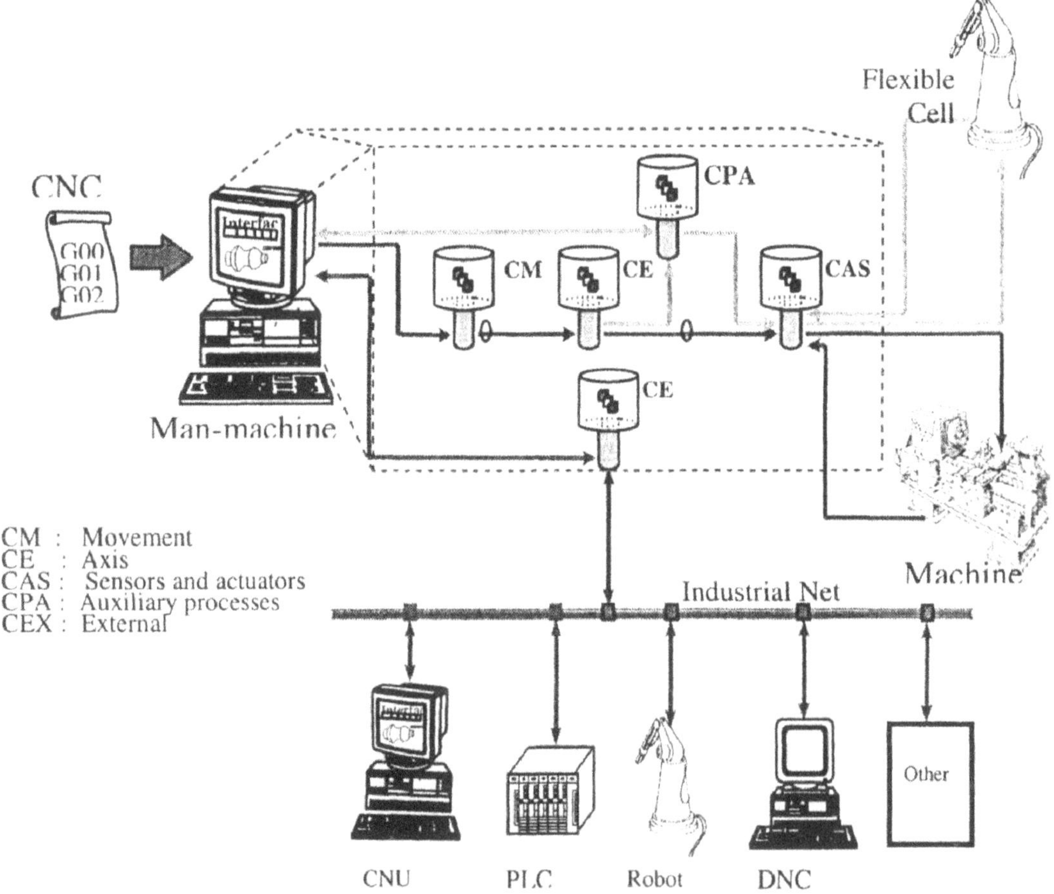

Figure 3. Information Flow in CNU Application.

The lathe was retrofitting mounting servomotor, limit switches, position sensors, a personal computer, ballscrews and data acquisition card. The CNC control implemented used unix platform because all software was developed with QNX real-time operating system. The use of real-time techniques let implemented the system in a standard PC with processor of 600 Mhz.

4. CONCLUSIONS

This paper focus on shows the use of reference architecture concept implemented with real-time operating system in order to design and implement any system to do by multidisciplinary teams.

The reference architecture let design and implement an engineering course in order to prove it as an educational tool. The main issues are:

a) The use of the reference architecture let the professor organized the course with flexibility and efficiency.
b) The student centered all his attention in a specific problem or area because the communication forms with others parts of the systems were established previously.
c) This educational tool had proved that is a efficient form to plan engineering courses where participate many persons with different professional profiles.
d) The cost of the implementation of control systems is less than implement the course with commercial platforms of software and expensive machines.

As a future line, the author proposes design and implement a system on the reference architecture relate with virtual organizations to build collaborative environments. Exist on the literature efforts using reference architectures on virtual organizations (Bernus et al., 2002), however, will be interesting to apply real-time items in order to get more control on the system behavior.

5. ACKNOWLEDGMENTS

The project has been accepted by the QNX Educational Programm of QNX Software Systems LTD, and therefore the QNX operating system has been given as a grant to our research group. The grant consist development software for the CNU project, the donation consist in the follow items: microkernel of the system, Watcom C++ compilator, Photom microGUI development kit; with a value of 4,200 USD.

6. REFERENCES

1. Bernus P., Baltrusch R., Vesterager J., Tolle M. "Fast tracking ICT infrastructure requirements and design, based on enterprise reference architecture and matching reference models". 1st. Edition, Colaborative business ecosystems and virtual enterprises, Kluwer Academic Publishers, 2002. p.p. 293-302.
2. Everett W.W. "Reliability and safety of real-time systems", Computer. May 1995. p.p. 13-16.
3. Phillips L., Valero J., Tijerina J. "Bienes de producción críticos en la industria manufacturera del estado de Nuevo León: el caso de los tornos de control numérico". Entorno económico Journal. Vol. XXXV. June 1997. p.p. 13-16.
4. Pritschow G., Altintas Y., Jovane F., Koren Y., Mitsuishi M., Takata S., Van Brussel H., Weck M., Yamazaki K. "Open Controller Architecture: Past, Present and Future. CIRP. 2001.

5. Ramírez M., "Algoritmos de interpolación matemáticos aplicados al corte de metal". Memories of the First meeting in Mathematics applied to the Engineer, computing and science, San José, Costa Rica. February 6-9, 2001.
6. Ramírez M., "Desarrollo de Geotecnología: El caso del control Numérico Universal". Memories of the IX seminario Latino-Americano de Gestión Tecnológica ALTEC 2001, San José, Costa Rica. October 17-19, 2001.
7. Ramírez M., Molina A., "Sofware based Computer Numerical Controller for Low Cost Automation in Small and Medium sized Metal-Processing Enterprises in Developing Countries". Memories of the VI IFAC Symposium on Cost Oriented Automation, Berlin, German. October 8-9, 2001.
8. IEEE 1003.0, Technical Committee of Open Systems of IEEE.

ACKNOWLEDGMENT

The editors would like to acknowledge the significant support they received from the following co-organizing and sponsoring institutions:

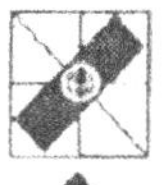

IFIP WG 5.3 AND WG 5.5

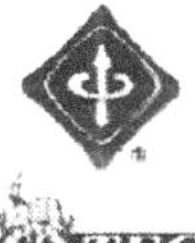

IEEE ROBOTICS AND AUTOMATION SOCIETY

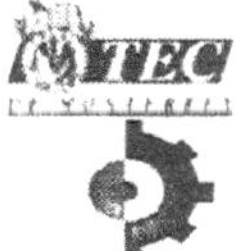

TEC DE MONTERREY – INSTITUTO TECHNOLÓGICO Y DE ESTUDIOS SUPERIORES DE MONTERREY, MÉXICO

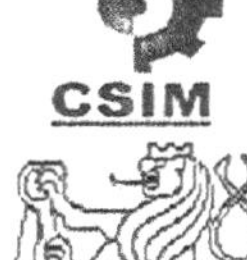

CSIM –CENTRO DE SISTEMAS INTEGRADOS DE MANUFACTURA, MONTERREY, MÉXICO

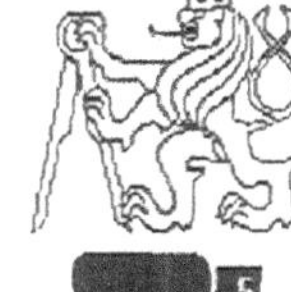

CTU – CZECH TECHNICAL UNIVERSITY IN PRAGUE, CZECH REPUBLIC

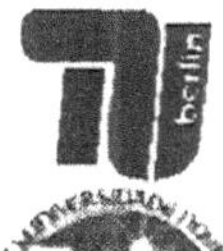

TU BERLIN – TECHNISCHE UNIVERSITAET, BERLIN, GERMANY

UNIVERSIDADE NOVA DE LISBOA, LISBON, PORTUGAL

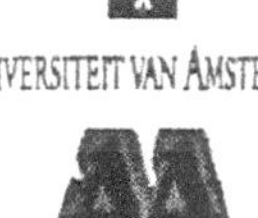

UNIVERSITY OF AMSTERDAM, THE NETHERLANDS

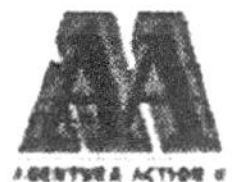

ACTION M AGENCY, PRAGUE, CZECH REPUBLIC

The editors are also grateful to many persons who helped them to prepare this volume, namely to Arturo Molina, Edwin H. van Leeuwen and Joao J. Pinto-Ferreira as well as to people who helped in communication with the contributors and in organizing/formatting the papers, namely to Jiří Lažanský, David Hromas, Jan Zach, Hana Krautwurmová, and Jindřich Recina.

AUTHORS INDEX

Z

GPSR Compliance
The European Union's (EU) General Product Safety Regulation (GPSR) is a set of rules that requires consumer products to be safe and our obligations to ensure this.

If you have any concerns about our products, you can contact us on

ProductSafety@springernature.com

In case Publisher is established outside the EU, the EU authorized representative is:

Springer Nature Customer Service Center GmbH
Europaplatz 3
69115 Heidelberg, Germany

www.ingramcontent.com/pod-product-compliance
Ingram Content Group UK Ltd.
Pitfield, Milton Keynes, MK11 3LW, UK
UKHW061831190726
13855UKWH00005B/1751

* 9 7 8 1 4 7 5 7 5 6 3 1 9 *